Methods in Comparative Effectiveness Research

Chapman & Hall/CRC Biostatistics Series

Editor-in-Chief

Shein-Chung Chow, Ph.D., Professor, Department of Biostatistics and Bioinformatics,
Duke University School of Medicine, Durham, North Carolina

Series Editors

Byron Jones, Biometrical Fellow, Statistical Methodology, Integrated Information Sciences,
Novartis Pharma AG, Basel, Switzerland

Jen-pei Liu, Professor, Division of Biometry, Department of Agronomy,
National Taiwan University, Taipei, Taiwan

Karl E. Peace, Georgia Cancer Coalition, Distinguished Cancer Scholar, Senior Research Scientist
and Professor of Biostatistics, Jiann-Ping Hsu College of Public Health,
Georgia Southern University, Statesboro, Georgia

Bruce W. Turnbull, Professor, School of Operations Research and Industrial Engineering,
Cornell University, Ithaca, New York

Published Titles

Published Titles

Biosimilars: Design and Analysis of Follow-on Biologics
Shein-Chung Chow

Biostatistics: A Computing Approach
Stewart J. Anderson

Cancer Clinical Trials: Current and Controversial Issues in Design and Analysis
Stephen L. George, Xiaofei Wang, and Herbert Pang

Causal Analysis in Biomedicine and Epidemiology: Based on Minimal Sufficient Causation
Mikel Aickin

Clinical and Statistical Considerations in Personalized Medicine
Claudio Carini, Sandeep Menon, and Mark Chang

Clinical Trial Data Analysis using R
Ding-Geng (Din) Chen and Karl E. Peace

Clinical Trial Methodology
Karl E. Peace and Ding-Geng (Din) Chen

Computational Methods in Biomedical Research
Ravindra Khattree and Dayanand N. Naik

Computational Pharmacokinetics
Anders Källén

Confidence Intervals for Proportions and Related Measures of Effect Size
Robert G. Newcombe

Controversial Statistical Issues in Clinical Trials
Shein-Chung Chow

Data Analysis with Competing Risks and Intermediate States
Ronald B. Geskus

Data and Safety Monitoring Committees in Clinical Trials
Jay Herson

Design and Analysis of Animal Studies in Pharmaceutical Development
Shein-Chung Chow and Jen-pei Liu

Design and Analysis of Bioavailability and Bioequivalence Studies, Third Edition
Shein-Chung Chow and Jen-pei Liu

Design and Analysis of Bridging Studies
Jen-pei Liu, Shein-Chung Chow, and Chin-Fu Hsiao

Design & Analysis of Clinical Trials for Economic Evaluation & Reimbursement: An Applied Approach Using SAS & STATA
Iftekhar Khan

Design and Analysis of Clinical Trials for Predictive Medicine
Shigeyuki Matsui, Marc Buyse, and Richard Simon

Design and Analysis of Clinical Trials with Time-to-Event Endpoints
Karl E. Peace

Design and Analysis of Non-Inferiority Trials
Mark D. Rothmann, Brian L. Wiens, and Ivan S. F. Chan

Difference Equations with Public Health Applications
Lemuel A. Moyé and Asha Seth Kapadia

DNA Methylation Microarrays: Experimental Design and Statistical Analysis
Sun-Chong Wang and Arturas Petronis

DNA Microarrays and Related Genomics Techniques: Design, Analysis, and Interpretation of Experiments
David B. Allison, Grier P. Page, T. Mark Beasley, and Jode W. Edwards

Dose Finding by the Continual Reassessment Method
Ying Kuen Cheung

Dynamical Biostatistical Models
Daniel Commenges and Hélène Jacqmin-Gadda

Elementary Bayesian Biostatistics
Lemuel A. Moyé

Empirical Likelihood Method in Survival Analysis
Mai Zhou

Exposure–Response Modeling: Methods and Practical Implementation
Jixian Wang

Frailty Models in Survival Analysis
Andreas Wienke

Methods in Comparative Effectiveness Research

Edited by

Constantine Gatsonis
Brown University, Providence, Rhode Island, USA

Sally C. Morton
Virginia Tech, Blacksburg, Virginia, USA

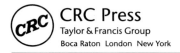

CRC Press
Taylor & Francis Group
Boca Raton London New York

CRC Press is an imprint of the
Taylor & Francis Group, an **informa** business

A CHAPMAN & HALL BOOK

CRC Press
Taylor & Francis Group
6000 Broken Sound Parkway NW, Suite 300
Boca Raton, FL 33487-2742

Printed on acid-free paper

International Standard Book Number-13: 978-1-4665-1196-5 (Hardback)

Library of Congress Cataloging-in-Publication Data

Names: Gatsonis, Constantine, editor. | Morton, Sally C., editor.
Title: Methods in comparative effectiveness research / Constantine Gatsonis, Sally C. Morton.
Description: Boca Raton : Taylor & Francis, 2017. | "A CRC title, part of the Taylor & Francis imprint, a member of the Taylor & Francis Group, the academic division of T&F Informa plc."
Identifiers: LCCN 2016039233 | ISBN 9781466511965 (hardback)
Subjects: LCSH: Clinical trials. | Medicine--Research--Statistical methods.
Classification: LCC R853.C55 G38 2017 | DDC 610.72/4--dc23
LC record available at https://lccn.loc.gov/2016039233

Visit the Taylor & Francis Web site at
http://www.taylorandfrancis.com

and the CRC Press Web site at
http://www.crcpress.com

Contents

Section I   Causal Inference Methods

Section II   Clinical Trials: Design, Interpretation, and Generalizability

Section III   Research Synthesis

Section IV   Special Topics

Contributors

Heather D. Anderson
Department of Clinical
 Pharmacy
University of Colorado
Aurora, Colorado

Michael Baiocchi
Department of Medicine
Stanford University
Stanford, California

Jeffrey A. Bridge
The Research Institute at
 Nationwide Children's Hospital
Columbus, Ohio

Bradley P. Carlin
Division of Biostatistics
School of Public Health
University of Minnesota
Minneapolis, Minnesota

Anna Chaimani
Department of Hygiene and
 Epidemiology
University of Ioannina School
 of Medicine
Ioannina, Greece

Jing Cheng
Department of Preventive and
 Restorative Dental Science
UCSF School of Dentistry
San Francisco, California

Jagpreet Chhatwal
MGH Institute for Technology
 Assessment
Harvard Medical School
Boston, Massachusetts

Jason T. Connor
Berry Consultants, LLC
Orlando, Florida

Issa J. Dahabreh
Department of Health Services,
 Policy and Practice
Center for Evidence Synthesis in
 Health
Brown University School of Public
 Health
Providence, Rhode Island

Orestis Efthimiou
Department of Hygiene and
 Epidemiology
University of Ioannina School of
 Medicine
Ioannina, Greece

Haoda Fu
Clinical Research Department
Eli Lilly and Company
Indianapolis, Indiana

Constantine Gatsonis
Department of Biostatistics
Brown University School of
 Public Health
Providence, Rhode Island

Joel B. Greenhouse
Department of Statistics
Carnegie Mellon University
Pittsburgh, Pennsylvania

Sebastien J-P.A. Haneuse
Department of Biostatistics
Harvard Chan School of Public
 Health
Boston, Massachusetts

Miguel A. Hernán
Departments of Epidemiology and
    Biostatistics
Harvard T.H. Chan School of
    Public Health
Harvard University
Cambridge, Massachusetts

Hwanhee Hong
Department of Mental Health
Johns Hopkins University
Baltimore, Maryland

Kelly J. Kelleher
The Research Institute at
    Nationwide Children's Hospital
Columbus, Ohio

David M. Kent
Predictive Analytics and
    Comparative Effectiveness
    Center
Tufts Medical Center
Boston, Massachusetts

Ken Kleinman
Department of Biostatistics and
    Epidemiology
University of Massachusetts
Amherst, Massachusetts

Lauren M. Kunz
Office of Biostatistics Research
National Heart, Lung, and Blood
    Institute
National Institutes of Health
Bethesda, Maryland

Eric B. Laber
Department of Statistics
North Carolina State University
Raleigh, North Carolina

Joseph Lau
Department of Health Services,
    Policy and Practice
Center for Evidence Synthesis
    in Health
Brown University School of
    Public Health
Providence, Rhode Island

Sandra Lee
Department of Biostatistics
    and Computational
    Biology
Dana-Farber Cancer Institute
    and Harvard Medical
    School
and
Department of Biostatistics
Harvard T.H. Chan School of
    Public Health
Boston, Massachusetts

Anne M. Libby
Department of Emergency
    Medicine
University of Colorado
Aurora, Colorado

Dimitris Mavridis
Department of Hygiene and
    Epidemiology
University of Ioannina School of
    Medicine
and
Department of Primary Education
University of Ioannina
Ioannina, Greece

Sally C. Morton
College of Science and Department
    of Statistics
Virginia Tech
Blacksburg, Virginia

Sharon-Lise T. Normand
Department of Health Care Policy
(Biostatistics)
Harvard T.H. Chan School of
Public Health
Boston, Massachusetts

Robert T. O'Neill
Office of Translational Sciences
Center for Drug Evaluation and
Research
Silver Spring, Maryland

Karen L. Price
Eli Lilly and Company
Indianapolis, Indiana

Min Qian
Department of Biostatistics
Columbia University
New York, New York

Mark S. Roberts
Department of Health Policy and
Management
University of Pittsburgh
Pittsburgh, Pennsylvania

James M. Robins
Departments of Epidemiology and
Biostatistics
Harvard T.H. Chan School of
Public Health
Harvard University
Cambridge, Massachusetts

Sherri Rose
Department of Health Care Policy
(Biostatistics)
Harvard T.H. Chan School of
Public Health
Boston, Massachusetts

Georgia Salanti
Faculty of Medicine
Institute of Social and Preventive
Medicine
University of Bern
Bern, Switzerland

Christopher H. Schmid
Department of Biostatistics
Center for Evidence Synthesis in
Health
Brown University School of
Public Health
Providence, Rhode Island

Susan M. Shortreed
Biostatistics Unit
Group Health Research Institute
Seattle, Washington

Dylan S. Small
Department of Statistics
The Wharton School of the
University of Pennsylvania
Philadelphia, Pennsylvania

Kenneth J. Smith
Department of Medicine
School of Medicine
University of Pittsburgh
Pittsburgh, Pennsylvania

Donna Spiegelman
Departments of Epidemiology,
Biostatistics, and Nutrition
Harvard T.H. Chan School of
Public Health
Boston, Massachusetts

Elizabeth A. Stuart
Department of Mental Health
Johns Hopkins University
Baltimore, Maryland

Thomas A. Trikalinos
Department of Health Services,
    Policy and Practice
Center for Evidence Synthesis in
    Health
Brown University School of
    Public Health
Providence, Rhode Island

Robert Valuck
Department of Clinical Pharmacy
University of Colorado
Aurora, Colorado

Marvin Zelen
Department of Biostatistics
Harvard T.H. Chan School of
    Public Health
Boston, Massachusetts

Introduction

What Is Comparative Effectiveness Research?

Comparative effectiveness research (CER) has emerged as a major component of health care and policy research over the past two decades. Several definitions of CER have been proposed. The most widely used is the definition provided by the Institute of Medicine (IOM; now the National Academy of Medicine) committee convened to define national priorities for CER in 2009. According to this definition, "Comparative effectiveness research (CER) is the generation and synthesis of evidence that compares the benefits and harms of alternative methods to prevent, diagnose, treat, and monitor a clinical condition or to improve the delivery of care" [1]. According to the IOM report, CER is conducted in order to develop evidence that will aid patients, clinicians, purchasers, and health policy makers in making informed decisions. The overarching goal is to improve health care *at both the individual and population levels.*

Insofar as the focus of CER is *on effectiveness*, the contrast with *efficacy* needs to be made. Efficacy refers to the performance of a medical intervention under "ideal" circumstances, whereas *effectiveness* refers to the performance of the intervention in "real-world" clinical settings. With efficacy and effectiveness defining the two ends of a continuum, actual studies typically occupy one of the intermediate points. However, effectiveness trials are expected to formulate their aims and design based on the realities of routine clinical practice and to assess outcomes that are directly relevant to clinical decisions. Such trials are often termed "pragmatic clinical trials" in the CER lexicon [2].

In order to maintain the focus on effectiveness, CER studies involve populations that are broadly representative of clinical practice. CER also calls for comparative studies, including two or more alternative interventions with the potential to be the best practice and assessing both harms and benefits. CER studies often involve multiple arms and rarely include placebo arms. Importantly, CER aspires to focus on the *individual* rather than the *average* patient. As a result, the goal of CER is to develop as granular information as possible, in order to assist medical decision making for individuals. Comparative results on subgroups are very important in the CER context.

Patient-Centered Research and PCORI

Among several entities that promote and fund studies of comparative effectiveness, a central role was given to the Patient-Centered Outcomes Research Institute (PCORI). This institute, a public–private partnership, was established and funded by the Patient Protection and Affordable Care Act (PPACA) to conduct CER and generate information needed for health care and policy decision making under PPACA. PCORI developed its own formulation of CER with an emphasis on patient-centeredness. In this formulation, an overarching goal of CER is to provide information that will address the following main questions faced by patients: (a) Given my personal characteristics, conditions, and preferences, what should I expect will happen to me? (b) What are my options, and what are the potential benefits and harms of those options? (c) What can I do to improve the outcomes that are most important to me? (d) How can clinicians and the healthcare delivery systems they work in help me make the best decisions about my health and health care? [3]. An important caveat here is that the class of patient-centered outcomes is not the same as the class of patient-reported outcomes. In addition, PCORI asks that studies include a wide array of stakeholders besides patients, including family members, informal and formal caregivers, purchasers, payers, and policy makers, but the patient remains the key stakeholder.

Evolution of CER

As Greenfield and Sox noted in summarizing the IOM CER Committee Report, "Research that informs clinical decisions is everywhere, yet a national research initiative to improve decision making by patients and their physicians is a novel concept" [4]. Healthcare reform, and particularly the establishment of PCORI and consequently targeted funding, accentuated CER. Notably, funding related to CER is not restricted to PCORI. Other agencies have adopted the CER paradigm in funding announcements and also recommend the involvement of stakeholders in studies [5].

CER has evolved in the 6 years since healthcare reform. Researchers and the patient advocacy community are designing and conducting CER studies, as well as developing the methodology to conduct such studies. The PCORI legislation required that methodological standards for conducting CER be established by the PCORI Methodology Committee. Forty-seven standards were constructed [6], with a current revision ongoing. These standards have increased the attention on methods, and the quality of CER studies. Methodological work is especially focused on trial design, for example, adaptive designs, as well as causal inference in the observational setting. As discussed in the next section, this book addresses these methodological issues and more.

The scientific literature has responded with several special issues devoted to CER, including *Health Affairs* in October 2010 and the *Journal of the American Medical Association* (*JAMA*) in April 2012. A journal devoted to CER, the *Journal of Comparative Effectiveness Research*, was established in 2012. The renewed focus on causal inference has increased methodological work and resulted in new journals as well, including *Observational Studies*, established in 2015.

In terms of data availability, particularly for the conduct of large pragmatic trials, PCORI has funded the construction of a national clinical data research network PCORnet to facilitate the analysis of electronic health records (EHRs) and claims [7]. Funding for training and education is now available, particularly via the Agency for Healthcare Research and Quality (AHRQ), which receives a portion of PCORI funding for such activities. AHRQ has funded a K12 Scholars Program on patient-centered outcomes research, for example. The interested reader may also wish to take advantage of the methodology standards curriculum [8] and the continuing medical education material [9] available at PCORI. Dissemination and implementation of CER results are still in their infancy, though the spotlight has now turned to these essential next steps.

Scope and Organization of This Book

CER encompasses a very broad range of types of studies. In particular, studies of comparative effectiveness can be experimental, notably randomized-controlled trials, or observational. The latter can be prospective studies, for example, involving registries and EHR databases, or postmarketing safety studies. They can also be retrospective, for example, involving the analysis of data from healthcare claims. Research synthesis occupies a significant place in CER, including the conduct of systematic reviews and meta-analyses. The use of modeling is increasingly important in CER given CER's focus on decision making, including decision analysis and microsimulation modeling. Although the legal framework of PCORI does not cover cost-effectiveness analysis, the area is an important dimension of CER in the eyes of many in the research and health policy communities.

The choice of material and organization of this book is intended to cover the main areas of methodology for CER, to emphasize those aspects that are particularly important for the field, and to highlight their relevance to CER studies. Although the coverage of topics is not encyclopedic, we believe this book captures the majority of important areas.

The book is organized into four major sections. The first three cover the fundamentals of CER methods, including (I) Causal Inference Methods, (II) Clinical Trials, and (III) Research Synthesis. The fourth section is devoted to more specialized topics that round out the book. Each section contains several chapters written by teams of authors with deep expertise and extensive track record in their respective areas. The chapters are cross-referenced and provide an account of both theoretical and computational issues, always anchored in CER domain research. The chapter authors provide additional references for further study.

The book is primarily addressed to CER methodologists, quantitative trained researchers interested in CER, and graduate students in all branches of statistics, epidemiology, and health services and outcomes research. The intention is for the material to be accessible to anyone with a masters-level course in regression and some familiarity with clinical research.

Acknowledgments

We thank our chapter authors and our publisher, particularly John Kimmel, for their contributions and patience. We thank our institutions, Brown University and Virginia Tech, and Dr. Morton's prior institution, the University of Pittsburgh, respectively, for their support. We hope that this book will help patients and their families make better healthcare decisions.

Constantine Gatsonis and Sally C. Morton

References

1. Initial National Priorities for Comparative Effectiveness Research. IOM Committee Report, 2009, http://www.nap.edu/read/12648/chapter/1
2. Thorpe KE, Zwarenstein M, Oxman AD, Treweek S, Furberg CD, Altman DG, Tunis S et al. A pragmatic-explanatory continuum indicator summary (PRECIS): A tool to help trial designers. *J Clin Epidemiol*. 2009;62(5):464–75. doi: 10.1016/j.jclinepi.2008.12.011.
3. http://www.pcori.org/research-results/patient-centered-outcomes-research; accessed April 9, 2016.
4. Sox HC, Greenfield S. Comparative effectiveness research: A report from the Institute of Medicine. *Ann Intern Med*. 2009;151(3):203–5.
5. Burke JG, Jones J, Yonas M, Guizzetti L, Virata MC, Costlow M, Morton SC, Elizabeth M. PCOR, CER, and CBPR: Alphabet soup or complementary fields

of health research? *Clin Transl Sci.* 2013;6(6):493–6. doi: 10.1111/cts.12064. Epub May 8, 2013.

6. PCORI (Patient-Centered Outcomes Research Institute) Methodology Committee. The PCORI Methodology Report, 2013, http://www.pcori.org/research-we-support/research-methodology-standards, accessed April 12, 2016.

7. Fleurence RL, Curtis LH, Califf RM, Platt R, Selby JV, Brown JS. Launching PCORnet, a national patient-centered clinical research network. *J Am Med Inform Assoc.* 2014;21(4):578–82. doi: 10.1136/amiajnl-2014-002747. Epub May 12, 2014.

8. http://www.pcori.org/research-results/research-methodology/methodology-standards-academic-curriculum, accessed April 12, 2016.

9. http://www.pcori.org/research-results/cmece-activities, accessed April 12, 2016.

Section I

Causal Inference Methods

1

An Overview of Statistical Approaches for Comparative Effectiveness Research

Lauren M. Kunz, Sherri Rose, Donna Spiegelman,
and Sharon-Lise T. Normand

CONTENTS

ABSTRACT   This chapter reviews key statistical tenets of comparative effectiveness research with an emphasis on the analysis of observational cohort studies. The main concepts discussed relate to those for causal analysis whereby the goal is to quantify how a change in one variable causes a change in another variable. The methodology for binary treatments and a single outcome are reviewed; estimators involving propensity score matching, stratification, and weighting; G-computation; augmented inverse probability of treatment weighting; and targeted maximum likelihood estimation are discussed. A comparative assessment of the effectiveness of two different artery access strategies for patients undergoing percutaneous coronary interventions illustrates the approaches. Rudimentary R code is provided to assist the reader in implementing the various approaches.

1.1 Introduction

Comparative effectiveness research (CER) is designed to inform healthcare decisions by providing evidence on the effectiveness, benefits, and harms of different treatment options [1]. While the typology of CER studies is broad, this chapter focuses on CER conducted using prospective or retrospective observational cohort studies where participants are not randomized to an intervention, treatment, or policy. We assume outcomes and covariates are measured for all subjects and there is no missing outcome or covariate information throughout; we also assume that the data are sampled from the target population—the population of all individuals for which the treatment may be considered for its intended purpose. Without loss of generality, we use the terms "control" and "comparator" interchangeably and focus on one nontime-varying treatment. The scope of methods considered are limited to linear outcome models—a single treatment assignment mechanism model and a single linear outcome model.

An example involving the in-hospital complications of radial artery access compared to femoral artery access in patients undergoing percutaneous coronary interventions (PCI) illustrates ideas. Coronary artery disease can be treated by a PCI in which either a balloon catheter or a coronary stent is used to push the plaque against the walls of the blocked artery. Access to the coronary arteries via the smaller radial artery in the wrist, rather than the femoral artery in the groin, requires a smaller hole and may, therefore, reduce access-site bleeding, patient discomfort, and other vascular complications. Table 1.1 summarizes information for over 40,000 adults undergoing PCI in all nonfederal hospitals located in Massachusetts. The data are prospectively collected by trained hospital data managers utilizing a standardized collection tool, sent electronically to a data coordinating center, and adjudicated [2]. Baseline covariates measured include age, sex, race, health insurance information, comorbidities, cardiac presentation, and medications given prior to the PCI. Overall, radial artery access (new strategy) compared to femoral artery access (standard strategy) is associated with fewer in-hospital vascular and bleeding complications (0.69% vs. 2.73%). However, there is significant treatment selection—healthier patients are more likely to undergo radial artery access compared to those undergoing femoral artery access. Patients associated with radial artery access have less prior congestive heart failure, less left main coronary artery disease, and less shock compared to those undergoing femoral artery access. The CER question is: *When performing PCI, does radial artery access cause fewer in-hospital complications compared to femoral artery access for patients with similar risk?*

The remainder of the chapter provides the main building blocks for answering CER questions in settings exemplified by the radial artery access example—a single outcome with two treatment options. We sometimes refer to the two treatment groups as treated and comparator, exposed and unexposed, or treated and control. Notation is next introduced and the statistical causal framework is described. We adopt a *potential outcomes* framework to causal inference [3]. The underlying assumptions required for CER are discussed. We restrict our focus to several major classes of estimators, and note that we do not exhaustively include all possible estimators for our parameter of interest. Approaches for assessing the validity of the assumptions follow and methods are illustrated here using the PCI data.

1.2 Causal Model Basics

Assume a population of N units indexed by i each with an outcome, Y_i. In the radial artery example, units are subjects, and $Y_i = 1$ if subject i had

TABLE 1.1

Population Characteristics Stratified by Type of Intervention

	Intervention	
	Radial	**Femoral**
Number of observations	5,192	35,022
Demographics		
Mean age [SD]	63 [12]	65 [12]
Female	25.3	29.8
Race		
White	89.6	89.4
Black	3.3	3.2
Hispanic	4.3	3.5
Other	2.8	3.9
Health insurance		
Government	46	50.3
Commercial	4.8	13.4
Other	49.2	36.3
Comorbidities		
Diabetes	33.1	32.7
Prior congestive heart failure	9.4	12.7
Prior PCI	2	34.3
Prior myocardial infarction (MI)	28.7	30.1
Prior coronary artery bypass surgery	8.4	15.7
Hypertension	79.6	80.7
Peripheral vascular disease	12.1	12.8
Smoker	24.8	23.1
Lung disease	13.7	14.4
Cardiac presentation		
Multivessel disease	10.3	10.9
Number of vessels >70% stenosis	1.49	1.58
Left main disease	3.7	7.2
ST-segment elevated MI	38.9	42.6
Shock	0.44	1.8
Drugs prior to procedure		
Unfractionated heparin	87.3	61.7
Low-molecular-weight heparin	3.83	4.27
Thrombin	25.5	54.9
G2B3A inhibitors	26.7	26.8
Platelet aggregate inhibitors	85.8	86.6
Aspirin	98.2	97.5
In-hospital complication (%)	0.69	2.73

Note: All entries are percentages with the exceptions of number of observations, age, and number of vessels with >70% stenosis.

TABLE 1.2

Notation for the Potential Outcomes Framework to Causal Inference

Notation	Definition
T_i	Binary treatment for unit i (1 = treatment; 0 = comparator)
Y_i	Observed outcome for unit i
Y_{0i}	Potential outcome for unit i if $T_i = 0$
Y_{1i}	Potential outcome for unit i if $T_i = 1$
X_i	Vector of pretreatment measured covariates for person i
μ_T	$E_X(E(Y \mid T = t, X))$, marginal expected outcome under t
Δ	$\mu_1 - \mu_0$, causal parameter

a complication after PCI and 0 otherwise. Assume a binary-valued treatment such that $T_i = 1$ if the patient received the new treatment (e.g., radial artery access) and 0 (e.g., femoral artery access) otherwise. Approaches for treatments assuming more than two values, *multivalued* treatments, generalize from those based on binary-valued treatments (see References 4 and 5). Variables that are not impacted by treatment level and occur prior to treatment assignment are referred to as covariates. Let X_i denote a vector of observed covariates, all measured prior to receipt of treatment. The notation is summarized in Table 1.2. Confounding occurs due to differences in the outcome between exposed and control populations even if there was no exposure. The covariates that create this imbalance are called confounders [6]. Another type of covariate is an *instrumental variable* that is independent of the outcome and correlated with the treatment (see Reference 7). A detailed discussion of methods for instrumental variables is provided in Chapter 2. Instrumental variables, when available, are used when important key confounders are unavailable; their use is not discussed here. In the radial artery example, X includes age, race, sex, health insurance information, and cardiac and noncardiac comorbidities. Because there are two treatment levels, there are two potential outcomes for each subject [8]. Only one of the two potential outcomes will be observed for a unit.

1.2.1 Parameters

The idea underpinning a causal effect involves comparing what the outcome for unit i would have been under the two treatments—the *potential outcomes*. Let Y_{1i} represent the outcome for unit i under $T_i = 1$ and Y_{0i} for $T_i = 0$. The causal effect of the treatment on the outcome for unit i can be defined in many ways. For instance, interest may center on an *absolute effect*, $\Delta_i = Y_{1i} - Y_{0i}$, the *relative effect*, $\Delta_i = Y_{1i}/Y_{0i}$, or on some other function of the potential outcomes. The fundamental problem of causal inference is that we only observe the outcome under the actual treatment observed for unit i, $Y_i = Y_{0i}(1 - T_i) + Y_{1i}(T_i)$. A variety of causal parameters are available with the choice dictated by the particular problem. We focus on the causal parameter on the difference scale, $\Delta = \mu_1 - \mu_0$, where μ_1 and μ_0 represent the true proportions of complications if all patients had undergone radial artery access and femoral artery access, respectively. The marginal mean outcome under treatment $T = t$ is defined as

$$\mu_T = E_X(E(Y \mid T = t, X)), \tag{1.1}$$

averaging over the distribution of X. The marginal expected outcome is found by examining the conditional outcome given particular values of X and averaging the outcome over the distribution of all values of X. The parameter μ_T is useful when interest rests on assessing population interventions. If the treatment effect is constant or homogeneous, then the marginal parameter is no different from the conditional parameter.

The average treatment effect (ATE) is defined as

$$E[Y_1 - Y_0] = E_X(E[Y \mid T = 1, X = x] - E[Y \mid T = 0, X = x]) \tag{1.2}$$

and represents the expected difference in the effect of treatment on the outcome if subjects were randomly assigned to the two treatments. The ATE includes the effect on subjects for whom the treatment was not intended, and therefore may not be relevant in some policy evaluations [9]. For example, to assess the impact of a food voucher program, interest rests on quantifying the effectiveness of the program for those individuals *who are likely to participate in the program*. In this case, the causal parameter of interest is the average effect of treatment on the treated (ATT)

$$E_X(E[Y \mid T = 1, X = x] - E[Y \mid T = 0, X = x] \mid T = 1). \tag{1.3}$$

The ATT provides information regarding the expected change in the outcome for a randomly selected unit from the treatment group.

Which causal estimand is of interest depends on the context. When randomized, on average, the treated sample will not be systematically different from the control sample, and the ATT will be equal to the ATE. Throughout this chapter, we focus on the ATE as the causal estimand of interest because (1) both radial and femoral artery access are a valid strategy for all subjects undergoing PCI and (2) we wish to determine whether fewer complications would arise if everyone had undergone radial artery access rather than femoral artery access.

1.2.2 Assumptions

The foremost is the explicit assumption of potential outcomes. The ability to state the potential outcomes implies that although an individual receives a particular treatment, the individual could have received the other treatment, and hence has the potential outcomes under both treatment and comparison conditions.

1.2.2.1 Stable Unit Treatment Value Assignment: No Interference and No Variation in Treatment

The stable unit treatment value assignment (SUTVA) consists of two parts: (1) no interference and (2) no variation in treatment. SUTVA is untestable and requires subject matter knowledge. The no interference assumption implies that the potential outcomes for a subject do not depend on treatment assignments of other subjects. In the radial artery example, we require that radial artery access in one subject does not impact the probability of an in-hospital complication in another subject. If a subject's potential outcomes depend on treatments received by others, then $Y_i(T_1, T_2, \ldots, T_N)$, indicating the outcome for subject i, depends on the treatment received by $T_1, T_2, \ldots, T_N$. SUTVA implies

$$Y_i(T_1, T_2, \ldots, T_N) = Y_i(T_i) = Y_{it}. \tag{1.4}$$

Under what circumstances would the assumption of no interference be violated? Consider determining whether a new vaccine designed to prevent infectious diseases—because those who are vaccinated impact whether others become infected, there will be interference. The radial artery access example may violate the no interference assumption when considering the *practice makes perfect* hypothesis. As physicians increase their skill in delivering a new technology, the less likely complications arise in subsequent uses, and the more likely the physician is to use the new technology. Conditioning physician random effects would make the no interference assumption reasonable.

The second part of SUTVA states that there are not multiple versions of the treatment (and of the comparator), or that the treatment is well defined and the same for each subject receiving it. In the radial artery access example, if different techniques are used to access the radial artery (or the femoral artery) by different clinicians, then the SUTVA is violated.

1.2.2.2 Ignorability of Treatment Assignment

The most common criticism of CER using observational cohort studies involves the unmeasured confounder problem—the assertion that an unmeasured variable is confounding the relationship between treatment and the outcome. Ignorability of the treatment assignment or *unconfoundedness* of the treatment assignment with the outcome assumes that conditional on observed covariates, the probability of treatment assignment does not depend on the potential outcomes. Hence, treatment is effectively randomized conditional on observed baseline covariates. This assumption is untestable and can be strong, requiring observation of all variables that affect both outcomes and treatment in order to ensure

$$(Y_0, Y_1) \perp T \mid X \quad \text{and} \quad P(T = 1 \mid Y_0, Y_1, X) = P(T = 1 \mid X). \tag{1.5}$$

In the radial artery access example, ignorability of treatment assignment may be violated if someone with subject matter knowledge demonstrated that we had omitted a key covariate from Equation 1.1 that is associated with the probability of receiving radial versus femoral artery access, as well as in-hospital complications. For instance, if knowledge regarding whether the patient experienced an ST-segment elevated MI (STEMI) prior to the PCI was not collected, then differences in outcomes between the two access strategies could be due to STEMI.

If the previous assumptions of SUTVA and ignorability of treatment assignment are violated, the causal parameters can be estimated statistically, but cannot be interpreted causally. The remainder of the assumptions can be statistically assessed (see Section 1.4).

1.2.2.3 Positivity

Positivity requires units at every combination of observed covariates,

$$0 < P(T = 1 \mid \mathbf{X}) < 1. \tag{1.6}$$

Structural violations of positivity occur when units associated with a certain set of covariates cannot possibly receive the treatment or control. The ATE and the ATT cannot be identified under structural violations of positivity. A treatment for use only in women, for example, requires exclusion of males. Practical violations of the positivity assumption may arise due to finite sample sizes. With a large number of covariates, there may not be subjects receiving treatment and control in strata induced by the covariate space. Positivity is a statistically testable assumption.

1.2.2.4 Constant Treatment Effect

A constant treatment effect conditional on X implies that for any two subjects having the same values of covariates, their observable treatment effects should be similar:

$$\Delta_i \mid X = \Delta_j \mid X \; i \neq j. \tag{1.7}$$

Under a constant treatment effect, the ATE may be interpreted both marginally and conditionally. While this assumption can be empirically assessed, guidelines regarding exploratory and confirmatory approaches to determination of nonconstant treatment effects should be consulted (see Reference 10).

1.3 Approaches

Under the assumptions described above, various approaches exist to estimate the ATE. The approaches are divided into three types: methods that model only the treatment assignment mechanism via regression, methods that model only the outcome via regression, and methods that use both the treatment assignment mechanism and outcome. Formulae are provided and general guidelines for implementation based on existing theory to assist the reader in deciding how best to estimate the ATE are described.

1.3.1 Methods Using the Treatment Assignment Mechanism

Rosenbaum and Rubin [11] defined the propensity score as the probability of treatment conditional on observed baseline covariates, $e(X_i) = P(T_i = 1 \mid X_i)$. The propensity score, $e(X)$, is a type of balancing score such that the treatment and covariates are conditionally independent given the score, $T \perp X \mid e(X)$. As a result, for a given propensity score, treatment assignment is random. The true propensity score in an observational study is unknown and must be estimated. Because of the large number of covariates required to satisfy the treatment ignorability assumption, the propensity score is typically estimated parametrically by regressing the covariates on treatment status and obtaining the estimated propensity score, $\widehat{e(X)}$. Machine-learning methods have been developed for prediction and have been applied to the estimation of the propensity score (see References 12–15). Variables included in the propensity score model consist of confounders and those related to the outcome but not to the treatment. The latter are included to decrease the variance of the estimated treatment effect [16]. Instrumental variables, those related to treatment but not to the outcome, should be excluded [17]. The rationale for the exclusion of instrumental variables under treatment ignorability relates to the fact that their inclusion does not decrease the bias of the estimated treatment effect but does increase the variance. Chapter 2 provides a detailed account of instrumental variables methodology.

By their construction, propensity scores reduce the dimensionality of the covariate space so that they can be utilized to match, stratify, or weight observations. These techniques are next described. Inclusion of the propensity score as a predictor in a regression model of the outcome to replace the individual covariates constitutes a simpler dimension reduction approach compared to other estimators that use both the complete outcome regression and treatment mechanism (see Section 1.3.3). However, if the distribution of propensity scores differs between treatment groups, there will not be balance [18] between treated and control units when using $\widehat{e(X)}$ as a covariate; subsequent results may display substantial bias [19]. Thus, methods that do not make use of the propensity score, such as G-computation (Section 1.3.2.2), still benefit from an analysis of the propensity score, including testing for empirical violations of the positivity assumption.

1.3.1.1 Matching

Matching methods seek to find units with different levels of the treatment but having similar levels of the covariates. Matching based on the propensity score facilitates the matching problem through dimension reduction. Several choices must be made that impact the degree of incomplete matching (inability to find a control unit to match to a treated unit) and inexact matching (incomparability between treated and control units). These considerations include determination of the structure of the matches (one treated matched to one control, one-to-k, or one-to-variable), the method of finding matches (greedy vs. optimal matching), and the closeness of the matches (will any match do or should only close matches be acceptable). The literature on matching is broad on these topics. We refer the reader to Rassen et al. [20] for discussion about matching structure, Gu and Rosenbaum [21] for a discussion on the comparative performance of algorithms to find matches, and Rosenbaum [22] for options for defining closeness of matches.

Let $j_m(i)$ represent the index of the unit that is m th closest to unit i among units with the opposite treatment to that of unit i, $\mathcal{J}_M(i)$ the set of indices for the first M matches for unit i, such that $\mathcal{J}_M(i) = j_1(i), \ldots, j_M(i)$, and $K_M(i)$ the number of times unit i is used as a match. Lastly, define $K_M(i) = \sum_{l=1}^{N} I i \in \mathcal{J}_M(l)$, where I is the indicator function. Then the ATE estimator and its corresponding variance are

$$\hat{\Delta}_{Matching} = \frac{1}{N} \sum_{i=1}^{N} \left[(2T_i - 1) \left(1 + \frac{K_M(i)}{M} \right) Y_i \right],$$

$$\text{Var}(\hat{\Delta}_{Matching}) = \frac{1}{N^2} \sum_{i=1}^{N} \left(1 + \frac{K_M(i)}{M} \right)^2 \hat{\sigma}^2(X_i, T_i), \qquad (1.8)$$

where the conditional variance $\hat{\sigma}^2(X_i, T_i)$ is estimated as $(J/(J+1))(Y_i - (1/J) \sum_{m=1}^{J} Y_{l_j(i)})^2$ and J is a fixed number of observations. This approach [23] is implemented in the Matching package in the R software system. The variance formula does not account for estimation of the propensity score, only the uncertainty of the matching procedure itself. While adjustment for the matched sets in computing standard errors is debated [18], we recommend that this design feature be accounted for in the analysis.

Much of the preceding discussion assumed a larger pool of controls to find matches for treated subjects—an estimator using this strategy provides inference for the ATT. Estimating the ATE additionally requires identification of treatment matches for each control group unit. Therefore, the entire matching process is repeated to identify matches for units in the control group.

The matches found by both procedures are combined and used to compute the ATE.

1.3.1.2 Stratification

Stratification methods, also referred to as subclassification methods, divide subjects into strata based on the estimated propensity score. Within each stratum, treatment assignment is assumed random. As with matching, sub-classification can be accomplished without using the propensity score, but this runs into problems of dimensionality. Commonly, subjects are divided into groups by quintiles of the estimated propensity score, as Rosenbaum and Rubin [24] showed that using quintiles of the propensity score to strat-ify eliminates approximately 90% of the bias due to measured confounders in estimating the absolute treatment effect parameter, $\Delta = Y_1 - Y_0$. The aver-age effect is estimated in each stratum as the average of the differences in outcomes between the treated and control:

$$\hat{\Delta}_q = \frac{1}{N_{1q}} \sum_{i \in T \cap I_q} Y_i - \frac{1}{N_{0q}} \sum_{i \in C \cap I_q} Y_i,$$

where N_{iq} is the number of units in stratum q with treatment i, and I_q indicates membership in stratum q, so $T \cap I_q$ would indicate that a subject in stratum q received the treatment. The overall average is computed by averaging the within-strata estimates based on their sample sizes:

$$\hat{\Delta}_{Stratification} = \sum_{q=1}^{Q} W_q \Delta_q; \quad W_q = \frac{N_{1q} + N_{0q}}{N},$$

$$\text{Var}(\hat{\Delta}_{Stratification}) = \Sigma_q W_q^2 v_q^2; \quad v_q^2 = \frac{v_{1q}^2 + v_{0q}^2}{2}, \quad (1.9)$$

where $v_{iq}^2 = s_{iq}^2 / N_{iq}$. Because individuals in each stratum do not have identi-cal propensity scores, there may be residual confounding (see Reference 25) and balance between treated and control units requires examination within strata.

1.3.1.3 Inverse Probability of Treatment Weighted (IPTW) Estimators

The intuition behind weighting is that units that are underrepresented in one of the treatment groups are upweighted and units that are overrepresented are downweighted. The ATE can be estimated as

$$\hat{\Delta}_{HT-IPTW} = \frac{1}{N} \sum_{i=1}^{N} \frac{T_i Y_i}{\widehat{e(X_i)}} - \frac{1}{N} \sum_{i=1}^{N} \frac{(1 - T_i) Y_i}{1 - \widehat{e(X_i)}} \quad (1.10)$$

using the estimated propensity score, $\widehat{e(X)}$. We denote this estimate HT-IPTW to acknowledge the Horvitz–Thompson [26] ratio estimator utilized in survey sampling. IPTW estimators solve an estimating equation that sets the estimating function to zero and aims to find an estimator that is a solution of the equation. For example, consider

$$\sum_{i=1}^{N} D(\hat{\Delta})(T_i, Y_i, X_i) = 0,$$

where $D(\Delta)(T_i, Y_i, X_i)$ defines the estimating function and $\hat{\Delta}$ is an estimator of the parameter that is a solution of the estimating equation. Robins et al. [27] derived variance estimators, but bootstrapping can also be used. Inverse propensity score weighting is sensitive to outliers. Treated subjects with a propensity score close to one or control subjects with a propensity score close to zero will result in large weights. The weights can be trimmed but doing so introduces bias in the estimation of the treatment effect [28]. Robins et al. [29] propose using stabilizing weights, such that

$$\hat{\Delta}_{S-IPTW} = \left(\sum_{i=1}^{N} \frac{T_i}{\widehat{e(X_i)}} \right)^{-1} \sum_{i=1}^{N} \frac{T_i Y_i}{\widehat{e(X_i)}} - \left(\sum_{i=1}^{N} \frac{1-T_i}{1-\widehat{e(X_i)}} \right)^{-1} \sum_{i=1}^{N} \frac{(1-T_i)Y_i}{1-\widehat{e(X_i)}}.$$

$$(1.11)$$

IPTW estimators are known to have problems with large variance estimates in finite samples. Inverse probability weights can be used to estimate parameters defined by a marginal structural model, which we do not discuss here (see Reference 29). See References 30 and 31 for details regarding deriving variances using the empirical sandwich method. Alternatively, a bootstrap procedure may be applied to the whole process, including estimation of the propensity score.

1.3.2 Methods Using the Outcome Regression

1.3.2.1 Multiple Regression Modeling

The ATE can be estimated by the treatment coefficient from regression of the outcome on the treatment and all of the confounders. The functional form of the relationship between the outcome and covariates needs to be correctly specified. The risk difference can be validly estimated by fitting an ordinary least squares regression model and using the robust variance to account for nonnormality of the error terms. This approach is exactly equivalent to fitting a generalized linear model for a binomial outcome with the identity link and robust variance.

In the case of no overlap of the observed covariates between treatment groups, the model cannot be fit as the design matrix will be singular. Therefore, erroneous causal inferences are prohibited by the mechanics of the estimation procedure in the case of complete nonoverlap. However, standardized differences should still be examined to see how the treated and control groups differ, even under the assumption of no unmeasured confounding. If there is little overlap, causal inferences would be based on extrapolations, and hence, on less solid footing.

1.3.2.2 G-Computation

G-computation (G-computation algorithm formula, G-formula, Generalized-computation) is completely nonparametric [32], but we focus on parametric G-computation, which is a maximum-likelihood-based substitution estimator [33]. Substitution estimators involve using a maximum-likelihood-type estimator (e.g., regression, super learning) for the outcome regression and plugging it into the parameter mapping that defines the feature we are interested in estimating—here, that feature is the average treatment effect $\mu_1 - \mu_0$. For further discussion and references, the reader can consult Chapter 3. Under ignorability of the treatment assignment, the G-computation formula permits identification of the distribution of potential outcomes based on the observed data distribution. In step 1, a regression model or other consistent estimator for the relationship of the outcome with treatment (and covariates) is obtained. In step 2, (a) set each unit's treatment indicator to $T = 1$ and obtain predicted outcomes using the fit from step 1 and (b) repeat step 2(a) by setting each unit's treatment indicator to $T = 0$. The treatment effect is the difference between $\hat{Y}_{1i}$ and $\hat{Y}_{0i}$ for each unit, averaged across all subjects. When there are no treatment covariate interactions, linear regression and G-computation that uses a parametric linear regression provide the same answer for a continuous outcome. We can define this as

$$\hat{\Delta}_{G-comp} = \frac{1}{N} \sum_{i=1}^{N} [\hat{E}(Y \mid T_i = 1, X_i) - \hat{E}(Y \mid T_i = 0, X_i)], \quad (1.12)$$

where $\hat{E}(Y \mid T_i = t, X_i)$ is the regression of Y on X in the treatment group $T = t$. Two points are worth noting. First, if the outcome regression is not estimated consistently, the G-computation estimator may be biased. Second, while positivity violations will not be obvious when implementing a G-computation estimator, they remain important to assess, and can lead to a nonidentifiable parameter or substantially biased and inefficient estimate.

1.3.3 Methods Using the Treatment Assignment Mechanism and the Outcome

Double robust methods use an estimator for both the outcome regression and the treatment assignment. Estimators in this class may be preferable because they are consistent for the causal parameters if either the outcome regression or treatment assignment regression is consistently estimated [34]. Two double robust methods include the augmented inverse probability of treatment-weighted estimator (A-IPTW) and the targeted maximum likelihood estimator (TMLE).

1.3.3.1 Augmented Inverse Probability Weighted Estimators

Like IPTW estimators, A-IPTW estimators are also based on estimating equations but differ in that A-IPTW estimators are based on the *efficient influence curve*. An efficient influence curve is the derivative of the log-likelihood function with respect to the parameter of interest. The efficient influence curve is a function of the model and the parameter, and provides double robust estimators with many of their desirable properties, including consistency and efficiency [35]. The A-IPTW for the ATE is

$$\hat{\Delta}_{A-IPTW} = \frac{1}{N} \sum_{i=1}^{N} \frac{[I(T_i = 1) - I(T_i = 0)]}{\widehat{e(X_i)}} (Y_i - \hat{E}(Y \mid T_i, X_i))$$

$$+ \frac{1}{N} \sum_{i=1}^{N} (\hat{E}(Y \mid T_i = 1, X_i) - \hat{E}(Y \mid T_i = 0, X_i)), \qquad (1.13)$$

where $\hat{E}(Y \mid T_i = t, X_i)$ is the regression of Y on X in the treatment group $T = t$, and $I()$ is an indicator function. The nuisance parameters in the estimating equation for the A-IPTW are the treatment assignment mechanism and the outcome regression. Further discussion of estimating equations and efficient influence curve theory can be found in References 15, 35, and 36. Of note, A-IPTW estimators ignore the constraints imposed by the model by not being substitution estimators. For example, an A-IPTW estimator for a binary outcome may produce predicted probabilities outside the range [0,1]. Thus, finite sample efficiency may be impacted, even though asymptotic efficiency occurs if both the outcome regression and treatment assignment mechanism are consistently estimated.

1.3.3.2 Targeted Maximum Likelihood Estimator

The TMLE has a distinct algorithm for estimation of the parameter of interest, sharing the double robustness properties of the A-IPTW estimator, but boasting additional statistical properties. TMLE is a substitution estimator; thus, unlike the A-IPTW, it does respect the global constraints of the model. There-fore, among other advantages, this improves the finite sample performance of the TMLE.

The TMLE algorithm for the ATE involves two steps. First, the out-come regression $E[Y \mid T, X]$ and the treatment assignment mechanism $e(X)$ are estimated. Denote the initial estimate $\hat{E}[Y \mid T, X] = \widehat{Q^0}(T, X)$ and the updated estimate

$$\widehat{Q^1}(T, X) = \widehat{Q^0}(T, X) + \hat{\epsilon} \left(\frac{T}{\widehat{e(X)}} - \frac{1 - T}{1 - \widehat{e(X)}} \right),$$

where ϵ is estimated from the regression of Y on $(T/(\widehat{e(X)})) - ((1 - T)/(1 - \widehat{e(X)}))$ with an offset $\widehat{Q^0}(T, X)$. The estimator for the ATE is the given by

$$\hat{\Delta}_{TMLE} = \frac{1}{N} \sum_{i=1}^{N} (\widehat{Q^1}(T = 1, X_i) - \widehat{Q^1}(T = 0, X_i)). \tag{1.14}$$

A parametric regression can be used to estimate both the outcome regres-sion and the treatment assignment mechanism. However, the targeted learn-ing framework allows for the use of machine-learning methods to estimate these components in an effort to achieve consistent estimators [15,37,38]. Confidence intervals for both the A-IPTW and TMLE can be constructed using influence curve methods or bootstrapping techniques [15,35,36].

1.4 Assessing Validity of Assumptions

In this section, we introduce ways to assess the assumptions outlined in Sec-tion 1.2.2. Methods for testing the assumptions given the data (or possibly additional data) are areas of active research and this section is not exhaus-tive. SUTVA and ignorability of treatment assignment are untestable, but empirical data can provide evidence for how tenable these assumptions are in practice. In contrast, positivity and constant treatment effect are statistical assumptions that can be directly tested with the data.

1.4.1 SUTVA

As previously mentioned, SUTVA is composed of two parts: (1) no interfer-ence and (2) no variation in treatment. SUTVA is generally argued heuris-tically, but recent research uses the data to assess the no interference por-tion, mainly in randomized studies. Hudgens and Halloran [39] introduce the terminology of direct and indirect effects where the direct effect is an individual's response to treatment and the response to interference is the indirect effect. Detecting indirect effects is a way to assess the first component of SUTVA. For the randomized setting, Aronow [40] presents a *post hoc* method to detect interference using a conditional randomization test to calculate the dependence between outcomes on the treatment of other units.

However, for the second component, no variation in treatment refers to the actual or levels of treatments or the precise treatment procedure, rather than the treatment effects. We cannot assess this from the data alone in any practical or feasible way. When treatment is a drug intervention, one might question whether the patient really took 10 mg or if they received another dose. If we had millions of dollars and could collect unlimited variables related to precisely how every procedure was performed, we could ensure that there is no variation in the actual treatment. For the radial versus femoral artery access example, perhaps we would measure how high the surgeon's hands were from the incision, the time in between sedation and the beginning of procedure, number of hours the surgeon had slept, and so on.

1.4.2 Ignorability

Ignorability of the treatment assignment is not directly testable and largely assessed by subject matter knowledge. Several strategies can bolster the viability of the assumption [41] however. Multiple control or comparison groups that differ with respect to an unmeasured confounder, if available, can be used. If outcomes between the two control groups do not differ, then this observation would support the argument that the unmeasured confounder is not responsible for any treatment–control outcome differences. Another option is to identify an outcome that is associated with an unmeasured covariate but where a treatment would not expect to have any effect. Such outcomes, referred to as *control* outcomes, provide a means to detect unobserved confounding. Tchetgen [42] proposes a method to correct estimates using control outcomes. Finally, Rosenbaum [22] provides approaches to perform a sensitivity analysis for an unobserved confounder through examination of a range of potential correlations between the unobserved confounder and the treatment assignment, and the unmeasured confounder and the outcome.

1.4.3 Positivity

Positivity or overlap can be measured through examination of the distributions of covariates for the treated and control subjects. While there are many measures of balance, the difference in average covariates scaled by the sample standard deviation, d, provides an intuitive metric. It is calculated as

$$d = \frac{\bar{x}_{1j} - \bar{x}_{0j}}{\sqrt{(s_{1j}^2 + s_{0j}^2)/2}}, \tag{1.15}$$

where $\bar{x}_{ij}$ is the mean of covariate j among those with treatment i and s_{ij} is the estimated standard deviation. The quantity d is interpreted as the number of standard deviations the treated group is above the control group. Mapping the standardized differences to percentiles provides a mechanism to describe the extent of nonoverlap between two groups. For instance, a standardized difference of 0.1 indicates 7.7% nonoverlap of the two normal distributions; a standardized difference of 0 indicates complete overlap of the two groups; and a standardized difference of 0.7 corresponds to 43.0% nonoverlap. Rules of thumb suggest that a standardized difference less than 0.1 is negligible [43]. Examination of the standardized differences alone characterizes only marginal distributions—the distribution of individual covariates. Because areas of weak overlap may exist, reviewing the distributions of the estimated propensity scores stratified by treatment groups is recommended.

1.4.4 Constant Treatment Effect

The assumption of a constant treatment effect may be explored by introducing interactions between the treatment and subgroup indicators, or by dividing the population into subgroups based on X_i, estimating an average causal effect within each subgroup, and comparing the constancy of subgroup-specific causal effects. Cases in which the treatment effect may not be constant should be identified *a priori* as well as the size of meaningful treatment effect heterogeneity in order to avoid multiple testing.

1.5 Radial versus Femoral Artery Access for PCI

We return to the PCI example introduced earlier to determine whether access via the radial artery reduces the risk of in-hospital complications compared to access via the femoral artery. Table 1.3 indicated imbalances between the radial and femoral artery-accessed subjects. For instance, the standardized difference for use of thrombin is -0.6285, indicating 40% nonoverlap between the distribution of thrombin use for those undergoing PCI via the radial artery and those via the femoral artery. Ten of the observed covariates have standardized differences greater than 0.1 or 7.7% nonoverlap.

1.5.1 Estimating Treatment Assignment: Probability of Radial Artery Access

The propensity score was estimated using logistic regression. The set of covariates initially considered were determined by conversations with cardiologists who perform PCI. A primary model specification was selected

TABLE 1.3

Population Characteristics Pre- and Postmatching Listed by Type of Intervention

	Prematch			Postmatch		
	Intervention		% Standardized Mean Difference	Intervention		% Standardized Mean Difference
	Radial	Femoral		Radial	Femoral	
Number of procedures	5,192	35,022		10,326	10,326	
Demographics						
Mean age [SD]	63 [12]	65 [12]	−15.68	63 [12]	63 [12]	0.29
Female	25.3	29.8	−9.88	25.4	25.0	0.91
Race						
White	89.6	89.4	0.66	89.7	89.2	1.83
Black	3.3	3.2	0.91	3.2	3.1	0.72
Hispanic	4.3	3.5	4.40	4.3	4.8	−2.50
Other	2.8	3.9	−6.74	2.7	2.9	−1.00
Health insurance						
Government	46	50.3	−8.65	46.2	46.1	0.23
Commercial	4.8	13.4	−30.09	4.8	5.6	−3.31
Other	49.2	36.3	26.24	48.9	48.3	1.24
Comorbidities						
Diabetes	33.1	32.7	0.85	33.1	33.8	−1.35
Prior CHF	9.4	12.7	−10.41	9.5	9.8	−1.08
Prior PCI	32	34.3	−4.75	32.1	33.3	−2.44
Prior MI	28.7	30.1	−3.24	28.7	29.2	−1.05
Prior bypass surgery	8.4	15.7	−22.68	8.4	9.3	−2.90

(Continued)

TABLE 1.3 (Continued)

Population Characteristics Pre- and Postmatching Listed by Type of Intervention

| | Prematch | | | Postmatch | | |
| | Intervention | | % Standardized | Intervention | | % Standardized |
	Radial	Femoral	Mean Difference	Radial	Femoral	Mean Difference
Hypertension	79.6	80.7	-2.81	79.7	79.8	-0.24
Peripheral vascular disease	12.1	12.8	-2.22	12.1	13.2	-3.21
Smoker	24.8	23.1	3.94	24.9	24.7	0.38
Lung disease	13.7	14.4	-2.04	13.8	14.1	-0.92
Cardiac presentation						
Multivessel disease	10.3	10.9	-2.21	10.2	9.9	0.97
Number of vessels >70% stenosis	1.49	1.58	-12.53	1.49	1.49	0.30
Left main disease	3.7	7.2	-15.21	3.8	4.1	-1.60
ST-segment elevated MI	38.9	42.6	-7.56	39.1	39.1	0.04
Shock	0.44	1.8	-13.08	0.4	0.7	-3.90
Drugs prior to procedure						
Heparin (unfractionated)	87.3	61.7	61.50	87.2	86.6	1.81
Heparin (low-molecular weight)	3.83	4.27	-2.21	3.8	3.6	1.33
Thrombin	25.5	54.9	-62.85	25.7	24.9	1.83
G2B3A inhibitors	26.7	26.8	-0.33	26.8	25.6	2.75
Platelet aggregate inhibitors	85.8	86.6	-2.20	86.2	86.4	-0.48
Aspirin	98.2	97.5	4.79	98.2	98.1	0.79
In-hospital complication (%)	0.69	2.73		0.69	2.09	

Note: All are reported as percentages, except the number of procedures, age, and number of vessels. Positive standardized difference indicates a larger mean in the radial artery group.

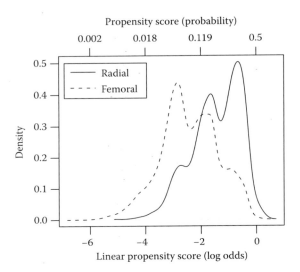

FIGURE 1.1

Density of estimated linear propensity scores, $\text{logit}(\widehat{e(X_i)})$, by artery access strategy. Larger values of the propensity score correspond to a higher likelihood of radial artery access. The upper horizontal axis gives the scale of the actual estimated probabilities of radial artery access.

for determining radial versus femoral artery access and included all covariates linearly as well as interactions (Appendix 1A.1). Visual examination of a density plot of the estimated linear propensity scores by treatment arm (Figure 1.1) provides insights into the observable differences between the radial and femoral groups. The overlap assumption may also be tested with a formal comparison test, such as the Kolmogorov–Smirnov nonparametric test. If there is little overlap, excluding subjects with extreme propensity score values may be necessary. For example, there are some subjects undergoing femoral artery-accessed PCI whose estimated linear propensity scores do not overlap with the linear propensity scores for radial artery-accessed subjects (Figure 1.1, density to the left of values of −5.0). Dropping subjects will make the estimates only valid for the region of common support. For the PCI example, visual inspection indicates that there are no patients who have a very high probability of radial treatment (on the probability scale, values near 1). The majority of subjects in both groups have low propensity scores, but those receiving radial artery access have higher propensity scores on average, as expected.

1.5.2 Approaches

Using the estimators described earlier, we determine the comparative effectiveness of radial artery access relative to femoral artery access. For comparability among estimates, all 95% interval estimates reported below are constructed using robust standard errors (1,000 bootstrap replicates or theoretical results).

1.5.2.1 Matching on the Propensity Score

Using the Matching program in R, we implement 1-1 matching without replacement to estimate the ATE. First, we identified femoral artery-accessed matches for each radial artery-accessed subject and next, found radial artery-accessed matches for each femoral artery-accessed subject. This resulted in 10,326 matched pairs using a caliper of 0.2 standard deviations of the linear propensity score. The caliper was necessary in order to reduce the standardized differences for all covariates to below 0.1. In the matched sample, 42 of the radial artery subjects were used only once, 5,142 were used twice, and 8 were not used; 7,084 of the femoral artery subjects were used once, 1,621 were used twice, and 26,317 were not used. After matching, the percent standardized mean differences (Table 1.3 and Figure 1.2) improved. The linear propensity scores for radial artery and femoral artery-accessed subjects in the matched sample overlap substantially (Figure 1.3).

The ATE estimated using matching and corresponding 95% confidence interval is

$$\hat{\Delta}_{Matching} = -0.0143(-0.0182, -0.0104), \qquad (1.16)$$

indicating subjects undergoing PCI via radial artery access were 1.43% less likely to have an in-hospital complication compared to those accessed via the femoral artery. Using a more stringent caliper moved the point estimate further from the null, and toward the estimate found by the other methods, but discarded more observations.

We note two additional facts. First, the estimate of the ATT is -0.0145 (standard error $= 0.0023$), a slightly larger benefit in those likely to undergo PCI via the radial artery. Second, because we created matched pairs, McNemar's test could also be used for inference. The number of pairs in which the in-hospital complication rates differed within members of the pairs was 285 (2.76% of the 10,326 matched pairs). Among the 285 discordant pairs, the number of pairs in which the radial artery-accessed member had an in-hospital complication was 70 (0.25 of discordant pairs). This value is lower than the null of 0.5 and indicates a benefit of radial artery access.

1.5.2.2 Stratification on the Propensity Score

The 40,214 subjects were grouped into five strata using estimated propensity scores (Table 1.4). In the lowest quintile ($q = 1$), 2.46% of subjects fell into the radial artery access group whereas, in the highest quintile, 31.8% of the subjects were accessed via the radial artery. If the propensity scores are balanced in each stratum, the covariates in each stratum should also be balanced. However, only using five strata did not result in balanced propensity scores for the

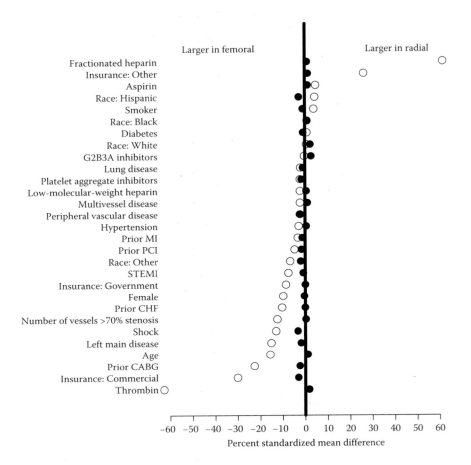

FIGURE 1.2
Percent standardized mean differences before (unfilled) and after matching (filled), ordered by largest positive percent standardized mean difference before matching.

PCI data. Two sample *t*-tests within strata showed significant differences in the propensity scores for the radial and femoral groups, although, visually, the linear propensity scores appear quite similar within strata (Figure 1.4). There was less balance in the extreme quintiles, as is often the case.

The stratum-specific estimates are consistent—in every quintile, radial artery-accessed patients were less likely to have complications compared to femoral artery-accessed patients. Quintile-specific estimates were combined to obtain an overall $\hat{\Delta}_{Stratification} = -0.0168(-0.0213, -0.0122)$ (Section 1.3.1.2), indicating that subjects undergoing PCI via radial artery access were 1.68% less likely to have in-hospital complications compared to those accessed via the femoral artery. Caution should be exercised in interpreting this estimate given the imbalance between treatment groups is still present

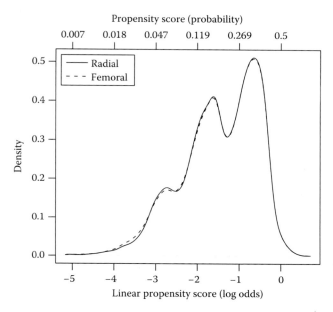

FIGURE 1.3

Density of estimated linear propensity scores, $\text{logit}(\widehat{e(X_i)})$, after matching by artery access strategy. Larger values of the propensity score correspond to a higher likelihood of radial artery access. The top axis gives the scale of the actual estimated probabilities of radial artery access.

TABLE 1.4

Properties of the Quintiles Based on the Propensity Score Where $q = 1$ Has the Smallest Values of the Propensity Score and $q = 5$ the Largest

	Radial		Femoral		Average
Stratum q	N_{1q}	%	N_{0q}	$\bar{y}_{1q} - \bar{y}_{0q}$	$\widehat{e(X)}$
1	198	2.46	7,845	−0.0135	0.0246
2	435	5.41	7,608	−0.0147	0.0529
3	753	9.36	7,289	−0.0217	0.0926
4	1,249	15.53	6,794	−0.0181	0.1588
5	2,557	31.79	5,486	−0.0158	0.3166
Overall	5,192	12.91	35,022	−0.0168	0.1291

Note: For each quintile, sample sizes, and percentages of subjects undergoing radial artery access, the difference in mean in risk of complications ($\hat{\Delta}_q$, Section 1.3.1.2) and the average estimated propensity score are reported.

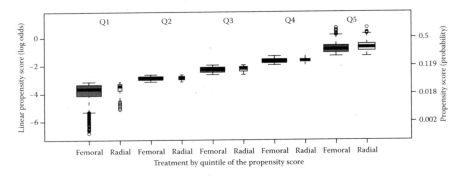

FIGURE 1.4
Boxplots of the linear propensity scores (log odds of radial artery access) by quintile. Boxplot widths are proportional to the square root of the samples sizes. The right axis gives the scale of the actual estimated probabilities of radial artery access.

within quintiles. Increasing the number of strata from 5 to 10 did not eliminate imbalance of the linear propensity scores between radial and femoral subjects within strata based on two sample t-tests (6 out of the 10 strata had p-values >0.05). Achieving balance requires modifying the logistic model for treatment assignment or eliminating subjects residing in areas of nonoverlap. In our example, we are unable to find a propensity score method that balances the data using stratification and thus conclude that this approach is unsuitable. Haviland et al. [44] found their treatment and control groups to be too dissimilar to warrant continued propensity score analysis.

1.5.2.3 Weighting by the Propensity Score

To implement weighting by the inverse probability, we estimate the weights as $1/\widehat{e(X)}$ for the radial subjects and $1/(1-\widehat{e(X)})$ for the femoral subjects. The weights are strongly right skewed having a maximum of 170 (radial artery-accessed subject) and median of 1.11 leading to $\hat{\Delta}_{HT-IPTW} = -0.0168(-0.0214, -0.0122)$. The stabilized point and interval estimates are $\hat{\Delta}_{S-IPTW} = -0.0169(-0.0214, -0.0124)$. The results are similar, both indicating a benefit of radial artery access. However, the maximum weight, even after stabilizing, remained large with a value of 22.

1.5.2.4 Multiple Regression

We estimate the ATE for a few different multiple regression models with robust standard errors. Adjusting for all measured covariates using indicators for quintiles of age and number of vessels with $>70\%$ stenosis, the ATE was $-0.0160(-0.0205, -0.0112)$. All potential confounders have events, so it is reasonable with our sample size to include all known and suspected risk factors in the multivariable model. A stepwise selected model with a liberal entry/exit criteria (p-value $= 0.2$) was also run where, when any variable where 1 or more levels were selected, all levels were forced into the final model. This model resulted in an ATE closer to the null value, $-0.0152(-0.0200, -0.0107)$.

1.5.2.5 G-Computation

G-computation does not use the model for the propensity score. To estimate the ATE using G-computation, we assume a linear relationship between in-hospital complications and all covariates and the treatment indicator. The estimated coefficients and standard errors are reported in Table 1.5. The key parameter is the coefficient of the term *Radial*, which is estimated as -0.016 (standard error $= 0.002$). Using all the estimated regression coefficients to obtain predictions and differencing yields $\hat{\Delta}_{G-comp} = -0.0160(-0.0189, -0.0127)$.

1.5.2.6 Augmented IPTW

The augmented IPTW uses the models for both the outcome and the propensity score (see Section 1.5.1 and Appendix Table 1A.1) for an estimate of $\hat{\Delta}_{AIPTW} = -0.0164(-0.0210, -0.0118)$. The risk of in-hospital complications is 1.64% lower in the radial group.

1.5.2.7 Targeted Maximum Likelihood Estimation

To estimate the ATE using TMLE, we utilize the tmle package in R. We supply parametric models for the outcome and the propensity score (see Section 1.5.1 and Appendix Table 1A.1) to compare results. The resulting treatment effect estimate is $\hat{\Delta}_{TMLE} = -0.0163(-0.0209, -0.0117)$. Inferences are similar to the earlier findings—a lower risk of in-hospital complications associated with radial compared to femoral artery access.

1.5.3 Comparison of Approaches

The results of the various approaches to the estimation of the effectiveness of radial artery access compared to femoral artery access for PCI are similar (Figure 1.5; Table 1.6). Each indicated a lower risk of in-hospital complications for the radial artery approach compared to the femoral approach. The only method that discarded subjects was matching on the propensity score, which may explain why the estimated risk difference for this method differed from the others. The ATE based on G-computation had the shortest confidence interval (width $= 0.62$), 2/3 the size of the largest.

TABLE 1.5

Estimated Coefficients (Standard Errors) of the Outcome Model

Covariate	Estimated Coefficient	Estimated Standard Error
Female	0.017	(0.002)
Diabetes	0.001	(0.002)
Smoker	0.001	(0.002)
Prior PCI	−0.004	(0.002)
Prior MI	0.0002	(0.002)
Prior CABG	−0.007	(0.003)
Prior CHF	0.027	(0.002)
Lung disease	0.006	(0.002)
STEMI	0.012	(0.002)
Race: Black	−0.008	(0.004)
Race: Hispanic	−0.003	(0.004)
Race: Other	−0.0002	(0.005)
Insurance: Commercial	0.005	(0.003)
Insurance: Other	−0.002	(0.002)
Shock	0.068	(0.006)
Left main disease	0.022	(0.003)
Age	0.001	(0.0001)
Multivessel disease	0.008	(0.003)
Number of vessels >70% stenosis	−0.001	(0.001)
Peripheral vascular disease	0.006	(0.002)
Hypertension	0.003	(0.002)
Aspirin	0.0002	(0.005)
Fractionated heparin	0.002	(0.002)
Low-molecular-weight heparin	0.001	(0.004)
G2B3A inhibitors	0.021	(0.002)
Platelet aggregate inhibitors	−0.006	(0.002)
Thrombin	−0.001	(0.002)
Radial access	−0.016	(0.002)
Constant	−0.034	(0.008)

Did we make reasonable assumptions? We indicated that the SUTVA may be violated as a consequence of (a) patients nested with physicians and (b) the practice makes perfect hypothesis. A reasonable next step would involve the inclusion of random physician effects. The positivity assumption is met for the matching estimator because of the restrictions we placed on identifying matches. However, there may be regions of imbalance for the other estimators using the estimated propensity scores—we observed residual confounding when using the stratified estimate. In terms of treatment assignment ignorability, we do not have a control outcome nor an

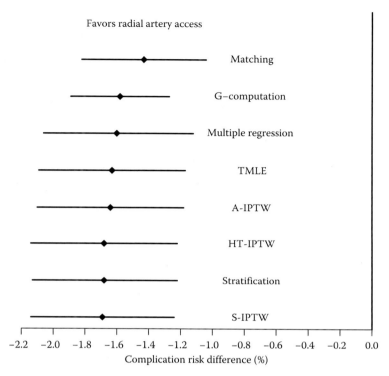

FIGURE 1.5

Comparison of results, ordered by size of ATE estimate. All methods use the same model for treatment assignment and outcome. All 95% confidence intervals are based on 1,000 bootstrap replicates. TMLE, targeted maximum likelihood estimation; A, augmented; HT, Horvitz–Thompson; S, stabilized; IPTW, inverse probability of treatment weighted.

TABLE 1.6

Model Results: Estimated Coefficient of the Treatment Effect, Radial versus Femoral Artery Access on Any In-Hospital Complications (Robust Standard Errors)

	Estimated	
Method	**Coefficient**	**Standard Error**
Matching	−0.0143	(0.0020)
Stratification	−0.0168	(0.0023)
IPTW	−0.0168	(0.0023)
Multiple regression	−0.0160	(0.0024)
G-computation	−0.0160	(0.0016)
A-IPTW	−0.0164	(0.0023)
TMLE	−0.0163	(0.0023)

additional comparison group. We did determine that to attribute the ATE to an unobserved confounder rather than to radial artery access, an unobserved confounder would need to produce a 2.5-fold increase in the odds of radial access (beyond that adjusting for the set of covariates we have already included). Is it plausible that such a confounder exists? Of course one could exist—to place the size of the unmeasured confounder into context, the odds associated with fractionated heparin is 7.1, and with no shock, it is 3.9. Finally, there is an *a priori* reason to believe that the effectiveness of radial versus femoral artery access may differ between males and females, that is, there may be a nonconstant treatment effect. Using matching estimators, we find a benefit of radial artery access in both males and females, with the ATE in females twice that of males: female ATE $= -0.0267$ (standard error $= 0.004317$) and male ATE $= -0.0100$ (standard error $= 0.001583$).

Although all patients considering PCI may wish to undergo radial access for their procedure, women may have fewer complications than men with radial versus femoral. Overall, had everyone undergone PCI via radial access versus femoral access, the risk of in-hospital complications would have been 1.6% lower. The number needed to treat (the reciprocal of the risk difference) is 49.1 with bootstrapped 95% CI from 46.7 to 51.0, meaning 49 people need to have PCI with radial access rather than femoral to prevent one additional in-hospital complication. The individual risks of in-hospital complications are quite low for the procedure overall with less than 1,000 patients experiencing complications in the entire cohort of over 40,000. As such, many patients may leave the choice up to their physician for the access site and the physician's level of comfort with the procedure is important for the patient outcome.

1.6 Concluding Remarks

As the need for CER grows, reliance on observational cohort studies will as well. Several estimators are available to researchers to infer the effect of interventions. Causal inference can be made from observational studies whenever there is no bias. In cross-sectional studies, standard multivariable modeling methods can be used to obtain causal estimates, but the model needs to include all confounders properly parameterized. Standard multivariate methods to adjust for confounding yielded the same results as those obtained from the other, more computationally intensive methods. Further research is needed to identify when causal inference requires more complex methods, and when standard approaches adjust sufficiently for bias due to confounding and can be used to obtain causal interpretations. For instance, double robust methods may be helpful if we have more knowledge about the model for treatment assignment than the model for the outcome. All involve statistical assumptions, and, as we have described, some fundamental causal assumptions that are not testable. In this chapter, we reviewed a selected set of estimators—our review is by no means comprehensive and is for cross-sectional data only. The reader is strongly encouraged to read the articles we have referenced. An example involving the choice of artery to utilize when unblocking clogged arteries illustrated the assumptions required, empirical evidence to support the assumptions when possible, and the estimates. The data involved over 40,000 subjects and the availability of many covariates. We focused on a single treatment assignment mechanism model and a single outcome model—clearly, more than one model may fit the data and meet the assumptions. As data acquisition technologies grow, researchers will be faced with making more analytical decisions when conducting empirical studies. These decisions should be made transparent to readers.

Acknowledgments

Dr. Normand's effort was supported by FDA/Chickasaw Nation Industries contract HHSF223201110172C (MDEpiNet Methodology Center) and by U01-FD004493 (MDEpiNet Medical Counter Measures Study). We gratefully acknowledge the Massachusetts Department of Public Health for permitting the use of the radial artery access example data.

Appendix 1A.1: Implementing Methods for Comparative Effectiveness Research

1A.1.1 Factors Associated with Radial Artery Access versus Femoral Artery Access

1A.1.1.1 R code

All analyses were performed with R software, version 2.14.1. The general code is provided for the case where Y is the binary outcome, T is the binary treatment, X is the vector of covariates, and PS is the estimated propensity score. All standard errors were computed by bootstrapping. The appendix of Ahern et al. [45] provides guidance for this procedure.

1A.1.1.1.1 Propensity Score Estimation
Denote the propensity score by PS and the linear propensity score by lPS.

```
PSmodel=glm(T ~ X,family=binomial(link="logit"),data=dataset)
                PS=predict(PSmodel,dataset,type="response")
                    lPS=predict(PSmodel,dataset)
```

TABLE 1A.1

Covariates Included in the Propensity Score Model

Linear Terms	Interaction Terms
Female	Smoker:race
Diabetes	Smoker:age
Smoker	Smoker:platelet aggregate inhibitors
Prior PCI	Prior CABG:peripheral vascular disease
Prior MI	Prior CHF:hypertension
Prior CABG	Prior CHF:G2B3A inhibitors
Prior CHF	Prior CHF:thrombin
Lung disease	Lung disease:left main disease
STEMI	Lung disease:hypertension
Race: white (baseline), black, Hispanic, other	Age^2
Insurance: government (baseline), commercial, other	STEMI:fractionated heparin
Shock	STEMI:low-molecular-weight heparin
Left main disease	STEMI:G2B3A inhibitors
Age	STEMI:platelet aggregate inhibitors
Multivessel disease	STEMI:thrombin
Number of vessels >70% stenosis	Insurance:race
Peripheral vascular disease	Insurance:age
Hypertension	Insurance:peripheral vascular disease
Aspirin	Insurance:hypertension
Fractionated heparin	Insurance:G2B3A inhibitors
Low-molecular-weight heparin	Insurance:thrombin
G2B3A inhibitors	Age:peripheral vascular disease
Platelet aggregate inhibitors	Age:hypertension
Thrombin	Age:platelet aggregate inhibitors
	Age:thrombin
	Age:fractionated heparin
	Age:low-molecular-weight heparin
	Peripheral vascular disease:fractionated heparin
	Peripheral vascular disease:low-molecular-weight heparin
	Fractionated heparin:G2B3A inhibitors
	Low-molecular-weight heparin:G2B3A inhibitors
	Fractionated heparin:platelet aggregate inhibitors
	Low-molecular-weight heparin:platelet aggregate inhibitors
	Fractionated heparin:thrombin
	Low-molecular-weight heparin:thrombin
	G2B3A inhibitors:thrombin

1A.1.1.1.2 Matching on the Propensity Score

Using the Matching package to perform 1-1 matching ($M = 1$), without replacement (replace = FALSE) and a caliper of 0.2 standard deviations of the propensity score (caliper = 0.2), to estimate the average treatment effect (estimand = "ATE"). Further options can be found in the manual for this package.

```
library(Matching)
runmatch=Match(Y=Y,Tr=T,X=1PS,
M=1,replace=FALSE,caliper=0.2,estimand="ATE")
runmatch$est # estimated ATE
runmatch$est-1.96*runmatch$se.standard # lower 95% CI limit
runmatch$est+1.96*runmatch$se.standard # upper 95% CI limit
```

The original data can be accessed to identify the matched pairs using:

```
matcheddata =
dataset[c(runmatch$index.treated,runmatch$index.control),]
```

1A.1.1.1.3 Stratification on the Propensity Score

First create the quintiles and then create a variable to indicate the stratum to which a subject belongs. The data may be divided into fewer or more quantiles by modifying the quantile() command. The balance within each stratum can be assessed with a *t*-test, where in the following "i" should be replaced by the stratum of interest. A loop can be used to quickly cycle through all of the strata.

```
breakvals=quantile(PS, prob=0:5*0.2)
strat=cut(PS, breaks=breakvals,
labels=c('1','2','3','4','5'),include.lowest=TRUE)
t.test(PS[strat==i&T==1],PS[strat==i&T==0])
```

To combine the results across strata, we wrote the following functions that can be called by plugging in the variables for the outcome (out), treatment (treat), and strata (str):

```
difference.means = function(out, treat)
{mean(out[treat==1],na.rm=TRUE)-mean(out[treat==0],na.rm=TRUE)}
```

```
SE = function(out,treat)
{sqrt(var(out[treat==1],na.rm=TRUE)/sum(treat==1)+var(out
[treat==0],na.rm=TRUE)/sum(treat==0))}
```

```
         strata.average = function(out, treat, str) {
Q = length(table(str)); n=length(out); differences=rep(NA,Q)
                    for (q in 1:Q) differences[q] =
        difference.means(out[str==q],treat[str==q])
                             weights=table(str)/n
      overall.difference = weights%*%differences
            return(list("Mean Difference within
                   Strata"=differences,"Average
  Weighted Mean Difference"=overall.difference))}

         strata.variance = function(out,treat,str)
{Q = length(table(str)); n=length(out); variances=rep(NA,Q)
for (q in 1:Q) variances[q]= SE(out[str==q],out[str==q])**2
                      weights = table(str)/n
           overall.variance = weights**2%*%variances
    return(list("Variance within Strata"=variances,"Overall
                                      Variance"=
   overall.variance,"Overall SE"=sqrt(overall.variance)))}

                        strata.average(Y,T,strat)
              strata.variance.average(Y,T,strat)
```

1A.1.1.1.4 Weighting by the Propensity Score

For the IPTW estimators, the point estimates are obtained using

```
       HT.IPTW = mean((T/PS-(1-T)/(1-PS))*Y)
  S.IPTW= sum(T*Y/PS)/sum(T/PS)-sum((1-T)*Y/(1-PS))/
                          sum((1-T)/(1-PS))
```

1A.1.1.1.5 G-Computation

G-computation performs the outcome regression and then predicts the outcome as if all subjects received treatment and also if all subjects received control. Without using MSM, the estimate of the ATE is the average of each individuals predicted Y_{1i} and Y_{0i}.

```
        outreg=lm(Y ~ T+X, data=dataset)
     all.pred=predict(outreg) # predicts Y
                                     T1.pred=
  predict(outreg,newdata=data.frame(dataset[,-"T"],T=1))
        # predictions when T=1 for all subjects
                                    T0.pred =
  predict(outreg,newdata=data.frame(dataset[,-"T"],T=0))
        # predictions when T=0 for all subjects
              G.comp = mean(T1.pred-T0.pred)
```

1A.1.1.1.6 Augmented IPTW

Augmented IPTW uses the same predictions of the outcome as G-computation and then combines the predictions to compute the point estimate.

```
A.IPTW=mean(((T/PS-(1-T)/(1-PS))*(Y-all.pred))+ mean
                                        (T1.pred-T0.pred)
```

1A.1.1.1.7 Targeted Maximum Likelihood Estimation

TMLE uses the `tmle` program and we demonstrate how to specify the parametric forms of the outcome and treatment regressions. Super learning is the default when Qform and gform are unspecified.

```
                                        library(tmle)
TMLE =tmle(Y=Y,A=T,W=X,Qform=Y~A+X,gform=A ~X)
                                        summary(TMLE)
```

References

1. What is comparative effectiveness research, http://effectivehealthcare.ahrq.gov/index.cfm/what-is-comparative-effectiveness-research1/, April 2014.
2. L. Mauri, T. S. Silbaugh, P. Garg, R. E. Wolf, K. Zelevinsky, A. Lovett, M. R. Varma, Z. Zhou, S.-L. T. Normand, Drug-eluting or bare-metal stents for acute myocardial infarction, *New England Journal of Medicine* 359, 2008, 1330–1342.
3. P. W. Holland, Statistics and causal inference, *Journal of the American Statistical Association* 81 (396), 1986, 945–960.
4. G. W. Imbens, The role of the propensity score in estimating dose-response functions, *Biometrika* 87 (3), 2000, 706–710.
5. B. Lu, E. Zanutto, R. Hornik, P. R. Rosenbaum, Matching with doses in an observational study of a media campaign against drug abuse, *Journal of the American Statistical Association* 96, 2001, 1245–1253.
6. S. Greenland, J. M. Robins, Identifiability, exchangeability, and epidemiological confounding, *International Journal of Epidemiology* 15 (3), 1986, 413–419.
7. G. W. Imbens, J. D. Angrist, Identification and estimation of local average treatment effects, *Econometrica* 62 (2), 1994, 467–475.
8. J. S. Sekhon, The Neyman–Rubin model of causal inference and estimation via matching methods, *The Oxford Handbook of Political Methodology*, edited by J. M. Box-Steffensmeier, H. E. Brady, and D. Collier, Oxford University Press Inc. New York, 2008, 271–299.
9. J. J. Heckman, H. Hidehiko, P. Todd, Matching as an econometric evaluation estimator: Evidence from evaluating a job training programme, *Review of Economic Studies* 64, 1997, 605–654.

10. The PCORI (Patient-Centered Outcomes Research Institute) methodology report, http://www.pcori.org/research-we-support/research-methodology-standards, November 2013.
11. P. R. Rosenbaum, D. B. Rubin, The central role of the propensity score in observational studies for causal effects, *Biometrika* 70, 1983, 41–55.
12. B. Lee, J. Lessler, E. A. Stuart, Improving propensity score weighting using machine learning, *Statistics in Medicine* 29, 2009, 337–346.
13. D. F. McCaffrey, G. Ridgeway, A. R. Morral, Propensity score estimation with boosted regression for evaluating causal effects in observational studies, *Psychological Methods* 9, 2004, 403–425.
14. S. Setoguchi, S. Schneeweiss, M. A. Brookhart, R. J. Glynn, E. F. Cook, Evaluating uses of data mining techniques in propensity score estimation: A simulation study, *Pharmacoepidemiology and Drug Safety* 17, 2008, 546–555.
15. M. J. van der Laan, S. Rose, *Targeted Learning: Causal Inference for Observational and Experimental Data*, Springer, New York, 2011.
16. D. B. Rubin, The design versus the analysis of observational studies for causal effects: Parallels with the design of randomized trials, *Statistics in Medicine* 26, 2007, 20–36.
17. M. A. Brookhart, S. Schneeweiss, K. J. Rothman, R. J. Glynn, J. Avorn, T. Sturmer, Variable selection for propensity score models, *American Journal of Epidemiology* 163, 2006, 1149–1156.
18. E. A. Stuart, Matching methods for causal inference: A review and a look forward, *Statistical Science* 25 (1), 2010, 1–21.
19. J. D. Y. Kang, J. L. Schafer, Demystifying double robustness: A comparison of alternative strategies for estimating a population mean from incomplete data, *Statistical Science* 22 (4), 2007, 523–539.
20. J. A. Rassen, A. A. Shelat, J. Myers, R. J. Glynn, K. J. Rothman, S. Schneeweiss, One-to-many propensity score matching in cohort studies, *Pharmacoepidemiology and Drug Safety* 21 (S2), 2012, 69–80.
21. X. Gu, P. R. Rosenbaum, Comparison of multivariate matching methods: Structures, distances, and algorithms, *Journal of Computational and Graphical Statistics* 2, 1993, 405–420.
22. P. R. Rosenbaum, *Observational Studies*, 2nd Edition, Springer, New York, 2002.
23. A. Abadie, G. W. Imbens, Large sample properties of matching estimators for average treatment effects, *Econometrica* 74, 2006, 235–267.
24. P. R. Rosenbaum, D. B. Rubin, Reducing bias in observational studies using subclassification on the propensity score, *Journal of the American Statistical Association* 79, 1984, 516–524.
25. P. C. Austin, M. M. Mamdani, A comparison of propensity score methods: A case study estimating the effectiveness of postami statin use, *Statistics in Medicine* 25, 2006, 2084–2106.
26. D. G. Horvitz, D. J. Thompson, A generalization of sampling without replacement from a finite universe, *Journal of the American Statistical Association* 47 (260), 1952, 663–685.
27. J. M. Robins, A. Rotnitzky, L. P. Zhao, Analysis of semiparametric regression models for repeated outcomes in the presence of missing data, *Journal of the American Statistical Association* 90, 1995, 106–121.

28. F. J. Potter, The effect of weight trimming on nonlinear survey estimates, in: *Proceedings of the Section on Survey Research Methods of American Statistical Association*, American Statistical Association, San Francisco, CA, 1993.

29. J. M. Robins, M. Hernan, B. Brumback, Marginal structural models and causal inference in epidemiology, *Epidemiology* 11 (5), 2000, 550–560.

30. J. K. Lunceford, M. Davidian, Stratification and weighting via the propensity score in estimation of causal treatment effects: A comparative study, *Statistics in Medicine* 23, 2004, 2937–2960.

31. L. A. Stefanski, D. D. Boos, The calculus of M-estimation, *The American Statistician* 56, 2002, 29–38.

32. J. M. Robins, A new approach to causal inference in mortality studies with sustained exposure periods: Application to control of the healthy worker survivor effect, *Mathematical Modelling* 7, 1986, 1393–1512.

33. J. M. Snowden, S. Rose, K. M. Mortimer, Implementation of G-computation on a simulated data set: Demonstration of a causal inference technique, *American Journal of Epidemiology* 173 (7), 2011, 731–738.

34. J. M. Robins, A. Rotnitzky, L. P. Zhao, Estimation of regression coefficients when some regressors are not always observed, *Journal of the American Statistical Association* 89, 1994, 846–866.

35. M. J. van der Laan, J. M. Robins, *Unified Methods for Censored Longitudinal Data and Causality*, Springer, New York, 2003.

36. M. J. van der Laan, D. B. Rubin, Targeted maximum likelihood learning, *The International Journal of Biostatistics* 2 (1), 2006, Article 11. DOI: 10.2202/1557-4679.1043.

37. M. J. van der Laan, E. C. Polley, A. E. Hubbard, Super learner, *Statistical Applications in Genetics and Molecular Biology* 6 (1), 2007, Article 25.

38. S. Rose, Mortality risk score prediction in an elderly population using machine learning, *American Journal of Epidemiology* 177 (5), 2013, 443–452.

39. M. G. Hudgens, M. E. Halloran, Toward causal inference with interference, *Journal of the American Statistical Association* 103, 2008, 832–842.

40. P. M. Aronow, A general method for detecting interference between units in randomized experiments, *Sociological Methods and Research* 41, 2012, 3–16.

41. P. R. Rosenbaum, The role of a second control group in an observational study, *Statistical Science* 2 (3), 1987, 292–316.

42. E. T. Tchetgen, The control outcome calibration approach for causal inference with unobserved confounding, *American Journal of Epidemiology* 175 (5), 2014, 633–640.

43. S.-L. T. Normand, M. B. Landrum, E. Guadagnoli, J. Z. Ayanian, T. J. Ryan, P. D. Cleary, B. J. McNeil, Validating recommendations for coronary angiography following acute myocardial infarction in the elderly: A matched analysis using propensity scores, *Journal of Clinical Epidemiology* 54, 2001, 387–398.

44. A. Haviland, D. Nagin, P. R. Rosenbaum, Combining propensity score matching and group-based trajectory analysis in an observational study, *Psychological Methods* 12 (3), 2007, 247–267.

45. J. Ahern, A. Hubbard, S. Galea, Estimating the effects of potential public health interventions on population disease burden: A step-by-step illustration of causal inference methods, *American Journal of Epidemiology* 169 (9), 2009, 1140–1147.

2

Instrumental Variables Methods*

Michael Baiocchi, Jing Cheng, and Dylan S. Small

CONTENTS

---

* The three authors contributed equally to this chapter.

ABSTRACT Comparative effectiveness seeks to determine the causal effect of one treatment versus another on health outcomes. Often, it is not ethically or practically possible to conduct a perfectly randomized experiment and instead an observational study must be used. A major difficulty with observational studies is that there might be unmeasured confounding, that is, unmeasured covariates that differ between the treatment and control groups before the treatment and that are associated with the outcome. Instrumental variables analysis is a method for controlling for unmeasured confounding. Instrumental variables analysis requires the measurement of a valid instrumental variable, which is a variable that is independent of the unmeasured confounding and encourages a subject to take one treatment level versus another, while having no effect on the outcome beyond its encouragement of a certain treatment level. This chapter discusses the types of causal effects that can be estimated by instrumental variables analysis; the assumptions needed for instrumental variables analysis to provide valid estimates of causal effects and sensitivity analysis for those assumptions; methods of estimation of causal effects using instrumental variables; and sources of instrumental variables in comparative effectiveness research studies.

2.1 Introduction

As noted in Chapter 1, the goal of comparative effectiveness research is to provide actionable information to patients, healthcare workers, and policy-makers about the comparative effects of one treatment versus another. As analysts, this requires specific attention to determining the causal impact of a given intervention on future outcomes. In order to justify a change in the way medicine is practiced, correlation is not sufficient; detecting and quantifying causal connections is necessary.

Medicine has relied on randomized-controlled studies as the gold standard for detecting and quantifying causal connections between an intervention and future outcomes. Randomization offers a clear mechanism for limiting the number of alternate possible explanations for what generates the differences between the treated and control groups. The demand for causal evidence in medicine far exceeds the ability to ethically conduct and finance randomized studies. Observational data offer a sensible alternative source of data for developing evidence about the implications of different medical interventions. However, for studies using observational data to be considered as a reliable source for evidence of causal effects, great care is needed to design studies in a way that limits the number of alternative explanations for observed differences in outcomes between intervention and control. This chapter will examine instrumental variables (IVs) as a framework for designing high-quality observational studies. A few of the common pitfalls to be aware of will be discussed.

2.1.1 Example: Neonatal Intensive Care Units

Medical care for premature infants (preemies) is offered within neonatal intensive care units (NICUs) of varying intensity of care. Higher-intensity NICUs (those classified as various grades of level 3 by the American Academy of Pediatrics) have more sophisticated medical machinery and highly skilled doctors who specialize in the treatment of tiny preemies.

While establishing value requires addressing questions of both costs and outcomes, our example will focus on outcomes, specifically estimating the difference in rates of death between the higher-level NICUs and the lower-level NICUs. Using data from Pennsylvania from the years 1995–2005, a simple comparison of death rates at high-level facilities to low-level facilities shows a higher death rate at high-level facilities, 2.26% compared to 1.25%; the death rate is for in-hospital mortality, which is either a death during the initial birth hospitalization (neonatal death) or a fetal death with a gestational age ≥ 23 weeks and/or a birth weight $>400\,g$ that meets a definition of a potentially preventable fetal death by care delivered at the hospital [1]. This higher death rate at high-level facilities is surprising only if one assumes preemies were randomly assigned to either a high- or low-level NICU, regardless of how sick they were. In fact, as in most health applications, the sickest patients were routed to the highest level of intensity. As a result, one cannot necessarily attribute the difference in outcomes between low-level (i.e., low intensity) NICUs and high-level (i.e., high intensity) NICUs to the difference in the intensity of these NICUs; some or all of the difference could be due to differences in the patients served between the two types of NICUs. Fortunately, our data provide a detailed assessment of baseline severity with 45 covariates, including variables such as gestational age, birth weight, congenital disorder indicators, parity, and information about the mother's socioeconomic status. Yet, even with this level of detail, our data cannot characterize the full set of clinical factors that a physician or family considers when deciding whether to route a preemie to a high-intensity care unit. As shall be discussed, these missing attributes will cause us considerable problems.

The causal effect of treatment at a high-level NICU versus a low-level NICU is the difference in probabilities of death if the same patients were served at both types of NICUs. This is different from what is estimated in the difference in raw rates of death between high-level NICUs and low-level NICUs. These concepts are formalized below.

2.1.2 Fundamentals

2.1.2.1 Potential Outcomes Framework

The literature has made great use of the potential outcomes framework (as described in References 2–4) as a systematic, mathematical description of the cause-and-effect relationship between variables. Although the framework is introduced already in Chapter 1, we recapitulate the notation and assumptions here for the convenience of the reader. Let us assume there are three variables of interest: the outcome of interest Y; the treatment variable T; and X as a vector of covariates. For most of this chapter, it will be assumed that there are only two treatment levels (e.g., the new intervention under consideration vs. the old intervention), though this assumption is only for simplicity's sake and treatments with more than two levels are permissible. These two levels will be referred to using the generic terms "treatment" and "control," without much discussion of what those two words mean aside from saying that they serve as contrasting interventions to one another. In the potential outcomes framework, the notion is that each individual has two possible outcomes—one that is observed if the person were to take the treatment and one if the person were to take the control. In practice, only one of these outcomes can be observed because taking the treatment often precludes taking the control and vice versa. Let subject i taking the treatment be denoted as $T_i = 1$ and subject i taking the control as $T_i = 0$. To formally denote the outcome subject i would experience under the treatment and control, write $Y(T_i = 1)$ and $Y(T_i = 0)$, respectively. To simplify the notation, let Y_{1i} and Y_{0i} denote the potential outcome under treatment and the potential outcome under control, respectively. In this chapter, Y will be thought of as a scalar, though it is possible to develop a framework where Y is a vector of outcomes. Excellent resources exist for reading up on the potential outcomes framework, for example, References 5–7.

The quantity of interest is the individual-level treatment effect, defined as

$$\Delta_i = Y_{1i} - Y_{0i}.$$

Thus, Δ_i denotes the difference in outcome, for subject i, between taking the treatment and control. If this quantity could be observed, then the benefit from intervention would be known explicitly. But, in practice, only one or the other of the potential outcomes is observed. To see this, write the observed outcome, denoted Y_i^{obs}, for the ith individual, as a function of the potential outcomes [3,4]:

$$Y_i^{obs} = T_i * Y_{1i} - (1 - T_i) * Y_{0i}.$$

Observing one of the potential outcomes precludes observing the other. In all but the most contrived settings, this problem is intractable. Both the treatment and control outcomes cannot be observed. So, other parameters of interest must be turned to.

2.1.2.2 Parameters of Interest

Assume that baseline characteristics of the study participants are available. It is important to stress that these should be baseline characteristics that reflect the state of the subject prior to the intervention and should not be posttreatment characteristics that are influenced by the treatment (see Section 2.4.2 of References 7 and 8). Controlling for posttreatment characteristics can bias the estimate of the treatment effect. For example, say a new drug is being tested for its ability to lower the risk of heart attack. High blood pressure is known to correlate with higher risk of heart attack, so it is tempting to control for this covariate. Controlling for blood pressure is likely to improve the precision of the estimate if a pretreatment blood pressure measure is used. However, it would be a mistake to control for a posttreatment measurement of blood pressure because this measurement may be affected by the drug and would thus result in an attenuated estimated causal effect. Intuitively, this is because the estimation procedure is limiting comparison in outcome not just between people who took the drug and who did not but between people who took the drug and then had a certain level of blood pressure and people who did not take the drug and had the same level of blood pressure. The impact from the drug may have already happened via the lowering of the blood pressure.

Let us denote these measured pretreatment characteristics as X_i for the ith subject. Further, the subjects are likely to have characteristics that were not recorded. Let us denote these unobserved characteristics as $\mathbf{U}_i$ for the ith subject. To keep things simple, assume that the covariates are linearly related to the outcomes like so

$$Y_{1i} = \mathbf{X}_i^T \beta^1 + \mathbf{U}_i^T \alpha^1,$$

$$Y_{0i} = \mathbf{X}_i^T \beta^0 + \mathbf{U}_i \alpha^0.$$

Note that the coefficients need to be indexed by the treatment level in order to account for interactions between the treatment level and the covariates.

Combining our equations for the observed outcome and the linear models, the observed outcome can be decomposed in terms of covariates, both observed and unobserved, as well as the treatment:

$$Y_i^{obs} = \mathbf{X}_i^T \beta^0 + T_i[(\mathbf{X}_i^T \beta^1 - \mathbf{X}_i^T \beta^0) + (\mathbf{U}_i^T \alpha^1 - \mathbf{U}_i^T \alpha^0)] + \mathbf{U}_i^T \alpha^0.$$

It is standard in econometrics to think of the above model as a regression, where the coefficient on the treatment variable comes from two sources of variation: the first source is the variation due to the observed covariates, $(\mathbf{X}_i^T \beta^1 - \mathbf{X}_i^T \beta^0)$, and the second is the variation due to the unobserved covariates, $(\mathbf{U}_i^T \alpha^1 - \mathbf{U}_i^T \alpha^0)$, where T_i may be correlated with U_i. It is common to interpret the first source of variation as the gains for the average person with covariate levels $\mathbf{X}_i$, and the second source of variation to be referred to as idiosyncratic gains for subject i. The idiosyncratic gains are the part of this model that allows persons i and j to differ in gains from treatment even when $\mathbf{X}_i = \mathbf{X}_j$.

2.1.2.3 Selection Bias

One of the biggest problems with observational studies is that there is selection bias. Loosely speaking, selection bias arises from how the subjects are sorted (or sort themselves) into the treatment or control groups. The intuition here is: the treatment group was different from the control group even before the intervention, and the two groups would probably have had different outcomes even if there had been no intervention at all. Selection bias can occur in a couple of different ways, but one way to write it is

$$f(\mathbf{X}, \mathbf{U}|T = 1) \neq f(\mathbf{X}, \mathbf{U}|T = 0),$$

that is, the joint distribution of the covariates for those who received the treatment is different than for those who received the control. If this is true, that there is selection bias, then

$$E[Y_1 - Y_0|\mathbf{X}] \neq E[Y_1|\mathbf{X}, T = 1] - E[Y_0|\mathbf{X}, T = 0].$$

This is problematic because the left-hand side of this equation is our unobservable quantity of interest but the right-hand side is made up of directly observable quantities. But it seems like the above equation is used in other settings, namely, experimentation. Why is that acceptable?

In an experiment, because of randomization, it is known that

$$(\mathbf{X}, U) \perp\!\!\!\perp T,$$

where $\perp\!\!\!\perp$ denotes independence. And it follows that

$$E[Y_1 - Y_0|\mathbf{X}] = E[Y_1|\mathbf{X}, T = 1] - E[Y_0|\mathbf{X}, T = 0].$$

Though it is often a dubious claim, many of the standard observational study techniques require an assumption that essentially says that the only selection between treated and control groups is on levels of the observed covariates, that is, $U \perp\!\!\!\perp T|\mathbf{X}$. This is sometimes referred to as overt selection bias. Typically, if overt selection bias is the only form of bias then either conditioning on observed covariates (for example by using a regression) or matching is enough to address overt bias. One particular assumption that is invoked quite often in the current health literature is the absence of omitted variables (i.e., only overt bias). In the NICU setting in Section 2.1.1, this would mean that the only variables that doctors and mothers use in deciding which type of NICU a baby is delivered at that also affect death rates are the 45 covariates we have in our data.

Hidden bias exists when there are imbalances in the unobserved covariates. Let's use the observed outcome formula again, rewriting it like so

$$Y_i^{obs} = \mathbf{X}_i^T \beta^0 + T_i E[\Delta|\mathbf{X}] + \mathbf{U}_i^T \alpha^0 + T_i(\mathbf{U}_i^T \alpha^1 - \mathbf{U}_i^T \alpha^0).$$

A least squares regression of Y on T based on the model above will tend to produce biased estimates for $E[\Delta|\mathbf{X}]$ when T is correlated with either $\mathbf{U}_i^T \alpha^0$ or $(\mathbf{U}_i^T \alpha^1 - \mathbf{U}_i^T \alpha^0)$. This can arise from unobserved covariates that influence both potential outcomes and selection into treatment. This bias is referred to as *hidden bias*. If the average treatment effects given $\mathbf{X}$, $E[\Delta|\mathbf{X}]$, and the hidden biases given $\mathbf{X}$, $E[\mathbf{U}_i^T \alpha^1|\mathbf{X}, T = 1] - E[\mathbf{U}_i^T \alpha^0|\mathbf{X}, T = 0]$, are the same for all $\mathbf{X}$, then the regression estimate of $E[\Delta|\mathbf{X}]$ is biased by

$$E[\mathbf{U}_i^T \alpha^1|\mathbf{X}, T = 1] - E[\mathbf{U}_i^T \alpha^0|\mathbf{X}, T = 0].$$

2.1.3 Methods to Address Selection Bias

In a randomized experiment setting, inference on the causal effect of treatment on the outcome requires no further assumption than that the subjects were randomized into treatment or control [9]. The randomization guarantees independence of assigned treatment from the covariates. This independence is for all covariates, both observed and unobserved. By observed covariates, we mean those covariates that appear in the analyst's data set, and by unobserved covariates, we mean all of those that do not. If the sample is large enough, then this independence means that the treatment group will almost surely have quite a similar covariate distribution as the control group. Therefore, any variation noted in the outcome is more readily attributed to the variation in the treatment level rather than variation in the covariates.

The primary challenge to observational studies is that selection into treatment is not randomly assigned. Usually, there are covariates, both observed and unobserved, which determine who receives treatment and who receives control. In the NICU example of Section 2.1.1, such observed covariates include gestational age (more premature babies are more likely to be delivered at high-level NICUs) and such unobserved covariates include fetal heart tracing results (if the fetal heart trace indicates potential problems, the doctor is more likely to recommend delivering at a high-level NICU). When there are covariates that affect who receives treatment and who receives control, variation in the outcome is not easily attributable to treatment levels because covariates are different between the different levels as well. There are techniques that were created to address this selection bias. These methods can be classified (roughly) into two groups: (1) those methods that address only the observed selection bias and (2) those methods that attempt to address selection bias on both the observed as well as unobserved covariates. Falling into the first category are techniques such as regression, Bayesian hierarchical modeling, propensity score matching, and inverse probability weighting. An account of such methods is provided in Chapter 1. The second category includes methods such as IV, regression discontinuity, and difference-in-differences.

2.1.3.1 Methods to Address Overt Selection Bias

Only through special justification should methods that address only overt bias be considered valid. Usually, this justification takes the form of an assumption. Informally, this assumption can be thought of as saying: selection into the treatment is occurring only on variables that are observed. Formally, this assumption is often written as

$$(Y_0, Y_1) \perp\!\!\!\perp T | \mathbf{X},$$

$$0 < pr(T = 1|\mathbf{X}) < 1,$$

where $\perp\!\!\!\perp$ denotes the conditional independence between the treatment and the joint distribution of the counterfactual outcomes given $\mathbf{X}$. Two random variables are conditionally independent given a third variable if and only if they are independent in their conditional distribution given the conditioning variable. The above assumption, essentially saying that all needed covariates are measured, has a few different names: strongly ignorable treatment assignment [10], selection on observables [11], conditional independence, no hidden bias (only overt bias due to X), no unmeasured confounders (in the epidemiology literature), or the absence of omitted variable bias (in the econometrics literature).

To assume strongly ignorable treatment assignment in many medical application is counterintuitive. In practice, the analyst often has access to only some subset of the recorded information from the patients' interaction with the health system. For example, many studies are based on administrative data (e.g., insurance claims) that are good for indicating the presence of a condition but not its severity, whereas medical decision makers have more information about the severity, for example, from the results of labs and biometric information. It is possible that as electronic health records become more readily available, this problem will diminish. But even when the health analyst does have access to electronic health records, the health analyst should be aware that medical practitioners are keen observers and intuitively adept at identifying issues that either may go unrecorded or may even be unquantifiable (e.g., practitioners will regularly refer to the frailty of a patient, which seems to be a generally understood yet unmeasurable quality of a patient). Given the additional information the medical decision makers have, and their desire to choose an optimal outcome, medical decision makers are actively working against the reasonableness of strongly ignorable treatment assignment.

It is unfortunate that methods that were designed only to address overt bias have become the default tools of choice in the literature. Given the complexity of health decision, it strains credibility that all variables that influence treatment and outcome are recorded and available to the analyst. The default for health analysts (and critically minded reviewers) should be to assume unobserved selection is occurring and to look for ways of mitigating it.

2.1.3.2 Instrumental Variables: A Framework to Address Overt Bias and Bias Due to Omitted Variables

Regression, propensity score matching, and any methods predicated on only overt bias do not address selection on unobserved covariates. It is important to be aware of this because a well-informed researcher needs to judge if available covariates are enough to make a compelling argument for the absence of omitted variables. This is often a dubious claim because (1) a clever reviewer will find several variables missing from your data set and/or (2) there are intangible variables that are difficult, or perhaps inconceivable, to measure. IV techniques are one way of addressing unobserved selection bias.

It is important to note IV techniques do not come for free and have their own assumptions. It is important to consider these assumptions carefully before deciding to use an IV analysis.

An IV design takes advantage of randomness that occurs in the treatment assignment to help address imbalances in the unobserved variables.

An instrument is a haphazard nudge toward acceptance of a treatment that affects outcomes only to the extent that it affects acceptance of the treatment. In settings in which treatment assignment is mostly deliberate and not random, there may nevertheless exist some essentially random nudges to accept treatment, so that use of an instrument might extract bits of random treatment assignment from a setting that is otherwise quite biased in its treatment assignments.

There have been many different formulations of IV, reflecting the diverse academic traditions that use IV. Though IVs existed in the literature for quite some time, Reference 12 used the potential outcomes framework to bring greater clarity to the math of IV. For the health analyst, perhaps Reference 2 offers the most intuitive introduction to IVs, framing IV as a randomized trial with noncompliance. The frameworks for IV discussed in References 2 and 12 enhance the classic econometric presentation of IVs where the focus is on correlation with the error term. Health analysts will likely find these introductions most engaging.

To illustrate IVs, consider the NICU example from earlier.

2.1.4 Instrumental Variables: NICU Example Revisited

NICUs have been established to deliver high-intensity care for premature infants (those infants born before 37 weeks of gestation). Considering all of the preemies that were delivered in Pennsylvania between 1995 and 2005, 2.26% of the preemies delivered at high-level NICUs died while only 1.25% of the preemies who were delivered at low-level NICUs died. No one believes the difference in outcomes reported above is solely attributable to the difference in level of intensity of treatment. People believe it is due to difference in covariates. Based on the observable covariates, this is plausible because the preemies delivered at high-level NICUs weighed almost 250 g less than the preemies that were delivered at low-level NICUs (2,454 at high-level NICUs vs. 2693 at low-level NICUs). Similarly, preemies delivered at high-level NICUs were born a week earlier than their counterparts at low-level NICUs on average (34.5 weeks vs. 35.5 weeks).

Unfortunately, complete medical records were not available for this study. Only birth and death certificates and a form, UB-92, that hospitals provide were available. It is quite likely that not all necessary covariates in our data set are available, so assuming only overt bias is likely to lead to biased estimates. To attempt to deal with this problem, References 1 and 13 used an IV approach. They used distance to treatment facility as an instrument, because travel time largely determines the likelihood that mother will deliver at a given facility but appears to be largely uncorrelated with the level of severity a preemie experiences.

To help visualize the problem, look at Figure 2.1. This is an example of a directed acyclic graph [6]. The arrows denote causal relationships. Read the relationship between variables T and Y like so: Changing the value of

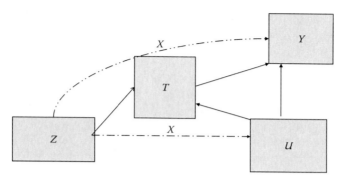

FIGURE 2.1
Directed acyclic graph for the relationship between an instrumental variable Z, a treatment T, unmeasured confounders U, and an outcome Y.

T causes Y to change. In our example, Y represents mortality. The variable T indicates whether or not a baby attended a high-level NICU. Our goal is to understand the arrow connecting T to Y. In order to keep the current example simple, assume there are no observed covariates (which would be denoted using an **X** in Figure 2.1). In general, IV techniques are able to adjust for variation in observed covariates (see Section 2.3.4).

The U variable causes consternation as it represents the unobserved level of severity of the preemie and it is causally linked to both mortality (sicker babies are more likely to die) and to which treatment the preemies select (sicker babies are more likely to be delivered in high-level NICUs). Because U is unobserved directly, it cannot be precisely adjusted for using statistical methods such as propensity scores or regression. If the story stopped with just T, Y, and U, then the effect of T on Y could not be estimated.

IV estimation makes use of an uncomplicated form of variation in the system. What is needed is a variable, typically called an instrument (represented by Z in Figure 2.1), that has very special characteristics. It takes some practice to understand exactly what constitutes a good IV.

Consider excess travel time as a possible instrument. Excess travel time is defined as the time it takes to travel from the mother's residence to the nearest high-level NICU minus the time it takes to travel to the nearest low-level NICU. If the mother lives closest to a high-level NICU, then excess travel time will take on negative values. If she lives closest to a low-level NICU, excess travel time will be positive.

There are three key features a variable must have in order to qualify as an instrument (see Section 2.3 for mathematical details on these features and additional assumptions for IV methods). The first feature (represented by the directed arrow from Z to T in Figure 2.1) is that the instrument causes a change in the treatment assignment. Women tend to deliver at hospitals near their home [14]. By selecting where to live, mothers assign themselves to be more or less likely to deliver in a high-level NICU. The fact that changes in the instrument are associated with changes in the treatment is verifiable from the data.

The second feature (represented by the crossed-out arrow from Z to U) is that the instrument is not associated with variation in unobserved variables U that also affect the outcome. That is, Z is not connected to the unobserved confounding that was a worry to begin with. In our example, this would mean unobserved severity is not caused by variation in geography. Since high-level NICUs tend to be in urban areas and low-level NICUs tend to be the only type in rural areas, this assumption would be dubious if there were high levels of pollutants in urban areas or if there were more pollutants in the drinking water in rural areas than in urban areas. The pollutants may have an impact on the unobserved levels of severity. The assumption that the instrument is not associated with variation in the unobserved variables, while most certainly an assumption, can at least be corroborated by looking at the values of variables that are perhaps related to the unobserved variables of concern (see Section 2.5.1).

The third feature (represented by the crossed-out line from Z to Y in Figure 2.1) is that the instrument does not cause the outcome variable to change directly. That is, it is only through its impact on the treatment that the IV affects the outcome. In our case, presumably a nearby hospital with a high-level NICU affects mortality only if the baby receives care at that hospital. That is, proximity to a high-level NICU in and of itself does not change the probability of death for a preemie, except through the increased probability of the preemie being delivered at the high-level NICU. This is referred to as the exclusion restriction (ER); see Reference 12 for discussion. In our case, the ER seems quite reasonable.

2.2 Sources of Instruments in Comparative Effectiveness Research Studies

In this section, common types of IVs that have been used in comparative effectiveness research studies will be described and issues to consider in assessing their validity will be discussed. Common types of IVs in comparative effectiveness research are summarized in Table 2.1. One way to study the effect of a treatment when that treatment cannot be controlled is to conduct a randomized encouragement trial. In such a trial, some subjects are randomly chosen to get extra encouragement to take the treatment and the rest of the subjects receive no extra encouragement [2]. For example, Permutt and Hebel [15] studied the effect of maternal smoking during pregnancy on an infant's birth weight using a randomized encouragement

TABLE 2.1

Common Sources of IVs in Comparative Effectiveness Studies

Source of Instrumental Variable	Example
Randomized encouragement	Pregnant women randomly assigned to receive extra encouragement versus usual encouragement to not smoke during pregnancy [16]
Distance	Difference between distance lived from nearest hospital that performs cardiac catheterization and nearest hospital that does not [17]
Preference of physicians	Preference of a patient's physician for using selective cyclooxygenase 2 inhibitors versus nonselective nonsteroidal anti-inflammatory drugs for treating GI problems [18]
Preference of hospitals	Preference of the hospital a patient is treated at for using surgery versus endovascular therapy for treating patients with a ruptured cerebral aneurysm [19]
Preference of geographic regions	Preference of geographic region a patient lives in for treating breast cancer with surgery plus irradiation versus mastectomy [20]
Calendar time	For studying the effect of hormone replacement therapy (HRT) on postmenopausal women, before 2002 versus after 2002 (when use of HRT dropped sharply) [21]
Genetic variation	For studying the effect of HDL cholesterol levels on cardiovascular disease, single nucleotide polymorphisms (SNPs) that are associated with high HDL levels but not associated with other cardiovascular disease biomarkers [22]
Timing of admission	For studying the effect of waiting time for surgery for hip fracture, whether patient was admitted on weekend versus weekday [23]
Insurance plan	For studying the effect of β-blocker adherence after hospitalization for heart failure, the drug copayment amount of the patient's insurance plan [24]

trial in which some mothers received extra encouragement to stop smoking through a staff person providing information, support, practical guidance, and behavioral strategies [16]. For a randomized encouragement trial, the randomized encouragement assignment (1 if encouraged, 0 if not encouraged) is a potential IV. The randomized encouragement is independent of unmeasured confounders because it is randomly assigned by the investigators and will be associated with the treatment if the encouragement is effective. The only potential concern with the randomized encouragement being a valid IV is that the randomized encouragement might have a direct effect on the outcome not through the treatment. For example, in the randomized encouragement trial to encourage expectant mothers to stop smoking, the encouragement could have a direct effect if the staff person providing the encouragement also encouraged expectant mothers to stop drinking alcohol during pregnancy. To minimize a potential direct effect of the encouragement, Sexton and Hebel [16] asked the staff person providing encouragement to avoid recommendations or information concerning other habits that might affect birth weight such as alcohol or caffeine consumption and also prohibited the discussion of maternal nutrition or weight gain.

When comparing two treatments, one of which is only provided by specialty care providers and one of which is provided by more general providers, the distance a person lives from the nearest specialty care provider has often been used as an IV. Proximity to a specialty care provider particularly enhances the chance of being treated by the specialty care provider for acute conditions. For less acute conditions, patients/providers have more time to decide and plan where to be treated, and proximity may have less of an influence on treatment selection. For treatments that are stigmatized such as substance abuse treatment, proximity could have a negative effect on the chance of being treated. A classic example of the use of distance as an IV is McClellan et al.'s study of the effect of cardiac catheterization for patients suffering a heart attack [17]; the IV used in the study was the difference in distance the patient lives from the nearest hospital that performs cardiac catheterization compared to the nearest hospital that does not perform cardiac catheterization. Another example is the study of the effect of high-level NICUs versus low-level NICUs [1] that was discussed in Section 2.1.4. Because distance to a specialty care provider is often associated with socioeconomic characteristics, it will typically be necessary to control for socioeconomic characteristics in order for distance to be potentially independent of unmeasured confounders. The possibility that distance might have a direct effect because the time it takes to receive treatment affects outcomes needs to be considered in assessing whether distance is a valid IV.

A general strategy for finding an IV for comparing two treatments A and B is to look for naturally occurring variation in medical practice patterns at the level of geographic region, hospital, or individual physician, and then use whether the region/hospital/individual physician has a high or low use of treatment A as the IV. Brookhart and Schneeweiss [25] termed these IVs "preference-based instruments" because they are derived from the assumption that different providers or groups of providers have different preferences or treatment algorithms dictating how medications or medical procedures are used. Examples of studies using preference-based IVs are Reference 20 that studied the effect of surgery plus irradiation versus mastectomy for breast cancer patients using geographic region as the IV, Reference 19 that studied the effect of surgery versus endovascular therapy for patients with a ruptured cerebral aneurysm using hospital as the IV, and Reference 18 that studied the benefits and risks of selective cyclooxygenase 2 inhibitors versus nonselective nonsteroidal anti-inflammatory drugs for treating gastrointestinal (GI) problems using individual physician as the IV. For the proposed preference-based IVs, it is important to consider that the patient mix may differ between the different groups of providers with different preferences, which would make the preference-based IV invalid unless patient mix is fully controlled for. It is useful to look at whether measured patient risk factors differ between groups of providers with different preferences. If there are measured differences, there are likely to be unmeasured differences as well; see Section 2.5 for further discussion. Also, for the proposed preference-based IVs, it is important to consider whether the IV has a direct effect; a direct effect could arise if the group of providers that prefers treatment A treats patients differently in ways other than the treatment under study compared to the providers who prefer treatment B. For example, Newman et al. [26] studied the efficacy of phototherapy for newborns with hyperbilirubinemia and considered the frequency of phototherapy use at the newborn's birth hospital as an IV. However, chart reviews revealed that hospitals that use more phototherapy also have a greater use of infant formula; use of infant formula is also thought to be an effective treatment for hyperbilirubinemia. Consequently, the proposed preference-based IV has a direct effect (going to a hospital with a higher use of phototherapy also means a newborn is more likely to receive infant formula even if the newborn does not receive phototherapy) and is not valid. The issue of whether a proposed preference-based IV has a direct effect can be studied by looking at whether the IV is associated with concomitant treatments such as use of infant formula [25]. A related way in which a proposed preference-based IV can have a direct effect is that the group of providers who prefer treatment A may have more skill than the group of providers who prefer treatment B. Also, providers who prefer treatment A may deliver treatment A better than those providers who prefer treatment B because they have more practice with it, for example, doctors who perform surgery more often may perform better surgeries. Korn and Baumrind [27] discuss a way to assess whether there are provider skill effects by collecting data from providers on whether or not they would have treated a different provider's patient with treatment A or B based on the patient's pretreatment records.

Another common source for an IV is calendar time. Variations in the use of one treatment versus another could result from changes in guidelines; changes in formularies or reimbursement policies; changes in physician preference (e.g., due to marketing activities by drug makers); release of new effectiveness or safety information; or the arrival of new treatments to the market [28]. For example, Shetty et al. [21] studied the effect of hormone replacement therapy (HRT) on cardiovascular health among postmenopausal women using calendar time as an IV. HRT was widely used among postmenopausal women until 2002; observational studies had suggested that HRT reduced cardiovascular risk, but the Womens' Health Initiative randomized trial reported opposite results in 2002, which caused HRT use to drop sharply. A proposed IV based on calendar time could be associated with confounders that change in time such as the characteristics of patients who enter the cohort, changes in other medical practices, and changes in medical coding systems [28]. The most compelling type of IV based on calendar time is one where a dramatic change in practice occurs in a relatively short period of time [28].

Another general source for potential IVs is genetic variants that affect treatment variables. For example, Voight et al. [22] studied the effect of high-density lipoprotein (HDL) cholesterol on myocardial infarction (MI) using as an IV the genetic variant LIPG 396Ser allele for which carriers have higher levels of HDL cholesterol but similar levels of other lipid and nonlipid risk factors compared to noncarriers. Another example is that Wehby et al. [29] studied the effect of maternal smoking on orofacial clefts in their babies using genetic variants that increase the probability that a mother smokes as IVs. The approach of using genetic variants as an IV is called *Mendelian randomization* because it makes use of the random assignment of genetic variants conditional on parents' genes discovered by Mendel and References 30 and 31 provide good reviews of Mendelian randomization methods. Although genetic variants are randomly assigned conditional on a parent's genes, genetic variants need to satisfy additional assumption to be valid IVs:

1. *Not associated with unmeasured confounders through population stratification.* Most Mendelian randomization analyses do not condition on parents' genes, creating the potential of the proposed genetic variant IV being association with unmeasured confounders through population stratification. Population stratification is a condition where there are subpopulations, some of which are more likely to have the genetic variant, and some of which are more likely to have the outcome through mechanisms other than the treatment being studied. For example, consider studying the effect of alcohol consumption on hypertension. Consider using the ALDH2 null variant, which is associated with alcohol consumption, as an IV (individuals who are homozygous for the ALDH2 null variant have severe adverse reactions to alcohol consumption and tend to drink very little [31]). The ALDH2 null variant is much more common in people with Asian ancestry than other types of ancestry [32]. Suppose ancestry was not fully measured. If ancestry is associated with hypertension through means other than differences in the ALDH2 null variant (e.g., through different ancestries tending to have different diets), then ALDH2 would not be a valid IV because it would be associated with an unmeasured confounder.

2. *Not associated with unmeasured confounders through genetic linkage.* Genetic linkage is the tendency of genes that are located near to each other on a chromosome to be inherited together because the genes are unlikely to be separated during the crossing over of the mother's and father's DNA [33]. Consider using a gene *A* as an IV where gene

A is genetically linked to a gene *B* that has a causal effect on the outcome through a pathway other than the treatment being studied. If gene *B* is not measured and controlled for, then gene *A* is not a valid IV because it is associated with the unmeasured confounder gene *B*.

3. *No direct effect through pleiotropy.* Pleiotropy refers to a gene having multiple functions. If the genetic variant being used as an IV affects the outcome through a function other than affecting the treatment being studied, this would mean the genetic variant has a direct effect. For example, consider the use of the APOE genotype as an IV for studying the causal effect of low-density lipoprotein cholesterol (LDLc) on MI risk. The ε2 variant of the APOE gene is associated with lower levels of LDLc but is also associated with higher levels of high-density lipoprotein cholesterol, less efficient transfer of very low-density lipoproteins and chylomicrons from the blood to the liver, greater postprandial lipemia and an increased risk of type III hyperlipoproteinemia (the last three of which are thought to increase MI risk) [31]. Thus, the gene APOE is pleiotropic, affecting MI risk through different pathways, making it unsuitable as an IV to examine the causal effect of any one of these pathways on MI risk.

Another source of IVs for comparative effectiveness research studies is timing of admission variables. For example, Reference 23 used the day of the week of hospital admission as an IV for waiting time for surgery to study the effects of waiting time on length of stay and inpatient mortality among patients admitted to the hospital with a hip fracture. Day of the week of admission is associated with waiting time for surgery because many surgeons only do nonemergency operations on weekdays, and therefore patients admitted on weekends for nonemergency surgery may have to wait longer for the surgery. In order for weekday versus weekend admission to be a valid IV, patients admitted on weekdays versus weekends must not differ on unmeasured characteristics (i.e., the IV is independent of unmeasured confounders) and other aspects of hospital care that affect the patients' outcomes besides surgery must be comparable on weekdays versus weekends (i.e., the IV has no direct effect). Another example of a timing of admission variable used as an IV is hour of birth as an IV for a newborn's length of stay in the hospital [34,35].

An additional general source of potential IVs for comparative effectiveness research studies is insurance plans, which may vary in the amount of reimbursement they provide for different treatments. For example, Reference 24 used drug copayment amount as an IV to study the effect of β-blocker adherence on clinical outcomes and healthcare expenditures after a hospitalization for heart failure. In order for variations in insurance plan like drug copayment amount to be a valid IV, insurance plans must have comparable patients after controlling for measured confounders (i.e., the IV is independent of unmeasured confounders) and insurance plans must not have an effect on the outcome of interest other than through influencing the treatment being studied (i.e., the IV has no direct effect).

2.3 IV Assumptions and Estimation for Binary IV and Binary Treatment

In this section, the simplest setting of a binary instrument and a binary treatment will be considered. The main ideas in IV methods are most easily understood in this setting and the ideas will be expanded to more complicated settings later.

2.3.1 Framework and Notation

The Neyman–Rubin potential outcomes framework will be used to describe causal effects [3,4]. Let Z_i denote the IV for subject i, where $Z_i = 0$ or 1 for a binary IV. Level 1 of the IV is assumed to mean the subject was encouraged to take level 1 of the treatment, where the treatment has levels 0 and 1. Let T_{zi} be the potential treatment received for subject i if she were assigned level z of the IV. $-T_{1i}$ is the treatment that subject i would receive if she were assigned level 1 of the IV and T_{0i} is the treatment that i would receive if she were assigned level 0 of the IV. The observed treatment received for subject i is $T_i \equiv T_{Z_i i}$. Let Y_{zti} be the potential outcome for subject i if she were assigned level z of the IV and level t of the treatment—there are four such potential outcomes $Y_{11i}, Y_{10i}, Y_{01i}, Y_{00i}$. However, only one of them will be observed in practice. The observed outcome for subject i is $Y_i \equiv Y_{Z_i T_i i}$. Let $\mathbf{X}_i$ denote observed covariates for subject i.

Reference 12 considered an IV to be a variable satisfying the following five assumptions:

1. *IV is correlated with the treatment received.* $E(T_{1i}|\mathbf{X}_i) > E(T_{0i}|\mathbf{X}_i)$.

2. *IV is independent of unmeasured confounders (conditional on covariates).*

   Z_i is independent of $(T_{1i}, T_{0i}, Y_{11i}, Y_{10i}, Y_{01i}, Y_{00i})|\mathbf{X}$.

3. *ER.* This assumption says that the IV affects outcomes only through its effect on treatment received: $Y_{zti} = Y_{z'ti}$. Under the ER, write $Y_{di} \equiv Y_{zdi}$ for any z, that is, Y_{1i} is the potential outcome for subject i if she were to receive level 1 of the treatment (regardless of her level of the IV) and Y_{0i} is the potential outcome if she were to receive level 0 of the treatment. This assumption is called the no direct effect assumption.

4. *Monotonicity assumption.* This assumption says that there are no subjects who are "defiers," who would only take level 1 of the treatment if not encouraged to do so, that is, no subjects with $T_{1i} = 0, T_{0i} = 1$.

5. *Stable unit treatment value assumption (SUTVA).* This assumption says that the treatment affects only the subject taking the treatment and the treatment effect is stable through time (see References 12 and 36 for details). The first part of this assumption, that the treatment affects only the subject taking the treatment, is called the no interference assumption.

The first three assumptions are the assumptions depicted in Figure 2.1.

The fourth assumption, monotonicity, plays a role in interpreting the standard IV estimate as a causal effect for a certain subpopulation. A subject in a study with binary IV and treatment can be classified into one of four latent compliance classes based on the joint values of potential treatment received [12]: C_i = never-taker (nt) if $(T_{0i}, T_{1i}) = (0,0)$; complier (co) if $(T_{0i}, T_{1i}) = (0,1)$; always-taker (at) if $(T_{0i}, T_{1i}) = (1,1)$, and defier (de) if $(T_{0i}, T_{1i}) = (1,0)$. Table 2.2 shows the relationship between observed groups and latent compliance classes. Under the monotonicity assumption, the set of defiers will be empty. The never-takers and always-takers do not change their treatment status when the instrument changes, so under the ER assumption, the potential treatment and potential outcome under either level of the IV ($Z_i = 1$ or 0) is the same. Consequently, the IV is not helpful for learning about the treatment effect for always-takers or never-takers. Compliers are subjects who change their treatment status with the instrument, that is, the subjects would take the treatment if they were encouraged to take it by the IV but would not otherwise take the treatment. Because these subjects change their treatment with the level of the IV, the IV is helpful for learning about their treatment effects. The average causal effect for this subgroup, $E(Y_{1i} - Y_{0i}|C_i = co)$, is called the complier average causal effect (CACE) or the local average treatment effect (LATE). It provides the information on the average causal effect of receiving the treatment for compliers. When

TABLE 2.2

Relation between Observed Groups and Latent Compliance Classes

Z_i	T_i		C_i	
1	1	Complier	or	Always-taker
1	0	Never-taker	or	Defier
0	0	Never-taker	or	Complier
0	1	Always-taker	or	Defier

Note: When the monotonicity assumption holds, there are no defiers.

monotonicity does not hold, the standard IV estimator (2.3) discussed in Section 2.3.2 estimates the quantity [12].

$$E(Y_{1i} - Y_{0i}|C_i = co) \times \frac{P(C_i = co)}{P(C_i = co) + P(C_i = de)} - E(Y_{1i} - Y_{0i}|C_i = de)$$
$$\times \frac{\dfrac{P(C_i = de)}{P(C_i = co) + P(C_i = de)}}{P(C_i = co) - P(C_i = de)}.$$

$$(2.1)$$

Equation 2.1 could potentially be negative even if the treatment has a positive effect for all subjects [12]. However, the IV method estimate of the CACE is not generally sensitive to small violations of the monotonicity assumption [12]. Additionally, if the treatment has the same effect for compliers and defiers, the monotonicity assumption is not needed as Equation 2.1 equals the CACE, $E(Y_{1i} - Y_{0i}|C_i = co)$ [37]. For further discussion of understanding the treatment effect that the IV method estimates, see Section 2.4.

The fifth IV assumption, SUTVA, also plays a role in interpreting what the standard IV method estimate (2.3) estimates. Consider in particular the no interference assumption part of SUTVA that subject A receiving the treatment affects only subject A and not other subjects. In the NICU study, the no interference assumption is reasonable—if preemie A is treated at a high-level NICU, this does not affect preemie B's outcome. If there were crowding effects (e.g., treating additional babies at a hospital decreases the quality of care for babies already under care at that hospital), this assumption might not be true. SUTVA is also not appropriate for situations like estimating the effect of a vaccine on an individual because herd immunization would lead to causal links between different people [38]. When no interference fails to hold, the IV method is roughly estimating the difference between the effect of the treatment and the spillover effect of some units being treated on those units left untreated (see Reference 39 for a precise formulation and details).

In economics, a latent index model is often considered for causal inference about the effect of a binary treatment based on a structural equation model or two-stage linear model, for example,

$$T_i^* = \alpha_0 + \alpha_1 Z_i + \varepsilon_{i1}$$
$$Y_i = \beta_0 + \beta_1 T_i + \varepsilon_{i2}$$

where

$$T_i = \begin{cases} 1 & \text{if } T_i^* > 0 \\ 0 & \text{if } T_i^* \leq 0 \end{cases}$$

$$Z_i \perp\!\!\!\perp \varepsilon_{i1}, \varepsilon_{i2}.$$

Vytlacil [40] shows that a nonparametric version of the latent index model is equivalent to Assumptions 1–5 above that Angrist et al. [12] use to define an IV.

2.3.2 Two-Stage Least Squares (Wald) Estimator

Let us first consider IV estimation when there are no observed covariates $\mathbf{X}$. For binary IV and treatment variable, Angrist et al. [12] show that under the framework and assumptions in Section 2.3.2, the CACE is nonparametrically identified by

$$E(Y_{1i} - Y_{0i}|C_i = co) = \frac{E(Y_i|Z_i = 1) - E(Y_i|Z_i = 0)}{E(T_i|Z_i = 1) - E(T_i|Z_i = 0)}, \qquad (2.2)$$

which is the intention-to-treat (ITT) effect divided by the proportion of compliers.

The standard IV estimator or two-stage least squares (2SLS) estimator is the ratio of sample covariances [41]

$$\begin{aligned} \hat{CACE}_{2SLS} &= \frac{\hat{cov}(Y_i, Z_i)}{\hat{cov}(T_i, Z_i)} \\ &= \frac{\hat{E}(Y_i|Z_i = 1) - \hat{E}(Y_i|Z_i = 0)}{\hat{E}(T_i|Z_i = 1) - \hat{E}(T_i|Z_i = 0)} \quad \text{for binary IV and treatment.} \end{aligned}$$

$$\tag{2.3}$$

The 2SLS estimator $\hat{CACE}_{2SLS}$, sometimes called the Wald estimator, is the sample analog of Equation 2.2 and consistently estimates the CACE. The asymptotic standard error for $\hat{CACE}_{2SLS}$ is given in Reference 42, Theorem 3.

The 2SLS estimator (2.3) can be used when information on Y, Z, and T are not available in a single data set, but one data set has Y and Z and the other data set has T and Z; this is called two-sample IV estimation [43,44]. For example, Kaushal [45] studied the effect of food stamps on body mass index (BMI) in immigrant families using differences in state responses to a change in federal laws on immigrant eligibility for the food stamp program as an IV. The National Health Interview Study was used to estimate the effect of state lived in on BMI and the Current Population Survey was used to estimate the effect of state lived in on food stamp program participation because neither data set contained all three variables.

2.3.3 More Efficient Estimation

Let $\mu^{c1} = E(Y_{1i}|C_i = co)$, $\mu^{c0} = E(Y_{0i}|C_i = co)$, $\mu^a = E(Y_i|C_i = at)$, $\mu^n = E(Y_i|C_i = nt)$, and π_a, π_c, and π_n denote the proportion of always-takers, compliers, and never-takers, respectively. Note that by Assumptions 1–5 and the mixture structure of the outcomes of the four observed groups shown in Table 2.2,

$$E(Y|Z_i = 1, T_i = 1) = \frac{\pi_c}{\pi_c + \pi_a}\mu^{c1} + \frac{\pi_a}{\pi_c + \pi_a}\mu^a, \tag{2.4}$$

$$E(Y|Z_i = 1, T_i = 0) = \mu^n,$$

$$E(Y|Z_i = 0, T_i = 0) = \frac{\pi_c}{\pi_c + \pi_n}\mu^{c0} + \frac{\pi_n}{\pi_c + \pi_n}\mu^n, \tag{2.5}$$

$$E(Y|Z_i = 0, T_i = 1) = \mu^a,$$

where the quantities on the left-hand side are expectations of observed outcomes and the quantities on the right-hand side are functions of expected potential outcomes and proportions for latent compliance classes. The 2SLS or standard IV estimator is to use the data in the $(Z_i = 1, T_i = 0)$ group to get $\hat{\mu}^n$ and then plug it into Equation 2.5 to get μ^{c0}, and use the data in the $(Z_i = 0, T_i = 1)$ group for $\hat{\mu}^a$ and then plug it into Equation 2.4 to get μ^{c1}. However, the data information in the mixture groups $(Z_i = 1, T_i = 1)$ and $(Z_i = 0, T_i = 0)$ is not used in the 2SLS estimator (2.3) even though it can be useful for estimating the average potential outcomes. Similarly, the 2SLS estimator uses only the information in the treatment group $(Z_i = 1)$ to estimate π_n and only the information in the control group $(Z_i = 0)$ to estimate π_a, but the mixture structure (see Table 2.1) implies that there is additional information in the control group for estimating π_n and additional information in the treatment group for estimating π_a.

Imbens and Rubin [46,47] proposed two approaches using mixture modeling to estimate the CACE. One approach assumes a parametric distribution (normal) for the outcomes and then estimates the CACE by maximum likelihood using the EM algorithm. This estimator provides considerable efficiency gains over the 2SLS estimator when the parametric assumptions hold. However, when the parametric assumptions are wrong, this estimator can be inconsistent, whereas the 2SLS estimator is consistent; see Table 4 of Reference 48 for finite-sample results. Imbens and Rubin's other approach to using mixture modeling to estimate the CACE is to approximate the density of the outcome distribution for each compliance class under each randomization group as a piecewise constant function, and then estimate the CACE by maximum likelihood [46]. This approach is in principle nonparametric as the number of constant pieces in each density function can be increased with the sample size. However, Reference 46 does not provide a systematic approach for choosing the number of and locations of the pieces.

To take into account the mixture structure in outcome distribution, Cheng et al. [48] developed a systematic and easily implementable approach for inference about the CACE using empirical likelihood [49]. Empirical likelihood profiles a general multinomial likelihood with support on the observed data points and therefore is an easily constructed random approximation to unknown distributions. Maximum empirical likelihood estimators have good properties. The maximum empirical likelihood estimator for the CACE is robust to parametric distribution assumptions since the empirical likelihood for a parameter such as the CACE is the nonparametric profile likelihood for the parameter. Cheng et al. [48] show that the maximum empirical likelihood estimator for the CACE provides substantial efficiency gains over the 2SLS estimator in finite samples.

In addition to the inference on CACE, Cheng et al. [50] developed a semiparametric IV method based on the empirical likelihood approach for distributional treatment effects for compliers and other general functions of the compliers' outcome distribution. They showed that their estimators are substantially more efficient than the standard IV estimator for treatment effects on outcome distributions (see Section 2.8.3 for more details).

2.3.4 Estimation with Observed Covariates

As discussed above, various methods have been proposed to use IVs to overcome the problem of selection bias in estimating the effect of a treatment on outcomes without covariates. However, in practice, instruments may be valid only after conditioning on covariates. For example, in the NICU study of Section 2.1.4, race is associated with the proposed IV excess travel time and race is also thought to be associated with infant mortality through mechanisms other than level of NICU delivery such as maternal age, previous cesarean section, inadequate prenatal care, chronic medical conditions, and other incompletely understood mechanisms such as social support and other contextual factors [51]. Consequently, in order for excess travel time to be independent of unmeasured confounders conditional on measured covariates, it is important that race be included as a measured covariate. Note that if race is associated with an unmeasured variable such as social support that affects infant mortality, then controlling for race in the IV analysis will control for the effect of social support as long as social support is only associated with excess travel time through race. See Figure 2.2.

To incorporate covariates into the 2SLS estimator, regress T_i on $\mathbf{X}_i$ and Z_i in the first stage to obtain $\hat{T}_i$ and then regress Y_i on $\hat{T}_i$ and $\mathbf{X}_i$ in the second stage. Denote the coefficient on $\hat{T}_i$ in the second-stage regression by $\hat{\lambda}^{2SLS}$. The estimator $\hat{\lambda}^{2SLS}$ estimates some kind of covariate-averaged CACE as we shall discuss [52]. Let (λ, ϕ) be the minimum mean squared error linear approximation to the average response function for compliers $E(Y|\mathbf{X}, T, C = co)$, that is, $(\lambda, \phi) = \arg\min_{\lambda^*, \phi^*} E[(Y - \phi^{*T}\mathbf{X} - \lambda^* T)^2 | C = co]$ (where $\mathbf{X}$ is assumed to contain the intercept). Specifically, if the CACE given $\mathbf{X}$ is the same for all $\mathbf{X}$ and the effect of $\mathbf{X}$ on the outcomes for compliers is linear (i.e., $E(Y|\mathbf{X}, T, C = co) = \phi^T\mathbf{X} + \lambda T$), then λ equals the CACE. The estimator $\hat{\lambda}^{2SLS}$ is a consistent (i.e., asymptotically unbiased) estimator of λ. Thus,

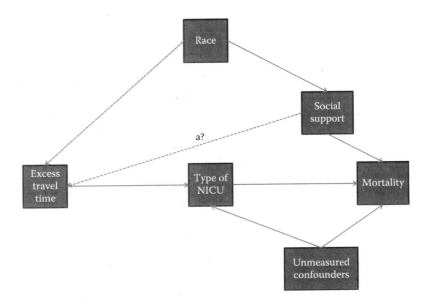

FIGURE 2.2
Directed acyclic graph for the NICU example, where it is assumed that the graph is conditional on measured confounders such as birth weight, gestational age, and so on. Suppose race is a measured covariate but social support is not measured. If the dashed line with a? between race and social support does not exist (i.e., no association between social support and excess travel time after controlling for race), then the IV analysis controlling for race will also effectively control for social support even though social support is unmeasured. However, if the dashed line with a? does exist, then the IV analysis will not fully control for social support and be biased.

if the CACE given $\mathbf{X}$ is the same for all $\mathbf{X}$ and the effect of $\mathbf{X}$ on the outcomes for compliers is linear, $\hat{\lambda}^{2SLS}$ is a consistent estimator of the CACE. The standard error for $\hat{\lambda}^{2SLS}$ is not the standard error from the second-stage regression but needs to account for the sampling uncertainty in using $\hat{T}_i$ as an estimate of $E(T_i|\mathbf{X}_i, Z_i)$; see References 53–55 and Chapter 8.8 of Reference 54. Other methods besides two-stage least squares for incorporating measured covariates into the IV model are discussed in References 48 and 56–62 among others. References 58 and 59 introduce covariates in the IV model of Reference 42 with distributional assumptions and functional form restrictions. Angrist and Imbens [57] consider settings under fully saturated specifications with discrete covariates. Without distributional assumptions or functional form restrictions, Abadie [56] develops closed forms for average potential outcomes for compliers under treatment and control with covariates. Cheng et al. [48] discuss incorporating covariates with the empirical likelihood approach of Section 2.3.3.

2.3.5 Robust Standard Errors for 2SLS

When there is clustering in the data, standard errors that are robust to clustering should be computed. For 2SLS, this can be done by using robust Huber–White standard errors [63]. For the NICU study, there is clustering by hospital.

Even when there is no clustering, we recommend always using the robust Huber–White standard errors for 2SLS as the nonrobust standard error's correctness requires additional strong assumptions about the relationships between the different compliance classes' outcome distributions and homoskedasticity while the robust standard error's correctness does not require these assumptions; see Theorem 3 in Reference 42 and Section 4.2.1 of Reference 52.

2.3.6 Example: Analysis of NICU Study

For the NICU study, Table 2.3 shows the 2SLS estimate for the effect of high-level NICUs using excess travel time as an IV and compares the 2SLS estimate to the estimate that does not adjust for any confounders and the multiple regression estimate that only adjusts for the measured confounders (those in Table 2.3 plus several other variables described in Reference 1). The unadjusted estimate is that high-level NICUs increase the death rate, causing 10.9 more deaths per 1,000 deliveries; this estimate is probably strongly biased by the selection bias that doctors and mothers are more likely to insist on babies being delivered at a high-level NICU if the baby is at a high risk of mortality. The regression estimate that adjusts for measured confounders is that high-level NICUs save 4.2 babies per 1,000 deliveries. The 2SLS estimate that adjusts for measured and unmeasured confounders is that high-level NICUs save even more babies, 5.9 babies per 1,000 deliveries.

As illustrated by Table 2.3, the multiple regression estimate of the causal effect will generally have a smaller confidence interval than the 2SLS

TABLE 2.3

Risk Difference Estimates for Mortality per 1,000 Premature Births in High-Level NICUs versus Low-Level NICUs

Estimator	Risk Difference	Confidence Interval
Unadjusted	10.9	(6.6, 15.3)
Multiple regression, adjusted for measured confounders	−4.2	(−6.8, −1.5)
Two-stage least squares, adjusted for measured and unmeasured confounders	−5.9	(−9.6, −2.2)

Note: The confidence intervals account for clustering by hospital through the use of Huber–White robust standard errors.

estimate. However, when the IV is valid and there is unmeasured confounding, the multiple regression estimate will be asymptotically biased whereas the 2SLS estimate will be asymptotically unbiased. Thus, there is a bias-variance trade-off between multiple regression and 2SLS (IV estimation). When the IV is not perfectly valid, the 2SLS estimator will be asymptotically biased, but the bias-variance trade-off may still favor 2SLS. Reference 64 develops a diagnostic tool for deciding whether to use multiple regression versus 2SLS.

2.4 Understanding the Treatment Effect That IV Estimates

2.4.1 Relationship between Average Treatment Effect for Compliers and Average Treatment Effect for the Whole Population

As discussed in Section 2.3, the IV method estimates the CACE, the average treatment effect for the compliers ($E[Y_1 - Y_0|C = co]$). The average treatment effect in the population is, under the monotonicity assumption, a weighted average of the average treatment effect for the compliers, the average treatment effect for the never-takers, and the average treatment effect for the always-takers:

$$E[Y_1 - Y_0] = P(C = co)E[Y_1 - Y_0|C = co] + P(C = at)E[Y_1 - Y_0|C = at]$$
$$+ P(C = nt)E[Y_1 - Y_0|C = nt].$$

The IV method provides no direct information on the average treatment effect for always-takers ($E[Y_1 - Y_0|C = at]$) or the average treatment effect for never-takers ($E[Y_1 - Y_0|C = nt]$). However, the IV method can provide useful bounds on the average treatment effect for the whole population if a researcher is able to put bounds on the difference between the average treatment effect for compliers and the average treatment effects for never-takers and always-takers based on subject matter knowledge. For example, suppose a researcher is willing to assume that this difference is no more than b, then

$$E[Y_1 - Y_0|C = co] - b[1 - P(C = co)] \leq E[Y_1 - Y_0] \leq E[Y_1 - Y_0|C = co]$$
$$+ b[1 - P(C = co)], \tag{2.6}$$

where the quantities on the left- and right-hand sides of Equation 2.6 other than b can be estimated as discussed in Section 2.3. For binary or other bounded outcomes, the boundedness of the outcomes can be used to tighten bounds on the average treatment effect for the whole population or other treatment effects [65,66]. Qualitative assumptions, such as that the average treatment effect is larger for always-takers than compliers, can also be used to tighten the bounds, for example, References 66–68.

2.4.2 Characterizing the Compliers

The IV method estimates the average treatment effect for the subpopulation of compliers. In most situations, it is impossible to identify which subjects in the data set are "compliers" because we only observe a subject's treatment selection under either $Z = 1$ or $Z = 0$, which means we cannot identify if the subject would have complied under the unobserved level of the instrument. So who are these compliers and how do they compare to noncompliers? To understand this better, it is useful to characterize the compliers in terms of their distribution of observed covariates [25,52]. Consider a binary covariate X that is part of $\mathbf{X}$. The prevalence ratio of X among compliers compared to the full population is

$$\text{Prevalence ratio} = \frac{P(X = 1 | C = co)}{P(X = 1)}.$$

The prevalence ratio can be written as

$$\frac{P(X = 1 | C = co)}{P(X = 1)} = \frac{P(C = co | X = 1)}{P(C = co)}$$

$$= \frac{\int [E(T | Z = 1, X = 1, \mathbf{X} = \mathbf{x}) - E(T | Z = 0, X = 1, \mathbf{X} = \mathbf{x})] f(\mathbf{x} | X = 1) d\mathbf{x}}{\int [E(T | Z = 1, \mathbf{X} = \mathbf{x}) - E(T | Z = 0, \mathbf{X} = \mathbf{x})] f(\mathbf{x}) d\mathbf{x}},$$

(2.7)

which can be estimated by

$$\frac{\frac{1}{\sum_{i=1}^{N} X_i} \sum_{i=1}^{N} X_i [\hat{E}(T | Z = 1, \mathbf{X} = \mathbf{x}_i) - \hat{E}(T | Z = 0, \mathbf{X} = \mathbf{x}_i)]}{\frac{1}{N} \sum_{i=1}^{N} [\hat{E}(T | Z = 1, \mathbf{X} = \mathbf{x}_i) - \hat{E}(T | Z = 0, \mathbf{X} = \mathbf{x}_i)]}.$$

(2.8)

Reference 56 provides an alternative approach to estimating the prevalence ratio.

Table 2.4 shows the mean of various characteristics X among compliers versus the full population, and also shows the prevalence ratio. Babies whose mothers are college graduates are slightly underrepresented (prevalence ratio = 0.85) and African-Americans are slightly overrepresented (prevalence ratio = 1.22) among compliers. Very low birth weight ($<1500\,\text{g}$) and very premature babies (gestational age ≤ 32 weeks) are substantially underrepresented among compliers, with prevalence ratios around 0.4; these babies are more likely to be always-takers, that is, delivered at high-level NICUs regardless of mother's travel time. Babies whose mothers' have comorbidities such as diabetes or hypertension are slightly underrepresented among

TABLE 2.4

Complier Characteristics for NICU Study

Characteristic X	Prevalence of X among Compliers	Prevalence of X in Full Population	Prevalence Ratio of X among Compliers to Full Population
Mother college graduate	0.22	0.26	0.85
African-American	0.20	0.16	1.22
Birth weight <1500 g	0.03	0.09	0.36
Gestational age ≤32 weeks	0.05	0.13	0.40
Gestational diabetes	0.05	0.05	0.92
Diabetes mellitus	0.01	0.02	0.74
Pregnancy-induced hypertension	0.09	0.10	0.82
Chronic hypertension	0.01	0.02	0.90

Note: The second column shows the estimated proportion of compliers with a characteristic X, the third column shows the estimated proportion of the full population with the characteristic X, and the fourth column shows the estimated ratio of compliers with X compared to the full population with X.

compliers. Overall, Table 2.4 suggests that higher-risk babies are underrepresented among the compliers. If high-level NICUs (compared to low-level NICUs) reduce the death rate more among higher-risk babies, then the IV estimate will underestimate the amount by which all premature babies being treated at high-level NICUs versus all premature babies being treated at low-level NICUs would reduce the death rate. This would mean that the 2SLS IV estimate in Table 2.3 that high-level NICUs reduce the death rate by 5.9 per 1,000 births is a lower bound on the estimated reduction in the death rate if all premature babies were delivered at high-level NICUs versus low-level NICUs.

2.4.3 Understanding the IV Estimate When Compliance Status Is Not Deterministic

For an encouragement that is uniformly delivered, such as patients who made an appointment at a psychiatric outpatient clinic are sent a letter encouraging them to attend the appointment [69], it is clear that a subject is a complier, always-taker, never-taker, or defier with respect to the encouragement. However, sometimes encouragements that are not uniformly delivered are used as IVs. For example, in the NICU study, consider the IV of whether the mother's excess travel time to the nearest high-level NICU is more than 10 min. If a mother whose excess travel time to the nearest high-level NICU was more than 10 min moved to a new home with an excess travel time less than 10 min, whether the mother would deliver her baby at a high-level NICU might depend on additional aspects of the move, such as the location and availability of public transportation at her new home [70] and the exact travel time to the nearest high-level NICU at her new home. Consequently, a mother may not be able to be deterministically classified as a complier or not a complier—she may be a complier with respect to certain moves but not others. Another example of nondeterministic compliance is when physician preference for one drug versus another is used as the IV (e.g., $Z = 1$ if a patient's physician prescribes drug A more often than drug B), whether a patient receives drug A may depend on how strongly the physician prefers drug A [25,71]. Another situation in which nondeterministic compliance status can arise is that the IV may not itself be an encouragement intervention but a proxy for an encouragement intervention. Consider the case of Mendelian randomization, in which the IV is often an SNP that might be part of a gene A. The SNP may be a marker for a gene B on the same chromosome that actually affects the level of the exposure T. The encouragement intervention is receiving the gene B that actually affects the level of the exposure T and the SNP is just a proxy for this encouragement. Consequently, even if a subject's exposure level would change as a result of a change in gene B, whether the subject is a complier with respect to a change in the SNP depends on whether the change in the SNP leads to a change in the gene B, which is randomly determined through the process of recombination [70].

Brookhart and Schneeweiss [25] provide a framework for understanding how to interpret the IV estimate when compliance status is not deterministic. Suppose that the study population can be decomposed into a set of $\kappa + 1$ mutually exclusive groups of patients based on clinical, lifestyle, and other characteristics such that within each group of patients, whether a subject receives treatment is independent of the effect of the treatment. All of the common causes of the potential treatment received T_1, T_0 and the potential outcomes Y_1, Y_0 should be included in the characteristics used to define these groups. For example, if there are L binary common causes of (T_1, T_0, Y_1, Y_0), then the subgroups can be the $\kappa + 1 = 2^L$ possible values of these common causes. Denote patient membership in these groups by the set of indicators $\mathbf{S} = \{S_1, S_2, \ldots, S_\kappa\}$. Consider the following model for the expected potential outcome:

$$E(Y_t|\mathbf{S}) = \alpha_0 + \alpha_1 t + \alpha_2^T \mathbf{S} + \alpha_3^T \mathbf{S}t.$$

The average effect of treatment in the population is $\alpha_1 + \alpha_3^T E[\mathbf{S}]$ and the average effect of treatment in subgroup j is $\alpha_1 + \alpha_{3,j}$. Under the IV Assumptions 1–3 and 5 in Section 2.3.1, that is, all the assumptions except monotonicity, the IV estimator estimates the following quantity:

$$\frac{E(Y|Z = 1) - E(Y|Z = 0)}{E(T|Z = 1) - E(T|Z = 0)} = \alpha_1 + \sum_{j=1}^{\kappa} \alpha_{3,j} E[S_j] w_j, \tag{2.9}$$

where

$$w_j = \frac{E(T|Z = 1, S_j = 1) - E(T|Z = 0, S_j = 1)}{E(T|Z = 1) - E(T|Z = 0)}.$$

The IV estimator (2.9) is a "weighted average" of treatment effects in different subgroups, where the subgroups in which the instrument has a stronger effect on the treatment get more weight. Note that when the compliance class is deterministic, then the subgroups can be defined as the compliance classes and Equation 2.9 just says that the IV estimator is the average treatment effect for compliers. In the NICU study, where compliance class may not be deterministic, Table 2.4 suggests that babies in lower-risk groups, for example, not very low birth weight or not very low gestational age, are weighted more heavily in the IV estimator. If there are subgroups for whom the instrument has no effect on their treatment level, then that subgroup gets zero weight. For example, mothers or babies with severe preexisting conditions may virtually always be delivered at a high-level NICU, so that the IV of excess travel time has no effect on their treatment level [1]. If there are subgroups for whom the encouraging level of the instrument makes them less likely to receive the treatment, then this subgroup would get "negative weight" and Equation 2.9 is not a true weighted average, potentially leading the IV estimator to have the opposite sign of the effect of the treatment. For example, Brookhart and Schneeweiss [25] discussed studying the safety of metformin for treating type 2 diabetes versus other antihyperglycemic drugs among patients with liver disease using physician preference as the IV ($Z = 1$ if a physician is more likely to prescribe metformin than other antihyperglycemic drugs). Metformin is contraindicated in patients with decreased liver disease, as it can cause lactic acidosis, a potentially fatal side effect. Brookhart and Schneeweiss [25] speculated that physicians who infrequently use metformin will be less likely to understand its contraindications and would therefore be more likely to misuse it. If this hypothesis is true, then for estimating the effect of metformin on lactic acidosis, the IV estimator could mistakenly make metformin appear to prevent lactic acidosis, as patients of physicians with $Z = 1$ are at lower risk of being inappropriately treated with metformin. When the compliance class is deterministic, a subgroup getting negative weight means that there are defiers, violating the monotonicity assumption.

2.5 Assessing the IV Assumptions and Sensitivity Analysis for Violations of Assumptions

2.5.1 Assessing the IV Assumptions

This section will discuss assessing the two key IV assumptions: (1) the IV is independent of unmeasured confounders; (2) the IV affects outcome only through treatment received (the ER).

One way of assessing whether the proposed IV is independent of unmeasured confounders conditional on measured confounders is to look at whether the proposed IV is associated with measured confounders. Although measured confounders can be controlled for, if the measured confounder is only a proxy for the true confounder, then an association between the proposed IV and the measured confounder suggests that there will be an association between the IV and the unmeasured part of the true confounder. If there are two or more sources of confounding, then it is useful to examine if the observable part of one source of confounding is associated with the IV after controlling for the other sources of confounding. These ideas will be illustrated using the NICU study described in Section 2.1.4. Table 2.5 shows the imbalance of measured covariates across levels of the IV. The racial composition is very different between the near ($Z = 1$) and far ($Z = 0$) babies, with near babies being much more likely to be African-American. Since race has a substantial association with neonatal outcomes [51,72], it is sensible to examine the association of other measured confounders with the IV after controlling for race. Table 2.6 shows the association of the IV with measured confounders for whites. The clinical measured confounders such as low birth weight, gestational age ≤32 weeks, and maternal comorbidities (diabetes and hypertension) are generally similar between near and far babies although there are some significant associations. This similarity between the clinical status of near and far babies and mothers after controlling for race provides some support that the IV is approximately, although not exactly, valid for whites. However, whether the mother is a college graduate differs substantially between white near and far mothers, suggesting that there may be residual confounding due to socioeconomic status. Table 2.7 shows the

TABLE 2.5

Imbalance of Measured Covariates across Levels of the Instrument for the NICU Data

Characteristic X	$P(X\|\text{Near})(\%)$	$P(X\|\text{Far})(\%)$	p-Value	Prevalence Difference Ratio
Birth weight <1500 g	9.4	7.7	<0.01	0.02
Mother college graduate	25.9	26.1	0.26	−0.04
African-American	25.6	4.6	<0.01	0.64
Gestational age ≤32 weeks	14.3	11.7	<0.01	0.23
Gestational diabetes	5.2	5.2	0.47	0.12
Diabetes mellitus	1.8	1.9	0.07	−0.16
Pregnancy-induced hypertension	10.6	10.1	<0.01	0.13
Chronic hypertension	1.9	1.3	<0.01	0.61

Note: The PDR is the ratio of the imbalance of the measured covariates across levels of the instrument to the imbalance across levels of the treatment. The estimated proportion of compliers is $P(T = 1|Z = 1) - P(T = 1|Z = 0) = 0.447$ so that a PDR less than 0.447 for an X indicates that there would be less bias in the IV method from failing to adjust for X than from OLS that failed to adjust for X.

TABLE 2.6

Imbalance of Measured Covariates across Levels of the Instrument for Babies Born to White Mothers in the NICU Data

Characteristic X	$P(X\mid\text{Near})(\%)$	$P(X\mid\text{Far})(\%)$	p-Value	Prevalence Difference Ratio
Birth weight <1500 g	7.5	7.2	0.07	0.04
Mother college graduate	34.4	26.8	<0.01	0.72
Gestational age ≤32 weeks	11.8	11.1	<0.01	0.07
Gestational diabetes	5.6	5.3	0.02	0.34
Diabetes mellitus	1.8	1.9	0.08	−0.17
Pregnancy-induced hypertension	10.6	10.1	<0.01	0.05
Chronic hypertension	1.6	1.3	<0.01	0.43

Note: The PDR is the ratio of the imbalance of the measured covariates across levels of the instrument to the imbalance across levels of the treatment. The estimated proportion of compliers is $P(T = 1\mid Z = 1, \text{white}) - P(T = 1\mid Z = 0, \text{white}) = 0.418$ so that a PDR less than 0.418 for an X indicates that there would be less bias in the IV method from failing to adjust for X than from OLS that failed to adjust for X.

association of the IV with measured confounders for African-Americans. For African-Americans, there are more substantial associations than for whites between near/far status and the important clinical status variables low birth weight and gestational age ≤32 weeks, raising more concern about whether the IV is approximately valid for African-Americans.

TABLE 2.7

Imbalance of Measured Covariates across Levels of the Instrument for Babies Born to African-American Mothers in the NICU Data

Characteristic X	$P(X\mid\text{Near})(\%)$	$P(X\mid\text{Far})(\%)$	p-Value	Prevalence Difference Ratio
Birth weight <1500 g	13.5	11.9	<0.01	0.41
Mother college graduate	8.0	10.7	<0.01	1.60
Gestational age ≤32 weeks	19.3	16.6	<0.01	0.48
Gestational diabetes	4.2	4.3	0.67	−0.70
Diabetes mellitus	1.9	2.6	<0.01	−1.35
Pregnancy-induced hypertension	11.8	10.0	<0.01	0.69
Chronic hypertension	2.8	2.4	0.12	0.34

Note: The PDR is the ratio of the imbalance of the measured covariates across levels of the instrument to the imbalance across levels of the treatment. The estimated proportion of compliers is $P(T = 1\mid Z = 1, \text{African-American}) - P(T = 1\mid Z = 0, \text{African-American}) = 0.503$ so that a prevalence difference ratio less than 0.503 for an X indicates that there would be less bias in the IV method from failing to adjust for X than from OLS that failed to adjust for X.

The last column of Tables 2.5 through 2.7 shows the *prevalence difference ratio* (PDR), a measure of how biased an IV analysis would be from failing to adjust from the confounder as compared to an ordinary least squares (OLS) analysis [25]. The below discussion of the PDR is drawn from Reference 25. Denote the confounder by U. Consider the following model for the potential outcome:

$$Y_t = \alpha_0 + \alpha_1 t + \alpha_2 U + \epsilon_t, \tag{2.10}$$

where $E(\epsilon_t | U) = 0$. The average treatment effect is $E[Y_1 - Y_0] = \alpha_1$. The observed data are

$$Y = \alpha_0 + \alpha_1 T + \alpha_2 U + \epsilon_0 + T(\epsilon_1 - \epsilon_0).$$

Assume that $E(\epsilon_t | T, U) = 0$ for $t = 0$ or 1. This assumption means that if U were controlled for, the parameters of Equation 2.10 could be consistently estimated by least squares. By iterated expectations, $E[\epsilon_0 + T(\epsilon_1 - \epsilon_0) | T] = 0$. Therefore,

$$E(Y|T = 1) - E(Y|T = 0) = \alpha_1 + \alpha_2(E[U|T = 1] - E[U|T = 0]),$$

so that an OLS analysis that did not adjust for U would be biased by $\alpha_2(E[U|T = 1] - E[U|T = 0])$. To evaluate the IV estimand, consider the further assumption that $E[\epsilon_0 | Z] = 0$ so that the proposed IV can be related to the observed outcome only through its effect on T or association with U; also assume that $E(\epsilon_1 - \epsilon_0 | C)$ is the same for all compliance classes C so that the CACE is equal to the overall average causal effect α_1. These assumptions together say that if U were controlled for, the IV estimator would consistently estimate the average treatment effect α_1. Under these assumptions, the probability limit of the IV estimator that does not control for U can be written as

$$\frac{E[Y|Z = 1] - E[Y|Z = 0]}{E[T|Z = 1] - E[T|Z = 0]} = \alpha_1 + \alpha_2 \frac{E(U|Z = 1) - E(U|Z = 0)}{E(T|Z = 1) - E(T|Z = 0)}.$$

The asymptotic bias of the IV estimator is thus

$$\text{Bias}(\hat{\beta}_1^{IV}) = \alpha_2 \frac{E(U|Z = 1) - E(U|Z = 0)}{E(T|Z = 1) - E(T|Z = 0)}. \tag{2.11}$$

The term $E(U|Z = 1) - E(U|Z = 0)$ is the difference in the prevalence of the risk factor U between levels of the IV. The total bias in the IV estimator is this difference multiplied by the excess risk of the outcome among patients with $U = 1$ divided by the strength of the IV. For the IV estimator to have less asymptotic bias than OLS, the following condition must hold [25]:

$$\frac{E[U|Z = 1] - E[U|Z = 0]}{E[U|T = 1] - E[U|T = 0]} < E(T|Z = 1) - E(T|Z = 0). \tag{2.12}$$

In other words, the difference in the prevalence of U between levels of Z relative to the difference in the prevalence of U between levels of T must be less than the strength of the IV [25]. The left-hand side of Equation 2.12 is called the PDR. In order for us to think that the IV analysis is likely to be less biased than OLS, the PDR should be less than the strength of the IV ($E[T|Z = 1] - E[T|Z = 0]$), particularly for those variables clearly related to the outcome. Table 2.6 shows that the PDRs are generally less than the strength of the IV (0.418) for whites, but the PDRs are often greater than the strength of the IV (0.503) for African-Americans, suggesting that the IV analysis reduces bias for whites compared to OLS but not for African-Americans.

A way of testing whether the two key IV assumptions (i.e., (i) the IV is independent of unmeasured confounders conditional on the measured confounders and (ii) the IV affects outcomes only through treatment received) hold is to find a subpopulation for whom the link between the IV and treatment received is thought to be broken and then test whether the IV is associated with the outcome in this subpopulation. The only way in which the IV could be associated with the outcome in such a subpopulation is if the IV was associated with unmeasured confounders or directly affected the outcome through a pathway other than treatment received. Figure 2.3 shows an example. Kang et al. [73] study the effect of children in Africa getting malaria on their becoming stunted (having a height that is two standard deviations below the expected height for the child's age) and consider the sickle cell

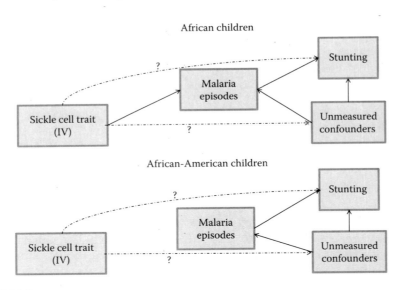

FIGURE 2.3
Causal diagrams for the effect of the sickle cell trait (the IV) and malaria episodes (the treatment) on stunting (the outcome) in African children and African-American children. If the sickle cell trait is a valid IV, then the dashed lines should be absent and the sickle cell trait will have no effect on stunting among African-American children.

trait as a possible IV. The sickle cell trait is that a person inherits a copy of the hemoglobin variant HbS from one parent and normal hemoglobin from the other. While inheriting two copies of HbS results in sickle cell disease and substantially shortened life expectancy, inheriting only one copy (the sickle cell trait) is protective against malaria and is thought to have little detrimental effect on health [74]. To test whether the sickle cell trait indeed does not affect stunting in ways other than reducing malaria and is not associated with unmeasured confounders, Kang et al. [73] considered whether the sickle cell trait is associated with stunting among African-American children; the sickle cell trait has high prevalence among African-Americans but does not affect malaria because malaria is not present in the United States. References 75 and 76 found no evidence that sickle cell trait is associated with growth and development in African-American children. This provides evidence that the dashed lines in Figure 2.3 are indeed absent, which would mean that the proposed IV of the sickle cell trait does indeed satisfy the two key IV assumptions of being independent of unmeasured confounders and affecting outcomes only through treatment received. Angrist and Krueger [77] also employed this strategy of finding a subpopulation for whom the link between the IV and treatment received is broken to test their IV of quarter of birth for studying the effect of education on earnings. The reason that quarter of birth is associated with education is that for students who plan to drop out of school as soon as they have reached the age at which they are no longer compelled to be in school (e.g., age 16), quarter of birth affects how much education these students will get before they drop out because children start school at different ages depending on their quarter of birth. However, for students who plan to go to college, quarter of birth does not affect their amount of schooling. Consequently, Angrist and Krueger [77] looked at whether there was an absence of an association between quarter of birth and earnings among students who went to college to test the IV assumptions.

Newcomers to IV methods often think that the validity of the IV can be tested by regressing the outcome on treatment received, the IV, and measured confounders, and testing whether the coefficient on the IV is significant. However, this is not a valid test as, even if the IV assumptions hold, the coefficient on the IV would typically be nonzero. One way to see this is that if there are no measured confounders, the test amounts to testing whether (i) $E[Y|Z = 1, T = 1] - E[Y|Z = 0, T = 1] = 0$ and (ii) $E[Y|Z = 1, T = 0] - E[Y|Z = 0, T = 0] = 0$. These are the differences between (i) the average potential outcome of the group of always-takers and compliers together when these subjects are encouraged to receive treatment and receive treatment versus those of always-takers alone when they are not encouraged to receive treatment but do receive treatment and (ii) the average potential outcome of never-takers when encouraged to receive treatment but do not receive treatment versus those of the group of never-takers and compliers when they are not encouraged to receive treatment and do not receive treatment. If the IV assumptions hold that the IV is not associated with unmeasured confounders and has no direct effect on the outcome other than treatment received, then (i) is equal to zero if and only if the average potential outcome of compliers and always-takers are the same when both groups receive treatment and (ii) is equal to zero if and only if the average potential outcomes of compliers and never-takers are the same when both groups do not receive treatment. Typically, the average potential outcome of compliers and always-takers (compliers and never-takers) will not be the same when both groups receive (do not receive) treatment even if the IV assumptions hold.

2.5.2 Sensitivity Analysis

A sensitivity analysis seeks to quantify how sensitive conclusions from an IV analysis are to plausible violations of key assumptions. Sensitivity analysis methods for IV analyses have been developed by References 12, 13, 25, 78, and 79 among others. Here, an approach will be presented to sensitivity analysis for violations of the assumption that the IV is independent of unmeasured confounders. Assume that the concern is that the IV may be related to an unmeasured confounder U, which has mean 0 and variance 1 and is independent of the measured confounders $\mathbf{X}$ (U can always be taken to the residual of the unmeasured confounder given the measured confounders to make this assumption plausible). Consider the following model:

$$Y_i^t = \alpha + \beta t + \gamma^T \mathbf{X}_i + \delta U_i + e_i,$$
$$U_i = \rho + \eta Z_i + v_i,$$
$$E(v_i|\mathbf{X}_i, Z_i) = 0, \quad E(e_i|\mathbf{X}_i, Z_i) = 0. \tag{2.13}$$

β is the causal effect of treatment. The sensitivity parameters are δ, the effect of a one standard deviation increase in the unmeasured confounder on the mean of the potential outcome under no treatment, and η, how much higher the mean of the unmeasured confounder U_i is in standard deviation units for $Z_i = 1$ versus $Z_i = 0$. Model (2.13) says that Z_i would be a valid IV if both the measured confounders $\mathbf{X}_i$ and the unmeasured confounder U_i were controlled for. Under model (2.13), the following holds:

$$Y_i = \alpha + \beta T_i + \gamma^T \mathbf{X}_i + \delta U_i + e_i,$$
$$Y_i - \delta \eta Z_i = \alpha + \delta \rho + \beta T_i + \gamma^T \mathbf{X}_i + e_i + \delta v_i,$$
$$E(v_i|\mathbf{X}_i, Z_i) = 0, \ E(e_i|\mathbf{X}_i, Z_i) = 0.$$

Consequently, a consistent estimate of and inferences for β can be obtained by carrying out a 2SLS analysis with $Y_i - \delta \eta Z_i$ as the outcome variable, T_i as the treatment variable, $\mathbf{X}_i$ as the measured confounders, and Z_i as the

TABLE 2.8

Estimates and 95% Confidence Intervals for β, the Risk Difference Effect of a Premature Baby Being Delivered in a High-Level NICU, for Different Values of the Sensitivity Parameters δ, the Effect of a One Standard Deviation Increase in the Unmeasured Confounder on the Mean of the Potential Outcome under No Treatment, and η, How Much Higher the Mean of the Unmeasured Confounder U_i Is in Standard Deviation Units for $Z_i = 1$ versus $Z_i = 0$

δ	η	$\hat{\beta}$	95% CI for β
0	0	−0.0059	(−0.0091, −0.0027)
−0.001	0.5	−0.0046	(−0.0079, −0.0014)
−0.005	0.5	0.0004	(−0.0029, 0.0036)
0.001	0.5	−0.0071	(−0.0104, −0.0039)
0.005	0.5	0.0121	(−0.0154, −0.0089)
−0.022	−0.093	−0.0110	(−0.0142, −0.0078)

IV. Table 2.8 shows a sensitivity analysis for the NICU study. If there was an unmeasured confounder U that decreased the death rate by 0.1% for a one standard deviation increase in U and was 0.5 standard deviations higher on average in subjects with $Z = 1$ versus $Z = 0$, then there would still be strong evidence that high-level NICUs reduce mortality substantially (lower end of 95% CI: 0.14% reduction). However, if there was an unmeasured confounder U that decreased the death rate by 0.5% for a one standard deviation increase in U and was 0.5 standard deviations higher in subjects with $Z = 1$ versus $Z = 0$, then there would no longer be strong evidence that high-level NICUs reduce mortality substantially. It can be useful to calibrate the effect of a potential unmeasured confounder U to that of a measured confounder. For example, an increase in gestational age from 30 to 33 weeks, which is a one standard deviation increase in gestational age, is associated with a reduction in the death rate of 2.2% and the mean gestational age is 0.093 standard deviations smaller among near ($Z = 1$) versus far ($Z = 0$) babies. For a comparable U that reduced the death rate by 2.2% for a one standard deviation increase in U and was 0.093 standard deviations smaller in babies with $Z = 1$ versus $Z = 0$, there would still be strong evidence that high-level NICUs reduce mortality substantially (see the last row of Table 2.8).

A sensitivity analysis for violations of the assumption that the IV has no direct effect on the outcome can be carried out as follows. Suppose that the IV has a direct effect of λ but the IV is independent of unmeasured confounders, that is,

$$Y_{zti} = \alpha + \beta t + \gamma^T \mathbf{X}_i + \lambda z + e_i,$$
$$E(e_i | \mathbf{X}_i, Z_i) = 0. \tag{2.14}$$

Then, a consistent estimate of and inferences for β can be obtained by carrying out a 2SLS analysis with $Y_i - \lambda Z_i$ as the outcome variable, T_i as the treatment variable, $\mathbf{X}_i$ as the measured confounders, and Z_i as the IV. When a proposed IV Z is thought to be independent of unmeasured confounders but there is concern that Z might have a direct effect on the outcome, Joffe et al. [80] proposed an extended IV strategy for obtaining an unbiased estimate of the causal effect of treatment that requires having a covariate W that interacts with Z in affecting treatment but for which the direct effect of Z does not depend on W.

2.6 Weak Instruments

The *strength* of an IV refers to how strongly the IV is associated with the treatment after controlling for the measured confounders $\mathbf{X}$. An IV is *weak* if this association is weak. When the IV is encouragement (vs. no such encouragement) to accept a treatment, the IV is weak if the encouragement only has a slight impact on acceptance of the treatment. The strength of the IV can be measured by the proportion of compliers or the partial R^2 when adding the IV to the first-stage model for the treatment after already including the measured confounders $\mathbf{X}$ [81,82].

Studies that use weak IVs face three problems:

1. *High variance.* The IV method is estimating the CACE and the only subjects that are contributing information about the CACE are the compliers. Thus, the weaker the IV (i.e., the smaller the proportion of compliers), the larger the variance of the IV estimate. One might think that for a sample of size N, the variance of the IV estimate would be equivalent to the variance from having a sample of $N \times P(C = co)$ known compliers. However, the situation is actually worse because additional variability is contributed from the always-takers and never-takers having different sample means in the encouraged and unencouraged groups, even though the population means are the same. Under the assumption that the variance of the outcomes for the always-takers, never-takers, compliers under treatment, and compliers under control is the same σ^2 for each group, the asymptotic variance of $\sqrt{N}(\hat{CACE}_{2SLS} - CACE)$, where $\hat{CACE}_{2SLS}$ is the 2SLS estimator (2.3), is [42]

$$\frac{\sigma^2 Var(Z)}{Cov(T, Z)} = \frac{\sigma^2}{[P(T = 1 | Z = 1) - P(T = 1 | Z = 0)]^2}. \tag{2.15}$$

Thus, for a sample of size N, the variance of the IV estimate is equivalent to the variance from having a sample of $NP(C = co)^2$

known compliers. For example, for a sample size of 10,000 with 20% compliers, the variance of the IV estimate is equivalent to that from a sample of 400 known compliers as could be obtained from a randomized trial of size 400 with perfect compliance. Thus, weak IVs can drastically reduce the effective sample size, resulting in high variance and potentially low power.

2. *Misleading inferences from 2SLS.* When the IV is weak enough, confidence intervals formed using the asymptotic standard errors for 2SLS, that is, Equation 2.15, may be misleading. Beginning with Reference 81, it has been recognized that the most common method of inference with IV, 2SLS, gives highly misleading inferences when the instrument is weak even when the instrument is perfectly valid. The 2SLS estimate can have substantial finite sample bias toward the OLS estimate and the asymptotic variance understates the actual variance. To see this, consider including a random number as an IV (the random number is not a valid IV because it is not correlated with the treatment received). Although the random number is theoretically unrelated to the unmeasured confounding variables, it will have some chance association with the unmeasured confounders in a sample and thus, some confounding will get transferred to the predicted value of the treatment. This will result in some unmeasured confounding getting transferred to the second-stage estimate of the treatment effect. Stock et al. [83] studied what strength of IV is needed to ensure that 2SLS provides reliable inferences. They suggested looking at the first-stage partial F statistic for testing that the coefficient on the IV(s) is zero. For one IV, if this first-stage partial F statistic is less than about 10, the 2SLS inferences are misleading in the sense that the type I error rate of a nominal 0.05 level is actually greater than 0.15. If more than one IV is used, then the first-stage partial F statistic needs to be larger to avoid misleading inferences, greater than 12 for 2 IVs, greater than 16 for 5 IVs, and greater than 21 for 10 IVs.

A number of methods have been developed that provide accurate inferences when the IV is weak. One method is to use the permutation inference developed in Reference 84 and illustrated in Reference 79. Another method developed by Reference 85 is to consider the conditional distribution of the likelihood ratio statistic, conditioning on the value of nuisance parameters. This method is implemented in a Stata program CLRv2.

3. *Highly sensitive to bias from unmeasured confounders.* Recall formula (2.11) for the bias in the IV estimator when the proposed IV is associated with an unmeasured confounder U. The numerator measures the association between the IV and the unmeasured confounder (multiplied by how much the unmeasured confounder affects the

outcome). The denominator is the proportion of compliers and reflects the strength of the IV. Thus, when the IV is weak (i.e., the proportion of compliers is small), the effect of the IV being invalid from being associated with an unmeasured confounder is greatly exacerbated and even a minor association between the IV and an unmeasured confounder can lead to substantial bias if the IV is weak [79,81].

In summary, when the IV is weak, the IV estimate may have high variance and if it is weak enough (i.e., partial F statistic less than 10), it is important to use inference methods other than 2SLS to provide accurate inferences. These inference methods may inform us that the confidence interval for the treatment effect is very wide, but it is possible that even when the IV is weak, if the treatment effect is large enough and the sample size is big enough, there may still be a statistically significant treatment effect assuming the IV is valid. The third problem with weak IVs is that they are very sensitive to bias from being slightly invalid, that is, being slightly correlated with unmeasured confounders. This problem does not go away with a larger sample size. A slightly biased but strong IV may be preferable to a less biased but weak IV [79].

2.7 Binary Outcomes

Often in comparative effectiveness research, the outcomes of interest take values that are not continuous, and thus are not amenable to common techniques such as 2SLS. In this section, methods appropriate for binary outcomes will be discussed. In the next section, methods appropriate for other noncontinuous outcomes settings will be introduced. For good general reviews of estimating IV effects in the binary outcome case, see References 86–88 (along with associated comments).

In 2SLS, one regression is run predicting the treatment, and then the estimated value of the treatment from this model is used and put into a second regression of the outcome on the covariates and the predicted treatment. This type of estimator, where the predictions from one model are substituted into a second model, is often referred to as a two-stage predictor substitution (2SPS).

When first encountering situations with binary outcomes, most analysts will recognize the regular 2SLS is problematic because it will not respect boundary conditions (i.e., the functional form imposes no constraints on parameter space, meaning 2SLS can produce logical absurdities such as probabilities greater than one or even negative). Through analogy to 2SLS, the naïve analyst may consider changing the second-stage regression to be a logistic model (or perhaps a probit) in lieu of the linear model. This would be a 2SPS. Unfortunately, in general, 2SPS models do not have the nice orthogonality properties of 2SLS and produce biased estimates [52,89]. Other approaches should be considered. These approaches include the parametric approaches of Reference 58 and the semiparametric approaches of References 56, 62, and 88. Two other widely used approaches (two-stage residual inclusion [2SRI] and a binary probit model) and a relatively new approach (effect ratios) will be considered in detail below.

2.7.1 Two-Stage Residual Inclusion

2SRI is a two-stage regression method that is equivalent to 2SPS when the outcome is continuous but differs when the outcome is binary. Consider the nonlinear model

$$E(Y|T, X, \mathbf{U}) = M(T\beta_T + \mathbf{X}^T \beta_X + \mathbf{U}^T \beta_U), \qquad (2.16)$$

where $M(\cdot)$ is a known function of the treatment T, a vector of observed covariates $\mathbf{X}$, and a vector of unobserved covariates $\mathbf{U}$. The unobserved covariates $\mathbf{U}$ are correlated with the treatment T when there is unmeasured confounding.

In a 2SPS model, the actual treatment is replaced by some predicted values, like so

$$E(Y|T, \mathbf{X}, \mathbf{U}) = M(\hat{T}\beta_T + \mathbf{X}^T \beta_X + \mathbf{U}^T \beta_U), \qquad (2.17)$$

where $\hat{T}$ is estimated using the IV. This is how 2SLS is done. If the model, $M()$, is linear, then—speaking loosely—2SLS makes use of the additivity of the terms on the right-hand side of the regression to separate the endogeneity of the treatment and allow unbiased estimation of the treatment effect. If $M()$ is nonlinear, though, generally 2SPS will not maintain the separability of the confounding variables through the substitution method.

Another approach here is to use a 2SRI model. The idea in a 2SRI is to model the unobserved covariates using the instrument, not the treatment, and thereby remove the endogeneity. The first stage in a 2SRI model is the same in that you model the treatment selection. But the difference is that in the second stage you substitute in the residuals from the first stage, not the predicted treatment. In formula, this is to say

$$E(Y|T, \mathbf{X}, \mathbf{U}) = M(T\beta_T + \mathbf{X}^T \beta_X + \mathbf{U}^T \hat{\beta}_U), \qquad (2.18)$$

where $\mathbf{U}^T \hat{\beta}_U$ is estimated as the difference between the actual treatment value and the predicted treatment value from the first stage (i.e., the residual). The difference between a 2SPS and a 2SRI is what information from the first stage is used in the second stage. 2SPS and 2SRI produce the same estimates for linear models but not for nonlinear models. For an introduction to

2SRI models and how they differ from 2SPS (of which 2SLS is a special case), see Reference 90. It was shown using simulation studies in Reference 91 that for the estimation of the causal odds ratio for compliers, the 2SPS and 2SRI models performed similarly; see also Reference 92 for an analytical comparison. The simulation studies of Reference 91 also showed that the generalized structural mean model (GSMM) in an IV framework with binary outcomes tended to perform quite well vis-a-vis 2SPS and 2SRI models. See Reference 88 for an introduction to GSMM in an IV framework.

2.7.2 Bivariate Probit Models

The bivariate probit model is a parameterized model that assumes an explicit functional form of the bivariate distribution of the error terms from the selection model and the error terms from the outcome model [93,94]. This model leans on the parametric assumptions of the error terms, leaving the conclusions sensitive to modifications of the assumptions. Additionally, these models suffer from difficulty in maximizing the likelihood functions and trouble with calculating appropriate standard errors [95].

2.7.3 Matching-Based Estimator: Effect Ratio

Coming out of a different tradition, a class of estimator has been proposed that is also capable of dealing with binary outcomes in an IV setting. Proposed by Baiocchi et al. [13], the "effect ratio" in a binary setting can be thought of as a risk difference estimator for the compliers. The effect ratio is predicated on having matched sets. In Reference 13, matched pairs were constructed using a study design-based approach called near–far matching. Near–far matching will be discussed in the next section.

First, the notation will be introduced that is required to discuss the effect ratio. Assume there are I matched pairs, $i = 1, \ldots, I$, with two subjects, $j = 1, 2$, one treated subject and one control, or $2I$ subjects in total. If the jth subject in pair i receives the treatment, write $Z_{ij} = 1$, whereas if this subject receives the control, write $Z_{ij} = 0$, so $1 = Z_{i1} + Z_{i2}$ for $i = 1, \ldots, I$. The matched pairs were formed by matching for an observed covariate $\mathbf{x}_{ij}$, but may have failed to control an unobserved covariate u_{ij}; that is, $\mathbf{x}_{ij} = \mathbf{x}_{ik}$ for all i, j, k, but possibly $u_{ij} \neq u_{ik}$.

For any outcome, each subject has two potential responses, one seen when the instrument encourages the subject to take the treatment, $Z_{ij} = 1$, the other seen when the instrument randomly assigns the subject to be encouraged to take the control, $Z_{ij} = 0$. Here, there are two responses, the potential outcomes $Y_{z=1,ij}, Y_{z=0,ij}$ and the potential treatment selections T_{1ij}, T_{0ij}. (Note that the potential outcome $Y_{z=1,ij}$ may differ from the potential outcome $Y_{1ij} = Y_{d=1,ij}$.)

The effect ratio, λ, is the parameter

$$\lambda = \frac{\sum_{i=1}^{I} \sum_{j=1}^{2} (Y_{z=1,ij} - Y_{z=0,ij})}{\sum_{i=1}^{I} \sum_{j=1}^{2} (T_{1ij} - T_{0ij})}, \tag{2.19}$$

where it is implicitly assumed that $0 \neq \sum_{i=1}^{I} \sum_{j=1}^{2} (T_{1ij} - T_{0ij})$. Here, λ is a parameter of the finite population of $2I$ individuals, and because $(Y_{z=1,ij}, Y_{z=0,ij})$ and (T_{1ij}, T_{0ij}) are not jointly observed, λ cannot be calculated from observable data, so inference is required.

To test the null hypothesis $H_0 : \lambda = \lambda_0$, construct the following statistics:

$$Q(\lambda_0) = \frac{1}{I} \sum_{i=1}^{I} \left\{ \sum_{j=1}^{2} Z_{ij} (Y_{ij} - \lambda_0 T_{ij}) - \sum_{j=1}^{2} (1 - Z_{ij}) (Y_{ij} - \lambda_0 T_{ij}) \right\}$$

$$= \frac{1}{I} \sum_{i=1}^{I} V_i(\lambda_0), \text{ say,} \tag{2.20}$$

where, because $Y_{ij} - \lambda_0 T_{ij} = Y_{z=1,ij} - \lambda_0 T_{1ij}$ if $Z_{ij} = 1$ and $Y_{ij} - \lambda_0 T_{ij} = Y_{z=0,ij} - \lambda_0 T_{0ij}$ if $Z_{ij} = 0$, write

$$V_i(\lambda_0) = \sum_{j=1}^{2} Z_{ij} (Y_{z=1,ij} - \lambda_0 T_{1ij}) - \sum_{j=1}^{2} (1 - Z_{ij}) (Y_{z=0,ij} - \lambda_0 T_{0ij}). \tag{2.21}$$

Also, define

$$S^2(\lambda_0) = \frac{1}{I(I-1)} \sum_{i=1}^{I} \{V_i(\lambda_0) - Q(\lambda_0)\}^2.$$

As shown in Reference 13, under reasonable conditions, the hypothesis $H_0 : \lambda = \lambda_0$ may be tested by comparing the test statistic $Q(\lambda_0)/S(\lambda_0)$ to the standard normal.

2.8 Multinomial, Survival, and Distributional Outcomes

2.8.1 Multinomial Outcome

Multinomial outcomes (i.e., nominal or ordinal outcomes) are common in comparative effectiveness research. For example, Bruce et al. [96] conducted a randomized trial to improve adherence to prescribed depression treatments among depressed elderly patients in primary care practices; the outcomes of interest included continuous outcomes as well as multinomial outcomes such as the number of depression symptoms, ranging from 0 to 9, and the depression class (major, minor, or no depression). There was noncompliance in this trial and Ten Have et al. [97] used random assignment as an IV to estimate the effect of receiving treatment on continuous outcomes. Cheng [98] considered how to estimate the effect of receiving treatment on the multinomial outcomes using random assignment as an IV.

For ordinal outcomes, the CACE is a function of coding scores and probabilities with respect to the categories:

$$CACE = E(Y_{1i} - Y_{0i}|C_i = co)$$

$$= \sum_j (W_j \times t_j) - \sum_j (W_j \times v_j)$$

$$= \sum_j (W_j \times t_j) - \frac{1}{\pi_c} \left[\sum_j (W_j \times q_j) - (1 - \pi_c) \sum_j (W_j \times s_j) \right],$$

where W_j is the coding score; t_j, v_j, and s_j are the probabilities for compliers under treatment and control, and never-takers, respectively; and q_j is the probability for observed group $Z_i = 0, T_i = 0$ for the jth category. For estimating the CACE for ordinal outcomes, the coding score needs to be chosen. Equally spaced scores or linear transformations of them, midranks, and ridit scores are among the options. A sensitivity analysis can be performed with different choices of scores to see how the results differ.

In addition to the CACE, Cheng [98] considered some other functions of outcome distributions for understanding the causal effect for ordinal outcomes, including the measure of stochastic superiority of treatment over control for compliers:

$$SSC = P(Y_{1i} > Y_{0i}|C_i = \text{complier}) + \frac{1}{2}P(Y_{1i} = Y_{0i}|C_i = \text{complier}). \quad (2.22)$$

$SSC = 0.5$ indicates no causal effect and $SSC > 0.5$ indicates beneficial effect of the treatment for compliers if a higher value of the outcome is a better result. Compared to the CACE, SSC is easy to interpret and avoids the problem of choosing scores W_j, but without use of weighting scores, it may not describe the strength of the effect well when some specific categories are known to be more important than other categories in measuring the treatment effect.

For nominal outcomes, it is difficult to get a summary measure of the causal effect such as the CACE or SSC for ordinal outcomes. Instead, the treatment effect on the entire outcome distributions of compliers with and without treatment can be evaluated, that is, to compare t_j to v_j, $j = 1, \ldots, J$ and test the equality of t_j and v_j, $j = 1, \ldots, J$. Cheng [98] estimated those causal effects with the likelihood method and proposed a bootstrap/double bootstrap version of a likelihood ratio test for the inference when the true values of parameters are on the boundary of the parameter spaces under the null.

2.8.2 Survival Outcome

Compared to trials with continuous, binary, and multinomial outcomes, randomized trials with survival outcomes often have an issue of administrative censoring in addition to noncompliance. For those studies, Robins and Tsiatis [99] considered a structural accelerated failure time model and developed semiparametric estimators for this model. Joffe [100] provided a good discussion of their approach and comparisons with other survival analysis methods. References 101 and 102 considered a structural proportional hazards model in which the hazard of the potential failure time under treatment for a certain group of subjects is proportional to the hazard of the potential failure time under control for these same subjects. Both the structural accelerated failure time model and the structural proportional hazards model are semiparametric models, where the effect of the treatment on the distribution of failure times is modeled parametrically.

Baker [103] extended the models and assumptions for discrete-time survival data and derived closed-form expressions for estimating the difference in the hazards at a specific time between compliers under treatment and control based on maximum likelihood. Baker's [103] estimator is analogous to the standard IV estimator for a survival outcome. Nie et al. [104] discussed this standard IV approach and parametric maximum likelihood methods for the difference in survival at a specific time between compliers under treatment and control.

Here, the standard IV approach of Reference 103 will be reviewed. Let $S_{c1}(V)$, $S_{c0}(V)$, $S_{at}(V)$, and $S_{nt}(V)$ be the potential survival functions at time V of compliers in the treatment and control groups and of always-takers and never-takers, respectively, $S_z(V)$ be the survival probabilities at time V for the group with assignment $Z = z$, and $S_{zt}(V)$ be the survival probabilities at time V for the group with assignment $Z = z$ and treatment received $T = t$. By Table 2.2, the following holds:

$$S_1(V) = \pi_c S_{c1}(V) + \pi_{at} S_{at}(V) + \pi_{nt} S_{nt}(V),$$

$$S_{11}(V) = \frac{\pi_c}{\pi_c + \pi_{at}} S_{c1}(V) + \frac{\pi_{at}}{\pi_c + \pi_{at}} S_{at}(V)$$

$$S_{10}(V) = S_{nt}(V),$$

$$S_0(V) = \pi_c S_{c0}(V) + \pi_{at} S_{at}(V) + \pi_{nt} S_{nt}(V),$$

$$S_{00}(V) = \frac{\pi_c}{\pi_c + \pi_{nt}} S_{c0}(V) + \frac{\pi_{nt}}{\pi_c + \pi_{nt}} S_{nt}(V)$$

$$S_{01}(V) = S_{at}(V).$$

Similar to the standard IV estimator for CACE, the standard IV estimator for the compliers difference in survival probabilities is

$$\hat{S}_{c1}(V) - \hat{S}_{c0}(V) = \frac{\hat{S}_1(V) - \hat{S}_0(V)}{\hat{E}(T|Z = 1) - \hat{E}(T|Z = 0)},$$

which is the difference of the observed survival probabilities at time V between compliers under treatment and control divided by the proportion of compliers. $\hat{S}_z(V)$ is the Kaplan–Meier estimator under assignment z. In addition to the five IV assumptions discussed in Section 2.3.1, an additional assumption is needed to ensure that the estimator based on Kaplan–Meier estimates is consistent:

Independence assumption of failure times and censoring times: The distributions of potential failure times and administrative censoring times are independent of each other. Type I censoring (i.e., censoring times are the same for all subjects) and random censoring are two special cases.

Although the standard IV estimator is very useful, it may give negative estimates for hazards and be inefficient because it does not make full use of the mixture structure implied by the latent compliance model. When the survival functions follow some parametric distributions, Nie et al. [104] used the EM algorithm to obtain the MLE on the difference in survival probabilities for compliers. However, the MLEs could be biased when the parametric assumptions are not valid. To address this concern, Nie et al. [104] developed a nonparametric estimator based on empirical likelihood that makes use of the mixture structure to gain efficiency over the standard IV method while not depending on parametric assumptions to be consistent.

2.8.3 Effect of Treatment on Distribution of Outcomes

As discussed in the previous sections, a large literature on methods of analysis for treatment effects focuses on estimating the effect of treatment on average outcomes, for example, the CACE [12,42]. However, in addition to the average effect, knowledge of the causal effect of a treatment on the outcome distribution and its general functions can often provide additional insights into the impact of the treatment and therefore can be of significant interest in many situations [105]. For example, in a study of the effect of school subsidized meal programs on children's weight, both low weight and high weight are adverse outcomes; therefore, knowing the effect of the program on the entire distribution of outcomes rather than just average weight is important for understanding the impact of the program. For an individual patient deciding which treatment to take, the patient must weigh the effects of the possible treatments on the distribution of outcomes, the costs of the treatments, and the potential side effects of the treatments [106]. Therefore, making the best decision requires information on the treatment's effect on the entire distribution of outcomes rather than just the average effect because a patient's utility over outcomes may be nonlinear over the outcome scale [107,108]. References 109–111 provide examples in HIV care, neonatal care, and cancer care, respectively.

For distributional treatment effects on nondegenerate outcome variables with bounded support, without any parametric assumption, Abadie [112] used the standard IV approach to estimate the counterfactual cumulative distribution functions (cdfs) of the outcome of compliers with and without the treatment and proposed a bootstrap procedure to test distributional hypotheses with the Kolmogorov–Smirnov statistic. However, References 46 and 112 pointed out that the standard IV estimates of the potential cdfs for compliers may not be nondecreasing functions:

$$\hat{H}_{c1}(y)^{SIV} = \frac{\hat{E}\{1(Y_i \leq y)T_i|Z_i = 1\} - \hat{E}\{1(Y_i \leq y)T_i|Z_i = 0\}}{\hat{E}(T_i|Z_i = 1) - \hat{E}(T_i|Z_i = 0)},$$

$$\hat{H}_{c0}(y)^{SIV} = \frac{\hat{E}\{1(Y_i \leq y)(1 - T_i)|Z_i = 1\} - \hat{E}\{1(Y_i \leq y)(1 - T_i)|Z_i = 0\}}{\hat{E}\{(1 - T_i)|Z_i = 1\} - \hat{E}\{(1 - T_i)|Z_i = 0\}},$$

where $\hat{H}_{c1}(y)^{SIV}$ and $\hat{H}_{c0}(y)^{SIV}$ are the standard IV estimators for compliers' cdf under treatment and control, respectively. Furthermore, as discussed in Section 2.3.3, the standard IV approach does not make full use of the mixture structure [46] implied by the latent compliance class model (see Table 2.2) and hence could be less efficient. Instead, Kaushal [46] proposed a normal approximation and two multinomial approximations to the outcome distributions. However, the estimator based on a normal approximation could be biased when the outcomes are not normal, and for the approach based on multinomial approximations, a systematic approach for choosing the multinomial approximations is needed.

Cheng et al. [50] developed a semiparametric IV method based on the empirical likelihood approach. Their approach makes full use of the mixture structure implied by the latent compliance class model without parametric assumptions on the outcome distributions as well as takes into account the nondecreasing property of cdfs and can be easily constructed based on data. Their method can be applied to general outcomes and general functions of outcome distributions. Cheng et al. [50] showed that their estimator has good properties and is substantially more efficient than the standard IV estimator.

For the mixture structure implied by the latent compliance model (see Table 2.2), Cheng et al. [50] adopted a density ratio model proposed by Anderson [113] to relate the densities of the latent compliance classes by an exponential tilt:

$$\frac{h_j(y)}{h_0(y)} = \exp(\alpha_j + \beta_j y), \quad j = 1, 2, 3, \tag{2.23}$$

where $h_0(y)$ is unspecified and $h_0(y) = P(Y_i = y | Z_i = 0, C_i = co)$, $h_1(y) = P(Y_i = y | C_i = nt)$, $h_2(y) = P(Y_i = y | Z_i = 1, C_i = co)$, $h_3(y) = P(Y_i = y | C_i = at)$ are the outcome density (mass) functions of the latent compliance groups: compliers under control, never-takers, compliers under treatment, and always-takers, respectively. The densities are modeled nonparametrically except for being related by a parametric "exponential tilt." The idea is similar to Cox's proportional hazards models and many conventional parametric families fall in the exponential tilt model category, including two normals with common variance but different means, two exponential distributions, and two Poissons. The exponential tilt model provides a good fit to the data when many conventional parametric models do not fit the data well.

Cheng et al. [50] show how to maximize the likelihood for $h_0(y)$, α_1, β_1, α_2, β_2, α_3, and β_3 using the EM algorithm. Once the maximum likelihood estimates for these parameters are obtained, the outcome densities (masses) of compliers under control $(h_0(y))$ and treatment $(h_2(y))$ are estimated by $\hat{h}_0(y_i)$ and $\hat{h}_0(y_i) \exp(\hat{\alpha}_2 + \hat{\beta}_2 y_i)$, respectively, and their corresponding cdfs $H_0(y)$ and $H_2(y)$ are estimated by $\hat{H}_0(y) = \sum_i \hat{h}_0(y_i) I(y_i \leq y)$ and $\hat{H}_2(y) = \sum_i \hat{h}_0(y_i) \exp(\hat{\alpha}_2 + \hat{\beta}_2 y_i) I(y_i \leq y)$, respectively. To examine the causal effect of actually receiving treatment on the outcome distribution for compliers, the equality of $h_0(y)$ and $h_2(y)$ can be tested by testing $H_0 : \alpha_2 = \beta_2 = 0$ by the semiparametric empirical likelihood ratio statistic that is described in detail in Reference 50.

In addition to investigating the distributional treatment effect, some function of the outcome distributions, $g(\eta)$, where g is a real valued function with nonzero first partial derivatives, can also be estimated. For example, under the semiparametric setting in Reference 50, the CACE can be estimated by using

$$\hat{CACE}^{SEM} = \sum_{i=1}^{n} y_i \hat{h}_0(y_i) \{ \exp(\hat{\alpha}_2 + \hat{\beta}_2 y_i) - 1 \}.$$

One can also compare the ι−quantiles of outcome distributions of compliers with and without treatment (marginal distributions of Y^1 and Y^0):

$$\hat{CQCE}^{SEM} = \hat{H}_2^{-1}(\iota) - \hat{H}_0^{-1}(\iota).$$

When $\iota = 0.5$, it is the difference of the medians for the compliers under treatment and control.

The goodness of fit of the density ratio model can be tested by comparing estimated outcome cdfs based on the density ratio model to the empirical distribution function estimates [114]:

$$\Delta_{zd} = \sup_{-\infty < y < \infty} \sqrt{n} |\hat{F}_{zt}(y) - \tilde{F}_{zt}(y)|, \quad z, d = 0, 1. \tag{2.24}$$

The *p*-value of the goodness-of-fit test can be estimated by a bootstrap *p*-value

$$\hat{P}_{zt}^B = \hat{P}_{zt}^B(\Delta_{zt}^* \geq \Delta_{zt}^{obs}), \tag{2.25}$$

where Δ_{zt}^{obs} is obtained from the actually observed data and Δ_{zt}^* is calculated from B bootstrap samples generated under the null hypothesis: the density ratio model (2.23) is true.

2.9 Study Design IV and Multiple IVs

2.9.1 Study Design IV: Near–Far Matching

Study design focuses attention on the data to be analyzed. The manner in which the data are structured largely determines the statistical procedures appropriate for analysis. The separation between study design and statistical analysis is quickly illustrated by considering a uniform randomized-paired analysis. The process of matching individual units of observation into pairs based on observed, pretreatment covariates, and then randomizing one unit within each pair to treatment and the other to control—this process is study design. The researcher constructs the pairs by carefully controlling the assignments to increase efficiency by decreasing within-pair variation (by constructing matched pairs) as well as to minimize unobserved bias (by randomization). These steps increase the validity of the results and go a long way toward reassuring the audience of the reliability of the reported conclusions. Only the manner in which the data are prepared has thus far been described. This is the design of the study.

Once the experiment is run and the data are recorded then the results need to be analyzed. Given the study design, most analysts would select a paired *t*-test, perhaps using Student's *t*. But that is not the only choice; one could justifiably use a permutation test or, with some additional assumptions, a model-based approach (e.g., regression) to adjust for potential covariate imbalances that routinely occur in finite sample randomizations. This is the statistical inference phase of the study. Statistical inference is distinct from, though predicated on and preceded by, the study design. The more well understood the study design, the more credibility the statistical inference is likely to have. This is true in experimentation and even truer in the observational setting.

In observational settings, data are often plentiful, especially compared to the experimental setting. The trouble with observational data is that estimates of treatment effects tend to be plagued by confounding by both observed and unobserved covariates. The goal of study design in the observational setting can be thought of as finding the subset of the data that will produce the best study given the limitations of the data (usually in the sense of internal validity).

In the literature, study design is also sometimes referred to as "preprocessing" [115]. For those new to study design, perhaps the most unintuitive insight is that the analysis can actually be improved by removing observations from consideration before performing the statistical inference. This is unintuitive because, loosely speaking, it seems like the study with the most observations is the most informative. This is a recognized problem in the observational literature. For example, it has become standard practice to use propensity scores to limit the analysis to only the observation units that have corresponding propensity score values in either the treated or control group, removing from inference the observational units with extreme values close to 1 or 0 [7,116].

Analogously for IVs, it is known that if the goal is to have greater power and results that are more robust to small violations of the IV assumptions, then a smaller data set with a stronger instrument is preferable to a larger data set with a weaker instrument [79]. The trade-off between bigger-but-weaker and smaller-but-stronger was thought to be informative, but not useful once the analyst has committed to using a particular data set. Contrary to this belief, Baiocchi et al. [13] demonstrated that even within a particular data set, the analyst may use near–far matching to go from a weaker-but-bigger study to a more robust smaller-but-stronger study.

There are two objectives in near–far matching. As in a randomized-controlled trial (RCT) with a matched pair design, one objective in near–far matching is to create matched pairs where the covariates are similar within a pair. Creating pairs with very similar covariate values (i.e., pairs that are near each other in covariate space) is used to improve efficiency. The other objective in near–far matching is to separate observations' instrument values within a matched pair. In the neonatal intensive care example outlined in the introduction, within a matched pair, one wants one mother to be highly encouraged to deliver at a high-level NICU and the other to be highly encouraged to deliver at a low-level NICU. This is similar to the matched pair design when there is the potential for noncompliance. If the level of encouragement can be varied, then it is preferential to have two mothers who are highly dissimilar (far) in their levels of randomly assigned encouragement because it is then more likely that within the pair, one mother will comply with the encouragement and take the treatment and the other will comply with the lack of encouragement and take the control. As outlined in Reference 13, algorithms exist that will construct pairs that maximize both of these objectives at the same time.

In most real-world examples there will be a trade-off between the "near" and the "far" part of the matching. The technical aspects of this trade-off, and how to construct such pairs, are context specific—for guidance, see References 13 and 117. The intuition is that as the analyst forces separation in the instrument values between pairs of patients, it becomes more difficult to find patients with quite dissimilar instrument values but very similar covariates. The Baiocchi et al. paper [13] outlines both theoretical arguments as well as practical reasons for designing studies with greater separation in the instrument.

It should be noted that pair matching is being referred to, but all of these arguments hold for larger block designs. Near–far matching would work with k:1 matching and other more exotic designs. The primary difference would be the optimization algorithm used to construct the sets.

This process is similar to propensity score matching, and other matching techniques in general. The goal is to prepare the data, by finding the parts of the data set that lend themselves to causal inference, so as to improve the reliability of the statistical analysis to be performed. Note that, just as with propensity score matching, the analyst may decide to use whichever appropriate statistical method of analysis post matching. That is, after performing near–far matching, the analyst may then decide to use a 2SRI model if that is appropriate for the given data set. But the selection of the statistical method must be made with justification, not out of convenience. This is why most analysts will decide to use the effect ratio (discussed in Section 2.7) after performing near–far matching as the study design leads naturally into the statistical analysis.

2.9.2 Multilevel and Continuous IVs

In some settings, the IV has multiple levels or is continuous. For example, in the neonatal intensive care example, the mother's excess travel time from the nearest high-level NICU compared to the nearest low-level NICU is continuous. Multiple levels of the IV provides us with the opportunity to identify a richer set of causal effects [118]. Suppose the IV is continuous and the following extended monotonicity assumption holds: $T_i^z \geq T_i^{z'}$ for all $z_i \geq z'_i$, that is, a higher level of the IV always leads to at least as high a level of the treatment. The limit of the treatment effect for subjects who would the take treatment if the IV was equal to z but not take the treatment if the IV was a little less than z is $\lim_{\epsilon \to 0} E[Y_{1i} - Y_{0i} | T_{zi} = 1, T_{z-\epsilon,i} = 0]$; Heckman and Vytlacil [119] refer to this as the marginal treatment effect at z. Treatment effects of interest can all be expressed as a weighted average of these marginal treatment effects [119]. For example, the treatment effect estimated by dichotomizing the IV as 1 or 0 according to whether the IV is above some cutoff or the treatment effect estimated by 2SLS using the continuous IV can be expressed as a weighted average of the marginal treatment effects. The average treatment effect over the whole population can also be expressed as a weighted average of the marginal treatment effects. Identification of the average treatment effect over the whole population requires identification of all the marginal treatment effects. In order for all the marginal treatment effects to be identified using the IV (and thus the average treatment effect identified), it is required that for large values of Z, $P(T = 1|Z)$ approaches 1 and for small values of Z, $P(T = 1|Z)$ approaches 0 [119]. Reference 120 shows how to estimate marginal treatment effects and the average treatment effect when this condition is satisfied.

2.9.3 Multiple IVs

In some settings, there may be multiple IVs available. For example, Reference 35 used IV methods to estimate the effect of longer postpartum stays on newborn readmissions. Reference 35 used two IVs: (1) hour of birth and (2) method of delivery (vaginal vs. cesarean section). Hour of birth influences length of stay because it affects whether a newborn will spend an extra night in the hospital; for example, Malkin et al. [35] found that newborns born in the a.m. have longer lengths of stay than newborns born in the p.m. Method of delivery influences length of stay because mothers need more time to recuperate after a cesarean section than following a vaginal delivery, and newborns are rarely discharged before their mothers. Each IV identifies the treatment effect for a different set of compliers. If treatment effects are heterogeneous, the CACEs may differ. For example, newborns who would only stay an extra day if born in the a.m. compared to the p.m. may differ in their risk characteristics compared to newborns who would only stay an extra day if delivered by cesarean section compared to vaginal delivery, and length of stay may have a different effect on newborns with different risk characteristics.

2SLS can be used to combine the IVs—in the first stage, regress T on both Z_1 and Z_2 (as well as **X**) and then use the predicted T as usual in the second stage. Under the assumption of homogeneous treatment effects and constant variance, the 2SLS estimate is the optimal way to combine the IVs [55]. When treatment effects are heterogeneous, 2SLS estimates a weighted average of the CACE for the IVs with stronger IVs getting greater weight [42,57]. When there are two or more distinct IVs, it is useful to report the estimates from the individual IVs in addition to the combined IVs since the IVs may be estimating treatment effects for different types of people.

When there are multiple IVs and treatment effects are homogeneous, the overidentifying restrictions test can be used to test the validity of the IVs [53,121]. The overidentifying restrictions test tests whether the estimates from the different IVs are the same. When treatment effects are homogeneous, if the estimates from two different IVs converge to different limits, this would show that at least one of the IVs is invalid. There are two problems with using the overidentifying restrictions test to test the validity of IVs. First, if treatment effects are heterogeneous, then the CACEs for the two IVs may be different even though both IVs are valid; in this case, the overidentifying restrictions test would falsely indicate that at least one of the IVs is invalid. Second, even if treatment effects are homogeneous, two IVs A and B may both be biased but in the same way so that the asymptotic limit of the estimators based on IV A and B, respectively, are the same; in this case, the overidentifying restrictions test would give false assurance that the IVs are valid [78].

2.10 Multilevel and Continuously Valued Treatments

The treatment under study may take on multiple or continuous values, for example, the dose of a medication. 2SLS can still be applied. Angrist and Imbens [57] present the following formula that shows that the 2SLS estimator converges to a weighted average of the effect of one-unit changes in the treatment level. Suppose the treatment can take on levels $0, 1, \ldots, \bar{t}$ and that monotonicity holds in the sense that $T_i^{z=1} \geq T_i^{z=0}$. Assume there are no covariates. Then, the 2SLS estimator converges to

$$\frac{E(Y_i|Z_i = 1) - E(Y_i|Z_i = 0)}{E(T_i|Z_i = 1) - E(T_i|Z_i = 0)} = \sum_{t=1}^{\bar{t}} \omega_t E[Y_t - Y_{t-1}|T_1 \geq t > T_0], \quad (2.26)$$

where $\omega_t = ((P(T_1 \geq t > T_0))/(\sum_{t=1}^{\bar{t}} P(T_1 \geq t > T_0)))$. The numerator of ω_t is the proportion of compliers at point t, that is, the proportion of individuals driven by the encouraging level of the IV from a treatment intensity less than t to at least t. The ω_t's are nonnegative and sum to one. The quantity $E[Y_t - Y_{t-1}|T_1 \geq t > T_0]$ in Equation 2.26 is the causal effect of a one-unit increase in the treatment from $t - 1$ to t for compliers at point t. Equation 2.26 shows that the 2SLS estimator converges to a weighted average of the causal effects of one-unit increases in the treatment from $t - 1$ to t for compliers at point t, where the points t at which there are more compliers get greater weight. The weights ω_t can be estimated since under monotonicity and the assumption that the IV is independent of the potential treatment received, $P(T_1 \geq t > T_0) = P(T_1 \geq t) - P(T_0 \geq t) = P(T \geq t|Z = 1) - P(T \geq t|Z = 0)$. See Reference 57 for an extension of these formulas to the setting where there are covariates $\mathbf{X}$ that are controlled for.

Researchers often times dichotomize multilevel or continuous treatments. However, using IV methods with a dichotomized continuous treatment can lead to an overestimate of the treatment effect. Let β denote the average causal effect (2.26) that the 2SLS estimator for a multilevel treatment converges to. Angrist and Imbens [57] show that if this treatment is dichotomized as $B = 1$ if $T \geq l$, $B = 0$ if $T < l$ for some $1 \leq l \leq \bar{t}$, then the 2SLS estimator using the binary treatment B converges to $\phi\beta$, where

$$\phi = \frac{E(T|Z = 1) - E(T|Z = 0)}{E(B|Z = 1) - E(B|Z = 0)} = \frac{\sum_{j=1}^{\bar{t}} P(T_1 \geq j > T_0)}{P(T_1 \geq l > T_0)} \geq 1.$$

The only situation when $\phi = 1$ is when the IV has no effect other than to cause people to switch from $T = l - 1$ to $T = l$. Otherwise, when a multilevel treatment is incorrectly parameterized as binary, the resulting estimate tends to be too large relative to the average per-unit effect of the treatment. The problem with dichotomizing a multilevel treatment is that the IV has a direct effect because the encouraging level of the IV can push a person to a higher level of treatment even if B is 1 under both the nonencouraging and encouraging levels of the IV. Although dichotomizing a continuous treatment results in a biased IV estimate, the sign of the treatment effect is still consistently estimated.

If the treatment effect for compliers is linear, that is, the causal effect of a one-unit increase in the treatment from $t - 1$ to t for compliers at point t is the same for all t, then the 2SLS estimator estimates this linear treatment effect. If the treatment effect is nonlinear, then with a binary IV, it is not possible to estimate anything other than the weighted treatment effect (2.26). If the IV is continuous, then the IV can be used to form multiple IVs (e.g., Z, Z^2, Z^3) and a nonlinear treatment effect can be estimated [122]. For example, suppose $Y^{T=t} = Y^0 + \beta_1 t + \beta_2 t^2$. Then, β_1 and β_2 can be consistently estimated with a continuous IV Z by using 2SLS where $\hat{T}$ is estimated by regressing T on Z and Z^2, $\hat{T}^2$ is estimated by regressing T^2 on Z and Z^2, and β_1 and β_2 are estimated by regressing Y on $\hat{T}$ and $\hat{T}^2$. Reference 123 discusses other estimation approaches for estimating nonlinear treatment effects.

A common setting is to have a treatment with three levels that may not be strictly ordered by dose. Cheng and Small [66] consider the setting of a treatment with three levels—control (0) and two active levels A and B, where A and B are not ordered by dose and some subjects may prefer A to B and some may prefer B to A. Subjects are randomly assigned to one of the three arms 0, A, and B, and then could either take the assigned treatment or not take it and receive the control (for the control arm, all subjects receive the control 0). The effect of treatment A versus control for subjects who would take treatment A if offered (i.e., compliers with treatment A) is identified by analyzing only subjects who were either assigned to the control arm or the treatment A arm. But for this setting, Reference 66 showed that the effect of treatment A for subjects who would take treatment A if assigned to it but not treatment B and the effect of treatment A for subjects who would take treatments A or B if assigned to A or B, respectively, is not point identified. However, the data provide information that can be used to narrow bounds on these treatment effects. These treatment effects are of interest for individuals making decisions about which treatment to take, for example, for a very compliant subject who knows she would take either treatment *A* or *B* if offered, she would like to know whether treatment *A* or *B* is better among very compliant subjects like herself; the treatment effects are also of interest for clinicians deciding which treatment to offer first and for health policymakers anticipating what would happen were the treatment(s) to be introduced into general practice in a setting in which compliance patterns are expected to differ from those of the trial [66].

2.11 IV Methods for Mediation Analysis

If a treatment has some effect, we would like to understand how the treatment works. Mediation analysis seeks to uncover the pathways through which a treatment works. These pathways can include measured intermediate biological, behavioral/social factors, or unmeasured intermediate variables. Mediation analysis helps us to understand the working mechanism of an intervention and consequently allows us to tailor the intervention for future research and applications in specific populations. For example, the PROSPECT study [96] was a randomized trial that evaluated an intervention for improving the treatment of depression in the elderly in primary care practices. The intervention consisted of having a depression specialist (typically a master's level clinician) closely collaborate with the depressed patient and the patient's primary care physician to facilitate patient and clinician adherence to a treatment algorithm and provide education, support, and ongoing assessment to the patient. The intervention significantly reduced depression (as measured by the Hamilton test) 4 months after baseline. Researchers of this study are interested in to what extent the effect of the intervention can be explained by its increasing use of prescriptive antidepressant medication as compared to other factors. Understanding the mechanism by which a treatment achieves its effects can help researchers and policymakers design more effective treatments [124]. For example, if the PROSPECT study intervention achieves its effects primarily through increasing use of antidepressants, then a more cost-effective intervention might be designed that has the depression specialist focus her time only on increasing use of antidepressants.

A widely used approach to mediation analysis [125,126], called the Baron–Kenny approach, makes a strong *sequential ignorability* assumption that, in addition to the intervention being randomly assigned conditional on measured confounding variables, the mediating variable (e.g., antidepressant use) is also effectively randomly assigned given the intervention and the measured confounding variables (i.e., the mediating variable is sequentially ignorable, meaning that there are no unmeasured confounders of the mediating variable–outcome relationship) [127]. In the PROSPECT study, potential unmeasured confounders of the mediating variable (antidepressant use)–outcome (depression) relationship include medical comorbidities during the follow-up period, which deter elderly depressed patients from taking antidepressant medications because of so many other medications that are necessitated by their medical comorbidities and also predispose patients to more depression [127]. To address such unmeasured confounding, Ten Have et al. [127] developed an IV approach to mediation analysis in which baseline covariate(s) $\mathbf{B}$ interacted with the treatment assignment T are assumed to be a valid IV(s). In order for the baseline covariates $\mathbf{B}$ interacted with the treatment assignment T to be valid IVs, the following assumptions must hold:

- (IV-MA-A1). The treatment assignment T must be independent of unmeasured confounders given the baseline covariates $\mathbf{B}$.
- (IV-MA-A2). The baseline covariates $\mathbf{B}$ must interact with the treatment assignment T in predicting the mediating variable M in a linear model for M.
- (IV-MA-A3). The baseline covariates $\mathbf{B}$ cannot modify the effect of the mediating variable M or the direct effect of the treatment T.

Let Y_{tm} be the potential outcome if the treatment is set to t and the mediating variable is set to m. Consider the following model:

$$Y_{t,m} = t\theta_T + m\theta_M + T\mathbf{B}^T\theta_{T\mathbf{B}} + M\mathbf{B}^T\theta_{M\mathbf{B}} + E(Y_{00}|\mathbf{B})$$
$$+ [Y_{00} - E(Y_{00}|\mathbf{B})]$$
$$E^*(M|T, \mathbf{B}) = \gamma_0 + T\gamma_T + \mathbf{B}^T\gamma_{\mathbf{B}} + T\mathbf{B}^T\gamma_{T\mathbf{B}}, \tag{2.27}$$

where $E^*(M|\mathbf{A}) = \arg\min_\lambda E(M - \lambda^T\mathbf{A})^2$ denotes the best linear predictor of M given $\mathbf{A}$. In model (2.27), for subjects with covariates $\mathbf{B}$, the direct effect of the treatment T is $\theta_T + \mathbf{B}^T\theta_{T\mathbf{B}}$ and the effect of the mediating variable M is $\theta_M + \mathbf{B}^T\theta_{M\mathbf{B}}$. In the context of Equation 2.27, assumption (IV-MA-A1) is that T is independent of $Y_{00} - E(Y_{00}|\mathbf{B})$; assumption (IV-MA-A2) is that $\gamma_{T\mathbf{B}} \neq 0$; and assumption (IV-MA-A3) is that $\theta_{T\mathbf{B}} = 0$ and $\theta_{M\mathbf{B}} = 0$.

Under assumptions (IV-MA-A1), (IV-MA-A2), and (IV-MA-A3), [127] used a g-estimation approach to estimate the direct effect of the treatment, $\theta_T + \mathbf{B}^T\theta_{T\mathbf{B}}$, and the effect of the mediating variable, $\theta_M + \mathbf{B}^T\theta_{M\mathbf{B}}$. References 80 and 128–130 show that 2SLS can also be used. The first stage is to regress the mediating variable M on the treatment T, baseline covariates $\mathbf{B}$, and the interaction between the baseline covariates and treatment, $T\mathbf{B}$. The second stage is to regress the outcome Y on the treatment, predicted value of the mediating variable from the first stage, and the baseline covariates $\mathbf{B}$. The illustrative code is provided in Section 2.12. Reference 130 presents a method of sensitivity analysis for violations of assumption (IV-MA-A3).

2.12 Software

The software for implementing IV analyses is available in R, SAS, and Stata. Here, we illustrate analyzing the NICU study using the ivpack package, freely downloadable from CRAN, in the freely available software R.

```
library(ivpack)
# y is the nx1 vector of the outcome (mortality)
# t is the nx1 vector of the treatment (1 if high level NICU,
  0 if low level NICU)
# xmat is the nxp matrix of observed covariates (e.g.,
  birthweight, gestational age, etc.)
# z is the IV
# (1 if excess travel time <=10 minutes, 0 if excess travel
  time greater than 10 minutes)

# Fit first stage model
first.stage.model=lm(t~ z+xmat)
# Calculate Partial F statistic for testing whether instrument
  has an effect
# in the first stage model
first.stage.model.without.z=lm(t~ xmat)
anova(first.stage.model.without.z,first.stage.model)
Analysis of Variance Table

Model 1: t ~ xmat
Model 2: t ~ z + xmat
 Res.Df  RSS Df Sum of Sq   F   Pr(>F)
1 192017 40737
2 192016 34964 1   5772.6 31702 < 2.2e-16 ***
# The partial F statistic is 31702, which is much greater
  than 10,
# so that IV is strong enough for two stage least squares
  inference to be reliable.

# Estimate proportion of compliers and proportion of compliers
  that are low birth weight
# E(T|Z,X) using a logistic regression model with interaction
  between Z and X z.times.xmat=z*xmat
treat.reg.est=glm(t~z+xmat+z.times.xmat,family=binomial)
# Matrix of covariates when z is set to 1
z1mat=cbind(rep(1,length(y)),rep(1,length(y)),xmat,xmat);
ev.tz1=expit(z1mat%*%matrix(coef(treat.reg.est),ncol=1));
# Matrix of covariates when z is set to 0
```

```
z0mat=cbind(rep(1,length(y)),rep(0,length(y)),xmat,
 matrix(rep(0,ncol(xmat)*length(y)),ncol=ncol(xmat)))
ev.tz0=expit(z0mat%*%matrix(coef(treat.reg.est),ncol=1))
# Proportion of compliers
prop.compliers=mean(ev.tz1-ev.tz0)
# Proportion of compliers given low birth weight
prop.compliers.given.low.birth.weight=
 mean(ev.tz1[low.birth.weight==1]-ev.tz0[low.birth.weight==1])
# Proportion with low birth weight among compliers
prop.low.birth.weight.in.compliers=
 (prop.compliers.given.low.birth.weight/prop.compliers)*mean
 (low.birth.weight)

# Bias ratio for low birth weight, see Table 6
bias.ratio.low.birth.weight=
ab,s(((mean(low.birth.weight[z==1])-mean(low.birth.weight
[z==0]))/(mean(t[z==1])-mean(dtz==0))))/
(mean(low.birth.weight[t==1])-mean(low.birth.weight[t==0]))));
bias.ratio.low.birth.weight
[1] 0.5157605

# Two stage least squares analysis
ivmodel=ivreg(y~ t+xmat|z+xmat)
# This summary gives the non-robust standard errors
summary(ivmodel)
Coefficients:
                Estimate  Std. Error t value Pr(>|t|)
(Intercept)      5.183e-01 1.019e-02 50.845 < 2e-16 ***
t               -5.888e-03 1.644e-03 -3.581 0.000342 ***
xmatbthwght      -6.298e-06 6.698e-07 -9.403 < 2e-16 ***
...
# We estimate that the effect of going to a high level NICU
  is to
# reduce the mortality rate for compliers by .005888 or 5.9
  babies
# per 1000 deliveries

# Standard errors that are robust for heteroskedasticity but
  not clustering robust.se(ivmodel)

# Huber-White standard errors that account for clustering
  due to hospital
# and are also robust to heteroskedasticity
# hospid is an identifier of the hospital the baby was
  delivered at
```

```
cluster.robust.se(ivmodel,hospid)
t test of coefficients:

                Estimate  Std. Error t value Pr(>|t|)
(Intercept)      5.1830e-01 2.7084e-02 19.1369 < 2.2e-16 ***
t               -5.8879e-03 1.9021e-03 -3.0955 0.0019653 **
xmatbthwght      -6.2983e-06 1.3268e-06 -4.7471 2.065e-06 ***
...


# Sensitivity Analysis for IV being associated with unmeasured
  confounders
# Second row of Table 10
delta=-1/1000
eta=.5;
adjusted.y=y-delta*eta*z;
sens.est=ivreg(adjusted.y~ t+xmat|z+xmat)
cluster.robust.se(sens.est,hospid)

t test of coefficients:
                Estimate  Std. Error t value Pr(>|t|)
(Intercept)      5.1780e-01 2.6995e-02 19.1818 < 2.2e-16 ***
t               -4.6396e-03 1.8678e-03 -2.4840 0.0129941 *
...


# Sensitivity Analysis for violation of exclusion restriction
lambda=.001 # having to travel far to a high level NICU
increases the
# death rate by 1 per 1000 deliveries
adjusted.y=y-lambda*(1-z)*t
sens.est=ivreg(adjusted.y~ t+xmat|z+xmat)
cluster.robust.se(sens.est,hospid)

t test of coefficients:
                Estimate  Std. Error t value Pr(>|t|)
(Intercept)      5.1733e-01 2.6922e-02 19.2159 < 2.2e-16 ***
d               -5.0945e-03 1.8550e-03 -2.7464 0.0060260 **
...
```

We will now illustrate using IVs in mediation analysis (Section 2.11). We use the PROSPECT study data set provided by Reference 127 under the Article Information link at the *Biometrics* website http://www.tibs.org/biometrics. The outcome (hamd) is the patient's Hamilton score (a measure of depression, with a higher score indicating more depression) 4 months after baseline. The treatment (interven) is having a depression specialist (typically a master's level clinician) closely collaborate with the depressed patient and the patient's primary care physician to facilitate patient and clinician adherence to a treatment algorithm and provide education, support, and ongoing assessment to the patient; interven=1 if the patient received the treatment, 0 if the patient received usual care. The mediating variable (medication) is an indicator for whether the subject used antidepressants during the period from baseline to 4 months after baseline. The baseline covariates are (i) an indicator of whether the subjects had used antidepressants in the past (scr01) and (ii) a baseline measure of antidepressant use (cad1) that ranges from 0 (no baseline use of antidepressants) to 4 (highest level of baseline use of antidepressants).

```
library(AER)
# scr01.interven = scr01*interven, cad1.interven=cad1*interven
model=ivreg(hamd~interven+medication+scr01+cad1|interven+scr01
+cad1+scr01.interven+cad1.interven)summary(model)

Call:
ivreg(formula = hamd ~ interven + medication + scr01 + cad1 |
   interven + scr01 + cad1 + scr01.interven + cad1.interven)

Residuals:
  Min    1Q Median    3Q    Max
-13.828 -5.944 -1.216  5.469 30.340

Coefficients:
       Estimate Std. Error t value Pr(>|t|)
(Intercept) 13.5308    1.0941 12.367  <2e-16 ***
interven    -0.9380    1.5184 -0.618   0.5372
medication  -2.8703    3.0735 -0.934   0.3511
scr01        1.3598    0.8174  1.664   0.0973 .
cad1         0.4655    0.4971  0.937   0.3498
---
Signif. codes: 0 *** 0.001 ** 0.01 * 0.05 . 0.1  1

Residual standard error: 7.911 on 292 degrees of freedom
Multiple R-Squared: 0.0219,    Adjusted R-squared: 0.008498
Wald test: 2.251 on 4 and 292 DF, p-value: 0.06372

# The treatment is estimated to have a direct effect of
   reducing the Hamilton score by 0.94 points
# and the mediating variable, antidepressant use, is estimated
   to be to reduce
# the Hamilton score by 2.87 points.
```

Acknowledgments

Jing Cheng and Dylan Small were supported by grant RC4MH092722 from the National Institute of Mental Health. Jing Cheng was also supported by grant NIH/NIDCR U54DE019285. The authors thank Scott Lorch for the use of the data from the NICU study.

References

1. S. Lorch, M. Baiocchi, C. Ahlberg, and D. Small, The differential impact of delivery hospital on the outcomes of premature infants, *Pediatrics*, 130, 2012, pp. 270–278.
2. P. Holland, Causal inference, path analysis, and recursive structural equations models, *Sociological Methodology*, 18, 1988, pp. 449–484.
3. J. Neyman, On the application of probability theory to agricultural experiments, *Statistical Science*, 5, 1990, pp. 463–480.
4. D. Rubin, Estimating causal effects of treatments in randomized and non-randomized studies, *Journal of Educational Psychology*, 66, 1974, pp. 688–701.
5. M. Hernán and J. Robins, *Causal Inference*, Chapman & Hall/CRC Press, Boca Raton, forthcoming.
6. J. Pearl, *Causality*, Cambridge University Press, New York, 2009.
7. P. Rosenbaum, *Observational Studies*, Springer Verlag, New York, 2002.
8. D. Cox, *Planning of Experiments*, Wiley, New York, 1958.
9. R. Fisher, *Design of Experiments*, Oliver and Boyd, Edinburgh, 1949.
10. P. Rosenbaum and D. Rubin, The central role of the propensity score in observational studies for causal effects, *Biometrika*, 70, 1983, pp. 41–55.
11. J. Heckman and R. Robb, Alternative methods for evaluating the impacts of interventions: An overview, *Journal of Econometrics*, 30, 1985, pp. 239–267.
12. J. Angrist, G. Imbens, and D. Rubin, Identification of causal effects using instrumental variables, *Journal of the American Statistical Association*, 91, 1996, pp. 444–455.
13. M. Baiocchi, D. Small, S. Lorch, and P. Rosenbaum, Building a stronger instrument in an observational study of perinatal care for premature infants, *Journal of the American Statistical Association*, 105, 2010, pp. 1285–1296.
14. C. Phibbs, D. Mark, H. Luft, D. Peltzman-Rennie, D. Garnick, E. Lichtenberg, and S. McPhee, Choice of hospital for delivery: A comparison of high-risk and low-risk women, *Health Services Research*, 28, 1993, p. 201.
15. T. Permutt and J. Hebel, Simultaneous-equation estimation in a clinical trial of the effect of smoking on birth weight, *Biometrics*, 45, 1989, pp. 619–622.
16. M. Sexton and J. Hebel, A clinical trial of change in maternal smoking and its effect on birth weight, *Journal of the American Medical Association*, 251, 1984, pp. 911–915.
17. M. McClellan, B. McNeil, and J. Newhouse, Does more intensive treatment of acute myocardial infarction in the elderly reduce mortality? Analysis using

instrumental variables, *Journal of the American Medical Association*, 272, 1994, p. 859.

18. M. Brookhart, P. Wang, D. Solomon, and S. Schneeweiss, Evaluating short-term drug effects using a physician-specific prescribing preference as an instrumental variable, *Epidemiology*, 17, 2006, pp. 268–275.

19. S. Johnston, Combining ecological and individual variables to reduce confounding by indication: Case study subarachnoid hemorrhage treatment, *Journal of Clinical Epidemiology*, 53, 2000, pp. 1236–1241.

20. J. Brooks, E. Chrischilles, S. Scott, and S. Chen-Hardee, Was breast conserving surgery underutilized for early stage breast cancer? Instrumental variables evidence for stage II patients from Iowa, *Health Services Research*, 38, 2004, pp. 1385–1402.

21. K. Shetty, W. Vogt, and J. Bhattacharya, Hormone replacement therapy and cardiovascular health in the United States, *Medical Care*, 47, 2009, pp. 600–606.

22. B. Voight, G. Peloso, M. Orho-Melander, R. Frikke-Schmidt, M. Barbalic, M. Jensen, G. Hindy, H. Hólm, E. Ding, T. Johnson et al., Plasma HDL cholesterol and risk of myocardial infarction: A Mendelian randomisation study, *Lancet*, 380, 2012, pp. 572–580.

23. V. Ho, B. Hamilton, and L. Roos, Multiple approaches to assessing the effects of delays for hip fracture patients in the United States and Canada, *Health Services Research*, 34, 2000, pp. 1499–1518.

24. J. Cole, H. Norman, L. Weatherby, and A. Walker, Drug copayment and adherence in chronic heart failure: Effect on costs and outcomes, *Pharmacotherapy*, 26, 2006, pp. 1157–1164.

25. M. Brookhart and S. Schneeweiss, Preference-based instrumental variable methods for the estimation of treatment effects: Assessing validity and interpreting results, *The International Journal of Biostatistics*, 3, 2007, p. 14.

26. T. Newman, E. Vittinghoff, and C. McCulloch, Efficacy of phototherapy for newborns with hyperbilirubinemia: A cautionary example of an instrumental variable analysis, *Medical Decision Making*, 32, 2012, pp. 83–92.

27. E. Korn and S. Baumrind, Clinician preferences and the estimation of causal treatment differences, *Statistical Science*, 13, 1998, pp. 209–235.

28. M. Brookhart, J. Rassen, and S. Schneeweiss, Instrumental variable methods in comparative safety and effectiveness research, *Pharmacoepidemiology and Drug Safety*, 19, 2010, pp. 537–554.

29. G. Wehby, A. Jugessur, L. Moreno, J. Murray, A. Wilcox, and R. Lie, Genetic instrumental variable studies of the impacts of risk behaviors: An application to maternal smoking and orofacial clefts, *Health Services and Outcomes Research Methodology*, 11, 2011, pp. 54–78.

30. V. Didelez and N. Sheehan, Mendelian randomization as an instrumental variable approach to causal inference, *Statistical Methods in Medical Research*, 16, 2007, pp. 309–330.

31. D. Lawlor, R. Harbord, J. Sterne, N. Timpson, and G. Smith, Mendelian randomization: Using genes as instruments for making causal inferences in epidemiology, *Statistics in Medicine*, 27, 2008, pp. 1133–1163.

32. H. Goedde, D. Agarwal, G. Fritze, D. Meier-Tackmann, S. Singh, G. Beckmann, K. Bhatia, L. Chen, B. Fang, and R. Lisker, Distribution of ADH2 and ALDH2 genotypes in different populations, *Human Genetics*, 88, 1992, pp. 344–346.

33. P. Sham, *Statistics in Human Genetics*, Arnold, London, 1998.

34. N. Goyal, J. Zubizarreta, D. Small, and S. Lorch, Length of stay and readmission among late preterm infants: An instrumental variable approach, *Hospital Pediatrics*, 3, 2013, 7–15.

35. J. Malkin, M. Broder, and E. Keeler, Do longer postpartum stays reduce newborn readmissions? Analysis using instrumental variables, *Health Services Research*, 35, 2000, pp. 1071–1091.

36. D. Rubin, Formal modes of statistical inference for causal effects, *Journal of Statistical Planning and Inference*, 25, 1990, pp. 279–292.

37. J. Robins and S. Greenland, A comment on Angrist, Imbens and Rubin: Identification of causal effects using instrumental variables, *Journal of the American Statistical Association*, 91, 1996, pp. 456–458.

38. M. Hudgens and M. Halloran, Towards causal inference with interference, *Journal of the American Statistical Association*, 103, 2008, pp. 832–842.

39. M. Sobel, What do randomized studies of housing mobility demonstrate? Causal inference in the face of interference, *Journal of the American Statistical Association*, 101, 2006, pp. 1398–1407.

40. E. Vytlacil, Independence, monotonicity, and latent index models: An equivalence result, *Econometrica*, 70, 2002, pp. 331–341.

41. J. Durbin, Errors in variables, *Revue de l'institut International de Statistique*, 22, 1954, pp. 23–32.

42. G. Imbens and J. Angrist, Identification and estimation of local average treatment effects, *Econometrica*, 62, 1994, pp. 467–475.

43. J. Angrist and A. Krueger, The effect of age at school entry on educational attainment: An application of instrumental variables with moments from two samples, *Journal of the American Statistical Association*, 87, 1992, pp. 328–336.

44. A. Inoue and G. Solon, Two-sample instrumental variables estimators, *The Review of Economics and Statistics*, 92, 2010, pp. 557–561.

45. N. Kaushal, Do food stamps cause obesity? Evidence from immigrant experience, *Journal of Health Economics*, 26, 2007, pp. 968–991.

46. G. Imbens and D. Rubin, Bayesian inference for causal effects in randomized experiments with noncompliance, *The Annals of Statistics*, 25, 1997, pp. 305–327.

47. G. Imbens and D. Rubin, Estimating outcome distributions for compliers in instrumental variables models, *The Review of Economic Studies*, 64, 1997, pp. 555–574.

48. J. Cheng, D. Small, Z. Tan, and T. Ten Have, Efficient nonparametric estimation of causal effects in randomized trials with noncompliance, *Biometrika*, 96, 2009, pp. 19–36.

49. A. Owen, *Empirical Likeliood*, Chapman & Hall/CRC Press, Boca Raton, 2002.

50. J. Cheng, J. Qin, and B. Zhang, Semiparametric estimation and inference for distributional and general treatment effects, *Journal of the Royal Statistical Society: Series B (Statistical Methodology)*, 71, 2009, pp. 881–904.

51. S. Lorch, C. Kroelinger, C. Ahlberg, and W. Barfield, Factors that mediate racial/ethnic disparities in us fetal death rates, *American Journal of Public Health*, 102, 2012, pp. 1902–1910.

52. J. Angrist and J.-S. Pischke, *Mostly Harmless Econometrics: An Empiricist's Companion*, Princeton University Press, Princeton, 2009.

53. R. Davidson and J. MacKinnon, *Estimation and Inference in Econometrics*, Oxford University Press, New York, 1993.

54. D. Freedman, *Statistical Models: Theory and Practice*, Cambridge University Press, Cambridge, 2009.
55. H. White, *Asymptotic Theory for Econometricians*, Academic Press, New York, 1984.
56. A. Abadie, Semiparametric instrumental variable estimation of treatment response models, *Journal of Econometrics*, 113, 2003, pp. 231–263.
57. J. Angrist and G. Imbens, Two-stage least squares estimation of average causal effects in models with variable treatment intensity, *Journal of the American Statistical Association*, 90, 1995, pp. 430–442.
58. K. Hirano, G. Imbens, D. Rubin, and X. Zhou, Assessing the effect of an influenza vaccine in an encouragement design, *Biostatistics*, 1, 2000, pp. 69–88.
59. R. Little and L. Yau, Statistical techniques for analyzing data from prevention trials: Treatment of no-shows using rubins causal model, *Psychological Methods*, 3, 1998, pp. 147–159.
60. R. Okui, D. Small, Z. Tan, and J. Robins, Doubly robust instrumental variables regression, *Statistica Sinica*, 22, 2012, pp. 173–205.
61. A. O'Malley, R. Frank, and S. Normand, Estimating cost-offsets of new medications: Use of new antipsychotics and mental health costs for schizophrenia, *Statistics in Medicine*, 30, 2011, pp. 1971–1988.
62. Z. Tan, Regression and weighting methods for causal inference using instrumental variables, *Journal of the American Statistical Association*, 101, 2006, pp. 1607–1618.
63. H. White, Instrumental variables regression with independent observations, *Econometrica*, 50, 1982, pp. 483–499.
64. A. Basu and K. Chan, Can we make smart choices between OLS and contaminated IV methods? *Health Economics*, 23, 2014, pp. 462–472.
65. A. Balke and J. Pearl, Bounds on treatment effects for studies with imperfect compliance, *Journal of the American Statistical Association*, 92, 1997, pp. 1171–1176.
66. J. Cheng and D. Small, Bounds on causal effects in three-arm trials with noncompliance, *Journal of the Royal Statistical Society, Series B*, 68, 2006, pp. 815–836.
67. J. Bhattacharya, A. Shaikh, and E. Vytlacil, Treatment effect bounds under monotonicity assumptions: An application to Swan-Ganz catheterization, *American Economic Review*, 98, 2008, pp. 351–356.
68. Z. Siddique, Partially identified treatment effects under imperfect compliance: The case of domestic violence, *Journal of the American Statistical Association*, 108, 2013, pp. 504–513.
69. J. Kitcheman, C. Adams, A. Prevaiz, I. Kader, D. Mohandas, and G. Brookes, Does an encouraging letter encourage attendance at psychiatric outpatient clinics? The Leeds prompts randomized study, *Psychological Medicine*, 38, 2008, pp. 717–723.
70. M. Joffe, Principal stratification and attribution prohibition: Good ideas taken too far, *International Journal of Biostatistics*, 7(1), 2011, pp. 1–22.
71. M. Hernán and J. Robins, Instruments for causal inference: An epidemiologist's dream? *Epidemiology*, 17, 2006, p. 360.
72. K. Demissie, G. Rhoads, C. Ananth, G. Alexander, M. Kramer, M. Kogan, and K. Joseph, Trends in preterm birth and neonatal mortality among blacks and whites in the United States from 1989 to 1997, *American Journal of Epidemiology*, 154, 2001, pp. 307–315.

73. H. Kang, B. Kreuels, O. Adjei, J. May, and D. Small, The causal effect of malaria on stunting: A Mendelian randomization and matching approach, *International Journal of Epidemiology*, 42, 2013, pp. 1390–1398.

74. M. Aidoo, D. Terlouw, M. Kolczak, P. McElroy, F. ter Kuile, S. Kariuki, B. Nahlen, A. Lal, and V. Udhayakumar, Protective effects of the sickle cell gene against malaria morbidity and mortality, *Lancet*, 359, 2002, pp. 1311–1312.

75. M. Kramer, Y. Rooks, and H. Pearson, Growth and development in children with sickle-cell trait, *New England Journal of Medicine*, 299, 1978, pp. 686–689.

76. N. Rehan, Growth status of children with and without sickle cell trait, *Clinical Pediatrics*, 20, 1981, pp. 705–709.

77. J. Angrist and A. Krueger, Does compulsory school attendance affect schooling and earnings? *Quarterly Journal of Economics*, 106, 1991, pp. 979–1014.

78. D. Small, Sensitivity analysis for instrumental variables regression with overidentifying restrictions, *Journal of the American Statistical Association*, 102, 2007, pp. 1049–1058.

79. D. Small and P. Rosenbaum, War and wages: The strength of instrumental variables and their sensitivity to unobserved biases, *Journal of the American Statistical Association*, 103, 2008, pp. 924–933.

80. M. Joffe, D. Small, S. Brunelli, T. Ten Have, and H. Feldman, Extended instrumental variables estimation for overall effects, *International Journal of Biostatistics*, 4, 2008, Article number 4.

81. J. Bound, D. Jaeger, and R. Baker, Problems with instrumental variables estimation when the correlation between the instruments and the endogenous explanatory variables is weak, *Journal of the American Statistical Association*, 90, 1995, pp. 443–450.

82. J. Shea, Instrument relevance in multivariate linear models: A simple measure, *Review of Economics and Statistics*, 79, 1997, pp. 348–352.

83. J. Stock, J. Wright, and M. Yogo, A survey of weak instruments and weak identification in generalized method of moments, *Journal of Business and Economic Statistics*, 20, 2002, pp. 518–529.

84. G. Imbens and P. Rosenbaum, Robust, accurate confidence intervals with weak instruments: Quarter of birth and education, *Journal of the Royal Statistical Society, Series A*, 168, 2005, pp. 109–126.

85. M. Moreira, A conditional likelihood ratio test for structural models, *Econometrica*, 71, 1990, pp. 463–480.

86. J. Angrist, Estimation of limited dependent variable models with dummy endogenous regressors, *Journal of Business and Economic Statistics*, 19, 2001, pp. 2–28.

87. P. Clarke and F. Windmeijer, Instrumental variable estimators for binary outcomes, *Journal of the American Statistical Association*, 107, 2012, pp. 1638–1652.

88. S. Vansteelandt, J. Bowden, M. Babnezhad, and E. Goetghebeur, On instrumental variables estimation of causal odds ratios, *Statisitcal Science*, 26, 2011, pp. 403–422.

89. J. Wooldridge, On two stage least squares estimation of the average treatment effect in a random coefficient model, *Economics Letters*, 56, 1997, pp. 129–133.

90. J. Terza, A. Basu, and P. Rathouz, Two-stage residual inclusion estimation: Addressing endogeneity in health econometric modeling, *Health Economics*, 27, 2008, pp. 527–543.

91. B. Cai, S. Hennessy, J. Flory, D. Sha, T. Ten Have and D. Small, Simulation study of instrumental variable approaches with an application to a study of the antidiabetic effect of bezafibrate, *Pharmacoepidemiology and Drug Safety*, 21, 2012, pp. 114–120.

92. B. Cai, D. Small, and T. Ten Have, Two-stage instrumental variable methods for estimating the causal odds ratio: Analysis of bias, *Statistics in Medicine*, 30, 2011, pp. 1809–1824.

93. J. Bhattacharya, D. Goldman, and D. McCaffrey, Estimating probit models with self-selected treatments, *Statistics in Medicine*, 25, 2006, pp. 389–413.

94. B. Muthen, A structural probit model with latent variables, *Journal of the American Statistical Association*, 74, 1979, pp. 807–811.

95. D. Freedman and J. Sekhon, Endogeneity in probit response models, *Political Analysis*, 18, 2010, pp. 138–150.

96. M. Bruce, T. Ten Have, C. Reynolds III, I. Katz, H. Schulberg, B. Mulsant, G. Brown, G. McAvay, J. Pearson, and G. Alexopoulos, Reducing suicidal ideation and depressive symptoms in depressed older primary care patients: A randomized trial, *Journal of the American Medical Association*, 291, 2004, pp. 1081–1091.

97. T. Ten Have, M. Elliott, M. Joffe, E. Zanutto, and C. Datto, Causal models for randomized physician encouragement trials in treating primary care depression, *Journal of the American Statistical Association*, 99, 2004, pp. 16–25.

98. J. Cheng, Estimation and inference for the causal effect of receiving treatment on a multinomial outcome, *Biometrics*, 65, 2009, pp. 96–103.

99. J. Robins and A. Tsiatis, Correcting for non-compliance in randomized trials using rank preserving structural failure time models, *Communications in Statistics, Theory and Methods*, 20, 1991, pp. 2609–2631.

100. M. Joffe, Administrative and artificial censoring in censored regression models, *Statistics in Medicine*, 20, 2001, pp. 2287–2304.

101. J. Cuzick, P. Sasieni, J. Myles, and J. Tyler, Estimating the effect of treatment in a proportional hazards model in the presence of non-compliance and contamination, *Journal of the Royal Statistical Society, Series B (Methodological)*, 69, 2007, pp. 565–588.

102. T. Loeys and E. Goetghebeur, A causal proportional hazards estimator for the effect of treatment actually received in a randomized trial with all-or-nothing compliance, *Biometrics*, 59, 2003, pp. 100–105.

103. S. Baker, Analysis of survival data from a randomized trial with all-or-none compliance: Estimating the cost-effectiveness of a cancer screening program, *Journal of the American Statistical Association*, 93, 1998, pp. 929–934.

104. H. Nie, J. Cheng, and D. Small, Inference for the effect of treatment on survival probability in randomized trials with noncompliance and administrative censoring, *Biometrics*, 67, 2011, pp. 1397–1405.

105. R. Poulson, G. Gadbury, and D. Allison, Treatment heterogeneity and individual qualitative interaction, *The American Statistician*, 66, 2012, pp. 16–24.

106. M. Hunink, P. Glasziou, J. Siegel, J. Weeks, J. Pliskin, A. Elstein, and M. Weinstein, *Decision Making in Health and Medicine: Integrating Evidence and Values*, Cambridge University Press, New York, 2001.

107. E. Karni, A theory of medical decision making under uncertainty, *Journal of Risk and Uncertainty*, 39, 2009, pp. 1–16.

108. J. Pliskin, D. Shepard, and M. Weinstein, Utility functions for life years and health status, *Operations Research*, 28, 1980, pp. 206–224.

109. J. Hogan and J. Lee, Marginal structural quantile models for longitudinal observational studies with time-varying treatment, *Statistica Sinica*, 14, 2004, pp. 927–944.

110. S. Saigal, B. Stoskopf, D. Feeny, W. Furlong, E. Burrows, P. Rosenbaum, and L. Hoult, Differences in preferences for neonatal outcomes among health care professionals, parents, and adolescents, *Journal of the American Medical Association*, 281, 1999, pp. 1991–1997.

111. B. D. Sommers, C. J. Beard, D. Dahl, A. V. D'Amico, I. P. Kaplan, J. P. Richie, and R. J. Zeckhauser. Decision analysis using individual patient preferences to determine optimal treatment for localized prostate cancer, *Cancer*, 110, 2007, pp. 2210–2217.

112. A. Abadie, Bootstrap tests for distributional treatment effects in instrumental variable models, *Journal of the American Statistical Association*, 97, 2002, pp. 284–292.

113. J. Anderson, Multivariate logistic compounds, *Biometrika*, 66, 1979, pp. 17–26.

114. J. Qin and B. Zhang, A goodness-of-fit test for logistic regression models based on case-control data, *Biometrika*, 84, 1997, pp. 609–618.

115. D. Ho, K. Imai, G. King, and E. Stuart, Matching as nonparametric preprocessing for reducing model dependence in parametric causal inference, *Political Analysis*, 15, 2007, pp. 199–236.

116. P. Rosenbaum, *Design of Observational Studies*, Springer Verlag, New York, 2009.

117. M. Baiocchi, D. Small, L. Yang, D. Polsky, and P. Groeneveld, Near/far matching: A study design approach to instrumental variables, *Health Services and Outcomes Research Methodology*, 12, 2012, pp. 237–253.

118. G. Imbens, Nonadditive models with endogenous regressors, in *Advances in Economics and Econometrics, Ninth World Congress of the Econometric Society*, R. Blundell, W. Newey, and T. Persson, eds., Cambridge University Press, New York, 2007.

119. J. Heckman and E. Vytlacil, Local instrumental variables and latent variable models for identifying and bounding treatment effects, *Proceedings of the National Academy of Sciences*, 96, 1999, pp. 4730–4734.

120. A. Basu, J. Heckman, S. Navarro-Lozano, and S. Urzua, Use of instrumental variables in the presence of heterogeneity and self-selection: An application to treatments of breast cancer patients, *Health Economics*, 16, 2007, pp. 1133–1157.

121. J. Sargan, The estimation of economic relationships using instrumental variables, *Econometrica*, 26, 1958, pp. 393–415.

122. H. Kelejian, Two-stage least squares and econometric systems linear in parameters but nonlinear in the endogenous variables, *Journal of the American Statistical Association*, 66, 1971, pp. 373–374.

123. Z. Tan, Marginal and nested structural models using instrumental variables, *Journal of the American Statistical Association*, 105, 2010, pp. 157–169.

124. H. Kraemer, G. Wilson, and C. Fairburn, Mediators and moderators of treatment effects in randomized clinical trials, *Archives of General Psychiatry*, 59, 2002, pp. 877–883.

125. R. Baron and D. Kenny, The moderator-mediator variable distinction in social psychological research: Conceptual, strategic, and statistical considerations, *Journal of Personality and Social Psychology*, 51, 1986, pp. 1173–1182.

126. D. MacKinnon, C. Lockwood, J. Hoffman, S. West, and V. Sheets, A comparison of methods to test mediation and other intervening variable effects, *Psychological Methods*, 7, 2002, pp. 83–104.
127. T. Ten Have, M. Joffe, K. Lynch, G. Brown, S. Maisto, and A. Beck, Causal mediation analyses with rank preserving models, *Biometrics*, 63, 2010, pp. 926–934.
128. J. Albert, Mediation analysis via potential outcomes models, *Statistics in Medicine*, 27, 2008, pp. 1282–1304.
129. G. Dunn and R. Bentall, Modeling treatment effect heterogeneity in randomised controlled trials of complex interventions (psychological treatments), *Statistics in Medicine*, 26, 2007, pp. 4719–4745.
130. D. Small, Mediation analysis without sequential ignorability: Using baseline covariates interacted with random assignment as instrumental variables, *Journal of Statistical Research*, 46, 2012, pp. 91–103.

3

Observational Studies Analyzed Like Randomized Trials and Vice Versa

Miguel A. Hernán and James M. Robins

CONTENTS

ABSTRACT Comparative effectiveness research is concerned with the causal effects of treatments and interventions on health outcomes. We conduct randomized trials and observational studies to estimate these comparative effects and help decision makers—patients, clinicians, payers, and policy makers—decide which interventions to implement. In fact, analyses of observational data for comparative effectiveness research can be viewed as an attempt to emulate a hypothetical randomized trial, which we will refer to as the *target trial*. This chapter uses the concept of the target trial to outline a unified framework for the analysis of longitudinal studies for comparative effectiveness research, regardless of whether they are randomized or observational.

3.1 Introduction

After briefly reviewing the concept of the target trial, we propose a taxonomy of causal effects that may be of interest when emulating a target trial, including intention to treat (ITT) and per-protocol (PP) effects. As we discuss, a valid estimation of those causal effects generally requires (i) data on time-varying prognostic factors that either predict loss to follow up or adherence to protocols of clinical interest or both, and (ii) appropriate adjustment for those time-varying factors using the so-called g-methods. It is precisely the development of g-methods that makes the concepts discussed here something more than a formal exercise: if data are available, the effects of interest can now be validly estimated. We finish with a discussion on the choice of time zero in follow-up studies and a brief conclusion. Detailed technical accounts of methods for causal inference are described in Chapters 1 and 2.

3.2 The Target Trial

Consider an open-label, parallel pragmatic randomized clinical trial to estimate the effect of estrogen plus progestin hormone therapy on the 5-year risk of breast cancer among postmenopausal women who will be randomly assigned to initiate and do not initiate hormone therapy at the start of follow-up (baseline) in a certain population, and will identify those who receive a diagnosis of breast cancer over the next 5 years. The women will be included only if, at baseline, they are within 5 years of menopause, have no history of cancer, and have not used hormone therapy for at least 2 years. The follow-up starts at the time of assignment and ends at diagnosis of breast cancer, death, loss to follow-up, or 5 years after baseline, whichever occurs earlier. During the follow-up period, some women will discontinue the hormone therapy they started at baseline, and others who were off therapy at baseline will start hormone therapy. Furthermore, some women will be lost to follow-up before the study ends.

When conducting this randomized trial is not a possibility, we may attempt to emulate it through the analysis of existing observational data. We refer to the trial as the target trial. For example, we can design an analysis of the observational data that adheres to the protocol of the target trial, except that no random assignment of treatment is possible. Rather, women in the observational analysis do or do not receive treatment according to her and her healthcare providers' decisions.

The protocol of randomized trials is usually explicit. Thus, we should be explicit about the protocol of the target trial we wish our observational analysis to emulate. To do so, we will need to specify the eligibility criteria, the start and end of follow-up, the interventions assigned at the start of follow-up, and the outcome of interest. The acronym PICO (population, intervention, comparator, and outcome) has been proposed to summarize some of these study characteristics (Richardson et al., 1995), which were briefly summarized for our target trial in the first paragraph of this section.

The protocol of a randomized trial is prespecified in a written document, but the protocol of a target trial is usually specified after the data are collected because data exploration may be needed to determine which target trials can be reasonably emulated. Note that, in principle, we may be able to emulate a target trial defined by a particular protocol by using data from an actual randomized trial that had a different protocol.

To fully characterize the protocol of the target trial, we need a detailed description of the interventions that are assigned at baseline. As a simplified example, our target trial can assign women to either the intervention "refrain from taking hormone therapy during the follow-up" or the intervention "initiate estrogen plus progestin hormone therapy at baseline and remain on it during the follow-up until a diagnosis of deep vein thrombosis, pulmonary embolism, myocardial infarction, or cancer."

Individuals outside blinded trials are usually aware of the treatment they receive. Therefore, the observational data cannot be used to emulate a target trial in which participants or their treating physicians are blinded to the intervention. This is not necessarily a limitation: when the goal of the study is to estimate realistic causal effects, it may actually be preferable to have nonblinded participants. Even with this goal, blinding of outcome ascertainment often remains a desirable feature. However, blinding of the outcome ascertainment cannot generally be emulated using observational data.

We still need to discuss an important component of the protocol of the target trial: the causal question of interest. The next section defines the causal effects that may be of interest in randomized trials, whether real or emulated.

3.3 A Taxonomy of Causal Effects in Randomized Trials

We often compare the effect estimates of randomized and observational studies. For example, observational studies and a large randomized trial reported similar estimates of the effect of hormone therapy on breast cancer; this congruence was widely interpreted as a proof that observational studies got it right. On the other hand, several observational studies and the randomized trial reported different estimates of the effect of hormone therapy on coronary heart disease than a large randomized trial; this discrepancy was interpreted by many as a proof that observational studies yielded biased estimates (Grodstein et al., 2003).

A logical implication of our direct comparisons of randomized and observational estimate is that we believe both types of studies can answer the same, or at least a closely related, causal question. What question might that be? Let us review three types of causal effects that may be of interest in a randomized trial:

1. *The effect of being assigned to the intervention, regardless of the treatment actually received.* This effect, commonly known as the ITT effect, is defined by a contrast of the outcome distribution under interventions of the sort:
   - Be assigned to treatment $A = 1$ at baseline and remain under study until the end of follow-up.
   - Be assigned to treatment $A = 0$ at baseline and remain under study until the end of follow-up.

   where, in our example, treatment $A = 1$ is hormone therapy and treatment $A = 0$ is no-hormone therapy. In some randomized trials, assignment to and initiation of the interventions occur simultaneously. That is, all individuals assigned to a given intervention start to receive the intervention, regardless of whether they continue it after baseline. In those cases, the ITT is not only the effect of assignment but also the effect of initiation of the intervention.

   The ITT effect is agnostic about any treatment decisions made after baseline, including discontinuation or initiation of the treatments of interest, use of concomitant therapies, or any other deviations from the protocol. This agnosticism implies that the magnitude of the ITT effect may heavily depend on the particular patterns of deviation from the protocol that occur during the conduct of each study. Two studies with the same protocol but conducted in different settings may have different ITT effect estimates with neither of them being biased.

2. *The effect of receiving the interventions as specified in the study protocol.* We refer to this effect as the PP effect. A first approximation to the PP effect would be defining it by a contrast of the outcome distribution under the interventions:
   - Receive treatment $A = 1$ continuously between baseline and end of follow-up.
   - Receive treatment $A = 0$ continuously between baseline and end of follow-up.

   However, sensible protocols will not mandate that treatment be continued when toxicity or contraindications arise. The PP effect is then more accurately defined by a contrast under the interventions:
   - Receive treatment $A = 1$ continuously between baseline and end of follow-up, unless otherwise clinically indicated.

- Receive treatment $A = 0$ continuously between baseline and end of follow-up, unless otherwise clinically indicated.

The above definition makes clear that the PP effect of sustained interventions generally involves the comparison of dynamic strategies ("do this, if X happens then do this other thing") rather than static strategies inherent to the ITT effect ("just assign to this treatment").

Sometimes, studies are explicitly designed to compare dynamic interventions. For example, the PP effect may be defined by a contrast of the sort:

- Receive treatment $A = 1$ continuously between baseline and the occurrence of event X, then switch to treatment $A = 0$ until the end of follow-up.
- Receive treatment $A = 0$ continuously between baseline and end of follow-up, unless otherwise clinically indicated.

where, in our example, event X might be endometrial cancer. There are many possible versions of PP effect: the control intervention (the one that starts with $A = 0$) may be dynamic too, dynamic interventions may involve several events X, Y, Z... that lead to treatment changes, treatment $A = 1$ may change to treatment $A = 2$ (e.g., another dose or type of hormone therapy), etc.

The PP effect is often the implicit target of inference. For example, often investigators question the fidelity of the interventions implemented in the study to the interventions described in the protocol, and say that there is bias (sometimes referred to as "performance bias" or "noncompliance bias"). This language indicates that the investigators are really interested in comparing the interventions implemented during the follow-up as specified in the protocol (i.e., the PP effect) and not in the effect of assignment to the interventions at baseline (i.e., the ITT effect) because noncompliance after baseline cannot possibly bias the effect of assignment at baseline.

Analogously, the PP effect cannot be biased by changes to the baseline treatment that are consistent with the protocol. For example, some study protocols intentionally let physicians make their own treatment decisions during the follow-up when toxicity or contraindications arise. Therefore, treatment decisions, including discontinuation of the originally assigned treatment or initiation of other treatments and use of concomitant therapies, because of toxicity or contraindications cannot possibly be considered a deviation from the protocol. These are not instances of noncompliance and should not be adjusted for when estimating the PP effect, for example, individuals who change treatments because of clinical reasons should not be censored (see below). Again, the PP effect is defined by a contrast of clinical strategies, not by an unrealistic, and possibly unethical, contrast of continuous treatment between baseline and the end of follow-up. PP effects are particularly relevant for comparative effectiveness research, which seeks to provide evidence for decisions in the "real world."

Ideally, to avoid confusions about what should or should not be deemed as noncompliance throughout the follow-up, the protocol would fully specify the clinical strategies of interest. Then, the PP effect would measure the comparative effectiveness of well-defined, rather than vaguely, or implicitly, defined strategies.

3. *The effect of receiving interventions other than the ones specified in the study protocol.* We continue the above discussion by now describing an example in which the interventions of interest differ from the ones in the protocol of the trial that was actually conducted.

An early randomized trial assigned human immunodeficiency virus (HIV)-infected patients to either high-dose or low-dose zidovudine (Fischl et al., 1990). The administration of prophylaxis therapy for *Pneumocystis* pneumonia, an opportunistic infection, was left to the physician's discretion. The ITT effect estimate suggested a survival benefit of low-dose zidovudine. However, individuals in the low-dose zidovudine group received significantly more prophylaxis therapy than those in the high-dose group (61% vs. 50%). By the time the trial ended, prophylaxis for *Pneumocystis* pneumonia had become the standard of care. At that point, the relevant clinical question was whether the low-dose group would still have had better survival than the high-dose group had all trial participants received prophylaxis. This question corresponds to neither the ITT effect nor the original PP effect. Rather, it is a question about the PP effect in a hypothetical trial in which individuals are randomized to both zidovudine dose and to prophylaxis, that is, a trial whose protocol is designed to estimate the direct effect of zidovudine dose that is not mediated through prophylaxis for *Pneumocystis* pneumonia.

This example illustrates how causal effects of interest that do not correspond to the original PP effect can be conceptualized as PP effects in target trials that can be emulated using the randomized trial data. Interestingly, if the interventions of interest differ from those in the actual trial, it is actually disadvantageous to have all participants in the actual trial adhere to the interventions specified in the protocol. Specifically, complete compliance implies that the trial data cannot be used to emulate a target trial with a different protocol (because of no individuals follow the protocol of the target trial in the actual data). For example, a randomized trial with full compliance in which HIV-infected individuals are assigned to different CD4 cell count thresholds at which to initiate antiretroviral therapy is of little use to emulate a trial in which individuals are assigned to either continuous treatment or no treatment, and vice versa. It is precisely the noncompliance that allows us to use the data from a given randomized trial to emulate other randomized trials that answer different, perhaps more relevant, causal questions.

3.4 A Taxonomy of Causal Effects in Observational Analyses That Emulate a Target Trial

The causal effects described above for randomized trials can be analogously defined for observational analyses that emulate a target trial.

The observational analog of the ITT effect is defined by a contrast of the outcome distribution under the hypothetical interventions:

- Initiate treatment $A = 1$ at baseline and remain under study until the end of follow-up.
- Do not initiate treatment $A = 1$ at baseline and remain under study until the end of follow-up (in head-to-head comparisons this would be "initiate another treatment $A = 2$").

This observational analog of the ITT effect in studies without randomization corresponds to the ITT effect in a target trial in which assignment to and initiation of the interventions occurs simultaneously. It differs slightly from the ITT effect in trials in which some individuals assigned to a particular intervention may never initiate it. In our example, we would estimate an observational analog of the ITT effect of hormone therapy by comparing women who initiate and do not initiate hormone therapy at baseline. This observational ITT effect differs from the ITT effect estimated of a target trial in which some women assigned to hormone therapy do not take any dose. Yet, a hypothetical intervention on initiation, as opposed to assignment, of treatment preserves the key feature of the ITT effect: interventions are defined solely by events occurring at baseline.

The observational analog of the PP effect is defined identically as that for the target trial. In randomized trials, we differentiated between the original PP effect and the PP effects in alternative target trials. In observational studies, this difference is unnecessary because, in the absence of a prespecified protocol, each PP effect corresponds to a particular target trial. Similarly to randomized trials, we can only use observational data to emulate target trials whose intended interventions are actually followed by at least some study subjects. If there are no such individuals, we say there is a positivity violation. An analyst may choose to use dose–response structural models to extrapolate to interventions for which positivity fails.

An advantage of defining the causal effects in observational studies in reference to those in the target trial is that we are then forced to be explicit about the interventions that are compared. Once we adopt this viewpoint, it is obvious that certain comparisons cannot be translated into a contrast between hypothetical interventions and therefore should be avoided, at least when the goal of the analysis is to help decision makers. For example, the highly publicized discrepancy between the estimates of the effect of postmenopausal hormone therapy on the risk of coronary heart disease in observational studies and a large randomized study was partly due to the use of a comparison of "current users" versus "never users" in the observational studies (Hernán et al., 2008). This comparison is rarely, if ever, used in randomized trials. A contrast of "prevalent users" versus "nonusers," with prevalent user status changing over the follow-up, does not generally correspond to the contrast of two interventions; furthermore, such a contrast may be particularly sensitive to selection bias.

Another advantage of an explicit definition of causal effects in observational studies is clarity. There is a widespread view that the ITT effect measures the effectiveness of treatment (loosely defined: the effect of treatment that would be observed under realistic conditions) in a given setting, whereas the PP effect measures efficacy (loosely defined: the effect of treatment that would be observed under perfect conditions). However, it is often difficult to argue that a PP effect of a sustained intervention in a realistic setting measures efficacy, or that the ITT effect in the presence of uncertainty about the benefits (or harms) of treatment measures the effectiveness after those benefits (or harms) are proven. The labels "effectiveness" and "efficacy" are ambiguous in settings with sustained interventions over long periods. An explicit definition of the interventions that define the causal effect of interest is more informative for comparative effectiveness research because specific decision makers need information about the effectiveness of well-defined causal interventions.

3.5 The Need for a Unified Analysis of Follow-Up Studies

Unifying the analysis of randomized and observational studies requires a common language to describe both types of studies. The concept of the target trial provides that common language. Other than baseline randomization, there are no other necessary differences between analysis of observational data that emulate a target trial and randomized trials. That is, a randomized trial can be viewed as a follow-up study with baseline randomization and the analyses of observational longitudinal data as a follow-up study without baseline randomization.

The similarities between follow-up studies with and without baseline randomization are increasingly apparent as a growing number of randomized trials attempt to estimate the effects of sustained interventions over long periods in real-world settings. These trials are a far cry from the short

TABLE 3.1

Confounding and Selection Biases to Estimate PP Effects in Studies with Treatments That May Vary over Time

	Randomized Trials	Observational Studies
Baseline confounding due to different risk factor distribution across treatment groups	Not expected	Possible
Postrandomization confounding due to time-varying risk factor distribution	Possible	Possible
Postrandomization selection bias due to loss to follow-up	Possible	Possible
Postrandomization selection bias due to competing risks	Possible	Possible

experiments in highly controlled settings that put randomized trials at the top of the hierarchy of study designs in the early days of clinical research. Randomized trials of sustained interventions over long periods, with their potential for substantial deviations from the protocol (e.g., imperfect adherence to the assigned intervention, initiation of concomitant interventions, and loss to follow-up), are subject to many of the biases that we have learned to associate exclusively with observational studies (Hernán et al., 2013). In particular, both randomized trials and observational studies may need adjustment for time-varying prognostic factors that predict dropout (selection bias) and treatment (confounding). Time-varying confounding in observational studies is a bias with the same structure as nonrandom noncompliance in randomized trials. Table 3.1 lists some biases in both randomized trials and observational studies that emulate target trials.

In fact, there are only three things that distinguish randomized data from observational data. In the randomized data, (i) no baseline confounding is expected, (ii) the randomization probabilities are known, and (iii) the randomization assignment (which arm the person was assigned to) is known for each individual. An observational analysis can emulate (i) if one measures and appropriately adjusts for a sufficient set of covariates, and (ii) if the model for treatment assignment is correctly specified. Interestingly, (iii) is not necessary for estimating the PP effect of the trial because efficient estimators (that are functions of the sufficient statistic) do not use this information; you can delete the randomization assignment from the dataset and conduct the analysis based on the received treatment when it happens that there is no confounding/selection given the covariates (Robins, 1986).

In view of the aforementioned similarities, one might expect that randomized trials and observational studies would be analyzed similarly (aside from the need for adjustment for baseline confounders in observational studies). In fact, the typical analysis of the two study types differs radically. The primary analysis of most randomized trials follows the "intention to treat" principle, whereas that of most observational studies follows the "as treated" principle. It is both problematic and perplexing that the analytic approaches differ so much. A unified approach based on g-methods, developed by Robins and collaborators, is both necessary and possible.

3.6 A Unified Analysis: G-Methods

The previous sections describe a classification of the effects of interest in follow-up studies, including the ITT and PP effects. A natural question is whether the ITT and PP *analyses* commonly used in randomized trials validly estimate the ITT and PP effects described above. In general, the answer is no.

A typical ITT analysis compares the distribution of outcomes between randomized groups without any form of adjustment for confounding or selection bias. Lack of adjustment for baseline confounding is justified by randomization: the randomized groups are comparable (or exchangeable) because they are expected to have the same risk of developing the outcome if either both groups received the same intervention. In our hormone therapy example, randomization ensures that the two groups of women are comparable because the assignment to each of the two interventions is done independently of each woman's risk of developing the outcome. No adjustment for postrandomization confounding (e.g., due to noncompliance) is required because, again, there cannot be postrandomization confounding for the effect of baseline assignment.

However, the interventions that define the ITT effect require that subjects remain in the study until their outcome variable can be ascertained. Thus, the ITT effect estimate may be affected by postrandomization selection bias if study participants are differentially lost to follow-up, and prognostic factors influence or are associated with loss of follow-up (this bias is sometimes referred to as "attrition bias"). Therefore, valid estimation of the ITT effect requires that the ITT analysis includes adjustment for postrandomization (time-varying) selection bias due to loss to follow-up (Little et al., 2012; Robins and Rotnitzky, 1992). Because baseline randomization cannot ensure comparability between those who are and are not lost to follow-up after randomization, we refer to a naïve ITT analysis that does not adjust for selection bias as a pseudo-ITT analysis (Toh and Hernán, 2008).

Adjustment for postrandomization, time-varying selection bias due to differential loss to follow-up requires measurement and adjustment of postrandomization, time-varying variables that may be themselves affected by the interventions of interest. For example, in a randomized trial of antiretroviral therapy among HIV patients, the probability of dropping out of the study may be influenced by the presence of toxicity, which is a consequence of the treatment itself. In those cases, an appropriate adjustment will require the use of inverse probability (IP) weighting or other techniques specifically designed to deal with time-varying factors (Little et al., 2012; Robins and Rotnitzky, 2004).

A typical PP analysis—also referred to as an "on treatment" analysis—only includes individuals who adhered to the instructions specified in the study protocol. For simple point interventions, the subset of trial participants included in a PP analysis, referred to as the PP population, includes only participants who were assigned to treatment and took it, and those who were not assigned to treatment and did not take it. A typical PP analysis then compares the distribution of outcomes between randomized groups in the PP population, typically without any form of adjustment for confounding or selection bias. For sustained interventions, in a typical PP analysis, individuals are censored at the first time they deviate from the protocol. That is, the remaining PP population at each time is the set of individuals who are still adhering to the protocol. Thus, a typical PP analysis is an ITT analysis restricted to the subset of the population who follow the protocol (the PP population) with no adjustment for covariates. Therefore, like an ITT analysis, a PP analysis needs to consider postrandomization selection bias due to differential loss to follow-up.

By restricting to the PP population, a PP analysis partly disregards the randomized groups and therefore the benefits of randomization because the subset of individuals who remain on protocol under one intervention may not be comparable with the subset on protocol under another intervention. That is, a PP analysis is akin to an observational analysis. Therefore, like any observational analysis, a PP analysis needs to consider bias due to postrandomization (time-varying) prognostic factors that affect the decision to stay on protocol (Hernan and Hernandez-Diaz, 2012; Robins, 1986). Again, when these postrandomization factors are affected by the interventions of interest, then, techniques specifically designed to deal with complex longitudinal data are required (Hernán et al., 2013; Robins, 1997). These methods, sometimes referred to as g-methods, include IP weighting, g-estimation, and the g-formula. Below, we provide a list of key references that describe these methods, including doubly robust versions that relax some of the modeling assumptions. Other methods, such as instrumental variable estimation (Greenland, 2000; Hernán and Robins, 2006; Robins, 1989, 1993), can sometimes be used to validly estimate PP effects without explicit adjustment for postrandomization factors, but the validity of these methods depends on having a valid instrument and on strong modeling assumptions. Some forms of instrumental variable estimation are a particular case of g-estimation.

Analogously to the adjusted ITT and PP analyses for randomized trials, we can conduct adjusted ITT and PP analyses for observational studies by using the above approach but now applied to the emulated trial. These observational analyses need generally be adjusted for both baseline and time-varying prognostic factors.

In summary, the analysis of randomized trials and observational studies should be similar. If we feel compelled to adjust for time-varying confounding and selection bias in the analysis of observational studies, we should feel equally compelled to adjust for postrandomization confounding and selection bias in the analysis of randomized trials. The only necessary difference between follow-up studies with and without baseline randomization is, precisely, baseline randomization. The only implication of this difference for the analysis is that no adjustment for baseline confounding is required in ITT analyses of randomized trials. However, adjustment for postbaseline (time-varying) factors will generally be necessary for both randomized trials and observational studies.

3.7 Time Zero in Follow-Up Studies without Baseline Randomization

A crucial component of the study protocol is the determination of the start of follow-up, also referred to as baseline or time zero. Eligibility criteria need to be met at that point but not later; study outcomes begin to be counted after that point but not earlier.

In randomized trials, the start of follow-up and the treatment assignment are generally simultaneous. Roughly speaking, the follow-up starts when the interventions start. Otherwise, the effect estimates would be hard to interpret and may often be biased. For example, consider a randomized trial to compare the risk of coronary heart disease for postmenopausal therapy versus placebo. Naturally, the start of follow-up is the time when treatment is assigned, which usually occurs shortly before, or at the same time as, treatment is initiated. We do not start the follow-up, say, 2 years before or after randomization. Starting before randomization would not be reasonable because treatment had yet to be assigned at that time and the eligibility criteria had not been defined, much less met; starting follow-up after randomization is potentially biased as cases of heart disease during the first 2 years of the trial would thereby be excluded from the analysis. If hormone therapy had a short-term effect on heart disease, it would be missed.

Even more problematic, starting 2 years after randomization would force us to exclude women who developed heart disease in the previous 2 years. If hormone therapy does indeed have a short-term effect on heart disease, then, by year 2, the hormone therapy group may be partly depleted of women susceptible to heart disease. The lower proportion of susceptible women in the hormone therapy group compared with the placebo group after 2 years destroys the baseline comparability achieved by randomization and opens the door to selection bias due to differential survival.

The same rules regarding time zero apply to observational analyses and randomized trials, and for the same reasons. Generally, the follow-up should start at the time the follow-up would have started in the emulated trial. Otherwise, the effect estimates (1) are hard to interpret, and (2) may be biased because of selection affected by treatment. As discussed above, the apparent failure of observational studies to correctly identify the effect of opposed estrogen therapy on the risk of coronary heart disease partly resulted from analyses that used current (prevalent) users, that is, analyses in which time zero was months or years after the initiation of hormone therapy.

We have argued that observational studies need to have the same time zero as the emulated trial but, as we next discuss, how to determine the start of follow-up of the emulated trial is not always obvious. There are two main scenarios, depending on how many times the eligibility criteria can be met throughout an individual's lifetime:

1. *Eligibility criteria can be met at a single time.* This is the simplest setting. Follow-up starts at the only time the eligibility criteria are met. Let us see some examples of such observational studies:

   - A study to compare various lifestyle interventions to reduce the 20-year risk of diabetes between June 1982 and June 2002 in a particular population. The follow-up of eligible individuals starts in June 1982 (Danaei et al., 2013a).

   - A study to compare high versus low epoetin doses among patients who have undergone 3 months of hemodialysis. The follow-up of eligible individuals starts after 3 months of hemodialysis (Zhang et al., 2011).

   - A study to compare initiating versus not initiating statin therapy for secondary prevention of coronary heart disease in patients discharged from the hospital after having suffered a myocardial infarction. The follow-up of eligible individuals starts at hospital discharge.

   - A study to compare immediate initiation of antiretroviral therapy when the CD4 cell count first drops below 500 cells/μL versus delayed initiation in HIV-infected patients. The follow-up of eligible individuals starts the first time their CD4 cell count drops below 500 (Cain et al., 2011).

2. *Eligibility criteria can be met at multiple times.* This is the setting that often leads to confusion. Let us see a paradigmatic example of an observational study in which eligibility criteria can be met multiple times:

   - A study to compare initiation versus no initiation of estrogen plus progestin hormone therapy among postmenopausal women with no history of chronic disease and no use of hormone therapy during the previous 2 years. Consider a woman who meets these eligibility criteria continuously between age 51 and 65 (note this implies that this woman could not have taken hormone therapy during those years). When should her follow-up start? At age 51, 52, 53…? In the emulated trial, a woman would be eligible to be recruited at multiple times during her lifetime, that is, she has multiple eligible times.

There are several alternatives to choose the time zero of each individual among her eligible times. One could choose as time zero:

a. the first eligible time

b. a randomly chosen eligible time

c. every eligible time

Strategy (c) requires emulating multiple nested trials, each of them with a different start of follow-up. The number of nested trials depends on the frequency with which data on treatment and covariates are collected:

- If fixed schedule for data collection at prespecified times (e.g., every 2 years, such as the Nurses' Health Study), then, emulate a new trial starting at each prespecified time.

- If subject-specific schedule for data collection (e.g., electronic medical records), then, choose a fixed time unit (e.g., a day, week, or month), and emulate a new trial starting at each time unit (Danaei et al., 2013b).

From a statistical standpoint, strategy (c) can be more efficient than the previous ones because it uses more of the available data. However, because individuals may be included in multiple emulated trials, appropriate adjustment of the variance of the effect estimate is required.

An issue closely related to the choice of the start of follow-up is the choice of the period during which the interventions may be initiated after the start of follow-up, that is, a grace period. In many randomized trials, the interventions start at the same time, or very shortly after, randomization. The time between assignment to the intervention and initiation of the intervention is essentially zero for all individuals: there is no grace period. Similarly, many observational studies may emulate trials with no grace period. In other cases, however, a grace period is necessary. For example, consider the study to compare immediate initiation of antiretroviral therapy when its CD4 cell count first drops below 500 cells/μL versus delayed initiation. One could assign those who start therapy on the same day as follow-up starts, that is, the first day their CD4 cell count is found to be below 500. However, such study would be unrealistic. In the real world, antiretroviral therapy cannot be started exactly on the same day the CD4 cell count is measured. Depending on the healthcare system, it may take weeks or even several months until the requisite clinical and administrative procedures are completed and patients are adequately informed. Therefore, investigators need to define "immediate initiation" by defining a grace period (say,

3 months) after baseline during which initiation is still considered to be immediate. Otherwise, the study would be estimating the effect of strategies that do not occur frequently in reality and, in fact, could not be successfully implemented in practice. Even in the unlikely event that you might want to know about the effects of such an unrealistic intervention, there would be too few people in the observational study whose data are consistent with the intervention to allow for statistically accurate inferences.

Grace periods need to be dealt with appropriately in the data analysis (Cain et al., 2010). A consequence of using a grace period is that, for the duration of the grace period, an individual's observed data are consistent with more than one strategy. For example, in the HIV trial described above, the introduction of a 3-month grace period implies that the interventions are redefined as "initiate therapy within 3 months after CD4 cell count first drops below 500 cells/μL" versus "initiate therapy more than 3 months after CD4 cell count first drops below 500 cells/μL." Therefore, an individual who starts therapy in month 3 after baseline has data consistent with both interventions during months 1 and 2. Had he died during those 2 months, to which arm of the emulated trial would we have assigned him? One possibility is to randomly assign him to one of the two arms.

Another possibility is to create two exact copies of this individual—clones—in the data and assign each of the two clones to a different arm. Clones are then censored at the time their data stop being consistent with the arm they were assigned to. For example, if the individual starts therapy in month 3, then, the clone assigned to "start after 3 months" would be censored at that time. The potential bias introduced by this likely informative censoring would need to be corrected by adjusting for time-varying factors via IP weighting. Importantly, if the individual had died in month 2, both the clones would have died and therefore the death would have been assigned to both arms. This double allocation of events prevents the bias that could arise if events occurring during the grace period were systematically assigned to one of the two arms only.

A consequence of using grace periods with cloning and censoring is that the ITT effect cannot be estimated because almost everyone will contribute a clone to each of the interventions. Because each individual is assigned to all interventions at baseline, a contrast based on baseline assignment (i.e., an ITT analysis) will compare groups with essentially identical outcomes. Therefore, analyses with grace period at baseline are geared toward estimating some form of PP effect.

A last note on the analysis of follow-up studies without baseline randomization. The approaches discussed here apply to both closed-cohort studies and to dynamic populations in which individuals may enter and exit the population repeatedly during the follow-up.

When defining the protocol of an emulated trial based on data from dynamic populations, person–time should not be confused with persons (a practice entrenched among epidemiologists who are taught to consider incidence rates as a primary target for inference). Eligibility criteria, interventions, start, and end of follow-up are defined for persons, not for person–time. Once an eligible person exits the dynamic population after baseline, the person is regarded as censored. Similarly, the approach discussed in this chapter can also be applied to case–control studies and other efficient sampling schemes. Investigators will first need to define the follow-up study from which cases and controls were sampled, and then the trial from which the follow-up study emulates.

3.8 Conclusion

Historically, randomized trials have been considered far superior to observational studies for the purpose of making causal inferences and aiding decision making. Unfortunately, randomized experiments are not always available. They may be too expensive, infeasible, or ethically inappropriate. Observational studies are what we do when we cannot conduct a randomized trial. (In the absence of practical and ethical constraints, reasonable people would always conduct a randomized experiment.) However, as much as we may like randomization, many decisions will need to be made with no evidence from randomized trials. It is therefore important to use a sound approach to design and analyze observational studies. Making the target trial explicit is one step in that direction. When the goal is to assist decision making, the analysis of existing data (e.g., observational studies) needs to emulate trials and be evaluated with respect to how well they emulate their target trial.

Randomization is indeed a powerful tool, but its advantages need to be carefully qualified.

In both randomized trials and observational studies, decisions about continued participation in the study and about treatment choices *after* baseline are not randomly assigned: Individuals may be differentially lost to follow-up, which may introduce selection bias, and individuals may change their treatment, which may introduce time-varying confounding, after baseline.

Follow-up studies with and without baseline randomization will need data on adherence to interventions, and often on confounders, after baseline. This type of information is not typically collected in the so-called large simple trials and pragmatic trials. It is time for randomized trial protocols to get serious about collecting the data needed for prespecified analysis plans that appropriately adjust for these biases.

Appendix 3A.1: Additional Papers That Describe g-Methods and Related Approaches

3A.1.1 Inverse Probability Weighting

- Robins, J. M. and Finkelstein, D. 2000. Correcting for non-compliance and dependent censoring in an AIDS clinical trial with inverse probability of censoring weighted (IPCW) log-rank tests. *Biometrics, 56*(3), 779–788.

- van der Laan, M. J., Hubbard, A. E., and Robins, J. M. 2002. Locally efficient estimation of a multivariate survival function in longitudinal studies. *Journal of the American Statistical Association, 97*(458), 494–507.

- Scharfstein, D. O., Rotnitzky, A., and Robins, J. M. 1999. Adjusting for non-ignorable drop-out using semiparametric non-response models. *Journal of the American Statistical Association, 94*, 1096–1120 (with discussion and rejoinder).

3A.1.2 Marginal Structural Models

- Robins, J. M. 1998. Marginal structural models. *1997 Proceedings of the American Statistical Association*, Alexandria, VA. Section on Bayesian Statistical Science, pp. 1–10.

- Robins, J. M. 1999. Marginal structural models versus structural nested models as tools for causal inference. In M. E. Halloran, and D. Berry (Eds.), *Statistical Models in Epidemiology: The Environment and Clinical Trials* (pp. 95–134). IMA Volume *116*, New York: Springer-Verlag.

- Petersen, M., Deeks, S., Martin, J. et al. 2007. History-adjusted marginal structural models for estimating time-varying effect modification. *American Journal of Epidemiology, 166*, 985–993.

- Joffe, M., Santanna, J., and Feldman, H. 2001. Partially marginal structural models for causal inference. *American Journal of Epidemiology, 153*(suppl), S261.

- van der Laan, M. J., Petersen, M. L., and Joffe, M. M. 2005. History-adjusted marginal structural models and statically-optimal dynamic treatment regimens. *International Journal of Biostatistics, 1*, article 4.

- Robins, J. M., Hernán, M. A., and Rotnitzky, A. 2007. Invited commentary: Effect modification by time-varying covariates. *American Journal of Epidemiology, 166*(9), 994–1002.

- Toh, S., Hernández-Díaz, S., Logan, R., Robins, J. M., and Hernán, M. A. 2010. Estimating absolute risks in the presence of nonadherence: An application to a follow-up study with baseline randomization. *Epidemiology, 21*(4), 528–539. PMCID: PMC3315056.

- Robins, J. M., Hernán, M. A., and Brumback, B. 2000. Marginal structural models and causal inference in epidemiology. *Epidemiology, 11*(5), 550–560.

- Hernán, M. A., Brumback, B., and Robins, J. M. 2000. Marginal structural models to estimate the causal effect of zidovudine on the survival of HIV-positive men. *Epidemiology, 11*(5), 561–570.

3A.1.3 Dynamic Regimes and Marginal Structural Models

- Murphy, S. A., Van der Laan, M. J., Robins, J. M., and CPPRG. 2001. Marginal mean models for dynamic regimes. *Journal of the American Statistical Association, 96*, 1410–1423.

- Hernán, M. A., Lanoy, E., Costagliola, D., and Robins, J. M. 2006. Comparison of dynamic treatment regimes via inverse probability weighting. *Basic and Clinical Pharmacology and Toxicology, 98*, 237–242.

- Robins, J. M. 1993. Analytic methods for estimating HIV treatment and cofactor effects. In D. G. Ostrow and R. Kessler (Eds.), *Methodological Issues of AIDS Mental Health Research* (pp. 213–290). New York: Plenum Publishing.

- Robins, J., Orellana, L., and Rotnitzky, A. 2008. Estimation and extrapolation of optimal treatment and testing strategies. *Statistical Medicine, 27*(23), 4678–4721.

- Orellana, L., Rotnitzky, A., and Robins, J. M. 2010. Dynamic regime marginal structural mean models for estimation of optimal dynamic treatment regimes, Part I: Main content. *International Journal of Biostatistics, 6*(2), Article 8.

- Orellana, L., Rotnitzky, A., and Robins, J. M. 2010. Dynamic regime marginal structural mean models for estimation of optimal dynamic treatment regimes, Part II: Proofs of results. *International Journal of Biostatistics, 6*(2), Article 9.

- Petersen, M. L., Deeks, S. G., and van der Laan, M. J. 2007. Individualized treatment rules: Generating candidate clinical trials. *Statistics in Medicine, 26*, 4578–4601.

- Lavori, P. W. and Dawson, R. 2004. Dynamic treatment regimes: Practical design considerations. *Clinical Trials, 1*, 9–20.

- Bembom, O. and van der Laan, M. J. 2007. Statistical methods for analyzing sequentially randomized trials. *Journal of the National Cancer Institute, 99*(21), 1577–1582.

3A.1.4 G-Estimation of Structural Nested Models

- Robins, J. M., Blevins, D., Ritter, G., and Wulfsohn, M. 1992. G-estimation of the effect of prophylaxis therapy for pneumocystis carinii pneumonia on the survival of AIDS patients. *Epidemiology, 3,* 319–336.

- Robins, J. M. and Greenland, S. 1994. Adjusting for differential rates of PCP prophylaxis in high- versus low-dose AZT treatment arms in an AIDS randomized trial. *Journal of the American Statistical Association, 89,* 737–749.

- Joffe, M. M. and Brensinger, C. 2003. Weighting in instrumental variables and G-estimation. *Statistics in Medicine, 22,* 1285–1303.

- Lok, J., Gill, R., van der Vaart, A., and Robins, J. 2004. Estimating the causal effect of a time-varying treatment on time-to-event using structural nested failure time models. *Statistica Neerlandica, 58*(3), 271–295.

- Chakraborty, B. and Moodie, E. E. M. 2013. Chapter 4. Statistical methods for dynamic treatment regimes. Reinforcement learning, causal inference, and personalized medicine. *Series: Statistics for Biology and Health, 76,* XVI, 204.

- Hernán, M. A., Cole, S. R., Margolick, J. B., Cohen, M. H., and Robins, J. M. 2005. Structural accelerated failure time models for survival analysis in studies with time-varying treatments. *Pharmacoepidemiology and Drug Safety, 14*(7), 477–491.

3A.1.5 G-Formula

- Robins, J. M. 1986. A new approach to causal inference in mortality studies with sustained exposure periods—Application to control of the healthy worker survivor effect. *Mathematical Modelling, 7,* 1393–1512 (errata in Computers and Mathematics with Applications 1987: 14:917–921).

- Robins, J. M. 1987. Addendum to a new approach to causal inference in mortality studies with sustained exposure periods—Application to control of the healthy worker survivor effect. *Computers and Mathematics with Applications, 14,* 923–945 (errata in Computers and Mathematics with Applications, 18:477).

- Robins, J. M. 1997. Causal inference from complex longitudinal data. In M. Berkane (Ed.), *Latent Variable Modeling and Applications to Causality* (pp. 69–117). *Lecture Notes in Statistics (120).* New York: Springer Verlag.

- Robins, J., Hernán, M. A., and Siebert, U. 2004. Effects of multiple interventions. In M. Ezzati, C. J. L. Murray, A. D. Lopez, and

A. Rodgers (Eds.), *Comparative Quantification of Health Risks: Global and Regional Burden of Disease Attributable to Selected Major Risk Factors* (pp. 2191–2230). Chapter 28; Vol 2. Geneva: World Health Organization.

- Young, J. G., Cain, L. E., Robins, J. M., O'Reilly, E., and Hernán, M. A. 2011. Comparative effectiveness of dynamic treatment regimes: An application of the parametric g-formula. *Statistics in Biosciences, 3,* 119–143.

3A.1.6 Doubly Robust Estimation

- Bang, H. and Robins, J. 2005. Doubly robust estimation in missing data and causal inference models. *Biometrics, 61,* 692–972.
- Robins, J. M., Sued, M., Lei-Gomez, Q., and Rotnitzky, A. 2007. Comment: Performance of doubly-robust estimators when "Inverse Probability" weights are highly variable. *Statistical Science, 22*(4), 544–559.
- van der Laan, M. J., and Robins, J. M. 2003. *Unified Methods for Censored Longitudinal Data and Causality.* New York: Springer-Verlag.
- Tsiatis, A. 2006. *Semiparametric Theory and Missing Data.* New York: Springer.
- van der Laan, M. J., and Rose, S. 2011. *Targeted Learning: Causal Inference for Observational and Experimental Data.* New York: Springer.

References

Cain, L. E., Logan, R., Robins, J. M., Sterne, J. A., Sabin, C., Bansi, L.,...Hernan, M. A. 2011. When to initiate combined antiretroviral therapy to reduce mortality and AIDS-defining illness in HIV-infected persons in developed countries: An observational study. *Annual International Medicine, 154*(8), 509–515.

Cain, L. E., Robins, J. M., Lanoy, E., Costagliola, D., and Hernán, M. A. 2010. When to start treatment? A systematic approach to the comparison of dynamic regimes using observational data. *International Journal of Biostatistics, 6*(2), Article 18.

Danaei, G., Pan, A., Hu, F. B., and Hernan, M. A. 2013a. Hypothetical midlife interventions in women and risk of type 2 diabetes. *Epidemiology, 24*(1), 122–128. doi:10.1097/EDE.0b013e318276c98a.

Danaei, G., Rodriguez, L. A., Cantero, O. F., Logan, R., and Hernan, M. A. 2013b. Observational data for comparative effectiveness research: An emulation of randomised trials of statins and primary prevention of coronary heart disease. [Comparative Study]. *Statistical Methods in Medical Research, 22*(1), 70–96. doi:10.1177/0962280211403603.

Fischl, M. A., Parker, C. B., Pettinelli, C., Wulfsohn, M., Hirsch, M. S., Collier, A.,... The AIDS Clinical Trials Group. 1990. A randomized controlled trial of a reduced daily dose of zidovudine in patients with the acquired immunodeficiency syndrome. *New England Journal of Medicine, 323*(15), 1009–1014.

Greenland, S. 2000. An introduction to instrumental variables for epidemiologists. *International Journal of Epidemiology, 29,* 722–729.

Grodstein, F., Clarkson, T. B., and Manson, J. E. 2003. Understanding the divergent data on postmenopausal hormone therapy. *New England Journal of Medicine, 348*(7), 645–650.

Hernán, M. A., Alonso, A., Logan, R., Grodstein, F., Michels, K. B., Willett, W. C.,...Robins, J. M. 2008. Observational studies analyzed like randomized experiments: An application to postmenopausal hormone therapy and coronary heart disease. *Epidemiology, 19*(6), 766–779. doi:10.1097/EDE.0b013e3 181875e61.

Hernán, M. A. and Hernández-Díaz, S. 2012. Beyond the intention-to-treat in comparative effectiveness research. *Clinical Trials, 9*(1), 48–55. doi:10.1177/ 1740774511420743.

Hernán, M. A., Hernández-Díaz, S., and Robins, J. M. 2013. Randomized trials analyzed as observational studies. [Research Support, N.I.H., Extramural]. *Annals of Internal Medicine, 159*(8), 560–562. doi:10.7326/0003-4819-159-8-201310150-00709.

Hernán, M. A. and Robins, J. M. 2006. Instruments for causal inference: An epidemiologist's dream? *Epidemiology, 17,* 360–372.

Little, R. J., D'Agostino, R., Cohen, M. L., Dickersin, K., Emerson, S. S., Farrar, J. T.,...Stern, H. 2012. The prevention and treatment of missing data in clinical trials. *The New England Journal of Medicine, 367*(14), 1355–1360. doi:10.1056/NEJMsr1203730.

Richardson, W., Wilson, M., Nishikawa, J., and Hayward, R. 1995. The well-built clinical question: A key to evidence-based decisions. *APC Journal Club, 123*(3), A12–A13.

Robins, J. M. 1986. A new approach to causal inference in mortality studies with a sustained exposure period—Application to the healthy worker survivor effect [published errata appear in Mathl Modelling 1987;14:917-21]. *Mathematical Modelling, 7,* 1393–1512.

Robins, J. M. 1989. The analysis of randomized and non-randomized AIDS treatment trials using a new approach to causal inference in longitudinal studies. In L. Sechrest, H. Freeman, and A. Mulley (Eds.), *Health Services Research Methodology: A Focus on AIDS* (pp. 113–159). Washington, DC: NCHRS, U.S. Public Health Service.

Robins, J. M. 1993. Analytic methods for estimating HIV treatment and cofactor effects. In D. G. Ostrow and R. Kessler (Eds.), *Methodological Issues of AIDS Mental Health Research* (pp. 213–290). New York: Plenum Publishing.

Robins, J. M. 1997. Causal inference from complex longitudinal data. In M. Berkane (Ed.), *Latent Variable Modeling and Applications to Causality. Lecture Notes in Statistics 120* (pp. 69–117). New York: Springer-Verlag.

Robins, J. M. and Rotnitzky, A. 1992. Recovery of information and adjustment for dependent censoring using surrogate markers. In N. Jewell, K. Dietz, and V. Farewell (Eds.), *AIDS Epidemiology —Methodological Issues* (pp. 297–331). Boston, MA: Birkhäuser.

Robins, J. M. and Rotnitzky, A. 2004. Estimation of treatment effects in randomised trials with non-compliance and a dichotomous outcome using structural mean models. *Biometrika*, 91(4), 763–783.

Toh, S. and Hernán, M. A. 2008. Causal inference from longitudinal studies with baseline randomization. *International Journal of Biostatistics*, 4(1), Article 22. doi:10.2202/1557-4679.1117.

Zhang, Y., Thamer, M., Kaufman, J. S., Cotter, D. J., and Hernan, M. A. 2011. High doses of epoetin do not lower mortality and cardiovascular risk among elderly hemodialysis patients with diabetes. *Kidney International*, 80(6), 663–669. doi:10.1038/ki.2011.188.

Section II

Clinical Trials: Design, Interpretation, and Generalizability

4

Cluster-Randomized Trials

Ken Kleinman

CONTENTS

ABSTRACT I review the cluster-randomized trial (CRT), a study design well suited to comparative effectiveness research, in that it often allows treatment under the study protocol to closely mimic the natural implementation of the study arms in practice. In addition, CRTs are often far cheaper per participant than traditional individually randomized trials (IRTs) and can be used in settings where individual randomization may be impossible, or would muddy, not clarify, the effect of the study arms. However, CRTs offer less power per participant so that an assessment of the trade-off of cost versus power may be necessary if both designs are plausible for the question under study. Alternatively, an increased sample size may be needed for a CRT to equal the power of an IRT for a given effect size. CRTs require more complex methods of data analysis than traditional trials, and power or sample size estimation is more complex and has received less methodological attention than traditional trials. I motivate the design and explain its suitability for effectiveness questions. I then provide several examples of specific CRTs, along with rationales for why a CRT was better than or necessary in preference to an IRT. Next, I provide heuristics for understanding the above assertions and discuss analysis methods and power/sample size methods for CRTs.

4.1 Introduction

The randomized controlled trial, which I will refer to here as the *individually randomized trial* (IRT), is generally recognized as the strongest study design available. Especially when coupled with sufficient blinding to prevent the expectation of research staff from biasing measurement, there is currently no better way to establish the effect of a treatment (which I describe more generally as an intervention) versus an alternate treatment (which I will describe as the control). A full discussion of the virtues of IRTs is beyond the scope of the chapter. Suffice it to say that a large, well-conducted IRT eliminates the most threatening sources of doubt that attend to lesser designs. If such a study is performed, then selection bias, confounding, competing secular trend, and so forth cannot be competing explanations of any observed results. A large community of professional "trialists" has emerged, and the science of implementing trials is highly refined.

However, some interventions cannot practically be assigned to individual patients. For example, consider an intervention to improve doctors' interpersonal skills. Because it is impossible in realistic settings to randomly assign patients to doctors, we cannot randomize patients. A related problem is "contamination," which occurs, to continue the example, when individual doctors treat both control and intervention patients: a given doctor's encounters with intervention patients may materially affect his or her interactions with patients in the control arm. A hypothetical but impracticable trial in which patients were randomly assigned to doctors would therefore allow only one patient per doctor, making costs very high.

The cluster-randomized trial (CRT), also known as a group-randomized trial, is a different design that allows researchers to avoid randomizing individuals and helps prevent contamination. CRTs can be cheaper than IRTs on a per-patient basis, though they have drawbacks that do not affect IRTs. In CRTs, groups or "clusters" of patients are all randomized together so that they are all in the treatment arm or all in the control arm. For example, in the hypothetical trial to improve physicians' interpersonal skills, we might randomize the patients of 20 doctors so that 10 doctors' patients were all in the control arm and 10 were in the intervention. In fact, we will randomly assign the doctors themselves to one treatment condition or the other, rather than randomizing the patients. We will also apply the intervention to the 10 randomized doctors. In general, we might randomize medical practices so that all the patients in each practice share an arm, or we might randomize hospitals, or communities, and so forth.

CRTs have become increasingly common in the scientific literature. Figure 4.1 shows the results of a simple Web of Science search for articles with the terms "cluster random*" or "group random*" in the title. The increase in the number of papers on this topic is rapid.

While IRTs are typically the strongest designs, when possible, they are not without flaws. Chapters 3 and 6 discuss the related topics of the relationship between trials and observational studies, and the generalizability of trial results, respectively. One example of a drawback of IRTs is that they are often conducted to establish efficacy, that is, the effect of an intervention for very homogeneous populations and under very controlled conditions. This is likely a function of their great cost and the commercial motives and regulatory environment in which they are often performed. Together, these

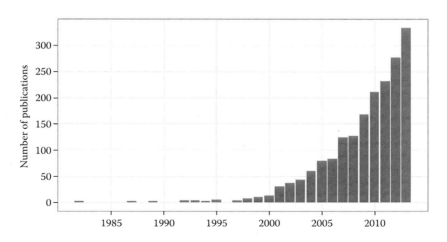

FIGURE 4.1
Articles with "cluster random" or "group random" in the title. (Retrieved from ISI Web of Science.)

features often mean that the subjects in an IRT do not comprise all the typical candidates for the treatment, threatening generalizability of the results. For example, if an IRT includes only healthy 40-year-olds, it is unknown whether the treatment will work among 80-year-olds with three chronic conditions. Strictly speaking, this homogeneity of population is not a requirement of IRTs, but in practice, it is a very common feature of IRT designs. In addition, the treatment environment may be very different for trial participants versus the general treatment population. If the IRT protocol requires a drug be administered every 3 h, it is unclear whether the results will apply to patients who sleep through the night.

In contrast, CRTs, by randomizing all the patients of a physician, clinic, hospital, and so forth, provide a setting in which it is natural to retain a more heterogeneous population, though investigators may choose to exclude some patients. Similarly, by allowing care to be provided in natural settings, they can often use protocols similar to those that might be followed by typical patients outside the study context. The effect of treatments in the general population and under typical use conditions is sometimes referred to as "effectiveness." While there is no scientific reason that IRTs should measure efficacy and CRTs should measure effectiveness, this is often the case.

There is, needless to say, a close relationship between effectiveness trials and comparative effectiveness research (CER). Simply stated, the more heterogeneous the population of a study and the more the study conditions resemble those which the treatment population will experience, the better the study results will be replicated outside the experimental context. That means that if an individual wants to know what to expect from a treatment, they should seek the results from an effectiveness trial. A CRT is likely to be one such trial.

The purpose of this chapter is to summarize the advantages and disadvantages of the CRT design, paying special attention to the settings in which they are useful. I also review the complications and special methods to address questions of data analysis and power and sample size. In Section 4.2, I provide some real-world examples of CRTs; in Section 4.3, I provide a brief heuristic review of some key distinctions between CRTs and IRTs, with an emphasis on the drawbacks and advantages. In Section 4.4, I review some methods for data analysis. In Section 4.5, I discuss the nuances of power and sample size calculation and discuss the practicalities of matching and stratification. In Section 4.6, I conclude the chapter.

4.2 Three CRT Case Studies

Here I briefly describe three CRTs. In each case, I review whether an IRT was possible or practical and also discuss effectiveness, efficacy, and CER.

4.2.1 The REDUCE Trial

Antibiotic-resistant microorganisms have attracted attention from both the popular press and the medical literature. One organism for which the problem has increasingly troubling impact is methicillin-resistant *Staphylococcus aureus* (MRSA). MRSA is resistant to many antibiotics and can cause skin infections in the community; in the hospital, it may lead to life-threatening bloodstream infections, pneumonia, and surgical site infections.

In recent years, some hospitals have adopted screening for and isolation of patients with MRSA at the time of admission. Screening means collecting samples and performing laboratory tests to determine if MRSA is present, and isolation typically means that the patient is assigned a private room and that those entering the room must use gowns, masks, and gloves. These steps are intended to decrease the spread of MRSA within hospitals. They are costly for hospitals and time-consuming for staff.

The Randomized Evaluation of Decolonization versus Universal Clearance to Eliminate MRSA (REDUCE) trial compared the effectiveness of three arms: (1) screening and isolation ("control"); (2) "targeted decolonization," in which patients were screened and those with identified MRSA were treated to remove the MRSA, but were not isolated; and (3) "universal decolonization," in which no patients were screened but all patients were treated with decolonization, as if MRSA were present. The main outcome of the study was time until infection with MRSA. The REDUCE trial was CER with the potential to improve the delivery of care and improve health at the population level. The main trial results have appeared in the peer-reviewed literature (Huang et al., 2013).

In the REDUCE trial, 45 hospitals were randomized and the assigned arm protocol was implemented across all intensive care units (ICUs) within the hospital. The existing hospital staff was not altered, and the intervention protocols were introduced as new standard practice for the hospital. The use of electronic medical records to determine the outcomes prevented the introduction of specialized data-collection instruments for the study.

Could an IRT have been performed? Suppose we had randomized individual patients. Since MRSA is spread by contact, in that hypothetical IRT it would be hard to interpret results when a control patient was lying in a bed next to a universal decolonization patient. Would an infection in one of these patients reflect a failure of the treatment they received or of the other treatment? Similarly, any noninfection that would otherwise have occurred is a benefit of the intervention that accrues not only to the treated patient but to those around them. So an IRT would have been very difficult to interpret.

In addition, the study treatment arms represent policies that hospital leadership might adopt as policy for all of their patients. The hospitals would not admit patients and then decide which of these routes is correct on a case-by-case basis. Thus, a trial that attempted to find the effect of the treatment arms on individuals would be of little interest. Only a trial that assesses the effectiveness of the arms as a hospital-wide policy has any salience in practice.

Finally, implementing the trial on individuals would have required additional staff in each hospital's ICUs. This would have disrupted the usual patterns of care in the ICU. In addition, it would have been extremely expensive. Both of these effects would diminish the effectiveness implications of the trial.

4.2.2 The REACH Trial

One cause of the increasing prevalence of antibiotic-resistant organisms is overprescribing by physicians, that is, the prescription of antibiotics when they are not needed. Overprescribing is thought to be partly driven by patients expecting or demanding antibiotics for their children. The Reducing Antibiotics for Children in Massachusetts (REACH) trial compared the effectiveness of a multipronged intervention to get parents to not demand antibiotics and to make pediatricians more cautious in prescribing them, to a control or "usual care" condition that got no intervention components. The REACH trial was CER with the potential to improve the delivery of care and improve health care at the population level.

In the REACH study, we randomized 16 communities to one of the two arms. In the intervention arm, we targeted mass media advertising, placed waiting room posters and pamphlets, and trained pediatricians through mailings, e-mail, and small-group meetings. The main outcome of the study was the probability of receiving a prescription for antibiotics, collected from health insurance claims. The main study results have been reported in the peer-reviewed literature (Finkelstein et al., 2008).

Could an IRT have been performed? Given the mass media, waiting room, and physician interventions, contamination, that is, exposure of the control group to the interventions, would have been very difficult to avoid. For example, in order to prevent families in the control communities from being exposed to the media parts of the intervention, it would have been necessary to isolate parents in the control group from all media carrying the advertisements. To prevent control group exposure to the waiting room posters and the contact with the pediatricians, it would have been necessary to control the choice of physician at the time of illness and possibly randomize only one patient to each physician, greatly increasing the cost. In addition, the intervention might well benefit from social contact between and among patients and physicians so that the effect observed in an IRT might be smaller than the one obtained if the intervention were implemented broadly. The investigators' interest was in the effectiveness of the whole intervention on the whole community, not on the efficacy of any particular aspect (e.g., advertising) of the intervention on a person in the absence of the other parts of the intervention. Together, these observations suggest that an IRT would not have been feasible or desirable.

4.2.3 The STAR Trial

The increasing prevalence of obesity in the United States and other countries is so alarming that it has been labeled an "epidemic." As weight and eating behaviors are entrained from childhood and difficult to modify in adults, it may be that interventions on children provide the highest likelihood for slowing or reversing the epidemic. Can pediatricians help steer overweight and obese children to treatment? If so, this might be a cost-effective way to help prevent adult obesity. The Study of Technology to Accelerate Research (STAR) study randomized 14 pediatric practices to compare the effectiveness of three treatment arms: electronic decision support to pediatricians through an existing electronic medical record system, decision support plus direct-to-parent outreach, or usual care. The main outcome was the child's weight, measured at the doctor's office. Publication of the main trial results is pending; design details have been published (Taveras et al., 2013). The STAR trial was CER with the potential to treat a clinical condition and improve health care at the individual level.

Could an IRT have been performed? As with the REACH study, many patients share pediatricians. To prevent contamination, we would have had to restrict the sample to one patient per pediatrician, though this seems less of a threat than in the REDUCE or REACH trials. Attempts to prevent contamination would have led to prohibitive costs for the study. So, individual randomization would at best have been impractical. In addition, the investigators were interested in the effectiveness of the decision support and outreach for real populations of patients, not in the efficacy of the prompts in changing physicians' behavior.

4.3 Insight into the Costs of CRTs

The CRT design offers both challenges and opportunities. In this section, I provide heuristic insight into the main challenges; details are included in the following sections.

4.3.1 Power

The primary cost is a loss of power, relative to an IRT with the same number of subjects. There are two sources of this loss of power.

4.3.1.1 Clustering

One source of power loss is the generally positive correlation or noninde-pendence among observations within each cluster. Loosely speaking, this correlation means that knowing the outcome for one subject in a cluster implies some knowledge about the outcome for every other subject in the cluster. For the purposes of power, this implies that each additional observa-tion in the cluster provides less information, and contributes less to power, than an uncorrelated observation would have.

4.3.1.2 Randomization

The second source of power loss is due to the randomization: the degrees of freedom for our main comparison must be based on the number of random-ized units, that is, the number of clusters, and not on the number of subjects (Cornfield, 1978). In CRTs, it is quite common to have fewer than 30 clusters randomized. In two of the three case studies described in Section 4.2, there are fewer than 20; the third, REDUCE, with 45 randomized clusters, is a fairly large CRT. The penalty incurred increases dramatically as the number of ran-domized units decreases below 30. With more than 30 degrees of freedom, the power improvements accruing to additional degrees of freedom are typi-cally negligible. Parenthetically, the association of power with the number of randomized units also occurs in IRT designs, but IRTs often have many more than 30 subjects.

4.3.2 Confounding and Balance

Since relatively few items are randomized, it is possible, and even likely, that some covariates will remain unbalanced after randomization. In an IRT of sufficient size, the possibility of this is so diminished that some trialists advocate not even assessing whether balance has been achieved. The reason to be concerned about balance is that in order for a putative causal effect to be an artifact of confounding, the confounder must both be a cause of the outcome and also have a different distribution in (be unbalanced across) intervention groups. Thus, if we achieve balance, then the result cannot be confounded.

Fortunately, in many cases, the administrative structure of CRTs often pro-vides a way to help address this problem. "Recruiting subjects" in a CRT means recruiting communities, physician practices, hospitals, and so forth. And the study intervention rarely, if ever, needs to be implemented before all clusters are recruited. Thus, it is often possible to collect data on some important confounders before randomization. For example, in the REDUCE study, it was possible to assess the baseline rate of MRSA infections among recruited hospitals before randomization. In the REACH and STAR stud-ies, it was possible to assess the racial/ethnic makeup of the communities and practices before randomization. This prerandomization information on potential confounders can then be used to stratify the randomization among clusters with similar values for the covariates. The stratified randomization is much more likely to result in balance between the arms than a naive randomization.

4.4 Data Analysis

The key difficulty with data analysis of CRTs is to account for the correlation within cluster. There are effectively two ways to address this problem. The first is to summarize within cluster, for example, by calculating the mean response, and then to perform an analysis of the within-cluster summaries. The other is to include all the data, but to account for clustering by modeling it explicitly, for example, with a mixed-effects model.

As a matter of intuitive appeal, it may seem attractive to summarize by unit, and in fact the lore in the community used to contain the supposed requirement that the "unit of analysis must match the unit of randomization." In addition, there may be settings in which only cluster summaries are available to the analyst. However, the mixed-model approach elegantly matches the conceptual model of the correlation that complicates the analysis. In addition, the mixed model can transparently accommodate variable cluster sizes and subject-level covariates. While methods exist to do this for the summarizing approach as well, at least for normally distributed outcomes, they become increasingly less general and more awkward. Nonetheless, as the summary methods are unbiased and have equal power compared to mixed-effects models in the settings where they apply, I will discuss them briefly. For a lengthier discussion, the reader is referred to the texts by Hayes and Moulton (2009) and Eldridge and Kerry (2012).

4.4.1 Cluster Summary Methods

Suppose that we observe outcome y_{ij} on subject j in cluster i ($i = 1, \ldots, N_g$, $j = 1, \ldots, M_i$) in treatment group g ($g = 1, \ldots, G$). For now, we assume $M_i = M$, for all i. Then the procedure is to:

1. Calculate some statistic for each cluster, such as the mean: $\bar{y} = \sum y_{ij}/M$.
2. Transform the statistic in Step 1, as necessary, to improve normality.
3. Perform a t-test (if $G = 2$) or an ANOVA (more generally) comparing the G groups.

The statistic calculated in Step 1 could also be the proportion with a dichotomous outcome, or the total count per total observed time, and so forth. In general, the t-test is extremely robust to departures from normality so that Step 2 may not be required, but it is possible that the data may have long enough tails that transformation may be desirable. The degrees of freedom for the test in Step 3 will be $\sum gN_g - G$. Confident limits and functions other than the difference, such as the risk ratio, can be calculated as if the means within cluster were the only data.

More generally, suppose not all $M_i = M$. Then the above algorithm would be "wrong," in the sense that it weights all clusters equally, while in fact there is unequal precision and variability of the observed statistic as an estimate of the true value. This is perhaps most obvious for dichotomous outcomes: a cluster with two observations can have observed proportions of only $0, 0.5,$ or 1, regardless of the true probability. A cluster with 100 observations is much more likely to have an observed proportion close to the true probability. One natural response to this observation is to weight the observed within-cluster statistics in a weighted t-test.

Due to the possibility of imbalance noted in Section 4.3.2, it may be more useful to adjust for potential confounders in CRTs than in IRTs. In addition, adjusting for covariates may result in greater precision even when confounding is not a threat. It is not immediately obvious how one might attempt to adjust for confounding, in a setting where a cluster summary analysis was desirable. Hayes and Moulton (2009) suggest extending the above algorithm as follows:

1. Estimate an unclustered, covariate-adjusted model for the whole population, ignoring intervention group status, for example, in a multivariable linear regression.
2. Within each cluster, calculate the average residual from the model in the previous step.
3. Perform a t-test (if $G = 2$) or an ANOVA (more generally) comparing the mean residuals between the G groups.

The residual in Step 2 might be the difference in means for a normal outcome, or a difference in probability for a dichotomous outcome, or a difference in rate for a count outcome. In the last case, we would divide the observed difference by the person-time of observation. Additionally, we might be interested in a ratio difference such as the rate ratio for count outcomes or the risk ratio for dichotomous outcomes. In those cases, the residual in Step 2 would be the sum of the observed values in the cluster divided by the sum of the expected value in the cluster. It is unclear whether this procedure underestimates the cost of estimating the additional parameters for the models in Step 1.

4.4.2 Methods Retaining Individual Data Elements

4.4.2.1 Mixed-Effects Models

In contrast to the two-step approach summarized in Section 4.4.1, mixed models, also known as random-effects models, incorporate all aspects of modeling into a single step (Laird and Ware, 1982, Breslow and Clayton, 1993). The generalized linear mixed model (GLMM) to describe the data can be written as

$$g\left(E\left[y_{ij}|b_i\right]\right) = \beta_0 + \sum_{g=2}^{G} \beta_g I(g_{ij} = g) + b_i \tag{4.1}$$

where $g_{ij} = g$ if subject j in cluster i is in treatment arm g, and typically it is assumed that $b_i \sim N\left(0, \sigma_b^2\right)$.

For the linear model, this is

$$y_{ij}|b_i = \beta_0 + \sum_{g=2}^{G} \beta_g I(g_{ij} = g) + b_i + e_{ij}$$

where $e_{ij} \sim N(0, \sigma^2)$, with the unconditional $Var(y_{ij}) = \sigma^2 + \sigma_b^2$, and $Cov(y_{ij}, y_{ij'}|j \neq j') = \sigma_b^2$ and $Cov(y_{ij}, y_{i'j'}|i \neq i') = 0$.

For dichotomous outcomes, $g(E[y_{ij}|b_i]) = \log it(Pr[y_{ij}|b_i] = 1)$ and y_{ij} has a binomial distribution while for count outcomes $g(E[y_{ij}|b_i]) = \log(E[y_{ij}|b_i])$ and y_{ij} has a Poisson or negative binomial distribution. In general, the negative binomial model is to be preferred; the cost of the negative binomial relative to a simpler Poisson model is modest, and the risk of overdispersion relative to the Poisson distribution is great.

For time-to-event outcomes, the analogous model is sometimes known as a shared frailty model (Ripatti and Palmgren, 2000). In essence, it is a proportional hazards regression model with random effects:

$$\lambda_{ij}(t) = \lambda_0(t)e^{\sum_2^G \beta_g I(g_{ij}=g)+b_i} \tag{4.2}$$

The "frailties" are defined as $\log(b_i) = u_i$, and writing the model in terms of these shows that the random effects modify the baseline hazard for each cluster by a constant multiplier:

$$\lambda_{ij}(t) = \lambda_0(t)u_i e^{\sum_2^G \beta_g I(g_{ij}=g)}$$

Regardless of the outcome distribution, inference is based on the estimated β_g.

While the methods in Section 4.4.1 can generate unbiased results and, under some conditions, equal power with the more complex methods described here, these more complex methods are more flexible. For example, incorporating potential confounders and other covariates is transparently simple. More importantly, they easily accommodate complicated designs.

One important complex design is the variety of crossover design used in the REDUCE study. The design called for a baseline period in which no intervention was introduced to any cluster, followed by an intervention period in which just one group received the intervention. In the mixed-model setting, it is simple to configure the equation for an appropriate difference-in-differences analysis:

$$\lambda_{ij}(t) = \lambda_0(t)u_i e^{\sum_{g=2}^{G} \beta_g I(g_{ij}=g) + \beta_3 I(t_{ij}=2) + \sum_{g=2}^{G} \beta_{(3+g)}[I(g_{ij}=g)I(t_{ij}=2)]} \qquad (4.3)$$

where we code the time period in which subject ij was observed 1 for the baseline and 2 for the intervention period, and subjects in "usual care" hospitals have $g_{ij} = 0$, those in the "targeted decolonization" have $g_{ij} = 1$, and those in the "universal decolonization" hospitals have $g_{ij} = 2$.

In the previous equation, e^{β_1} is the relative hazard for the targeted decolonization group in the baseline period, relative to the usual care group, and e^{β_2} is the hazard ratio for the universal decolonization group. The value e^{β_3} is the relative hazard for the usual care group in the intervention period relative to the baseline. Our main interest centers on e^{β_4} and e^{β_5}, which describe how the change between periods in the two intervention arms differs from the change in the usual care arm. A joint test to assess the null hypothesis that these two parameters are both 0 is the main test for the trial.

While the symbolic description and motivation for the model and the analysis are elegant, fitting the model is sometimes complicated. For example, it is sometimes necessary to try several maximum-finding techniques before discovering the one that will successfully iterate to a maximum. For some complex models, for example, frailty models with different frailty variance per group or with multiple levels of clustering, it may not be possible to find standard software for the analysis.

For models such as those shown in Equation 4.1, SAS PROC GLIMMIX (SAS Institute, 2014) or the R functions in the nlme (Pinheiro et al., 2014) or lme4 (Bates et al., 2014) packages can be used to fit the models. For frailty models such as those described in Equations 4.2 and 4.3, SAS PROC PHREG or the survival package (Therneau, 2014) in R can be used.

4.4.2.2 Generalized Estimating Equations

Another way of allowing clustering in a model without violating model assumptions is to use generalized estimating equations (GEEs) (Liang and Zeger, 1986, Zeger and Liang, 1986).

Briefly, GEEs treat the correlation within cluster as a nuisance parameter, without specifying a model from which this correlation might have arisen.

The parameter estimates are generated under the assumption of no correlation, but the standard errors of the estimates are corrected to account for the clustering. An attractive option is to further protect against an incorrectly specified correlation structure by using the "sandwich" estimator, which modifies the standard error. GEEs have the same modeling advantages that GLMMs have.

While GEEs are less commonly used in CRTs than GLMMs are, some authors suggest that when there are small numbers of clusters, the parametric assumptions associated with mixed-effects models may not be dependable. In such cases, they suggest that GEEs may be a viable alternative. While for normal outcomes, this may be acceptable, it pays to be cautious when using GEEs for dichotomous or count variables, as described in Section 4.4.3.

4.4.3 Interpretation

Interpretation of the two-stage approach is simple: either a difference in the means of the statistics was found or it was not. Interpretation of the model parameters depends on the outcome; a mean difference for normal outcomes, a log odds ratio for dichotomous outcomes, a log risk ratio for count outcomes.

However, there is a subtle but important difference between the GLMM and GEE approaches to modeling, often described as the difference between subject-specific and population average models. In nonlinear models, the two approaches are actually estimating different quantities. For example, the odds ratio estimated in the GLMM is the odds ratio *for a subject in an average cluster*. (Average here meaning average among the clusters in the analysis.) In other words, $e^{\beta_{GLMM}}$ estimates the relative odds a subject would experience if their cluster was moved from, for example, the control arm to the intervention arm. This is the subject-specific effect. In contrast, the odds ratio estimated from a GEE is the relative odds attributable to the intervention *for an average subject* in the population, averaging across the various clusters. This is the population average effect. It may be helpful in understanding this to recall that the GEE estimate is the same estimate as would be obtained from the model ignoring cluster. The GLMM estimate is not.

The difference is demonstrated in Figure 4.2 using a continuous covariate. The solid lines are the predicted probabilities in each cluster, while the dotted line is the population average. The solid lines have different random intercepts but share the same within-cluster effect of the covariate x. The observed relationship in this case, that the subject-specific slopes are steeper, can be proven mathematically to always be the case (McCulloch and Searle, 2001). However, it would be incorrect to claim that either of the estimates is biased. Instead, both are unbiased estimates, but of different underlying population characteristics.

In many cases, the subject-specific effect is a more appropriate estimate for CRTs. Since subjects will always experience the intervention within a cluster,

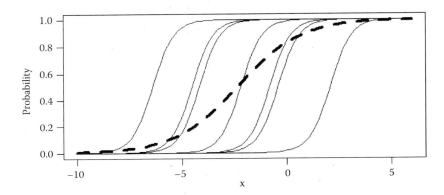

FIGURE 4.2
Demonstrating the difference between subject-specific effects (in the solid lines) and population average effects (in the dashed line). The solid lines reflect an odds ratio, within cluster, of 7.4; the population average odds ratio is 1.95.

we are often interested in the effects within clusters. From a clinician's perspective, for example, we want to know the effect of the drug on this patient, who belongs to a particular cluster, rather than for some generic average patient, averaged across the whole population. In the REDUCE study, our main interest is in what the effect on patients *in a hospital* will be, if we introduce, for example, the "universal decolonization" practice to the hospital. On the other hand, the population average effect may be interesting from a policy perspective, as is often the case in health services research. For example, in the REACH study, we may be interested in the global effect across the population if we make efforts to reduce antibiotic prescribing everywhere.

4.4.4 Accommodating Matching or Stratification

As discussed in Section 4.5.2, there are often reasons to stratify clusters before randomization. In the extreme, it may be desirable to match clusters into N groups of G clusters and assign one member of each cluster to each of the arms. Many discussions of this question focus on the cost, in degrees of freedom, of matching or stratifying, compared to the benefit in precision of estimates. In these discussions, it is assumed that an additional degree of freedom must be expended for each matched set or strata. The rationale for this lies in the two-stage approach and the analogy to the paired t-test.

Since there are often few clusters, this cost can seem prohibitive, which leads some practitioners away from stratification or matching. For example, if there are 10 clusters and 2 treatment groups, matching using this logic reduces the degrees of freedom from 8 to 4 and increases the t-statistic needed to reject the null from 2.3060041 to 2.7764451! An alternative approach is to break the matches, that is, to ignore the matching when doing the data analysis as if the matching had never occurred (Proschan, 1996, Diehr et al., 1995). In the example, rather than adjusting for each matched set, or actually taking the difference within pair and performing a paired t-test on the five differences, we would do a two-group t-test on the original 10 values. The citations provided above give simulation-based and analytic demonstrations that this procedure both maintains an appropriate alpha level and can be more powerful than retaining the matches in analysis.

4.5 Planning CRTs

Planning CRTs, from the statistician's perspective, comprises mainly an assessment of power and sample size and considerations of stratification in the randomization.

4.5.1 Power

At the most basic level, the difference between models for nonclustered data and models for clustered data is extra terms that define the clustering. So, analytic power calculations for these models depend on the usual parameters, plus these parameters. The expression of the degree of clustering most often used in power calculations is the intracluster correlation coefficient (ICC).

4.5.1.1 Intracluster Correlation Coefficient

For normal outcomes, the correlation between two subjects within any cluster is $\sigma_b^2 / (\sigma_b^2 + \sigma^2)$, using the notation from Section 4.4.2.1. This quantity is defined as the ICC and denoted ρ. In words, the ICC is the proportion of the total variability that is due to variability between clusters. In general, the ICC is not limited, though in particular areas of research typical values may be gleaned by experience. In health services research with large cluster sizes, ICCs larger than 0.1 are rarely observed, for example.

Note, however, that the definition as the ratio of two variance quantities makes sense mostly in the context of linear models in which the variance attributed to individuals within clusters (σ^2) and the variance attributable to the differences between clusters (σ_b^2) are independent and can be easily and sensibly separated. This is not true for logistic and Poisson outcomes, for example, since the mean and the variance depend on the same parameter.

It is possible to take the verbal definition and interpret it in the context of other distributions. For example, the total variability for dichotomous outcomes is $p_T(1 - p_T)$, where p_T is the average probability of the outcome across the population. And the variability between the clusters could be expressed as $\text{Var}(p_i)$, where p_i is the probability of the outcome within each cluster i. Following this logic, the ICC could be calculated as $\text{Var}(p_i)/(p_T(1-p_T))$.

From the perspective of the typical modeling framework, however, this seems awkward. In that light, we have, with two groups,

$$\log \text{it}(y_{ij}|b_i) = \beta_0 + \beta_1 I(g_{ij} = 1) + b_i$$

From this, we can see that the probability for a subject in cluster i, when i has $g_{ij} = 0$, is $\Pr(y_{ij}|b_i) = p_i = e^{\beta_0+b_i}/(1+e^{\beta_0+b_i})$. The variance for a subject in cluster i is $p_i(1-p_i)$. But for a subject in cluster i', the variance is $p_{i'}(1-p_{i'})$. There is simply not "a" variance within clusters to mimic the role of σ^2 in the model for normal outcomes. The importance of this difference is magnified if we consider the treatment arms. Clusters where $g_{ij} = 1$ clearly have a different within cluster *and* overall variance from those with $g_{ij} = 0$, if the study intervention has any effect. There is no known closed-form relationship between $\text{Var}(p_i)$ and σ_b^2, though an approximation has been proposed (Turner et al., 2001).

In contrast, in the normal setting, the conditional variance given the cluster, for all subjects, is σ^2.

Further complicating matter is the existence of a second definition of the ICC in dichotomous settings. This definition is based on the formulation that there is a latent, logistic-distributed variate that is dichotomized at some unknown cut-point to generate the observed dichotomous outcome. If this were the case, the total variance conditional on cluster would be $\Pi^2/3$ for any cluster, and the ICC would be $\sigma_b^2/(\sigma_b^2 + (\Pi^2/3))$. This at least depends on the model parameters. However, the two definitions do not approximate one another. And while authors sometimes report the ICC, it is often unclear which definition is reported (Eldridge et al., 2009).

Similar difficulties occur for count and survival outcomes, though these have not been so well explored. For these reasons, the focus on ICC as the central metric for assessing the impact of clustering in every setting seems misplaced.

4.5.1.2 *The Design Effect and Effective Sample Size*

The design effect D_{eff}, first discussed by Kish (1965), is defined as $1 + (M - 1)\rho$. In words, the D_{eff} is an approximate factor by which the variance has been artificially deflated, when the clustering has been ignored. Thus, it can be used to generate the "effective sample size," $\sum_{g,i} M_i/D_{\text{eff}}$. Using the effective sample size, power calculation can be performed using methods for uncorrelated data. The approximation can be surprisingly good in some cases, as shown in Figure 4.3. However, there are no strong arguments for using it in anything but preliminary stages. Also, note that the definition of design effect depends on equal cluster sizes.

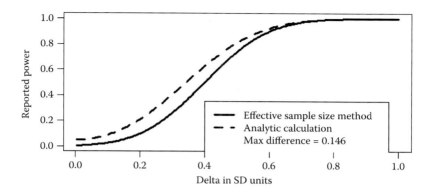

FIGURE 4.3
Comparing power estimated using the design effect and analytically, with ICC = 0.05, N = 5 clusters/arm, and M = 100 subjects/cluster, and alpha = 0.05.

4.5.1.3 Analytic Calculations

For some settings, such as normal outcomes with equal cluster sizes, analytic solutions to the power and sample size relationships exist. For example, for two groups with normal outcomes, there is a closed-form solution:

$$W = P\left(t_{df,\lambda} < t_{df}^{-1}\left(\frac{\alpha}{2}\right)\right) + P\left(t_{df,\lambda} > t_{df}^{-1}\left(\frac{1-\alpha}{2}\right)\right)$$

where $df = 2(N-1)$, $\lambda = d/[2(1+(N-1)\rho)/MN]^{1/2}$, $d = (\mu_1 - \mu_2)/\sigma$, μ_g is the mean in group g, and N is the number of clusters in each group (Donner and Klar, 1996). Also, $t_{k,\lambda}$ is a variate from the noncentral t, distribution with k degrees of freedom and noncentrality parameter λ, and $t_k^{-1}(a)$ is the ath quantile from the central t distribution with k degrees of freedom. The central role of ρ in this expression is why so much effort and discussion is devoted to the ICC.

It may be interesting to compare the resulting analytic power to the approximation based on the effective sample size discussed in Section 4.5.1.2. An example of the relationship is shown in Figure 4.3. In general, as the number of clusters increases, the approximation quickly improves. It worsens, slightly, as M increases and ρ decreases.

The accuracy of the effective sample size approximation and the role of the ICC provide a way to quickly grasp the difficulty of the power calculation for CRTs. With as few as 1000 subjects per cluster, increasing the ICC from 0.001 to 0.002 results in a 33% loss of effective sample size. In contrast, the confidence limits for estimated ICC are likely to be much broader than 0.001. Cluster sizes of 1,000 or greater are common in trials involving health delivery systems or communities, such as the REDUCE and REACH trials described in Section 4.2.

Approximate closed-form analytic results are available for dichotomous outcomes. These are effectively normal-approximation results of the design effect approach outlined in Section 4.5.1.2. Thus, they are less likely to be useful, despite their presence in common power assessment packages. Further approximation allows an analytic result for count data, assuming a Poisson distribution for the outcome (Hayes and Bennett, 1999, Donner and Klar, 2000).

Note, however, that each of these analytic approaches depends on D_{eff}, which is undefined when cluster size varies. In addition, as noted above, the ICC, an integral part of D_{eff}, does not have an agreed definition except for normal outcomes. Finally, there may not be analytic results, approximate or exact, for time-to-event outcomes.

One way to avoid these problems is to use a within-cluster summary approach to power calculation. Analogous to Section 4.4.1, assume a t-test or ANOVA with N_g observations (of the summary statistic) in each group. This approach is more dependent on the requirement of equal sample sizes and requires estimates of the variability of the summary statistics. Such estimates may be difficult to obtain from a literature focused on estimates of the ICC.

Another approach is to attempt to accommodate the variability of M_i in analytic calculations. Several approaches to this have been made for various settings (Manatunga et al., 2001, Kong et al., 2003, Eldridge et al., 2006, Teerenstra et al., 2012, Hemming and Marsh, 2013). However, the full distribution of M_i would appear to have some bearing on the power and may not be fully accounted for in methods that rely on just the mean and variance.

4.5.1.4 Power Estimation by Simulation

When the outcome is not normal, or when the clusters differ widely in size, a useful alternative is to estimate power by simulation. Since it is quite common for one of these situations to obtain, it may be worthwhile to use a simulation method by default.

Briefly, the routine is to simulate data under the alternative, evaluate whether the null hypothesis was rejected, and repeat. The proportion of observed rejections is an estimate of the power. This is an immensely flexible technique. While it does require some coding ability, it is not especially difficult. And this approach has the extremely desirable feature that the power assessment can mirror the proposed analytic technique as precisely as desired. The R package clusterPower (Reich et al., 2012) implements this approach for normal, dichotomous, and Poisson data.

A basic algorithm for a simulation assessment of power for a normal outcome, for two groups, is as follows:

1. Sample cluster sizes M_i.
2. Sample random effects b_i.

3. For each cluster i:
   a. Sample residual error e_{ij} from a normal distribution.
   b. Calculate $y_{ij} = \beta_0 + \beta_1 I(g_{ij} = 1) + \cdots + b_i + e_{ij}$.
4. Perform planned data analysis; record whether the null hypothesis was rejected.
5. Repeat previous steps K times.

The power is estimated by $\sum r_k/K$, where $r_k = 1$ if the null was rejected in iteration k. We can then calculate confidence interval (CI) for $\sum r_k/K$ based on properties of the binomial distribution. The key element here in specifying the alternative is the choice of β_1 in Step 3b. Note also that differing cluster sizes can be accommodated through Step 1. The process can easily be adapted to dichotomous data by omitting the e_{ij} and by calculating $y_{ij} = 1$ if a uniform random variate is less than the expit of $\beta_0 + \beta_1 I(g_{ij} = 1) + \cdots + b_i$. In this case, the intercept β_0 can be specified as the logit of the proportion with the outcome in the control or usual care group. Similarly, for a count outcome, omit e_{ij} and draw y_{ij} as a Poisson or negative binomial random variate.

As with the other approaches to power, it is necessary to estimate the association within cluster, here through the distribution of the b_i in Step 2. Typically, this will be modeled by a normal distribution with mean 0. In that case, it would make sense to simulate it that way as well so that we need to estimate the variance σ_b^2. This is less commonly reported than the ICC, unfortunately. So, finding a plausible value in the literature may be difficult.

4.5.1.5 Power via Resampling

If it is possible to obtain extensive data prior to the power assessment, it may be possible to use resampling methods to estimate power. This resembles the simulation approach described in the previous section, but instead of simulating values from various distributions, we draw them, either explicitly or implicitly, from our best guess at their actual distributions, namely, from observed data. This is most likely to be useful in projects that rely on electronic medical records or billing data.

With such data in hand, a resampling algorithm for power would be as follows:

1. Within each cluster i, resample M_i observations.
2. Randomize the clusters to intervention groups.
3. Alter the y_{ij} values in some groups to reflect the alternative.
4. Perform the planned data analysis on the resampled data.
5. Record whether the null was rejected or not.
6. Repeat.

Power can then be estimated as in Section 4.5.1.4 (Kleinman and Huang, 2014).

When the data are available, this approach has many advantages. Briefly, it easily maintains the actual distribution of cluster sizes, avoids the need to estimate either ICC or σ_b^2, and incorporates variability likely to be observed in σ_b^2 or ρ. It can easily include covariates and do so with faithfulness to the true relationships within the data. Potential confounders can be used to match the clusters according to the planned method for the trial (see Section 4.5.2).

Perhaps most importantly, it can accommodate any planned analysis, meaning that accurate power assessment is possible using this method when analytic results are not available and when it may be difficult to simulate data for the approach described in Section 4.5.1.4.

For example, in a follow-up project to the REDUCE trial described in Section 4.2.1, we plan to assess a similar intervention applied more broadly across the hospital. Fortunately, the data collected for the REDUCE trial include very similar data. The planned analysis will use the frailty model described in Equation 4.3. There exists no analytic approach to a power calculation for this model, as far as we know. In addition, the sizes of the hospitals vary widely; any analytic solution depending on a constant sample size would be inappropriate. We could conceivably simulate to estimate power. However, the distribution of time to infection and the distribution of censoring time do not conform to any common distributions. Rather than attempt to mimic them mathematically, the resampling approach described above seems likely to improve accuracy and save time.

The algorithm in this case is more complicated, since there is a baseline period followed by an intervention period, and the planned analysis is a difference in differences. The study leaders anticipated preventing 20% of the infections they would have otherwise expected. The algorithm is as follows:

1. Within each cluster i, resample M_i observations to serve as the baseline period data.

2. Randomize the clusters to intervention groups.

3. Within each cluster i, resample a new set of M_i observations to serve as the intervention period data.

4. Randomize some clusters to be in the "intervention" arm.

5. Alter the y_{ij} values of subjects in the intervention clusters: select 20% of them at random to change their events to be censored instead; these represent infections prevented by the intervention.

6. Fit the frailty model to the resampled data as in Equation 4.3.

7. Repeat.

4.5.2 Stratification or Matching

Another important aspect of planning CRTs is the question of whether and how to stratify or, in the extreme, to match. I will refer to "matching," intending to include stratification as well. Many discussions of matching refer to the power cost of matching, following, for example, Martin et al. (1993). However, there are nonpower gains to be made, and the power cost of matching is nil if the strategy of breaking the pairs (see Section 4.4.4) is followed.

A useful perspective on matching is to recall that while there may be many experimental units in a CRT, there are fewer randomization units. In general, it is as unrealistic to assume covariate balance will be achieved by a simple randomization in a CRT of 20 clusters as in an IRT of 20 individuals. Thus, it will likely be important to use matching to help prevent possible confounding. It is certainly true that readers of CRTs will seek information about whether balance was achieved on known confounders and will be concerned about lack of balance.

The typical design and process of CRTs means that it may be possible to use refined matching techniques not possible in IRTs that randomize patients as they enroll. In IRTs, it may be impossible to stratify randomization by more than one or two factors within site. In contrast, in CRTs, there is often extensive information about each cluster available before the trial begins. Thus, it is possible to use matching to seek balance on many possible confounders simultaneously.

But how should this be done? For example, in the REDUCE trial, it was desirable to ensure balance on the baseline prevalence of MRSA, and also on the capacity or patient volume of the hospital. Both were deemed important, but not equally so: baseline prevalence could well be a confounder if imbalanced, while baseline hospital probably less so. A natural thought for a statistician would be to make pairs that minimized the average Euclidean distance or Mahalanobis distance between pairs. But the need for matching is informal enough that there is no particular need to treat an absolute unit or a standardized unit difference as the "correct" distance to minimize. For example, if prevalence is very important, one could weigh differences on this factor more than differences in volume.

In fact, an infinite variety of weights exist, and matching schemes need not be based so directly on distance. What is needed is a way to compare matching schemes before randomization. To do this, I suggest the following procedure. First, construct matches via several plausible methods. Then, perform a faux "randomization" using those pairs; that is, randomly assign each cluster to a treatment arm, knowing that this is not the actual study assignment. Next, assess the balance as it will be assessed in the trial reports: for example, calculate the mean of each factor in each group and take the difference between the arms. Repeat this "randomization" many times. The result is a set of balance assessments for each factor that can be plotted, showing the range and distribution of differences that are likely to be achieved.

In the REDUCE trial, we tried several schemes: (a) match only on baseline prevalence; (b) match only on volume; make strata of (c) 6, (d) 9, or (e) 12 hospitals with similar prevalence, then match within strata by volume; and (f) match on the product of prevalence and volume. The result was six scatterplots, from which the investigators were able to select the one they felt best balanced the risk of imbalance and potential for confounding.

In the follow-up trial, we wanted to balance eight different factors. For that trial, I tried matching on the six-dimensional Euclidean distance, but also assessed different weighting schemes. I compared the results using a parallel coordinates plot.

Results are shown in Figures 4.4 through 4.6. Each axis plots the absolute value of the mean difference between two arms, on a scale of 0–1 standard deviation. Without dwelling on the features we wanted to balance, it is clear that matching only on all-pathogen bacteremia (the second axis), as shown in Figure 4.6, achieves better balance on this factor than either of the other matching strategies. However, the balance achieved does not appear to be markedly better for this strategy than it was when matching on Euclidean distance (Figure 4.5). And matching on Euclidean distance was much superior for all of the other factors. In this case, matching on Euclidean distance was acceptable to the investigators. In other settings, the investigators might use the same information to choose the strategy shown in Figure 4.6.

Another option for ensuring balance is "restricted randomization": limiting acceptable randomizations to those that meet some balance criteria. When using this approach, care must be taken to ensure that each cluster, and each pair of clusters, has approximately equal arm assignment probabilities (Moulton, 2004). Typically, with greater restrictions on acceptable randomizations, there are increasingly unequal arm assignment probabilities. In addition, it is unclear what an acceptable amount of inequality across

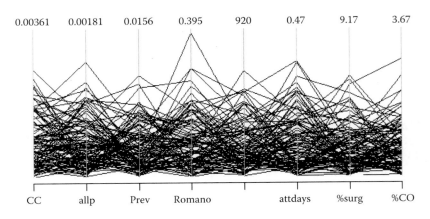

FIGURE 4.4
No matching: simple randomization.

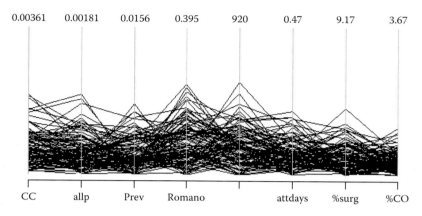

FIGURE 4.5
Match to minimize Euclidean distance.

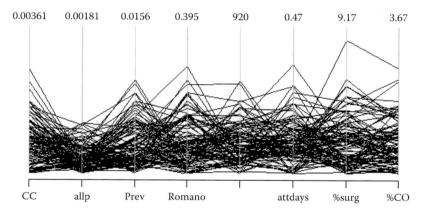

FIGURE 4.6
Match to minimize difference in prevalence of all-pathogen bacteremia, the second axis.

the arms may be. Unless inequality is very slight, it seems safer to use some sort of matching scheme.

4.6 Discussion

CRTs can be inexpensive compared to IRTs of similar sizes, especially if the opportunity to relax protocols and data collection are seized upon. These can result in natural comparative effectiveness trials that measure how a treatment or other intervention is likely to affect a typical patient in a typical setting. In the limit, CRTs can be *pragmatic* trials, in which the machinery of the trial interferes minimally with the implementation of care under the intervention. The REDUCE trial is a good example of a pragmatic CER trial.

In this chapter, I presented case studies of CRTs and reviewed some aspects of analysis and planning of CRTs. I have not attempted to survey the entire literature. In addition to the mentioned texts by Eldridge and Kerry (2012), Hayes and Moulton (2009), and Donner and Klar (2000), the reader is referred to the excellent foundational work by Murray (1998), to which I owe my own introduction and interest in this area.

References

Bates, D., Maechler, M., Bolker, B., Walker, S. 2014. *lme4: Linear Mixed-Effects Models Using Eigen and S4*. R package version 1.1-7.

Breslow, N.E., Clayton, D.G. 1993. Approximate inference in generalized linear mixed models. *Journal of the American Statistical Association*. 88:9–25.

Cornfield, J. 1978. Randomization by group: A formal analysis. *American Journal of Epidemiology*. 108:100–102.

Diehr, P., Martin, D.C., Koepsell, T.D., Cheadle, A. 1995. Breaking the matches in a paired t-test for community interventions when the number of pairs is small. *Statistics in Medicine*. 14:1491–1504.

Donner, A., Klar, N. 1996. Statistical considerations in the design and analysis of community intervention trials. *Journal of Clinical Epidemiology*. 49:435–439.

Donner, A., Klar, N. 2000. *Design and Analysis of Cluster Randomization Trials in Health Research*. Wiley, Chichester.

Eldridge, S., Kerry S. 2012. *A Practical Guide to Cluster Randomised Trials in Health Services Research*. Wiley, Chichester.

Eldridge, S.M., Ashby, D., Kerry, S. 2006. Sample size for cluster randomized trials: Effect of coefficient of variation of cluster size and analysis method. *International Journal of Epidemiology*. 35:1292–1300.

Eldridge, S.M., Ukoumunne, O.C., Carlin, J.B. 2009. The intra-cluster correlation coefficient in cluster randomized trials: A review of definitions. *International Statistical Review*. 77:378–394.

Finkelstein, J.A., Huang, S.S., Kleinman, K., Rifas-Shiman, S.L., Stille, C.J., Daniel, J., Schiff, N. et al. 2008. Impact of a 16-community trial to promote judicious antibiotic use in Massachusetts. *Pediatrics*. 121:e15–e23.

Hayes, R.J., Bennett, S. 1999. Simple sample size calculation for cluster-randomized trials. *International Journal of Epidemiology*. 29:319–326.

Hayes, R.J., Moulton, L.H. 2009. *Cluster Randomized Trials*. Chapman & Hall/CRC, Boca Raton.

Hemming, K., Marsh, J. 2013. A menu-driven facility for sample-size calculations in cluster randomized controlled trials. *The Stata Journal*. 13:114–135.

Huang, S.S., Septimus, E., Kleinman, K., Moody, J., Hickok, J., Avery, T.R., Lankiewicz, J. et al. 2013. Targeted versus universal decolonization to prevent ICU infection. *New England Journal of Medicine*. 368:2255–2265.

Kish, L. 1965. *Survey Sampling*. Wiley, New York.

Kleinman, K.P., Huang, S.S. 2014. *Calculating Power by Bootstrap, with an Application to Cluster-Randomized Trials*. arXiv:1410.3515 [stat.AP].

Kong, S.-H., Ahn, C.W., Jung, S.-H. 2003. Sample size calculation for dichotomous outcomes in cluster randomization trials with varying cluster size. *Therapeutic Innovation and Regulatory Science*. 37:109–114.

Laird, N. M., Ware, J. H. 1982. Random effects models for longitudinal data. *Biometrics*. 38:963–974.

Liang, K. Y., Zeger, S. L. 1986. Longitudinal data analysis using generalized linear models. *Biometrika*. 73:13–22.

Manatunga, A.K., Hudgens, M.G., Chen, S.D. 2001. Sample size estimation in cluster randomized studies with varying cluster size. *Biometrical Journal*. 43:75–86.

Martin, D.C., Diehr, P., Perrin, E.B., Koepsell, T.D. 1993. The effect of matching on the power of randomized community intervention studies. *Statistics in Medicine*. 12:329–338.

McCulloch, C.E., Searle, S.R. 2001. *Generalized, Linear, and Mixed Models*. Wiley, New York.

Moulton, L.H. 2004. Covariate-based constrained randomization of group-randomized trials. *Clinical Trials*. 1:297–305.

Murray, D.M. 1998. *Design and Analysis of Group-Randomized Trials*. Oxford University Press, New York.

Pinheiro, J., Bates, D., DebRoy, S., Sarkar, D., R Core Team. 2014. *nlme: Linear and Nonlinear Mixed Effects Models*. R package version 3.1-117.

Proschan, M.A. 1996. On the distribution of the unpaired t-statistic with paired data. *Statistics in Medicine*. 15:1059–1063.

Reich, N.G., Myers, J.A., Obeng, D., Milstone, A.M., Perl, T.M. 2012. Empirical power and sample size calculations for cluster-randomized and cluster-randomized crossover studies. *PLoS One*. 7(4):e35564.

Ripatti, S., Palmgren, J. 2000. Estimation of multivariate frailty models using penalized partial likelihood. *Biometrics*. 56:1016–1022.

SAS Institute. 2014. Cary, NC.

Taveras, E.M., Marshall, R., Horan, C.M., Gillman, M.W., Hacker, K., Kleinman, K.P., Koziol, R., Price, S., Simon, S.R. 2013. Rationale and design of the STAR randomized controlled trial to accelerate adoption of childhood obesity comparative effectiveness research. *Contemporary Clinical Trials*. 34:101–108.

Teerenstra, S., Eldridge, S., Graff, M., de Hoop, E., Borm, G.F. 2012. A simple sample size formula for analysis of covariance in cluster randomized trials. *Statistics in Medicine*. 31:2169–2178.

Therneau T. 2014. *A Package for Survival Analysis in S*. R package version 2.37-7.

Turner, R.M., Omar, R.Z., Thompson, S.G. 2001. Bayesian methods of analysis for cluster randomized trials with binary outcome data. *Statistics in Medicine*. 20:453–472.

Zeger, S.L., Liang, K.Y. 1986. Longitudinal data analysis for discrete and continuous outcomes. *Biometrics*. 42:121–130.

5

Bayesian Adaptive Designs

Jason T. Connor

CONTENTS

ABSTRACT   Bayesian analysis facilitates the incorporation of information from many sources and is particularly well suited for the ongoing learning character of comparative effectiveness research. This chapter discusses the use of Bayesian analysis in comparative effectiveness research and focuses on the design and analysis of studies using adaptive designs.

5.1 Bayesian Analysis and Comparative Effectiveness Research

Blaise Pascal, one of the first probabilists, once apologetically wrote to a friend, "I would have written a shorter letter, but I did not have the time." Clinical trials are much like letters—they are frequently inefficient because we often fail to put enough time and thought into their planning. Also like a poorly written letter, a poorly planned clinical trial may fail to convey the right message.

The Agency for Healthcare Research and Quality (AHRQ) cites two key methods by which evidence is found for comparative effectiveness research (CER). The first is "researchers look at all of the available evidence about the benefits and harms of each choice for different groups of people from existing clinical trials, clinical studies, and other research." The second is "researchers conduct studies that generate new evidence of effectiveness or comparative effectiveness of a test, treatment, procedure, or health-care service" [1]. This chapter focuses on the latter—when new research is designed to provide comparative effectiveness evidence and why the Bayesian approach is ideally suited to this context.

We describe first how the tenets of Bayesian analysis can be used to synthesize information in an intuitive comparative effectiveness manner. We then illustrate two Bayesian adaptive trial design features suitable for CER trials. Because many CER trials have more than two arms, we describe adaptive randomization, which may offer greater statistical power and, on average, lead to a greater proportion of patients receiving safer and/or more efficacious therapies. We also describe adaptive sample size or early stopping, which may offer efficiency by using only the patient resources and time necessary to answer the primary clinical question. Finally, we describe platform trials as a CER trial methodology for rapidly screening drugs for the same indication in a preapproval setting. While we describe methods for comparative effectiveness trials that, like a good letter, may require greater forethought and planning than most clinical trials, they offer the promise of shorter, more efficient trials that treat patients both in the trial and on the horizon better. This chapter assumes a working knowledge of Bayesian analysis. For a thorough review of Bayesian analysis, see Berry and Stangl [2], Krushke [3], Gelman et al. [4], or Carlin and Louis [5]. Lilford and Braunholtz provide a succinct discussion of why Bayesian analysis is well suited for public policy [6].

5.2 Bayesian Analysis

The synthesis of all available information is a hallmark of Bayesian analysis. Bayesian analyses can formally incorporate existing high-quality evidence (the prior distribution) while also allowing for the prospective trial to adapt to accumulating information (the posterior distribution).

Bayesian posterior probabilities reflect prior and current evidence and today's posterior distribution is tomorrow's prior distribution. The posterior can be sequentially updated as new evidence becomes available, and is independent of a particular experimental design. The frequentist or classical approach is less adept at synthesizing various data sources and explicitly dependent upon experimental design [7].

Bayesian inference is also ideally suited for CER because it allows competing treatment strategies or healthcare services to be ranked probabilistically rather than classical methods, which rely heavily on hypothesis testing. A frequentist analysis might consider the confidence interval around the treatment effect estimates. Inference would be based on whether the interval contains the null. On the other hand, a Bayesian analysis might calculate the probability each of many competing treatment strategies offers the highest proportion of responders, or the probability each treatment has the lowest adverse event rate. Furthermore, utility functions could be constructed to weigh various efficacy, safety, and quality of life metrics, so rankings can consider various outcomes simultaneously.

Imagine the simplest case where 300 patients are evenly randomized to three competing treatments: a device, a drug, and instructions for a behavioral change. After randomization and treatment, we observe 57/100 responders in the device group, 50/100 responders in the drug group, and 43/100 responders in the behavioral change group. A standard 2 d.f. chi-square test yields p-value = 0.14 and a decision that we cannot reject the hypothesis that all three treatments truly have the same response rate. That, however, is an unsatisfying conclusion for a physician needing to choose between one of these three treatments for a patient. She may reasonably conclude, other factors such as safety signals and cost being equal, to choose the treatment with the highest observed rate. But how good a decision is that? Or how should the doctor answer if a patient asks, "How sure are you this is the best option, doc?"

With the same data, a Bayesian analysis with uniform (flat/noninformative) priors on the response rates produces the inference that the device has a 83% chance of offering the highest response rate, the drug has a 16% chance of having the highest response rate, and the behavior change has a 1% chance of having the highest response rate. Instead of a flat prior, historical data could also be used to additionally inform this inference.

5.3 Bayesian Adaptive Designs

When comparative effectiveness analyses lead to ambiguous comparisons, we might desire more evidence in hopes of reaching a definitive conclusion. The highest-quality new information is typically acquired via prospective, randomized-controlled clinical trials.

A challenge of comparative effectiveness trials is that the difference between two efficacious therapies is typically smaller than the difference between either therapy and a placebo. Furthermore, many argue that CER trials are best conducted in a pragmatic fashion [8,9], which more appropriately reflects actual clinical practice but also increases within-trial variability.

Searching for a smaller effect size amidst greater trial variability requires much larger sample sizes and longer trials.

Another challenge is that comparative effectiveness trials most often focus on commercially available treatments, and therefore study participation is not usually necessary to receive a particular treatment (as opposed to preapproval trials where a study drug may not be available outside the trial). In such cases, a patient need not submit to a trial in order to receive the therapy she and her doctor identify as best for her. Furthermore, in lengthy trials, new evidence from other trials or case series may become available during the course of the study. If randomization is fixed throughout the course of the trial, this new information may upset study equipoise, accrual rates may slow down, and the trial may be difficult to complete. We describe adaptive randomization and adaptive sample size (early stopping) as methods to combat these challenges.

5.4 Adaptive Randomization

Too often, clinical practice and clinical research are at odds. This is particularly true in comparative effectiveness research when several approved and available therapies are compared. In a traditional protocol with fixed randomization, patients will continue to be randomized to treatments as evidence accumulates both within the trial and potentially from other studies (randomized-controlled trials or case series published during the course of the CER trial). And while we perform randomized clinical trials to eventually treat patients better, convention holds that patients within the trial rarely reap this benefit. In a trial with adaptive randomization, as the study progresses, patients and their clinicians will know they have a higher likelihood of being randomized to a treatment identified as being most beneficial. Furthermore, in a multiarm trial, focusing randomization to the best few treatment strategies increases statistical power. Imagine 100 additional patients are to be randomized in the simple three-arm trial described above. The behavioral therapy is performing poorly, but according to a standard 2 d.f. statistical test it is not demonstrably worse, and therefore a data monitoring board may not terminate accrual to that arm. However, continuing with equal randomization, one-third, or 33 patients, may be randomized to an inferior arm (providing them with little benefit). If the additional patients are randomized only to the drug and device arms, it would increase the study's power to discern between the two best treatment options.

To implement adaptive randomization, the trialists must consider (1) the aggressiveness of adaptive randomization and (2) when to conduct the first and each subsequent update to the adaptive randomization probabilities.

One general option for adaptive randomization is probability-weighted adaptive randomization, letting the randomization probabilities, R_D, in the next stage take the form

$$R_D \sim \frac{\theta_D^k}{\sum_{D=1}^{3} \theta_D^k}$$

where $k = 0$ would lead to fixed randomization, $R_D = 1/3$ throughout the trial, $k = 1$ would have the randomization probabilities match the probability each drug offers the highest response rate, $R_D = \theta_D$, and $k = \infty$ would randomize all patients in the next wave to the drug most likely to be the best—even if only marginally so at an interim analysis. Therefore, the coefficient k reflects the aggressiveness of the randomization, with higher values of k representing more aggressive adaptive randomization. Another choice is to let $k = n/N$, where n is the current sample size at an interim analysis and N is the maximum trial size. This results in a more conservative adaptive randomization early (closer to equal randomization) and allows it to become more aggressive as the trial progresses.

Another possible randomization function is information-based adaptive randomization where the randomization probability is also a function of each treatment's standard error and sample size:

$$R_D \sim \sqrt{\frac{\theta_D Var(p_D)}{n_D + 1}}$$

where θ_D remains the probability each arm, D, is the best, $Var(p_D)$ is the variance of each treatment effect, and n_D is the current sample size on each treatment arm. The R_D's are reweighted so that the probabilities sum to 1.

The consequence of including the effect size, variance, and sample size is that if a dose has a lower randomization probability at an early stage (leading to fewer patients being randomized to that treatment, a smaller sample size at subsequent analyses, and hence a higher variance) but appears more similar at a later interim, this randomization function assigns more patients to that treatment so it will catch up in total sample size.

At prespecified times—either based on number of patients enrolled, number of patients with outcomes, or calendar time—the unblinded trial team can perform interim analyses to update adaptive randomization probabilities. There is no single optimal choice for timing, though current technology allows for the selection of update frequency to be very rapid, including updating randomization for every single patient such as the ASTIN stroke trial [10].

In many trials, the question of when to conduct the adaptive randomization updates is a function of accrual rate and the time at which the primary outcome is observed. For example, if a trial enrolls 100 patients per month and the trial is a 90-day outcome, then 300 patients will be enrolled before any patient's primary outcomes are known. Therefore, adaptive randomization works best in settings where there is primary endpoint information to adapt to, those with slower accrual and/or short-term primary or surrogate outcomes.

A published CER trial example is the established status epilepticus treatment trial (ESETT) [11,12] comparing three frequently used therapies for patients not responding to first-line seizure medications. The primary outcome is a dichotomous responder endpoint: cessation of seizures within 20 min of the start of study drug infusion without recurrent seizures or a serious adverse event within 1 h. Therefore, the primary outcome, the response rate in each group, can be modeled as a probability, p_D, for $D \in \{1, 2, 3\}$.

While each of the three drugs included are commonly used for status epilepticus, there is little published evidence that includes this composite outcome. Therefore, the trial will use uninformative uniform priors for each study drug

$$p_D \sim Beta(1, 1)$$

Once x_D responses are observed in N_D patients randomized to drug D, the posterior probability for each response rate is

$$p_D | x_D, N_D \sim Beta(1 + x_D, 1 + N_D - x_G)$$

The probability that drug 1 then offers the highest response rate is

$$\theta_1 = Pr\,(p_1 = \max(p_1, p_2, p_3))$$

$$= \int_0^1 \int_0^{p_1} \int_0^{p_1} f(p_1|x_1, N_1) f(p_2|x_2, N_2) f(p_3|x_3, N_3) dp_3 dp_2 dp_1$$

where $f(p_D|x_D, N_D)$ is the pdf of the beta distribution.

In ESETT, the primary response is known within hours. Therefore, when considering the time for the first interim analysis, for example, simulating alternatives and exploring operating characteristics can be used to compare various trade-offs. Performing the first interim sooner will result, on average, in more patients being randomized to the best treatment, but it will also result in a higher probability (albeit rare) that the truly best arm is considered poor and receives fewer subsequent patients. There is no optimal choice of k, or analytical solution for k. Rather, one must simulate trials using various choices of k and their corresponding operating characteristics and individual trials. The earlier the first interim analysis, the less data available and the greater the natural variability. Therefore, there is a chance the best treatment will look worse, its randomization probability—especially with a high choice of k—will be closer to zero, and it never has a "second chance to make first impression." It can be combatted with a more conservative choice of k and/or a later first interim analysis. Later first looks may slightly decrease study power and decrease the proportion of patients randomized to the best treatment(s). In ESETT, the first update to adaptive randomization occurs when 300 out of the maximum 800 patients are enrolled and updates to adaptive randomization occur after every additional 100 patients are enrolled.

5.5 Adaptive Sample Size

A second adaptive trial design feature particularly well suited to CER trials is adaptive sample size or early stopping—terminating the trial as soon as we realize it is futile to continue, or as soon as the results are scientifically credible to report. Because many CER trials require large sample sizes and are lengthy to conduct, medical advances continue to be developed, studied, and published during the blinded phase of the CER trial. A large CER trial can be irrelevant by the time their results are announced [13]. Therefore, the faster the results are reported, the greater impact they can have on clinical practice.

Group sequential trials are well established and commonly used but tend to be conservative in their stopping rules in order to conserve power at the trial's end. Also, many group sequential stopping rules are based upon events or patients reaching final outcomes. Therefore, when an interim analysis is conducted, many patients may be enrolled but not contribute to the analysis. If the trial ends, the trial incurred the cost of enrolling patients without allowing the patients to contribute to the primary analysis.

Bayesian adaptive trials may incorporate group sequential-like boundaries [14] but more tend to base their stopping on predictive probabilities [15,16]. Here, instead of calculating a test statistic at an interim analysis, we can calculate two predictive probabilities: P_n = the probability of obtaining a statistically significant result with the currently enrolled patients if enrollment were to stop and all patients followed to their final outcomes and P_{max} = the probability of obtaining a statistically significant result if the trial enrolls to the maximum sample size.

Then, at an interim analysis if P_n is greater than some predetermined threshold, for example, 90%, accrual can stop for predicted success. Patients are followed to their primary outcomes (e.g., 90-day mortality) and the final analysis is performed. This is similar to powering a trial at 90% but rather than basing the power calculation on pilot data or expert opinion, the accrual stops once 90% the probability of trial success is validated from internal trial data.

This provides the advantage that all enrolled patients provide evidence toward the primary analysis and allows for lower sample sizes. The analysis plan asks, "Are enough patients currently enrolled to provide credible evidence?" In contrast, the typical group sequential trials that ask, "Are there enough patients through their final outcomes to provide credible evidence?" Furthermore, less type I error is spent at interim analyses, and hence less type I error adjustment is necessary. In a group sequential trial, a random high may result in a type I error; to limit these errors, the bar is set quite high to stop a trial early. When using predictive probabilities, if an erroneous random high leads to stopping for predicted success, then, many times, the final analysis fails to achieve its goal due to regression to the mean with the outstanding patients. These do not result in type I errors. Whereas if a treatment effect is truly present, then the data will continue to be positive and the trial will be successful. Therefore, a smaller multiplicity adjustment is necessary than in group sequential trials. The shorter the follow-up and fewer the outstanding patients, the more similar the two methods become. But for longer follow-up times and faster accrual, less adjustment for multiplicity is necessary. This may in turn allow for more frequent interim analyses for early stopping.

Similarly, if P_{max} is smaller than some predetermined value at an interim analysis, for example, less than 10%, the trial would stop for futility. It should be established *a priori* whether hitting such a futility bound is automatically a cause for futility stopping, or whether a data monitoring board has discretion whether to allow the trial to continue.

We call this combination of stopping rules the Goldilocks adaptive sample size algorithm because the aim is to get the sample size just right [15]. The predictive probabilities are most easily calculated via simulation by the following [16]:

1. Calculate current posteriors.
2. Calculate the predictive distribution for outstanding patients (enrolled but not at final outcomes for P_n and additionally patients on the horizon for P_{max}).
3. Based upon "complete" imputed data set, calculate the final test statistic and compare it to the established critical value.

Repeating steps 1–3 many (e.g., 10,000) times will estimate these predictive probabilities of trial success.

One key advantage of predictive probabilities is that they are more easily interpretable compared to p-values at interim analyses. For example, consider a simple one-sample trial with a dichotomous outcome. If the historical response rate is 50%, the trial may need to show that the response rate of the new treatment is greater than 50%. In a fixed, 100-patient Bayesian trial with a uniform, Beta(1,1) prior on the response rate, we might declare success if the posterior probability $Pr(p > 50\%) > 0.95$. This threshold would be the frequentist test at the $\alpha = 0.05$ level, observing 59/100 successes is needed to yield p-value < 0.05).

Now consider 3 interim analysis for futility stopping. At the first interim analysis, we see 12 responders in 20 patients. This produces a *p*-value of 0.25. At the second interim analysis, we see 28 responders in 50 patients. This produces a *p*-value of 0.24. At the third interim analysis, we see 41 responders in 75 patients. This produces a *p*-value 0.24.

At the first interim, the observed success rate is 60%, on pace for the necessary 59% for a successful trial. At the second analysis, the observed response rate is 56%, and we would have to see an improved 62% response rate in the final 50 patients to be a successful trial. The observed response rate is 55% at the third interim, and we would need to observe 18 responses in the 25 remaining patients (72%) to have a successful trial. These are, intuitively, getting increasingly less probable, though the *p*-values at each interim analysis are equal.

Similarly, imagine a fourth interim analysis with 50 responders in 92 patients, a 54.3% response rate. Even if all eight outstanding patients are responders at best, we observe 58 responders in 100 patients, failing to meet the 59/100 to achieve the primary aim. Yet the *p*-value for 50/92 is also 0.23, on par with our previous analyses. Basically, *p*-values, unlike predictive probabilities, fail to account for how much information is outstanding.

Predictive probabilities consider the amount of data that remain to be observed. Furthermore, they account for both the variability in the current parameter estimates and the natural variability in the remaining patients. While *p*-values are similar at each interim analysis, the predictive probabilities of trial success become increasingly smaller, representing that the trial is less and less likely to achieve its primary aim (Table 5.1).

We can extend this to multiple arms and stopping for both success and futility. In ESETT, because outcomes are rapidly known, trial success is known immediately at each interim analysis. Predictive probability for trial success is not useful in this context. Rather, ESETT uses a more group sequential-like success boundary: if the posterior probability that one treatment is the best is ever greater than 0.975, the trial stops for success.

TABLE 5.1

Predictive Probabilities versus *p*-Values for Four Interim Analyses

n	*x*	Obs %	% Needed	*p*-Value	Predictive Probability
20	12	60.0	58.8	0.25	0.54
50	28	56.0	62.0	0.24	0.30
75	41	54.7	72.0	0.24	0.086
92	50	54.3	112.5	0.23	0.00

Note: Obs % is the current proportion of responders; % Needed is the smallest proportion of responders needed to be observed to meet the success criteria at 100 patients.

TABLE 5.2

Operating Characteristics Comparing Adaptive Trial to Fixed Randomization

Scenario	Trial	Mean N	% to Best	Power
All equal	Adaptive	508	N/A	0.017
0.50 0.50 0.50	Fixed	499	N/A	0.023
One better	Adaptive	484	47	0.90
0.50 0.50 0.65	Fixed	492	33	0.87
One worse	Adaptive	684	83	0.11
0.50 0.65 0.65	Fixed	686	67	0.45
One worse, one better	Adaptive	592	47	0.49
0.50 0.575 0.65	Fixed	597	33	0.45

However, we can use predictive probabilities for futility stopping. A predictive probability is calculated to determine if the trial is likely to ever identify a best or worst treatment (posterior probability of having the lowest response rate >0.975) at the maximum sample size. If this predictive probability is ever less than 5%, then the trial stops for futility.

Table 5.2 shows operating characteristics for ESETT, including both information-based adaptive randomization and early stopping rules to a fixed 1:1:1 randomization with the same early stopping rules. This is based on 100,000 simulations for four different scenarios. These range from all three drugs offering equal response rates, one being 15% better, two being 15% better, and a scenario with rates of 50%, 57.5%, and 65%.

In the null scenario, "all equal," the sample size is slightly higher, but in the three cases with differences in response rates, adaptive stopping offers lower sample sizes. The proportion of patients randomized to the best treatment increases dramatically with adaptive randomization. In the "one good" scenario when one drug is 15% better than the other two, 47% of patients, on average, are randomized to the best drug, compared to 33% in a fixed trial. When two are equally effective with the third worse, then 83% instead of 67% are randomized between the best two drugs.

Finally, power in the two positive scenarios when one drug is truly superior is higher with adaptive randomization: 90% versus 87% in the "one good" scenario. Even when the best treatment is only slightly better than the second best, 65% versus 57.5% versus 50%, power increases from 45% to 49% with adaptive randomization. This illustrates how the combination of adaptive randomization with early stopping simultaneously leads to trials with lower mean sample size, a higher probability of patients randomized to the best therapy, and higher power. While we do trials in order to provide credible evidence to doctors and eventually treat patients better, we can use the accruing information to treat patients better within trials as well without sacrificing study power.

5.6 Simulation

Few software packages offer simple calculations of the operating characteristics for these methods, in part because these trials are typically specially tailored to the clinical situation. Therefore, operating characteristics are best calculated by simulation. Simulation also allows a means to select the adaptive design parameters.

Trial teams can best choose trial parameters by simulating trials and showing example trials and trial operating characteristics to the trial team and key stakeholders for discussion. Example trials step through a single simulated trial, showing the results of each interim analysis to illustrate the behavior of the trial. Example trials with both successful and unsuccessful results should be reviewed. Operating characteristics represent the average behavior of the trial and include average trial size, the proportion of patients randomized to the drug that is truly best, the trial's power, as well as other factors of interest to the study team.

The null scenario should be thoroughly simulated to determine the type 1 error. Trial designers may also give greater consideration to the choice of type I error rates during the design stage in CER because the clinical consequences of a type I error may be smaller in CER than in a placebo-controlled trial. In a CER trial comparing active therapies or treatment strategies, if one is erroneously chosen to be better among equals, patients would still receive an effective treatment, that is, if two treatments are truly similar, but one is erroneously ruled superior, subsequent patients still receive an effective therapy. This form of type I error may be less consequential than a situation in which a treatment is erroneously determined to be better than a placebo and patients pay for and receive an ineffective therapy while also being exposed to its adverse events and costs.

5.7 Platform Trials

In 1995, describing the frustration of breast cancer patients trying to learn about the many disjoint trials offered by various pharmaceutical companies, patient advocate Gracia Buffelben said, "Dying people don't have time or energy. We can't keep doing this one woman, one drug, one company at a time" [17]. Yet, nearly 20 years later, the research and development process typically is just that: one drug at a time, one company at a time.

While drugmakers understandably like to keep close control over their research, there are numerous advantages offered by platform trials in which multiple sponsors provide one or more drugs that are tested simultaneously.

With I-SPY 2, the Foundation of the National Institutes of Health collaborated with academic researchers, the National Cancer Institute, the U.S. Food and Drug Administration, and the pharmaceutical and biotechnology industry to introduce platform trials, a trial design methodology. A platform trial has an adaptive clinical trial infrastructure and *a priori* statistical rules that allow new drugs to be added, tested, and then they may be dropped from the trial for futility or graduate from the trial for success [18,19]. A new drug can then be added. Because dropping or graduating arms and then adding new arms may be ongoing for an indefinite period of time, platform trials are really better described as a process rather than a singular trial.

Many sponsors may pursue the development of drugs with similar chemical structures and biologic mechanisms. To further the collaborative nature of the project and increase drug development efficiency, I-SPY 2 collaborators have agreed to include just one drug per class. The trade-off is that the collaborators have agreed that data will be released to all partners who have a drug in that same class [19].

While comparing multiple competing drugs is typical in comparative effectiveness trials, CER trials tend to be Phase 4 trials and are often funded by government or payers. Platform trials, on the other hand, may have their initial infrastructure funded by third parties, but are additionally funded, at lower cost than an independent trial, by the drugmakers. Furthermore, they can be designed so even though drugs from different sponsors participate in the same trial, the primary aim is to identify how a company's drug compares to a placebo or standard of care, not against one another. Thus, they are defined as precompetitive trials.

Even in this precompetitive setting, there are many efficiencies largely related to the economy of scale of control groups because many different drugs are compared against a common control arm rather than each drug being randomized versus its own control. Figure 5.1 shows the typical

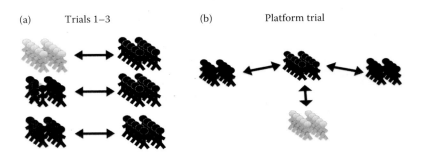

FIGURE 5.1
(a) Three separate trials, each versus placebo. (b) One platform trial with a common placebo group.

parallel drug development process. For example, three different pharmaceutical companies with compounds for the same disease may each run a similar but separate trial each with slightly different inclusion/exclusion criteria, endpoints, and study timing. Each trial (shown in separate rows) is a randomized-controlled trial of a compound (patients randomized to different company's compounds shown as different colors) to a placebo (patients randomized to placebo shown in black). The result is that many patients who choose to participate in a trial never receive a potentially helpful treatment. Furthermore, each pharmaceutical company has to pay for the entire trial infrastructure and to enroll, dose, and follow its own control group.

Figure 5.1b shows a simple platform trial. Here, each active arm is compared to a common placebo group. Even in the three-drug setting, the platform trial halves the proportion of patients randomized to placebo. Furthermore, the drugmakers can share the cost of the trial infrastructure and control patients.

A new compound could join the process and use only control patients enrolled during randomization to it. Or it could take advantage of similar historical controls. For example, one could start a new compound in the middle of the process, in year 3, and enroll for another 2 years. Patients would be randomized to this new treatment as well as other drugs within the platform trial and the control group. Patients randomized to this new drug arm could be simply compared to controls from years 3 and 4, or we could compare these 2 years of controls to earlier control group patients (via their demographics, their baseline disease states, and their outcomes), and if similar, we could also include the first 2 years of controls in the comparison to the new compound. If controls seem to be similar before and after this new drug entered the platform trial, then we can calculate a better estimate of the new compound's treatment effect.

By joining an ongoing platform trial, the drugmaker can decrease the start-up time of the new trial. The only regulatory hurdle is about the compound, not about the study design, which is preapproved. Posttrial regulatory review can also be expedited because the data have been generated by a well-understood trial process.

In the CER setting, as payers require more postmarket evidence, such trials may offer head-to-head comparisons of various competing drugs, or allow direct comparisons of drugs to devices to lifestyle changes. A drawback is a loss of autonomy. Pharmaceutical companies may not have entire control, for example, they may lack the ability to use a different or nonstandard endpoint, or choose their own data monitoring board members if they join an ongoing platform trial. They may still elect to explore more restrictive inclusion/exclusion criteria and compare their patients to just the control patients meeting their criteria.

In order to maintain privacy between competitors, early-stage trials, for example, I-SPY 2, are constructed so that when a drug graduates or terminates for futility, companies only see their own drug's data plus control data.

For postmarket CER trials, the level of data disclosure should be included in the protocol so sponsors understand the final uses of their data.

5.8 Personalized Medicine

Larger platform trials such as I-SPY 2 may also provide evidence toward personalized medicine and lead to smaller subsequent confirmatory trials. The I-SPY 2 trial, in addition to combining drugs and gaining the efficiency just described, also seeks to identify which drugs work best for which women suffering from breast cancer. Five drugs are compared to an active control in the trial and patients are adaptively randomized based on the genetic makeup of their tumor types. When patients in one genetic profile tend to do better on a particular drug, then future patients of the same tumor type will have an increased probability of being randomized to that drug.

Patients reap the obvious benefit from this real-time learning. However, patients are denied this benefit when different sponsors are running separate, although parallel, blinded trials. Identifying the subpopulation in which their drug works best offers huge advantages to sponsors, too.

Imagine, as shown in Figure 5.2, a case where a current treatment works in only 40% of a patient population (light gray). The new compound works in all those patients plus an additional 10% (medium gray). Neither of the drugs works in the remaining half of patients (dark gray). Of course, we rarely know which patients will benefit and which will not before treatment.

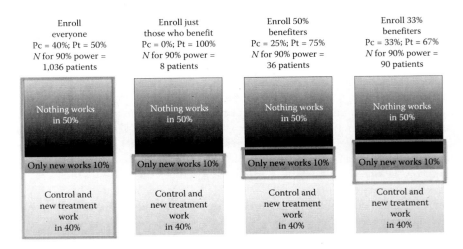

FIGURE 5.2
Statistical power as the effective subpopulation is identified.

If all patients with the disease are enrolled in a pivotal trial shown by thick outline surrounding everyone in the first panel in Figure 5.2, then 1,036 patients are needed to have 90% power to show that the new drug (50% efficacy) is superior to the standard of care (40% efficacy).

However, if an early-stage trial phase can identify the appropriate subpopulation who benefits from the new therapy, the inclusion criteria shown by the thick outline perfectly surrounding the medium gray patients in panel 2 in Figure 5.2 then just eight patients are necessary for 90% power. Of course, perfect prediction is unlikely. Even if the platform trial is less than perfect, for instance, producing an algorithm that requires enrolling two patients to obtain one patient that perfectly fits the profile, shown by the thick outline in panel 3, then just 36 patients are necessary for 90% power. In this case, the control would work in 25% of patients versus 75% in the treatment group. And if we enroll three patients to obtain one patient for whom there is benefit beyond control (control efficacy 33%, treatment efficacy 67%), then just 90 patients are necessary for 90% power.

By better identifying a drug's ideal patient population, dramatically smaller confirmatory trials are possible. Of course, such identification is difficult, but recent genetic advances provide the foundation for such efforts. At the very least, it is the path between our current one-size-fits-most healthcare delivery strategies and truly personalized medicine. Platform trials as described here could have advantages in many different indications. For instance, genetic variations might be explored in Alzheimer's disease, or different drugs with different biological mechanisms may work better in early-stage versus later-stage Alzheimer's disease.

Platform trials offer important advantages to patients. The obvious advantages are that fewer patients need to be randomized to placebo and that the platform trial learns as it progresses and can adaptively randomize patients to treatments that best match their particular type of disease or genetics. But they are also easier to navigate. Currently, the most educated, proactive patients may seek out numerous competing trials, attempt to discern from what little information is easily publicly available which trial is the most appropriate fit, and then work to find a convenient participating site. A less-informed patient may have access only to the trial his physician recommends, which is likely tied to a single drugmaker and single compound and is more likely to be a match of convenience than one of based on science. Constructing a broader platform trial with access across a range of clinical sites provides greater access to patients, and requires less homework by patients. The trial design itself can lead to patients receiving good medicine rather than the patient himself needing to guess which trial might match him with the best medicine. The expansion of platform trials, both geographic expansion to better represent the overall population and expanding participation from academic centers to community-based practices, will increase access to patients and provide improved care to patients less involved in their clinical care. Furthermore, adaptive randomization will ensure the most up-to-date care, even in the premarket setting to all trial-eligible patients.

In CER, an advantage of platforms trials may be to help address heterogeneity of disease and focus on personalized medicine. By comparing drugs post market in a formal, large, real-time platform trial setting, we may be more rapidly able to understand which drugs perform best in which types of patients.

Currently, such comparisons are often made post market from observational studies, error rates are unknown, and multiplicities abound. In a platform trial setting, trends within a certain subpopulation may be observed within the trial, then further validated as that subpopulation receives a higher randomization probability toward the seemingly optimal therapy. If the trend is spurious, a rapid increase in randomization probability will provide for quick regression to the mean in that subtype and the trial may revert to near equal randomization again. Whereas if the trend is real, the change in randomization probability in that patient subtype leads to increased power and a higher rate of patients in the trial being treated well.

A challenge for platforms trials in the postmarket/CER setting may be incentivizing sponsors to let their drugs compete scientifically and statistically against competitors as opposed to letting them compete via marketing.

5.9 Frequentist Adaptive Designs

While this chapter focuses on Bayesian adaptive designs, many adaptive techniques are based upon frequentist or classical statistics, too. The most common adaptive pivotal trials are group sequential trials that allow for early stopping and sample size reestimation analyses.

Group sequential trials are pivotal or confirmatory trials, usually with two arms, that predefine critical values for early stopping [20,21]. A key benefit of such trials is that they provide analytical control of type I error. A drawback is that they tend to be conservative, and only recently have designs been created that allow for formal consideration of patients who are enrolled but have not yet provided final outcome data at the time of the stopping analysis [22]. Shih provides a thorough survey of sample size reestimation analyses in which an interim analysis is performed to verify and potentially correct assumptions that went into a trial design, for example, event rate or variability [23].

5.10 Summary

Bayesian analysis is a natural fit for an ongoing learning environment such as comparative effectiveness research. The Bayesian machinery also allows for including data from many sources, such as historical data and data from meta-analyses. Building off this machinery and then incorporating Bayesian decision rules prospectively can allow for clinical trials to adapt to accruing clinical information and altering key trial attributes to change randomization probabilities to increase study power and increase the number of patients randomized to the better-performing therapies. Also stopping rules can be used to terminate trials or arms as soon as we are sufficiently confidant in a treatment's success or futility.

By incorporating these analytical and clinical trial tools, then simulating them in the context of a prospective trial, we can "tune" the trial's parameters and optimize its operating characteristics. Reference 24 is a thorough review paper of many Bayesian and adaptive techniques in CER.

One drawback to Bayesian adaptive trials is typically the need for custom software. Most designs require tailored software written to simulate patient accrual, patient randomization, patient outcomes data, each interim analysis, the adaptations that would occur in response to accumulating at data, and the possible stopping rules. The primary analysis is performed on the simulated data set. This process is completed thousands of times in "null" and various efficacious scenarios to calculate a trial's operating characteristics. Therefore, the time required to design such a trial is longer, and more sophisticated programming skills are needed. But with that comes much greater flexibility to tailor a trial and its decisions rules to each specific clinical effectiveness scenario. Furthermore, such clinical trial simulations allow for realistic sensitivity analyses, including sensitivity to accrual rates, nonuniform dropout patterns between treatment groups, and nonrandom missingness.

Simulating trials also allows designers to illustrate precisely how a trial would work to collaborators, investigators, data-monitoring boards, and institution review boards. Effectively, all stakeholders can observe precisely how the trial might go many times before the actual trial is initiated.

Many other sophisticated adaptive techniques have been used in earlier phase trials, especially dose-finding, that may be less applicable to CER trials [25,26].

Clinical trials based upon classical hypothesis tests are best suited for regulatory settings that inevitably end with a dichotomous approval or do not approve decision; such trials answer the question "Does this treatment work better than a placebo or control?" When more clinically driven questions are relevant, such as "Which of the competing therapies are best suited for this patient?," Bayesian adaptive trials that can rank competing treatments and formally incorporate data from a variety of sources may best inform clinicians and patients. Furthermore, Bayesian adaptive trials can be prospectively planned such that key clinical trial attributes such as randomization probabilities, inclusion criteria, and sample size mimic the real-world learning process.

Furthermore, platform trials based on Bayesian methodology [27] formally incorporate multiple competing therapies and can be design to include new therapies once they become approved or gain clinical acceptance, thus creating an ongoing process to evaluate and rank-order treatments' efficacy.

Acknowledgment

This chapter benefitted from comments by Kristine Broglio.

References

1. Agency for Healthcare Research and Quality. What is comparative effectiveness research? Rockville, MD. Available at: http://www.effectivehealthcare.ahrq.gov/index.cfm/what-is-comparative-effectiveness-research1/ (accessed November 17, 2014).
2. Berry D.A. and Stangl D.K. 1996. *Bayesian Biostatistics*. CRC Press, Boca Raton, FL.
3. Krushke J. 2011. *Doing Bayesian Data Analysis: A Tutorial with R and BUGS*. Elsevier, Oxford.
4. Gelman A. et al. 2013. *Bayesian Data Analysis*, 3rd ed. Chapman & Hall, London.
5. Carlin B. and Louis T. 2008. *Bayesian Methods for Data Analysis*. Chapman & Hall, New York.
6. Lilford L.J. and Braunholtz D. 1996. The statistical basic of public policy: A paradigm shift is overdue. *BMJ*, 313:603–607.
7. Berger J.O. and Berry D.A. 1988. Statistical analysis and the illusion of objectivity. *American Statistician*, 2:159–165.
8. Mullins C.D. et al. 2010. Generating evidence for comparative effectiveness research using more pragmatic randomized controlled trials. *PharmacoEconomics*, 28:969–976.
9. Tunis S.R., Stryer D.B., and Clancy C.M. 2003. Practical clinical trials increasing the value of clinical research for decision making in clinical and health policy. *JAMA*, 290:1624–1632.
10. Krams M. et al. 2003. Acute stroke therapy by inhibition of neutrophils (ASTIN): An adaptive dose-response study of UK-279,276 in acute ischemic stroke. *Stroke*, 34:2543–2548.
11. Connor J.T., Elm J.J., and Broglio K.R. 2013. Bayesian adaptive trials offer advantages in comparative effectiveness trials: An example in status epilepticus. *Journal of Clinical Epidemiology*, 66:S130–S137.
12. Cock H.R. and the ESETT Group. 2011. Established status epilepticus treatment trial (ESETT). *Epilepsia*, 52:50–52.
13. Luce B.R., Kramer J.M., Goodman S.N., Connor J.T., Tunis S., Whicher D., and Schwartz, J.S. 2009. Rethinking randomized clinical trials for comparative effectiveness research: The need for transformational change. *Annals of Internal Medicine*, 151:206–209.

14. Connor J.T. et al. 2013. Do Bayesian adaptive trials offer advantages for comparative effectiveness research? Protocol for the RE-ADAPT study. *Clinical Trials*, 10:807–827.

15. Broglio K.R., Connor J.T., and Berry S.M. 2014. Not too big, not too small: A Goldilocks approach to sample size selection. *Journal of Biopharmaceutical Statistics*, 3:685–705.

16. Saville B.R. et al. 2014. The utility of Bayesian predictive probabilities for interim monitoring of clinical trials. *Clinical Trials*, 11:485–493.

17. Evans N. and Peterson P. 1995. Dying for compassion. *Breast Cancer Action Newsletter*, August 1995.

18. Esserman L.J. and Woodcock J. 2011. Accelerating identification and regulatory approval of investigational cancer drugs. *JAMA*, 306:2608–2609.

19. Barker A.D. et al. 2009. I-SPY 2: An adaptive breast cancer trial design in the setting of neoadjuvant chemotherapy. *Clinical Pharmacology & Therapeutics*, 86:97–100.

20. Pocock S.J. 1977. Group sequential methods in the design and analysis of clinical trials. *Biometrika*, 64:191–199.

21. O'Brien P.C. and Fleming T.R. 1979. A multiple testing procedure for clinical trials. *Biometrics*, 35:549–556.

22. Hampson L.V. and Jennison C. 2013. Group sequential tests for delayed responses. *JRSS B*, 75:3–54.

23. Shih W.J. 2001. Sample size re-estimation—Journey for a decade. *Statistics in Medicine*, 20:515–518.

24. Berry D.A. 2011. Bayesian approaches for comparative effectiveness research. *Clinical Trials*, 9:37–47.

25. Gallo P. et al. 2006. Adaptive designs in clinical drug development—An executive summary of the PhRMA working group. *Journal of Biopharmaceutical Statistics*, 16:275–283.

26. Biswas S. et al. 2009. Bayesian clinical trials at MD Anderson. *Clinical Trials*, 6:205–216.

27. Berry S.M., Connor J.T., and Lewis R.L. 2015. The platform trial: An efficient strategy for evaluating multiple therapies. *JAMA*, 313:1619–1620.

6

Generalizability of Clinical Trials Results

Elizabeth A. Stuart

CONTENTS

ABSTRACT   Randomized trials are seen as the gold standard for estimating the effects of interventions because, when implemented well, they provide unbiased estimates of treatment effects in the sample at hand. However, recent years have seen an increased understanding of their limitations in providing evidence that is more broadly applicable and relevant for real-world practice, known as "generalizability." A lack of generalizability may be a particular problem for comparative effectiveness research (CER), which aims to help clinicians and policymakers make informed decisions for individuals and populations. This chapter outlines recent advances in methods to assess and enhance the generalizability of randomized trials in CER, discussing both design and analysis strategies. A case study is provided of a weighting approach that reweights the trial sample to reflect the target population with respect to effect modifiers. Recommendations for further research and the practical use of the methods discussed are also provided.

6.1 Introduction

Randomized trials are seen as the gold standard for estimating the effects of interventions because, when implemented well, they provide unbiased estimates of treatment effects in the sample at hand. However, recent years have seen an increased understanding of their limitations in providing evidence that is more broadly applicable and relevant for real-world practice (Rothwell, 2005; Zimmerman et al., 2005; Insel, 2006). In particular, as currently designed, randomized trials often enroll individuals who are quite different from those who may receive the drug or intervention of interest in general clinical practice. However, the generalizability of results is crucial for many policy and practice recommendations. This idea of generalizability or external validity ties directly into comparative effectiveness research (CER), and is reflected in the definition of CER laid out by the Institute of Medicine: "The purpose of CER is to assist consumers, clinicians, purchasers, and policymakers to make informed decisions that will improve health care at both the individual and population levels" (Institute of Medicine, 2009, p. 13). Generalizability is particularly inherently related to CER Characteristic 1: "CER has the objective of directly informing a specific clinical decision from the patient perspective or a health policy decision from the population perspective," Characteristic 3: "CER describes results at the population and subgroup levels," and Characteristic 6: "CER is conducted in settings that are similar to those in which the intervention will be used in practice" (Institute of Medicine, 2009, p. 37–39). This interest in population inferences that relate to how interventions will be used in practice requires careful thinking about the generalizability of randomized trials. We need to have some understanding of how well randomized trial results may generalize in order to base decisions on the results from those trials. This chapter discusses current ways of thinking about generalizability as well as design and analysis tools to increase the generalizability of randomized trial results.

The idea of generalizing from one sample or population to another, or of considering how much information about population effects we can deduce from a randomized trial, goes by a number of different terms. Shadish et al. (2002, p. 20) define external validity as "inferences about whether the causal relationship holds over variation in persons, settings, treatment, and measurement variables." In the medical literature, the GRADE* Working Group

(2004) terms it "directness" and discusses generalizability in relation to both the characteristics of patients and to the comparability of the treatments being investigated. Bareinboim and Pearl use a more precise term for the type of generalization we are generally concerned with in this chapter, defining "transportability" as a particular form of generalization, "defined as a license to transfer causal effects learned in experimental studies to a new population, in which only observational studies can be conducted" (Bareinboim and Pearl, 2013, p. 107). However, this chapter is also concerned with situations in which an experiment *could be* conducted in the target ("new") population, but has not yet been.

Concerns regarding generalizability (or the lack thereof) of clinical trial results have been becoming more visible and more vigorously discussed in recent years. This is true in medicine, education (e.g., Olsen et al., 2013), and international development settings (e.g., Deaton, 2009). In medical settings, potential lack of generalizability of results has been of concern especially in cases where interventions appear effective in trials but then when rolled out "in the real world" show less strong effects; although there could be many explanations for that, one explanation in some cases is changes in the patient populations, and thus differences in effects (e.g., Gheorghe et al., 2013).

When thinking about generalizability, there needs to be a target population of interest; the first step is to be clear about the group or setting to which one is trying to generalize. It is also important to note that policymakers may be interested in generalizing from one randomized trial to multiple target populations. For example, the National Center for Medicare & Medicaid Services may be interested in a target population of all Medicaid enrollees across the country, but state Medicaid officers may be more interested in a target population that is the Medicaid enrollees in their particular state. So, when talking about generalizability, one needs to be clear regarding the target population, and acknowledge, for example, that a particular study may have very good generalizability with respect to one target population but poor generalizability with respect to another.

6.1.1 Threats to Generalizability

There are many threats to the generalizability of randomized trial results. We will define external validity bias as the difference between the true treatment effect in the population and the estimated effect (e.g., the effect estimated in a randomized trial). This is formalized further below. Shadish et al. (2002) lay out a series of threats to generalizability (i.e., factors that will lead to external validity bias). These include (p. 87, Table 3.2):

1. "Interaction of the causal relationship with units"
2. "Interaction of the causal relationship over treatment variations"
3. "Interaction of the causal relationship with outcomes"

4. "Interactions of the causal relationship with settings"

5. "Context-dependent mediation"

In this chapter, we focus primarily on threat #1 and how to adjust for observed differences in characteristics between individuals in the trial and in the population of interest, with some discussion of threat #4 and how to adjust for differences in settings. Threat #2 relates to the possibility of variation in the treatments that individuals receive, discussed further in VanderWeele and Hernán (2003). We assume that the intervention and comparison conditions being studied in the trial are the same as those that will be implemented in the population. Threat 3 refers to differences that may arise if other outcomes are considered (e.g., that an effect on a self-reported depression scale may differ from the effect on a clinician's diagnosis). Threat #5 relates to different mediation mechanisms in the trial sample and the population; see Frangakis (2009) for one example of how to handle this threat, in particular settings where take-up or compliance rates may differ between a trial and a target population. This complication may happen if, for example, compliance rates change once a medication has received FDA approval; this issue of differences in compliance rates is also related to threat #2 and the "doses" of treatment individuals may receive.

Of particular concern in CER is the trial inclusion and exclusion criteria, which often yield randomized trial samples that are not representative of the target population of potential patients. Many randomized trials are designed to detect a large effect size, while minimizing potential risks to patients. This means that the trials often enroll individuals who are expected to particularly benefit from the intervention, and that those who are likely to increase costs or who are likely to have poor outcomes are often excluded (Pressler and Kaizar, 2013). This means in practice that individuals with multiple comorbidities, children, and women of childbearing age are often excluded from trials. This is of particular concern given that CER is meant to inform clinical practice, and that when there is treatment effect heterogeneity, results for those included in the trial may not reflect results that would be seen in other groups (expressed in the Institute of Medicine CER characteristic #3 cited above), as formalized below.

There are a number of studies that have looked specifically at the types of patients who enroll in clinical trials, and how they compare to the general patient population. Humphreys et al. (2005) found that exclusion criteria were commonly used in alcohol treatment research studies, and that the number of exclusion criteria used increased over time and varied depending on the study design as well as the funder. Likewise, Braslow et al. (2005) found that most studies of psychiatric treatment enrolled unrepresentative samples, with minorities underrepresented, and that those studies rarely reported on the representativeness of their samples in their reports. Using the STAR*D study, Wisniewski et al. (2009) also found large differences between those enrolled in that large-effectiveness trial and patients who would have been enrolled in a more limited efficacy trial. Finally, Hoertel et al. (2013) used a standard set of exclusion criteria for studies of treatment for bipolar depression or mania and found that more than 5 of 10 individuals with bipolar depression or mania in the National Epidemiologic Survey on Alcohol and Related Conditions (NESARC; a nationally representative sample) would have been excluded from a typical randomized trial. Having a high risk for suicide was the most common criterion excluding individuals with bipolar disorder, while having a diagnosis of alcohol abuse or dependence was the criterion that excluded the highest percentage of individuals with mania. Using a similar design strategy, Hoertel et al. (2012) found that over 7 out of 10 individuals with generalized anxiety disorder (GAD) would have been excluded from a typical trial of treatment for GAD. In a nonmental health setting, Ezekowitz et al. (2012) found similar concerns regarding differences between individuals in a randomized trial for acute heart failure and a comparable registry, and Koog et al. (2013) found differences between individuals enrolled in knee osteoarthritis clinical trials and the general patient population. Finally, Unger et al. (2013) found that individuals of lower socioeconomic status were less likely to choose to enroll in randomized trials in oncology.

It is, however, important to note that trials do not always enroll unrepresentative samples. Stevens et al. (2006) found that the MTA trial of multimodal treatment of attention-deficit hyperactivity disorder (ADHD) enrolled individuals who looked similar on average to large epidemiologic cohorts of individuals with ADHD. In fact, the MTA trial was designed to have as few exclusion criteria as possible. Similarly, Go et al. (2003) found that results on the effectiveness of anticoagulation therapy for stroke prevention in atrial fibrillation translated well into clinical practice (Go et al., 2003).

However, the potential lack of generalizability is not limited to studies with formal inclusion and exclusion criteria. For example, in education research, where there is often not strict inclusion or exclusion criteria, there is evidence that the types of schools that participate in large evaluations differ from the national population of schools (Stuart et al., 2016) and that this can lead to external validity bias (Bell et al., 2016).

Focusing on external validity bias due to differences in the composition of patients in a randomized trial and in a target population, some researchers have laid out formal models for the extent of external validity bias. Bareinboim and Pearl (2013) and Pearl and Bareinboim (2013) provide a framework for determining when results are "transportable," which requires positing a selection diagram that lays out the structure (e.g., the variables under investigation and how they relate to one another) and what factors do (and do not) remain consistent between a sample and the unit for which impact estimates are desired (e.g., the target population). When that structure is known (or hypothesized), its framework can be used to determine the implied generalizability (or transportability).

6.1.2 Notation and Setting

To formalize the discussion, we use the Neyman–Rubin causal model, which has been presented in Chapters 1 and 2 (Rubin, 1974; Holland, 1986). In that model, each individual in some target population (e.g., all Medicaid patients) is posited to have two potential outcomes (e.g., cholesterol levels)—one (Y_{1i}) that is observed if they receive the intervention of interest (e.g., a new cholesterol-lowering medication) and one (Y_{0i}) if they do not. The impact of the intervention for individual i is defined as the difference between these two potential outcomes: $\Delta_i = Y_{1i} - Y_{0i}$. We are interested in estimating the population average treatment effect (PATE), Δ; the average Δ_i across all N individuals in the target population:

$$\Delta = 1/N \sum_{i=1}^{N} \Delta_i.$$

Now, consider a randomized experiment that randomizes patients to receive the intervention or not. First, let S_i denote membership in the randomized trial sample ($S_i = 1$ for patients who participated in the clinical trial and $S_i = 0$ for those who did not). Let T_i denote treatment assignment in the trial ($T_i = 1$ for intervention, $T_i = 0$ for control). If treatment assignment is randomized, the difference in potential outcomes between the observed treatment and control groups $\hat{\Delta} = E(Y_{1i} \mid S_i = 1, T_i = 1) - E(Y_{0i} \mid S_i = 1, T_i = 0)$ provides an unbiased estimate of the treatment effect in the trial sample: $E(Y_{1i} \mid S_i = 1, T_i = 1) - E(Y_{0i} \mid S_i = 1, T_i = 0) = E(\hat{\Delta} \mid S_i = 1)$, but there is concern that the impact in the population may differ from that in the sample. We define the external validity bias as the difference between the impact estimated in the evaluation sample and the true population impact, $\hat{\Delta} - \Delta$. The goal of the methods described below is to reduce the size of that bias through either better design of the trial or adjustment of the randomized trial results. Many of the methods rely on having data on the population of interest, either characteristics or, sometimes, outcome data, which can be used to help adjust the trial results to relate to the population. These methods and data requirements are discussed further below.

   In an attempt to start thinking about external validity and the trade-offs of different study designs when estimating population treatment effects, Imai et al. (2008) decompose the bias in estimates obtained from a variety of study designs. In particular, Imai et al. decompose the overall bias when estimating population treatment effects (Δ) into four components: $\hat{\Delta} = (\Delta_{SX} + \Delta_{SU}) + (\Delta_{TX} + \Delta_{TU})$, where the subscript "$S$" refers to selection bias (unrepresentative samples from the population), "T" refers to treatment imbalance (treatment and comparison groups that are dissimilar; e.g., as happens in a nonexperimental study), "X" refers to observed characteristics, and "U" refers to unobserved characteristics. These characteristics (in both "X" and "U") may include both individual-level characteristics and characteristics of their broader contexts such as hospitals, providers, neighborhoods, and communities. As described in Imai et al. (2008), when interest is in population treatment effects, the standard beliefs about the pros and cons of different study designs may not always apply; for example, a small and nonrepresentative randomized trial may have larger external validity (or generalizability) bias, even if it has no treatment selection bias, than a well-done, nonexperimental study using a representative sample. Put more simply, when population treatment effects are of interest, internal validity may not be the only consideration. Imai et al. (2008) provide a framework for these ideas and trade-offs.

In some simple settings, one can also obtain analytic expressions for the size of external validity bias. To make ideas concrete, Cole and Stuart (2010) considered a setting with a randomized trial of an intervention T. Also, assume that the outcome Y is a linear function of binary treatment status T, a binary covariate Z, and the interaction between T and Z (implying treatment effect heterogeneity across levels of Z): $E(Y_i) = b_0 + b_T T_i + b_Z Z_i + b_{ZT} Z_i T_i$. In this case, the bias in estimating a PATE by just considering the effect estimate in the randomized trial sample at hand can be expressed as

$$b_{ZT} \left[\frac{P(Z=1)}{P(S=1)} [P(S=1|Z=1) - P(S=1)] \right].$$

In other words, the external validity bias is a function of the size of the treatment effect heterogeneity (b_{ZT}), the prevalence of the "heterogeneity characteristic" (Z) in the population, the proportion of the population enrolled in the trial ($P(S=1)$), and the association between Z and participation in the trial (S), expressed as $P(S=1|Z=1) - P(S=1)$. This expression for the bias also shows that there will be no external validity bias if there is no treatment effect heterogeneity ($b_{ZT} = 0$), if Z is unrelated to participation in the trial, so then $P(S=1|Z=1) = P(S=1)$, or if the randomized trial is done using everyone in the population ($P(S=1) = 1$). Olsen et al. (2013) provide a similar expression for the bias, for the context where sites (e.g., schools or hospitals) are the unit of selection for the trial, and then random assignment is done within the site.

6.2 Design Methods to Improve Generalizability

There are three main design strategies used to increase the generalizability of randomized trial results: (1) actual random sampling from the target population of interest, (2) trials with broad populations in real-world settings, such as practical clinical trials or pragmatic trials (e.g., Chalkidou et al., 2012),

TABLE 6.1

Randomized Trial Designs to Enhance Generalizability

Method	Main Idea	Pros	Cons
D-1 representative samples	Carry out trial in a random sample from the population of interest	• Allows formal statistical generalization, unbiased estimation of PATE	• Often difficult to carry out in practice • Requires knowledge of target population in advance
D-2 large trials of broad populations in real-world settings	Carry out trial in a broad set of patients, across a range of settings	• More likely to yield results that generalize	• Does not allow formal generalization • Study may still not represent full population of ultimate interest
D-3 doubly randomized preference trials	Randomize all patients in the population to participate in the trial, and then randomize treatments within those in the trial arm	• Allows estimation of the PATE • Allows calibration of the effect seen in trial arm to the effect seen in the nontrial arm	• Sometimes difficult to carry out • Requires knowledge of target population in advance • Few examples

which aim to enroll a more representative sample from the start, and (3) doubly randomized preference trials (e.g., Marcus, 1997; Marcus et al., 2012), which allow researchers to estimate the effect of randomization itself. We discuss each of these approaches in more detail here; Table 6.1 provides an overview of these design approaches.

6.2.1 D-1 Trials in Representative Samples

Perhaps the most obvious and ideal (but also most difficult) way to increase generalizability is to start out with a randomized trial sample that is formally representative of the population of interest. For example, in evaluations of government programs, it is sometimes possible to enroll a representative set of sites in the study, and then randomly assign eligible applicants to those sites to the intervention group or a control group. This was done in national evaluations of the Job Corps program (Schochet et al., 2008), Upward Bound (U.S. Department of Education, 2009), and Head Start (U.S. Department of Health and Human Services, 2010). However, this is more difficult in many CER settings since it requires having a listing of the target population at the beginning of the study. However, it may be feasible in studies carried out, for example, by large healthcare providers, who have a listing of all their members. However, a challenge that will still occur even in that setting is that the people selected to participate may decline such participation. As summarized by Shadish (1995, p. 424), "In general, however, formal sampling is inadequate to the task because a) it is rarely possible to even identify the population of treatments, outcomes, settings, persons, or times from which sampling should occur, and b) even when it is possible, randomly sampled units often refuse to be in the study or refuse to be randomly assigned to conditions."

6.2.2 D-2 Trials with Broad Populations in Real-World Settings

Effectiveness trials (Flay et al., 2005) are often a step closer to generalizability by virtue of their design being implemented in more real-world settings. Relatedly, a design coming more into favor in medical fields is that of practical clinical trials, also known as pragmatic trials (e.g., Sachs et al., 2003; Rush et al., 2004; Insel, 2006; Chalkidou et al., 2012). These types of trials are becoming more and more common and desired (e.g., through recent funding announcements from the Patient Centered Outcomes Research Institute). They are designed to enroll a broad spectrum of individuals, and thus at least potentially increase generalizability, but they can be very expensive and difficult to carry out. Large simple trials are another design increasing in use, which aim to enroll large samples of individuals, with broad eligibility criteria, using a simple design and at relatively low cost (e.g., utilizing existing electronic health records; Roehr, 2013). However, although these types of trials aim to enroll a more representative set of people, they generally still do not allow formal generalization to the target population, and there may be concerns that the types of people who choose to enroll in a trial may differ from patients in standard clinical practice, even if the trials sample from a broader distribution of settings and contexts. Tipton et al. (2014) formalize the process of selecting subjects to participate in an effectiveness or pragmatic trial, providing a method for selecting a representative sample using stratification on key variables.

6.2.3 D-3 Doubly Randomized Preference Trials

A design potentially more useful in medical settings, which allows formal statements of generalizability (or lack thereof) but is infrequently used, is a doubly randomized preference trial (Marcus et al., 2012). These trials enroll individuals into the study but then randomize them into two arms: (1) a randomized arm, in which individuals are randomly assigned to treatment conditions, and (2) a nonexperimental (observational) arm, where individuals are allowed to select their treatment condition. This double randomization allows researchers to compare the individuals in the randomized arm with the nonexperimental arm to investigate the effects of randomization itself.

This then gives a sense of the bias that may exist in the randomized trial due to the act of randomization itself. A less-rigorous version of this design can also be used sometimes, when it is not possible to randomize individuals into the randomized arm versus nonexperimental arm, but when there is the ability to follow a cohort of individuals who were not eligible for (or did not consent to be in) the randomized trial.

6.3 Analysis Methods to Assess and Enhance Generalizability

In many cases, however, researchers do not have the ability to modify the design of a trial (e.g., it has already been carried out), but there is interest in determining how well the results apply to some target population. To answer these sorts of questions, there are also a growing number of methods to assess and enhance the generalizability of randomized trials that have already been conducted. See Table 6.2 for a summary of these analysis approaches.

6.3.1 A-1 Broad Assessment of Similarity

One strategy for documenting factors that may affect the generalizability of study results is the "Reach Effectiveness Adoption Implementation Maintenance" (Re-AIM) framework by Green and Glasgow (2006). Re-AIM provides simple summary measures of external validity, covering a wide range of areas (such as the percentage of individuals who participate, measures of attrition, and quality of implementation) but with relatively little focus on the particular issue considered in this chapter—that of differences in the characteristics of individuals in a trial sample and a target population.

6.3.2 A-2 Comparison of Characteristics and Outcomes between Trial and Population

In this approach, the first step in assessing generalizability is to compare the characteristics of the individuals in the trial to those in a target population of interest. A step beyond this, as done in Greenhouse et al. (2008), Stuart et al. (2011), and Weisberg et al. (2009), and presented in the case study below, is to compare the outcomes observed in the target population with the outcomes in the control arm of the trial. When the control condition in the randomized trial is comparable to the "usual care" received by individuals in the target population, this allows a test of whether the groups are similar with respect to their prognosis under the control condition. Worse (or better) outcomes in the control arm of the trial may indicate that those individuals who enroll in

TABLE 6.2

Analysis Methods to Enhance Generalizability

Method	Data Needed	Pros	Cons
A-1 broad assessment of similarity and representativeness	• Summary measures of participation rate, quality of implementation, etc. in the trial	• Covers a broad spectrum of study characteristics	• Does not estimate PATE
A-2 comparison of characteristics and outcomes in the trial and population	• In trial X, T, and Y • In population Y, ideally Y	• Especially if outcome(s) available in the population, can provide quantitative evidence of similarity of the trial and population	• Assumes that the effect moderators are observed • Does not estimate PATE
A-3 investigation of effect heterogeneity	• In trial X, T, and Y • In population: nothing	• Generalizability is only a problem if effects vary, so understanding effect heterogeneity is crucial	• Trials often have limited power to detect effect heterogeneity • Does not estimate PATE
A-4 flexible outcome models	• In trial X, T, and Y • In population X, ideally Y	• Can work well if ignorability holds	• Accounts only for observed differences between the trial and population
A-5 combining experimental and nonexperimental data	• Multiple studies with X, T, and Y (experimental and nonexperimental)	• Can combine all available information • Can account for biases in different study designs	• Multiple studies on the same topic required • Complex methods with few examples • Can be sensitive to weight model
A-6 poststratification or weighting	• In trial X, T, and Y • In population X	• Can work well if ignorability holds	• Accounts only for observed differences between the trial and population

the trial are sicker (or healthier) than those who do not, which could limit the generalizability of the trial results.

6.3.3 A-3 Investigation of Effect Heterogeneity in the Trial

As discussed above, external validity bias arises when treatment effects are correlated with participation in the trial. At one extreme, if there is no treatment effect heterogeneity (i.e., if the treatment effect is constant for all individuals), there will be no external validity bias. Thus, an assessment of generalizability should also include investigation of the extent of effect heterogeneity in the trial, for example, by estimating subgroup effects or using new methods to examine the distribution of treatment effects (Imai and Ratkovic, 2013; Kraemer, 2013). A challenge, however, in these investigations is that of statistical power; randomized trials are generally designed to estimate the overall (main) treatment effect; the sample size needed to detect variation in treatment effects across subgroups is often four times as large as is needed to detect the main effect. Thus, failure to reject the null that there is no treatment effect variability may be just a result of limited statistical power rather than an actual lack of effect heterogeneity. A full discussion of methods for assessing treatment effect heterogeneity is beyond the scope of this chapter; for more details, see Kent et al. (2010), as well as Imai and Ratkovic (2013), which presents a new method for identifying treatment effect heterogeneity, including an illustration of how to then use the results to extrapolate treatment effects to a target population.

6.3.4 A-4 Flexible Outcome Models

A recently developed method that has not been used much in practice but has been found to work well in simulations (Hill, 2011; Kern et al., 2016) is Bayesian Additive Regression Trees (BART), which fits a flexible model of the outcomes as a function of treatment status in the trial, and then extrapolates that model to the population to estimate population effects. This can be thought of as a more flexible way of assessing treatment effect heterogeneity in the trial, as compared to, for example, linear models that simply include a number of treatments by covariate interactions. In particular, BART generates a predicted potential outcome under control and a predicted potential outcome under treatment for each individual in the population, and uses the difference in those average outcomes to estimate the PATE. Although simple regression models such as linear regression models would generally not be appropriate for this task because of the risk of model extrapolation, flexible models such as BART seem to work well, since they allow for complex relationships between covariates, treatment assignment, and outcomes and take into account the uncertainty when making predictions of outcomes for those outside the original trial sample. This approach does not require outcome data in the target population but does work better if it is available, as it allows the calibration of models to the potential outcomes in the population.

6.3.5 A-5 Combining Experimental and Nonexperimental Evidence

Another set of methods is useful when there are multiple studies available on a particular topic, so that there multiple estimates of the treatment effect. (These approaches thus require outcome data across all studies.) These include meta-analysis, research synthesis approaches, and the confidence profile method. The main idea behind meta-analysis is to combine results from multiple studies; often used in settings where multiple randomized trials have been done on roughly the same research question and population (Hedges and Olkin, 1985; Sutton and Higgins, 2008). Meta-analysis typically takes just one result from each study, for example, the treatment effect size, and combines those results across studies, either assuming that the effect sizes from the different studies are all estimating some common effect (a fixed effects model), or allowing variation in the effects across studies (a random effects model). The drawback with traditional meta-analysis is that it does not necessarily answer the question of interest for this chapter, especially if the set of trials were all conducted on similar types of subjects, who may not be representative of the population. Traditional meta-analysis puts relatively little focus on assessing how similar the individuals in the trials are to the target population. Individual-patient-data (IPD) meta-analysis (Riley et al., 2010) has the potential to be more helpful for assessing generalizability, but its use for estimating treatment effects in a target population has not been investigated, and it may suffer from the same limitations as standard meta-analysis if the trials did not enroll a broad set of patients.

A broader class of methods called cross-design synthesis involves similar ideas as meta-analysis but is potentially more able to explicitly address the question of generalizability. Cross-design synthesis enables the combination of results from randomized and nonrandomized studies (Prevost et al., 2000; Kaizar, 2011), and thus, for example, can be used to combine information on program effects from a randomized trial with information from an observational study, which may contain a more representative sample. Cross-design synthesis does this by modeling multiple parameters from each study and through the incorporation of study characteristics. Brown et al. (2008) used this method to model variation in impacts across trials and outcomes. A common strategy for cross-design synthesis is to fit a Bayesian hierarchical model that includes a level for study type. A Bayesian approach allows the incorporation of beliefs regarding the relative merits of the multiple sources of evidence (e.g., Turner et al., 2009). For example, a Bayesian model can incorporate the belief that a randomized design yields a less-biased estimate of the average treatment effect in the trial sample as compared to a nonrandomized design, but that the nonrandomized design may provide more information about population effectiveness. However, more work needs to be done to fully investigate the potential use of cross-design synthesis to answer the question of generalizability of interest in this chapter, as estimating population effects is not always the explicit goal of these methods. For example, cross-design synthesis approaches do not have formal ways of examining how similar subjects in a trial (or trials) are to individuals in a target population. These methods are discussed in detail in Chapter 7 of this book.

Pressler and Kaizar (2013) present a particular approach for combining experimental and nonexperimental data in order to assess what they term "generalizability bias" due to strict inclusion or exclusion criteria in the randomized trial. One important point is that their method for assessing generalizability bias does not require individual-level data from the trial, which makes the approach useable in many settings where the individual-level trial data may be impossible, or very difficult, to obtain. In particular, they use a nonexperimental data source and nonexperimental methods such as propensity scores to separately estimate the effect of the treatment among the people included in and excluded from the trial. They can then compare the nonexperimental estimate for the people who would have been included to the "true" impact seen in the trial to estimate the bias from a nonexperimental comparison, then use that to adjust the nonexperimental effect estimate obtained for those excluded from the trial. They thus use a combination of the experimental and nonexperimental evidence to estimate the treatment effect among those who would have been excluded from the trial; not just relying on the nonexperimental estimate, but also bringing in information from the experiment to make that estimate more robust. The approach, however, does rely on an assumption that the bias in effect estimates obtained using the nonexperimental data is the same for those included and those excluded from the randomized trial; it is not clear how common this would be in practice. See Frank and Min (2007) for another method that can be used to judge the ability to extrapolate from a study sample to an excluded population.

6.3.6 A-6 Poststratification and Weighting

A final type of approach involves adjusting the trial sample to resemble the population on a set of observed characteristics. This approach requires covariate and outcome data from the trial, and at least covariate data on the target population of interest. As detailed below, outcome data in the population can also be useful for assessing the validity of the approaches. A simple example of this is a variation on poststratification, which is commonly used in survey contexts to make a survey sample match the population distribution of certain key variables (e.g., by race, sex, and state of residence; Holt and Smith, 1979). This is similar to the idea of standardization in demography and epidemiology (Kitagawa, 1964). A very simple example of this in the generalizability context would involve, for example, estimating treatment effects separately by racial groups and then estimating the population treatment effect by averaging those subgroup-specific effects by the proportion of each race in the population.

A challenge in the use of standardization is that limited sample sizes, and low power to detect subgroup-specific treatment effects in randomized trials, make it hard to implement standardization. To avoid this problem, researchers have moved toward a version of standardization that involves using something like the propensity score (a summary measure of the covariates) as the dimension of standardization. Thus, instead of forming strata based on a cross-tabulation of individual variables (e.g., age 30–35, male, 1–2 comorbidities, African American), the strata are formed on the basis of the propensity score, as a scalar combination of the individual covariates. Propensity scores are traditionally used in nonexperimental studies to balance treatment and comparison groups on the set of observed covariates (Rosenbaum and Rubin, 1983; Stuart, 2010). In this context of generalizability, the "propensity score" instead models the probability of being in the randomized trial (vs. the population as a whole), but it still uses the key properties of the propensity score in terms of its ability to balance two groups. For generalizability, the balancing serves to make the randomized trial sample balance (or look like) the target population, at least with respect to the observed covariates. Hartman et al. (2013), O'Muircheartaigh and Hedges (2014), Stuart et al. (2011), and Tipton (2013), all present applications of this approach, as well as discussion of the underlying assumptions and details of the method. The primary assumption that allows generalization from the sample to the population is called "sample ignorability" by Tipton (2013), and it has two components: (1) that there are no unobserved variables associated with impacts and with selection into the trial sample, and (2) that there are no individuals in the population with a selection probability of 0; that is, every individual in the population had some positive probability of being in the trial.

Tipton (2013) estimates the PATE of a mathematics software for middle-school students by subclassifying the 92 schools that participated in a randomized trial (using 26 covariates in the model of participation, and sub-classifying based on predicted probabilities of participation, the propensity scores) of the software, and reweighting subclass-specific treatment effects by the proportion of target population schools in each subclass. An alternative to subclassification is reweighting, which weights subjects participating in the trial by one over their probability of participating, thus reweighting the trial sample to the target population (again, similar to sample selection and nonresponse adjustments in sample surveys; Horvitz and Thompson, 1952). A case study of such reweighting is presented in Section 6.4, with details of the approach.

These poststratification and reweighting approaches can be used when outcomes are not available. One benefit of these approaches is that, when outcomes under the control condition are available in the population, they can be used as a "placebo check" to examine the plausibility of generalizing from the trial to the population, as discussed by Stuart et al. (2011) and Hartman et al. (2013). In particular, if the observed characteristics are sufficient to account for the differences between the sample and the population, then the population-weighted control group outcomes from the trial should match the average outcomes seen in the population. (Or, if some individuals in the target population receive the treatment, then the population-weighted treatment group outcomes should match the outcomes of those individuals in the population who got the treatment.) Failure of these values to match may indicate some unobserved difference between the trial and population, which makes the outcomes differ even when receiving the same treatment condition and even after adjusting for the observed covariates. Hartman et al. (2013) describe the formal conditions for this test and provide some examples.

6.4 Case Study: Generalizing the Effects of HAART to a National Population

As a case study of the reweighting approach (A-6), we now present a summary of Cole and Stuart (2010), which used the reweighting approach described briefly above in order to estimate PATEs, combining data from a randomized trial and a target population of interest. (See Hartman et al., 2013, for an example from cost-effectiveness research.) Following a seminal human immunodeficiency virus (HIV) treatment trial that showed that highly active antiretroviral therapy (HAART) was effective at reducing mortality, Cole and Stuart (2010) were interested in determining what the effects of HAART would be if given to all individuals newly infected with HIV in the United States. In particular, Cole and Stuart (2010) used data from the ACTG 320 trial, which randomly assigned 1,156 eligible patients to HAART or a comparison combination therapy. Patients were followed for up to 1 year, with the primary endpoints of acquired immunodeficiency syndrome (AIDS) or death. HAART was found to reduce AIDS or death, with a hazard ratio of 0.51. As a target population, Cole and Stuart (2010) obtained data from the Centers for Disease Control and Prevention (CDC) on all individuals newly infected with HIV in 2006. Individual-level data were not available, but the joint distribution of age, sex, and race groups was available and was used to create a target population.

Of importance in terms of the ability to generalize the ACTG 320 results to the target population, the trial sample and the target population vary on a number of characteristics (Table 6.3, adapted from Table 1 of Cole and Stuart, 2010). And, importantly, some of those characteristics were also moderators of the treatment effect. In particular, as shown in the top half of Table 6.4,

TABLE 6.3

Characteristics of HIV-Infected Patients in the AIDS Clinical Trial Group (ACTG) 320 Study in 1996–1997 Followed for 1 Year and of the Estimated HIV-Infected Individuals in the United States in 2006

Characteristic[a]	Trial Patients ($n = 1,156$)	U.S. Population ($n = 54,220$)
Age, years	38 (33, 44)	NA
Age group, years[b]	%	%
13–29	09	34
30–39	45	31
40–49	34	25
≥ 50	13	10
Male sex	83	73
Race	%	%
White, non-Hispanic	54	36
Black, non-Hispanic	28	46
Hispanic	18	18
CD4 count (cells/mm^3)[c]	75 (33, 137)	NA

Source: Adapted from Cole, S. R. and Stuart, E. A. 2010. *American Journal of Epidemiology*, 172(1): 107–115, Table 1.

Abbreviations: AIDS, acquired immunodeficiency syndrome; HIV, human immunodeficiency virus; NA, not available.

[a] Values are expressed as median (quartiles) or percentage; percentages may not sum to 100 because of rounding.

[b] Youngest and oldest patients in the trial were aged 16 and 75 years, respectively.

[c] CD4 cell count was missing for one trial patient.

there were larger effects for young people, and some indication of stronger effects for blacks. Note that the trial tended to enroll older individuals and those of white race or Hispanic ethnicity.

To estimate the PATE, Cole and Stuart (2010) first fit a logistic regression model predicting participation in the trial as a function of age, sex, race, and their two- and three-way interactions. Each person in the trial receives a weight equal to $W_i = P(S_i = 1)/P(S_i = 1|Z_i)$, where the numerator $P(S = 1)$ is the overall probability of being in the trial (the marginal probability), and the denominator $P(S = 1|Z)$ is each individual's probability of being in the trial, given their covariates Z. Individuals in the trial but who actually had a small probability of being in the trial (small $P(S = 1|Z)$) will receive a large weight, reflecting the fact that they provide a lot of information about population effects. To estimate the PATE, an inverse probability of selection-weighted Cox proportional hazards model is then fit using the data from the randomized trial and individuals' weights.

The bottom half of Table 6.4 presents the PATE estimates, when the trial has been reweighted to match the age, sex, and race distributions of the target

TABLE 6.4

Hazard Ratios and 95% Confidence Limits for Incident AIDS or Death within 1 Year for Patients in the ACTG 320 Study in 1996–1997 and for the Population of Individuals Infected with HIV in 2006, the United States

	Hazard Ratio	95% CL	CL Ratio
Trial results			
Intent to treat[a]	0.51	0.33, 0.77	2.33
Age-group stratified, years[b,c]			
13–29	1.87	0.34, 10.2	
30–39	0.21	0.09, 0.48	
40–49	0.84	0.41, 1.70	
≥ 50	0.59	0.24, 1.45	
Sex stratified[d]			
Male	0.47	0.29, 0.74	
Female	0.76	0.28, 2.10	
Race stratified[e]			
White, non-Hispanic	0.59	0.34, 1.01	
Black, non-Hispanic	0.30	0.11, 0.83	
Hispanic	0.54	0.22, 1.36	
Population results			
Age weighted	0.68	0.39, 1.17	3.00
Sex weighted	0.53	0.34, 0.82	2.41
Race weighted	0.46	0.29, 0.72	2.48
Age–sex–race weighted	0.57	0.33, 1.00	3.03

Source: Adapted from Cole, S. R. and Stuart, E. A. 2010. *American Journal of Epidemiology,* 172(1): 107–115, Table 3.

Note: CL ratio included for rows that aim to estimate the PATE.

Abbreviations: AIDS, acquired immunodeficiency syndrome; CL, confidence limit; HIV, human immunodeficiency virus.

[a] The age-group-adjusted hazard ratio was 0.50 (95% CL: 0.33, 0.77).
[b] P for homogeneity across age-group strata = 0.0348.
[c] Youngest and oldest patients in the trial were aged 16 and 75 years, respectively.
[d] P for homogeneity across sex strata = 0.3930.
[e] P for homogeneity across race strata = 0.5396.

population. To talk through the intuition for one of the findings, we see that the race-weighted effect is stronger than the main trial effect. This is because the trial selected against blacks and the treatment effect is larger for blacks; upweighting blacks to better represent the U.S. population then increases the expected effect. When accounting for the age, sex, and race distribution in the U.S. population, the estimated PATE is 0.57, just slightly weaker than the 0.51 hazard ratio observed in the trial. We also note that the standard errors for all of the PATE estimates are larger than the intent-to-treat estimates from the trial, which is expected given the extrapolation from the trial sample to the target population.

It is important to acknowledge the key underlying assumption of these PATE estimates, which is that we have measured and appropriately modeled the factors that influence selection into the trial and treatment effects. One limitation of the data used, for example, is that CD4 cell counts are not available for the U.S. population of newly infected individuals. This precludes us from being able to adjust for this important clinical characteristic that may moderate treatment effects. The approach is likely to work best when a large set of potential effect moderators are observed in the trial sample and the population. The method also assumes that the selection model has been correctly specified. Sensitivity analysis should consider different specifications of the weight model (e.g., as in Cole and Hernan, 2008). Finally, given the different underlying modeling assumptions, it may make sense to estimate the PATE using the reweighting approach as well as one of the flexible outcome modeling approaches, such as BART (A-4), to assess robustness of the results. As discussed further below, there are many potential areas for further research, as well as many methodological questions.

6.5 Conclusions

Recent years have seen an increased interest in determining the generalizability of randomized trials to target populations and estimating population treatment effects when possible. This is true especially given recent increases in data available on broad populations (e.g., claims data, registries), which give researchers more ability to start thinking about generalizability.

With recent movements toward personalized medicine, some may say that generalizability to a broad "target population" is less important, and that what really matters is determining "what works for whom" (not "what works for everyone."). While identifying the best treatments for individuals is important, for many questions, it is still important to understand what impacts would be in a broad target population. This includes studies of interventions that may be potentially applied to a full population, for example, whether the general population should be screened for melanoma (Helfand et al., 2001), or new guidance on when highly antiretroviral therapy should be started, as well as for when decision makers need to make decisions regarding, for example, whether a new intervention or treatment should be covered by insurance or Medicare. We also highlight that sometimes the "target population" may be a particular subpopulation of interest; for example, perhaps a decision maker is interested in determining whether a given randomized trial can be informative for decisions regarding a particular subpopulation at high risk or of primary interest (e.g., those with a particular comorbidity, or a disadvantaged sample). As stated by Goodman, "Comparative effectiveness research (CER) is still an evolving framework for which much needs to be done to improve the ability of randomized controlled trials (RCTs) to supply the necessary evidence. Perhaps, most important is to start with a clearly specified decision and decision maker in mind when the RCTs are designed" (2012, p. 22).

As detailed above, if effects truly are constant across individuals in the population, then there will be no problems with generalizability. It is when effects vary across individuals (or schools or communities) that generalizability may be more limited. This implies that as we move more toward "personalized medicine," with its underpinning in nonconstant treatment effects, we may need to be even more cautious regarding generalizability. This also points to a need to understand treatment effect heterogeneity and better methods for assessing variation in treatment effects, especially since trials are generally underpowered to detect effect heterogeneity. Alemayehu (2011) provides an overview of some of the considerations when assessing effect heterogeneity in CER.

It is also crucial to understand the mechanisms through which interventions work, and thus the factors that may moderate treatment effects; this is related to the selection diagrams of Bareinboim and Pearl (2013) and laying out formal diagrams of which factors and associates generalize and which do not. As stated by the GRADE* Working Group, "To determine whether important uncertainty exists, we can ask whether there is a compelling reason to expect important differences in the size of the effect" (2004, p. 5 of electronic version). One example of this is provided by Goodman (2012), who describes the Extracranial–Intracranial (ECIC) Bypass Study. Clinicians raised concerns about the lack of generalizability of that study because of concerns that the trial had not enrolled a sample that was representative of all patients at risk for stroke. However, as stated by Goodman, "the trial results turned out to be broadly generalizable because the pathophysiology of the involved system was the most generalizable element" (2012, p. 24).

The newness of methods for assessing generalizability also highlights the need for more investigation of those methods and of diagnostics for when generalization is feasible and when it is not. Some preliminary work shows limited success of methods for generalizing effects (Orr et al., 2012; Kern et al., 2016); further work needs to be done to determine which methods work best and when. If in fact analysis procedures are not promising, then new designs that are also feasible to implement are needed, perhaps through smart combining of experimental and nonexperimental evidence of treatment effects.

In summary, assessing generalizability is an exciting area that has the potential to help answer questions regarding treatment effects in target populations, making clinical trial results potentially more relevant for policy questions. However, there are still many questions regarding when it is possible to make such generalizations, and the best methods to use when doing so. This chapter has presented some of the statistical methods that can be used to assess generalizability, as well as many directions for further research in these areas.

Acknowledgements

Dr. Stuart's time on this work was supported by the Patient Centered Outcomes Research Institute (PCORI), Grant ME-1502-27794 (PI: Dahabreh and Stuart), and the US Department of Education Institute of Education Sciences (R305D150003; PIs: Stuart and Olsen).

References

Alemayehu, D. 2011. Evaluation of heterogeneity of treatment effects in comparative effectiveness research. *Journal of Biometrics and Biostatistics*, 2(5): 1000125.

Bareinboim, E. and Pearl, J. 2013. A general algorithm for deciding transportability of experimental results. *Journal of Causal Inference*, 1(1): 107–134.

Bell, S.H., Olsen, R.B., Orr, L.L., and Stuart, E.A. 2016. Estimates of external validity bias when impact evaluations select sites nonrandomly. *Educational Evaluation and Policy Analysis*, 38(1): 1–18.

Braslow, J. T., Duan, N., Starks, S. L., Polo, A., Bromley, E., and Wells, K. B. 2005. Generalizability of studies on mental health treatment and outcomes, 1981–1996. *Psychiatric Services*, 56(10): 1261–1268.

Brown, C. H., Wang, W., and Sandler, I. 2008. Examining how context changes intervention impact: The use of effect sizes in multilevel mixture meta-analysis. *Child Development Perspectives*, 2(3): 198–205.

Chalkidou, K., Tunis, S., Whicher, D., Fowler, R., and Zwarenstein, M. 2012. The role for pragmatic randomized controlled trials (pRCTs) in comparative effectiveness research. *Clinical Trials*, 9: 436–446.

Cole, S. R. and Hernan, M. A. 2008. Constructing inverse probability weights for marginal structural models. *American Journal of Epidemiology*, 168: 656–664.

Cole, S. R. and Stuart, E. A. 2010. Generalizing evidence from randomized clinical trials to target populations: The ACTG-320 trial. *American Journal of Epidemiology*, 172(1): 107–115.

Deaton, A. 2009. Instruments of development: Randomization in the tropics, and the search for the elusive keys to economic development. *NBER Working Paper 14690*.

Ezekowitz, J. A., Hu, J., Delgado, D., Hernandez, A. F., Kaul, P., Leader, R., Proulx, G. et al. 2012. Acute heart failure: Perspectives from a randomized trial and a simultaneous registry. *Circulation: Heart Failure*, 5(6): 735–741.

Flay, B. R., Biglan, A., Boruch, R. F., Castro, F. G., Gottfredson, D., Kellam, S., Mościcki, E. K., Schinke, S., Valentine, J. C., and Ji, P. 2005. Standards of evidence: Criteria for efficacy, effectiveness, and dissemination. *Prevention Science*, 6(3): 151–175.

Frangakis, C. E. 2009. The calibration of treatment effects from clinical trials to target populations. *Clinical Trials*, 6: 136–140.

Frank, K. and Min, K.-S. 2007. Indices of robustness for sample representation. *Sociological Methodology*, 37(1): 349–392.

Gheorghe, A., Roberts, T. E., Ives, J. C., Fletcher, B. R., and Calvert, M. 2013. Centre selection for clinical trials and the generalisability of results: A mixed methods study. *PLoS One*, 8(2): e56560.

Go, A. S., Hylek, E. M., Chang, Y., Phillips, K. A., Henault, L. E., Capra, A. M., Jensvold, N. G., Selby, J. V., and Singer, D. E. 2003. Anticoagulation therapy for stroke prevention in atrial fibrillation: How well do randomized trials translate into clinical practice? *Journal of the American Medical Association*, 290(20): 2685–2692.

Goodman, S. N. 2012. Quasi-random reflections on randomized controlled trials and comparative effectiveness research. *Clinical Trials*, 9: 22–26.

The GRADE* Working Group. 2004. Grading quality of evidence and strength of recommendations. *British Medical Journal*, 328(7454): 1490–1494.

Green, L. W. and Glasgow, R. E. 2006. Evaluating the relevance, generalization, and applicability of research: Issues in external validation and translation methodology. *Evaluation and the Health Professions*, 29: 126–153.

Greenhouse, J., Kaizar, E. E., Seltman, H., Kelleher, K., and Gardner, W. 2008. Generalizing from clinical trial data: A case study. The risk of suicidality among pediatric antidepressant users. *Statistics in Medicine*, 27(11): 1801–1813.

Hartman, E., Grieve, R., Ramsahai, R., and Sekhon, J. S. 2015. From sample average treatment effect to population average treatment effect on the treated. Combining experimental with observational studies to estimate population treatment effects. *Journal of the Royal Statistical Society Series A: Statistics in Society*, 178(3): 757–778.

Hedges, L. V. and Olkin, I. 1985. *Statistical Methods for Meta-Analysis*. Academic Press, Orlando.

Helfand, M., Mahon, S., and Eden, K. 2001. *Screening for Skin Cancer. Systematic Evidence Review No 2*. Agency for Healthcare Research and Quality, Rockville, MD.

Hill, J. L. 2011. Bayesian nonparametric modeling for causal inference. *Journal of Computational and Graphical Statistics*, 20(1): 217–240.

Hoertel, N., LeStrat, Y., Blanco, C., Lavaud, P., and Dubertret, C. 2012. Generalizability of clinical trial results for generalized anxiety disorder to community samples. *Depression and Anxiety*, 29(7): 614–620.

Hoertel, N., LeStrat, Y., Lavaud, P., Dubertret, C., and Limosin, F. 2013. Generalizability of clinical trial results for bipolar disorder to community samples: Findings from the national epidemiologic survey on alcohol and related conditions. *The Journal of Clinical Psychiatry*, 74(3): 265–270.

Holland, P. W. 1986. Statistics and causal inference. *Journal of the American Statistical Association*, 81(396): 945–960.

Holt, D. and Smith, T. M. F. 1979. Post stratification. *Journal of the Royal Statistical Society Series A*, 142(1): 33–46.

Horvitz, D. and Thompson, D. 1952. A generalization of sampling without replacement from a finite universe. *Journal of the American Statistical Association*, 47: 663–685.

Humphreys, K., Weingardt, K. R., Horst, D., Joshi, A. A., and Finney, J. W. 2005. Prevalence and predictors of research participant eligibility criteria in alcohol treatment outcome studies, 1970–1998. *Addiction*, 100: 1249–1257.

Imai, K., King, G., and Stuart, E. A. 2008. Misunderstandings between experimentalists and observationalists about causal inference. *Journal of the Royal Statistical Society Series A*, 171: 481–502.

Imai, K. and Ratkovic, M. 2013. Estimating treatment effect heterogeneity in randomized program evaluation. *The Annals of Applied Statistics*, 7(1): 443–470.

Insel, T. R. 2006. Beyond efficacy: The STAR*D trial. *The American Journal of Psychiatry*, 163: 5–7.

Institute of Medicine. 2009. *Initial National Priorities for Comparative Effectiveness Research*. The National Academies Press, Washington, DC.

Kaizar, E. E. 2011. Estimating treatment effect via simple cross design synthesis. *Statistics in Medicine*, 30(25): 2986–3009.

Kent, D. M., Rothwell, P. M., Ioannidis, J. P. A., Altman, D. G., and Hayward, R. A. 2010. Assessing and reporting heterogeneity in treatment effects in clinical trials: A proposal. *Trials*, 11: 85.

Kern, H. L., Stuart, E. A., Hill, J., and Green, D. P. 2016. Assessing methods for generalizing experimental impact estimates to target populations. *Journal of Research on Educational Effectiveness*, 9(1): 103–127.

Kitagawa, E. M. 1964. Standardized comparisons in population research. *Demography*, 1: 296–315.

Koog, Y. H., Wi, H., and Jung, W. Y. 2013. Eligibility criteria in knee osteoarthritis clinical trials: Systematic review. *Clinical Rheumatology*, 32(11): 1569–1574.

Kraemer, H. C. 2013. Discovering, comparing, and combining moderators of treatment on outcome after randomized clinical trials: A parametric approach. *Statistics in Medicine*, 32(11): 1964–1973.

Marcus, S. M. 1997. Assessing non-constant bias with parallel randomized and nonrandomized clinical trials. *Journal of Clinical Epidemiology*, 50: 823–828.

Marcus, S. M., Stuart, E. A., Wang, P., Shadish, W. R., and Steiner, P. M. 2012. Estimating the causal effect of randomization versus treatment preference in a doubly-randomized preference trial. *Psychological Methods*, 17(2): 244–254. PMC Journal—In Progress. PMID: 22563844. http://www.ncbi.nlm.nih.gov/pubmed/22563844

Olsen, R., Bell, S., Orr, L., and Stuart, E. A. 2013. External validity in policy evaluations that choose sites purposively. *Journal of Policy Analysis and Management*, 32(1): 107–121.

O'Muircheartaigh, C. and Hedges, L. V. 2014. Generalizing from experiments with nonrepresentative samples. *Journal of the Royal Statistical Society, Series C*, 63: 195–210.

Orr, L. L., Olsen, R., Bell, S., and Stuart, E. A. 2012. Assessing methods to reduce the external validity bias due to purposive site selection. *Presentation at the Association for Public Policy Analysis and Management Fall Research Conference*. Washington, DC. https://appam.confex.com/appam/2012/webprogram/Paper2745.html

Pearl, J. and Bareinboim, E. 2013. External validity: From do-calculus to transportability across populations. UCLA Cognitive Systems Laboratory, Technical Report (R-400), First version: May 2012: Last revision: September 2013. Submitted, *Statistical Science*. Available at http://ftp.cs.ucla.edu/pub/stat_ser/r400.pdf

Pressler, T. R. and Kaizar, E. E. 2013. The use of propensity scores and observational data to estimate randomized controlled trial generalizability bias. *Statistics in Medicine*, 32(20): 3552–3568.

Prevost, T. C., Abrams, K. R., and Jones, D. R. 2000. Hierarchical models in generalized synthesis of evidence: An example based on studies of breast cancer screening. *Statistics in Medicine*, 19(24): 3359–3376.

Riley, R. D., Lambert, P. C., and Abo-Zaid, G. 2010. Meta-analysis of individual participant data: Rationale, conduct, and reporting. *British Medical Journal*, 340: c221.

Roehr, B. 2013. The appeal of large simple trials. *British Medical Journal*, 346: f1317.

Rosenbaum, P. R. and Rubin, D. B. 1983. The central role of the propensity score in observational studies for causal effects. *Biometrika*, 70(1): 41–55.

Rothwell, P. M. 2005. External validity of randomised controlled trials: "To whom do the results of this trial apply?" *The Lancet*, 365(9453): 82–93.

Rubin, D. 1974. Estimating causal effects of treatments in randomized and nonrandomized studies. *Journal of Educational Psychology*, 66(5): 688–701.

Rush, A. J., Fava, M., Wisniewski, S. R., Lavori, P. W., Trivedi, M. H., Sackeim, H. A., Thase, M. E. et al. and STAR*D Investigators Group. 2004. Sequenced treatment alternatives to relieve depression (STAR*D): Rationale and design. *Controlled Clinical Trials*, 25(1): 119–142.

Sachs, G. S., Thase, M. E., Otto, M. W., Bauer, M., Miklowitz, D., Wisniewski, S. R., Lavori, P. et al. 2003. Rationale, design, and methods of the Systematic Treatment Enhancement Program for Bipolar Disorder (STEP-BD). *Biological Psychiatry*, 53: 1028–1042.

Schochet, P. Z., Burghardt, J., and McConnell, S. 2008. Does job corps work? Impact findings from the national job corps study. *American Economic Review*, 98(5): 1864–1886.

Shadish, W. R. 1995. The logic of generalization: Five principles common to experiments and ethnographies. *American Journal of Community Psychology*, 23(3): 419–428.

Shadish, W. R., Cook, T. D., and Campbell, D. T. 2002. *Experimental and Quasi-Experimental Designs for Generalized Causal Inference*. Houghton Mifflin, Boston.

Stevens, J., Kelleher, K., Greenhouse, J., Chen, G., Xiang, H., Kaizar, E., Jensen, P. S., and Arnold, L. E. 2006. Empirical evaluation of the generalizability of the sample from the Multimodal Treatment Study for ADHD. *Administration and Policy in Mental Health*, 34: 221–232.

Stuart, E. A. 2010. Matching methods for causal inference: A review and a look forward. *Statistical Science: A Review Journal of the Institute of Mathematical Statistics*, 25(1): 1–21.

Stuart, E. A., Cole, S., Bradshaw, C. P., and Leaf, P. J. 2011. The use of propensity scores to assess the generalizability of results from randomized trials. *Journal of the Royal Statistical Society Series A*, 174(2): 369–386.

Stuart, E. A., Bell, S. H., Ebnesajjad, C., Olsen, R. B., and Orr, L. L. 2016. Characteristics of school districts that participate in rigorous national educational evaluations.

Journal of Research on Educational Effectiveness. Published online June 30, 2016. http://dx.doi.org/10.1080/19345747.2016.1205160

Sutton, A. J. and Higgins, J. P. 2008. Recent developments in meta-analysis. *Statistics in Medicine*, 27(5): 625–650.

Tipton, E. 2013. Improving generalizations from experiments using propensity score subclassification: Assumptions, properties, and contexts. *Journal of Educational and Behavioral Statistics*, 38: 239–266.

Tipton, E., Hedges, L. V., Vaden-Kiernan, M., Borman, G. D., Sullivan, K., and Caverly, S. 2014. Sample selection in randomized experiments: A new method using propensity score stratified sampling. *Journal of Research on Educational Effectiveness*, 7(1): 114–135.

Turner, R. M., Spiegelhalter, D. J., Smith, G. C. S., and Thompson, S. G. 2009. Bias modelling in evidence synthesis. *Journal of the Royal Statistical Society Series A*, 172(1): 21–47.

Unger, J. M., Hershman, D. L., Albain, K. S., Moinpour, C. M., Petersen, J. A., Burg, K., and Crowley, J. J. 2013. Patient income level and cancer clinical trial preparation. *Journal of Clinical Oncology*, 31(5): 536–542.

U.S. Department of Education. 2009. *The Impacts of Regular Upward Bound on Postsecondary Outcomes Seven to Nine Years after Scheduled High School Graduation.* Office of Planning, Evaluation and Policy Development, Policy and Program Studies Service, Washington, DC.

U.S. Department of Health and Human Services. 2010. *Head Start Impact Study Final Report.* Office of Planning, Evaluation and Policy Development, Administration for Children and Families, Policy and Program Studies Service, Washington, DC.

VanderWeele, T. J. and Hernán, M. A. 2013. Causal inference under multiple versions of treatment. *Journal of Causal Inference*, 1: 1–20.

Weisberg, H. I., Hayden, V. C., and Pontes, V. P. 2009. Selection criteria and generalizability within the counterfactual framework: Explaining the paradox of antidepressant-induced suicidality? *Clinical Trials*, 6(109): 109–118.

Wisniewski, S., Rush, A., Nierenberg, A., Gaynes, B., Warden, D., Luther, J., McGrath, P. J. et al. 2009. Can phase III trial results of antidepressant medications be generalized to clinical practice? A STAR*D report. *American Journal of Psychiatry*, 166(5): 599–607.

Zimmerman, M., Chelminski, I., and Posternak, M. A. 2005. Generalizability of antidepressant efficacy trials: Differences between depressed psychiatric outpatients who would or would not qualify for an efficacy trial. *American Journal of Psychiatry*, 162(7): 1370–1377.

7

Combining Information from Multiple Data Sources: An Introduction to Cross-Design Synthesis with a Case Study

Joel B. Greenhouse, Heather D. Anderson, Jeffrey A. Bridge, Anne M. Libby, Robert Valuck, and Kelly J. Kelleher

CONTENTS

ABSTRACT A goal of comparative effectiveness research is to help stakeholders reach consensus about the benefits and harms of medical interventions, at both the individual and population levels. The Institute of Medicine and others have recognized that to advance comparative effectiveness research, it will be necessary to use evidence from data sources other than randomized-controlled clinical trials. Different sources of evidence, such as randomized trials, observational studies, and meta-analyses, however, have strengths and weaknesses. Therefore, to help stakeholders reach consensus about the effectiveness of medical interventions, we argue it will be necessary not only to generate, but also to synthesize and weigh evidence from multiple data sources. In this chapter, we illustrate and refine an approach for using information from multiple data sources called cross-design synthesis. Cross-design synthesis is a way of thinking about and framing comparative effectiveness questions such that multiple data sources can be used together to help answer those questions. We briefly review the strengths and weaknesses of evidence generated from different study designs, introduce cross-design synthesis, and illustrate the use of cross-design synthesis with a case study investigating whether the initiation of the use of antidepressants increases the risk of suicidal behavior in depressed children and adolescents.

7.1 Introduction

A goal of comparative effectiveness research is to help stakeholders, such as patients, providers, payers, and policy makers, reach consensus about the benefits and harms of medical interventions, at both the individual and population levels. Questions that are key to effectiveness research include, for example, whether a treatment effect is homogeneous and replicable in a specific population and whether it is generalizable to other populations and settings; are there identifiable subgroups more likely to benefit or to be harmed by an intervention; and what are the gaps in understanding about the effectiveness of interventions and about practice variations in the delivery of care? Clearly, the scope of comparative effectiveness research is quite broad. The Institute of Medicine (IOM) and others have recognized that to advance comparative effectiveness research, it will be necessary to use evidence from data sources other than randomized-controlled clinical trials (Sox and Greenfield 2009). As discussed in several chapters in this volume, different sources of evidence, such as randomized trials, observational studies, and meta-analyses, however, have strengths and weaknesses. Therefore, to help stakeholders reach consensus about the effectiveness of medical interventions, we believe it will be necessary not only to generate, but also to synthesize and weigh evidence from multiple data sources (Greenhouse and Kelleher 2005).

In this chapter, we illustrate and refine an approach for using information from multiple data sources called *cross-design synthesis* (Droitcour et al. 1993). Cross-design synthesis is not a single methodology but rather a way of thinking about and framing comparative effectiveness questions such that multiple data sources can be used together to help answer those questions. Utilizing state-of-the-art statistical, epidemiological, and computational methods, cross-design synthesis uses evidence from complementary studies to help answer questions about whether a treatment works across the full range of patients, providers, and settings. The reader can consult Chapter 6 for a general discussion of generalizability of results from clinical trials.

The organization of this chapter is as follows. In the next section, we briefly review the strengths and weaknesses of evidence generated from different study designs. Section 7.3 introduces cross-design synthesis and provides a formal framework for thinking about the approach. We then illustrate the use of cross-design synthesis with a case study investigating whether the initiation of the use of antidepressants increases the risk of suicidal behavior in depressed children and adolescents. We conclude the chapter with a summary and a discussion of the role of cross-design synthesis in comparative effectiveness research.

7.2 Sources of Evidence for Comparative Effectiveness Research

Randomized clinical trials (RCTs) are traditionally considered the gold standard for evaluating the efficacy of medical interventions. The RCT design permits researchers to enforce high levels of internal validity, in part, through a tightly controlled process of participant selection. Eligibility criteria for an RCT typically aim to generate a homogeneous sample of participants for whom the treatment is both safe and likely to demonstrate a beneficial effect if one exists. However, a restrictive selection process can create tension between the objectives of internal validity and generalizability. The assessment of the generalizability of RCT results is critical to help determine which interventions are most effective and safe for which patients.

Observational data, such as those obtained from health surveys, epidemiology databases, and administrative claims, are larger in size and typically more representative of the target population of interest than data from RCTs. However, the results from observational studies are often distrusted because of the concern that treatment groups are noncomparable due to selection effects. Nevertheless, observational studies are important for studying rare adverse events due to the larger size of such studies, and for assessing the generalizability of findings from academic and pharmaceutical company research to practice in the community. Methods for the analysis of observational studies are discussed in Chapters 1 through 3.

Since a single study, either an RCT or observational study, is rarely sufficient to convincingly establish a cause-and-effect relationship, especially for questions concerning the effectiveness and/or safety of drugs or medical devices, it is necessary to use methods that combine evidence from multiple sources. As discussed in the Chapters 10 through 12 on Research Synthesis, meta-analysis of RCTs has become a key methodology for the formal accumulation and evaluation of evidence. Combining information from a number of similar randomized trials, however, often suffers from the same limitations of evidence generated from a single randomized trial, such as restrictive study inclusion/exclusion criteria, limitations on generalizability, and narrowly focused questions (see, e.g., Rothwell 2005). In addition, it is important to recognize that any meta-analysis is itself an observational study, even meta-analysis of RCTs, and therefore the evidence from a meta-analysis needs to be subjected to the same scrutiny as any observational study (see, e.g., Hammad et al. 2011).

7.3 Cross-Design Synthesis

7.3.1 Background

Concerned with the difficulties of applying results from RCTs to clinical practice, the Congress in 1992 requested the U.S. Government Accountability Office (GAO) to develop a new strategy for evaluating the effectiveness and generalizability of medical interventions. The GAO called this approach *cross-design synthesis* (GAO 1992; Droitcour et al. 1993). Our interest in using cross-design synthesis in comparative effectiveness research is motivated in part by the recognition that evidence about patient outcomes is available from both RCTs and observational studies, and that neither data source is perfect, in the sense that RCTs may be rigorous but restricted and observational studies more general but may be biased. Cross-design synthesis uses evidence from complementary studies to help answer questions about whether a treatment works across the full range of patients, providers, and settings. The challenge of this approach is to extract information from different kinds of research by capturing the strengths and minimizing the weaknesses of the different designs. Using state-of-the-art statistical and computational methods, we believe cross-design synthesis is a valuable methodological approach that will help advance comparative effectiveness and patient-centered outcomes research, especially when there is concern about generalizability, concern about treatment heterogeneity, and/or concern about rare adverse effects that may be undetected in usual RCT designs.

In this chapter, we illustrate the use of cross-design synthesis in the context of a case study that (i) investigates the generalizability of results from a set of RCTs and (ii) investigates the independent replication of study results across different settings and populations. First, however, we outline the broad steps for doing a cross-design synthesis.

The four major steps in using evidence from studies with complementary designs are (GAO 1992):

1. Specify the question(s) of interest and identify the target population of interest. Identify data sources, both experimental and observational, that might provide evidence about the question of interest, including RCTs, health surveys, epidemiological studies, and large administrative databases.

2. Assess existing randomized studies for generalizability, that is, external validity, across the full range of relevant patients. Evaluate studies for quality and "combinability." Using expert judgment and methods from meta-analysis, this step requires careful review of each study with respect to its design, methods, patient selection process, and patient representativeness.

3. Assess nonexperimental or observational studies for "imbalanced comparison groups." This step requires careful review of existing studies with respect to relevance to the question of interest and the degree of balance or imbalance of patient characteristics across the groups being compared. Then, formal methods for statistical adjustment, such as matching, linear models, weighting, and propensity scores, are used to reduce bias resulting from any imbalance in the comparison groups. Again, evaluate studies for quality and "combinability."

4. Before synthesizing studies, adjust the results of each randomized study and each observational study, compensating for biases as needed. The methodology for this step is similar to the ones used in steps 2 and 3.

5. Address the comparative effectiveness or patient-centered outcome question of interest, whether it is synthesizing evidence for the effectiveness of an intervention, identifying adverse effects of interventions, assessing the generalizability of a result, or investigating treatment heterogeneity. Typically, in a cross-design synthesis, we will not be interested in a single summary measure, but in a systematic quantification of the evidence along with a description of variability. Formal statistical methods for combining information from diverse studies will be based on the use of Bayesian hierarchical models and methods for sensitivity analyses to assess the robustness of conclusions to the various model assumptions (e.g., Greenhouse and Iyengar 2009).

The GAO (1994) used cross-design synthesis to address the following question: Even though RCTs had shown that breast cancer patient survival rates following mastectomy and breast conservation therapy were equivalent, were the results similar in day-to-day medical practice—with its less certain more variable quality of care? They first examined the 5-year survival results separately for single-center and multicenter randomized studies; next, they examined database records (drawn from the SEER database) for breast cancer patients treated outside of randomized studies, and performed an analysis on a set of cases that had been selected to be comparable to the kinds of patients covered in the randomized studies; the final step consisted of quantitative comparisons across study designs and a consideration of the strength of the evidence. They found that the 5-year survival results were similar across the three study types, suggesting that the treatment effect is homogeneous with respect to setting. Despite this early case study, cross-design synthesis is an idea that has had limited application.

7.3.2 Conceptual Framework for Cross-Design Synthesis

The motivation for cross-design synthesis is based on (i) an appreciation that evidence about a question of interest is available from multiple data sources, and (ii) the recognition that different study designs have different strengths, and that it cannot be assumed in combining their study results, that their strengths will be preserved while their weaknesses are eliminated. We have found that a useful statistical framework for thinking about cross-design synthesis is to conceptualize the problem of combining evidence across different study designs using the language of response surface methodology.

The original concept for cross-design synthesis, we believe, can be traced to Rubin (1990, 1992). Rubin proposed a different perspective on meta-analysis, which is useful to consider in general and is at the intellectual heart of cross-design synthesis. The idea is that the objective of combining information across studies is to build and extrapolate response surfaces in an attempt to estimate "true effects" from ideal studies rather than estimate effects as averages of effects from some population of "flawed" studies. In this approach, each study can be classified by two types of characteristics: S, which are variables of scientific interest (e.g., class of antidepressant, dose, diagnosis, participant age), and D, which are design variables (e.g., sample size, whether the study was randomized or not, investigator characteristics). If Y represents the observed outcome for each study, then in principle a response surface model can be built for Y given (S,D) using the observed studies. However, the region where the observed data can fall is not necessarily of primary scientific interest because it reflects the various choices that were made by necessity about values of D. Interest would be in the extrapolated response surface, $E(Y|S, D = D_0)$ with D fixed at specified ideal values, say D_0. Building a response surface model is a standard, though not necessarily easy, statistical task.

Rubin speculates on a number of intriguing practical implications that follow from this perspective. For example, there is no need to be selective about which studies to include in a research synthesis since all studies contribute to the estimate of the response surface and modeling will automatically downweight poorer studies. Also, this approach will provide guidance in the choice of new studies to add to the database based on choosing studies, that is, values of **S** and **D**, which increase the precision of estimation of the response surface, E(Y|**S, D**). Finally, this framework readily allows focus to be moved to patient-centered inference by examining the response surface where the scientific values **S** are set at individual patient-relevant values.

The basis for this conceptualization is grounded in ideas underlying response surface methodology, hierarchical statistical models, and statistical methods for causal inference and missing data. As far as we know, this response surface approach has not been used in practice and we appreciate that a number of details of implementation remain to be developed. Many of these details, however, will be context specific.

7.4 Case Study

One possible explanation for differences in results between RCTs and observational studies could be due to the fact that these studies are sampling from different patient populations. A strategy for assessing the generalizability of samples obtained in randomized trials is to compare study samples to target populations on measured characteristics that might directly modify outcomes or are correlated with unmeasured variables that might modify outcomes (Greenhouse et al. 2008). If the treatment interacts with some characteristic to produce an outcome that depends on the treatment-by-characteristic combination, a situation called treatment heterogeneity, then generalizing results from a single study to the larger target population may not be appropriate (Longford 1999). Thus, if such a comparison shows that the study population is "similar" to the target population, then we would be more confident in making inferences from the former to the latter. If, however, the two populations are shown to be dissimilar and there is treatment heterogeneity, there would be reason to be cautious about generalizing the study results.

In the following case study, we will describe and illustrate how we can use cross-design synthesis to make what we call generalizability judgments. Specifically, we are concerned with the generalizability of results from RCTs and the identification of subpopulations that either benefit or are harmed by an intervention. The case study is concerned with the evidence for an increased risk of suicidal behavior in depressed children and adolescents who are treated with antidepressants. Our goal is to illustrate the practice of evidence synthesis from multiple data sources in the context of this real and compelling question about the harmful effects of a medical intervention. (For other examples, see Horwitz et al. 1990; Hernán et al. 2008).

7.4.1 Background

In 2004, the Food and Drug Administration (FDA) issued a black box warning advising physicians and patients that antidepressant use is associated with an increased risk of suicidality, that is, suicidal ideations or suicidal behavior, in youths. The basis for the black box warning was a meta-analysis of 24 randomized placebo-controlled efficacy trials for different psychiatric disorders, involving nearly 4,600 children and adolescents. Although the FDA found that youths receiving antidepressants were twice as likely to have suicidal ideation and behaviors as youths receiving placebo (Hammad et al. 2006) and concluded that "[T]here is a causal link between the newer antidepressants and pediatric suicidality" (Leslie et al. 2005), these conclusions and the box warning have been controversial.

Concerns related to the strength of evidence from the FDA meta-analysis included the choice of outcome and the exclusion of high-risk cases from the randomized trials. Specifically, critics noted that there is only weak evidence for an association in this age group between suicidal ideation, a component of the FDA primary composite outcome they called suicidality, and suicidal behavior (either attempts or suicides) (Klein 2006; Baldessarini et al. 2006). In addition, all but one of the primary trials used in the FDA meta-analysis excluded patients who had serious comorbidities and/or were at high risk of suicide, raising questions about the generalizability of the FDA results (Posner et al. 2007; Greenhouse et al. 2008; Weisberg et al. 2009).

Attempts to replicate the FDA finding have been mixed. Because suicide and suicide attempts are rare, randomized trials designed to examine the safety of antidepressants in children and adolescents are prohibitively costly and may now be unethical. As a result, many investigators have turned to observational studies for evidence about the safety of antidepressants. For example, a case–control study using national Medicaid data on depressed inpatients found that antidepressants increased the risk of suicide attempts and suicide in children and adolescents (Olfson et al. 2006), a result similar to the FDA's finding. Further, a meta-analysis of five observational studies that reported completed or attempted suicide in depressed youth found a nearly twofold increase in risk among selective serotonin reuptake inhibitor (SSRI) users, a specific class of antidepressants (Barbui et al. 2009). Valuck et al. (2004), however, using a propensity-adjusted retrospective cohort study of over 24,000 newly diagnosed depressed adolescents from a managed care database, found that treatment with SSRIs was not significantly associated with risk of suicide attempt. Others, using claims data, found that the period of greatest risk for suicide and suicide attempt appeared to be in the month before starting antidepressant treatment and that risk decreased following the initiation of treatment (Gibbons et al. 2007; Simon et al. 2006; Simon and Savarino 2007).

Clearly, there are many challenges to assessing the safety of antidepressant use in youth with respect to suicidal outcomes. Experimental studies are typically not sufficiently generalizable, whereas observational studies, while much larger in size, often suffer from noncomparable treatment groups due to selection effects (Horwitz et al. 1990). Since there is a lack of consensus about the harmful effects of antidepressants in youth and to address issues raised by critics of the FDA findings, we have investigated the evidence for an increased risk of suicidal behavior in youth using cross-design synthesis. One motivation for our cross-design synthesis is the concern about the generalizability of the findings from the FDA's meta-analysis due to the explicit exclusion of patients at high risk of suicide from nearly all of the randomized trials, a critical subset of the population affected by the black box warning. To the degree that these exclusion criteria restricted the representativeness of the study samples resulting in a biased estimate of risk, generalizations to the larger target population could be limited.

Our cross-design synthesis uses a subset of studies from the database of randomized-controlled clinical trials used by the FDA as the source of evidence for the 2004 black box warning, and the IMS LifeLink Health Claims database, the largest commercially available U.S. database of longitudinal healthcare claims (IMS LifeLink® 2009). Our work consists of three phases corresponding to three complementary sources of evidence:

Phase I. We conduct a new meta-analysis using (i) just the subset of depression trials from the FDA RCT database and (ii) suicidal behavior, not suicidality, as the outcome of interest. This phase will provide us with a database from which we can characterize the patients who participated in the randomized trials and obtain an estimate of risk that will help inform the analysis of the observational data.

Phase II. Using the observational IMS LifeLink claims data, we investigate the risk of suicide attempt due to antidepressant use in depressed youths. The IMS LifeLink database is representative of the commercially insured pediatric population affected by the FDA's black box warning (Libby et al. 2007).

Phase III. Finally, we select a nonrandom subset of patients from the IMS LifeLink cohort based on exclusion criteria typically used to identify patients for participation in antidepressant RCTs. We simulate a randomized trial using the claims data by excluding patients who would typically be ineligible for an antidepressant trial, balancing treatment groups using propensity score adjustment, and finding an estimate of risk using regression models. In addition, to assess the selection effect of the trial exclusion criteria, we compare the estimate of risk from Phase III to the risk obtained in the unrestricted IMS LifeLink cohort in Phase II. To investigate the convergence of evidence from the different data sources and analyses, we also compare the risk estimate obtained from the meta-analysis of the RCT data in Phase I to the estimates of risk found in the claims data in Phases II and III.

In summary, the goal of our case study is to investigate the replicability and the generalizability of the FDA meta-analysis of the harmful effects of antidepressant medication in children and adolescents that resulted in a black box warning.

7.4.2 Methods

7.4.2.1 Phase I: Meta-Analysis

Details about the 24 pediatric antidepressant-randomized trials used in the FDA meta-analysis and the results of the FDA analyses have been published elsewhere (Hammad et al. 2006). Table 7.1 presents features of the primary studies in the original FDA meta-analysis. To align these RCT studies with the outcome typically available from observational studies, our primary outcome is *suicidal behavior* and not *suicidality*. Because there were no completed suicides in the primary RCT studies, the FDA defined *suicidal behavior* to be the union of the Columbia code 1 "suicide attempt" and code 2 "preparatory actions toward imminent suicidal behavior" (Posner et al. 2007). In addition, we also restrict our meta-analysis to the subset of 16 depression trials. We limited our meta-analysis to the depression RCTs included in the FDA database to ensure reliability of the outcome, as assessed by the Columbia group (FDA Report 2004), and comparability with Hammad et al. (2006). Our data source is the FDA Report (2004).

7.4.2.1.1 Data Analysis

We calculated a fixed-effects, Mantel–Haenszel estimate of the relative risk of suicidal behavior for antidepressant use versus placebo and its confidence

TABLE 7.1

FDA Meta-Analysis: Study-Level Characteristics

Drug Class	Number of Studies	Diagnosis	Number of Studies
SSRI	16	MDD	16
Celexa	2	OCD	4
Luvox	1	Anxiety	3
Paxil	5	ADHD	1
Prozac	5		
Zoloft	3		
		Trial Length (4–16 Weeks)	
Atypical	8	≤8 weeks	13
Effexor	4	≥9 weeks	11
Remeron	1		
Serzone	2		
Wellbutrin	1		

interval (Woodward 2005). For comparability, we follow the FDA's analytic approach and added 0.5 to all cells of studies that had events in only one arm. The FDA approach, however, excluded information from the five studies that had no events. We replicated all analyses using alternative measures of risk, including the odds ratio and the incidence rate ratio. As a sensitivity analysis that allowed us to use the results from all 16 studies, we also calculated a Bayes estimate of risk and a 95% credible interval using several different prior distributions (Kaizar et al. 2006). This analysis also takes into account any between-study variability.

7.4.2.2 Phase II: LifeLink Cohort

The observational data for this study were drawn from the IMS LifeLink Health Plan Claims Database, the largest commercially available database of longitudinal healthcare claims in the United States. The data included integrated medical, specialty, facility, and pharmacy paid claims from January 1998 to December 2008 for more than 95 managed care plans and represent approximately 42 million covered lives. Data were unidentified and anonymous, and therefore an expedited review was obtained from the Colorado Multiple Institutional Review Board.

Using the IMS LifeLink data, we created a cohort of subjects with new episodes of depression based on the following specifications of the National Committee for Quality Assurance Health Plan and Employer Data and Information Set: (1) an ICD-9 diagnostic code of 296.2, 296.3, 300.4, or 311 (major depressive disorder, single or recurrent episode; neurotic depression; and depression not otherwise specified, respectively); (2) at least 90 days prior to the depression diagnosis with no claims for an antidepressant; and (3) at least 120 days prior to the depression diagnosis with no claims with a depression-related diagnosis (Scholle 2005). Subjects aged 18 years and older were excluded, resulting in a pediatric cohort of subjects aged 5–17 years. Only depression episodes between January 1, 1999 and June 30, 2008 were included. For each subject, the earliest depression episode during this time period was identified as the index depression episode. Subjects were required to have at least 12 months of eligibility prior to their depression episode and 6 months of eligibility following their depression episode. The resulting pediatric depressed cohort, which we call the *LifeLink cohort*, included 52,293 subjects aged 5–17 years.

7.4.2.2.1 Treatment Groups

Treatment groups were defined based on receipt of an antidepressant, SSRI or other, and/or psychotherapy following the index depression episode. SSRI monotherapy treatment was defined as one or more fills of the same SSRI, with the first fill being within 30 days of the index depression episode start. Psychotherapy treatment was defined as two or more psychotherapy visits within 90 days of the index depression episode start. Using these definitions, five mutually exclusive treatment groups were identified:

1. "SSRI, No-psychotherapy" included subjects who received SSRI treatment but no psychotherapy treatment.
2. "SSRI + Psychotherapy" included subjects who received both SSRI treatment and psychotherapy.
3. "Psychotherapy, No-antidepressant" included subjects who received psychotherapy but no antidepressants during the follow-up period.
4. "No-treatment" included subjects who did not receive psychotherapy and received no antidepressant treatment during follow-up.
5. "Other-antidepressant" treatment included subjects who received a non-SSRI antidepressant during follow-up or received their first SSRI more than 30 days after the index depression episode start.

7.4.2.2.2 Suicide Attempt

The first suicide attempt was identified using the Centers for Disease Control and Prevention (2011) recommended framework of E-code groupings for self-inflicted injury: ICD-9 codes E950-E959 and ICD-10 codes X60-X84 and Y87.0. The use of these codes, we believe, will provide a conservative estimate of suicidal behavior. Furthermore, any bias due to the use of these codes should be evenly distributed among treatment groups.

7.4.2.2.3 Study Period

Each subject's study period began with the start of their index depression episode and ended 6 months later or when the first claim indicating an attempt was seen, whichever came first. In an attempt to emulate a randomized trial intent-to-treat analysis, subjects remained assigned to their initial treatment group throughout their 6-month study period.

7.4.2.2.4 Data Analysis

Because of its size and representativeness, we consider the IMS LifeLink cohort to be our population of interest. The crude rate ratios in this cohort are then the parameters that represent the associations of interest.

7.4.2.3 Phase III: Restricted Cohort

The five most common exclusion criteria for trial participation found in almost all of the 16 FDA depression-randomized trials were (1) lifetime suicidal tendencies, risk, ideation, or self-inflicted injury; (2) current schizophrenia diagnosis; (3) current or lifetime history of drug or alcohol dependence diagnosis; (4) current bipolar I or II diagnosis; and (5) currently pregnant or sexually active females not using medically accepted means of contraception. We defined "current" as occurring during the 12 months prior to or 6 months following the index depression episode and lifetime as occurring at any time prior to the index depression episode.

To create the *Restricted cohort*, that is, a cohort of subjects who were similar to the patients who participated in the RCTs, subjects from the IMS LifeLink cohort who met any of the above five criteria were excluded ($n = 12,823$). Also excluded were subjects who had a claim for a suicide attempt within 7 days of their index depression episode ($n = 74$), in part, because the suicide attempt would have excluded them from participation in an RCT, and because the timing of medication and suicide attempt is uncertain. After these exclusions, there were 39,396 subjects in the Restricted cohort.

7.4.2.3.1 Data Analysis

The distributions of demographic characteristics in the Restricted cohort were compared statistically to the corresponding characteristics in the unrestricted LifeLink cohort for the SSRI-only and the No-treatment groups. We used large, one-sample tests for proportions and for means, treating the LifeLink cohort parameters as fixed and known.

Our primary comparison of interest was the "SSRI, No-psychotherapy" group versus the "No-treatment" group. A secondary comparison of interest was the "Other-antidepressant" treatment group versus "No-treatment." To address the issue of nonrandom allocation to treatment group, a two-stage propensity analysis approach was used to estimate adjusted rate ratios for the Restricted cohort (Rubin 1997). First, we estimated the propensity to be in a particular treatment group compared to its referent group using logistic regression. These propensity models were adjusted for age, gender, region, Medicaid status, number of SSRI trials during the 12 months prior to the index depression episode (one or more vs. none), and a linear and quadratic term for year relative to 2003 (FDA's first risk communication regarding increased suicide risk in pediatric patients). We assessed the fit of the models using the Hosmer–Lemeshow test, and the success of the models to balance treatment groups using propensity score stratification. Next, we used Poisson regression models to estimate the propensity-adjusted risk of suicide attempt, adjusting for propensity score, age, gender, region, and Medicaid status (D'Agostino 1998; Rubin 2010). All data manipulations and statistical analyses used SAS version 9.2 (2008).

7.5 Results

7.5.1 Phase I: Meta-Analysis

Figure 7.1 displays a forest plot for the meta-analysis of the depression trials. Each row in the top part of the figure presents a study-wise estimate of the relative risk and its 95% confidence interval. For the five studies that had no

RCT data: Phase I[*]

Study name	Relative Risk (95% Cl)	Events/Total Treated	Placebo
Citalopram 94404	2.90 (0.60–14.10)	6/124	2/120
Citalopram CIT-MD-18	0.91 (0.06–14.39)	1/93	1/85
Fluoxetine HCCJ	0.30 (0.01–7.02)	0/21	1/19
Fluoxetine X065	5.00 (0.25–101.48)	2/48	0/48
Fluoxetine TADS	5.14 (0.25–105.78)	2/109	0/112
Paroxetine 329	4.73 (0.23–97.25)	2/93	0/88
Paroxetine 377	1.32 (0.26–6.67)	5/180	2/95
Paroxetine 701	4.90 (0.24–100.93)	2/104	0/102
Sertraline A0501001	2.82 (0.12–68.26)	1/97	0/91
Sertraline A0501017	0.51 (0.05–5.48)	1/92	2/93
Venlafaxine 384	2.77 (0.11–67.10)	1/102	0/94
Overall fixed effects	2.00 (1.01–3.96)		
Bayes	2.10 (0.96–4.12)[**]		

Observational data: Phases II–III

Restricted cohort	2.29 (1.10–5.10)
Lifelink cohort = ▲	2.69

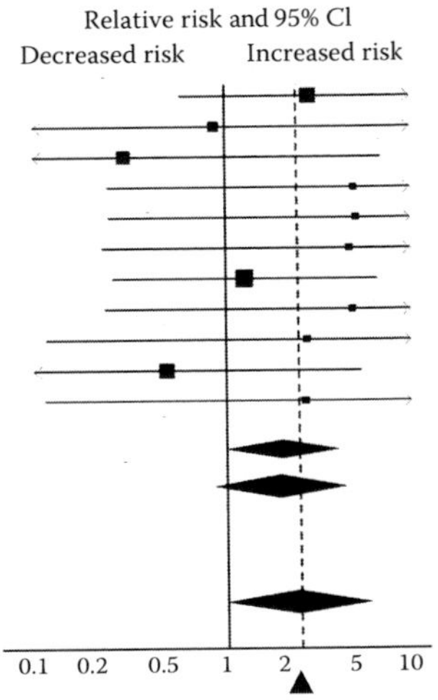

Relative risk and 95% Cl — Decreased risk — Increased risk

Scale: 0.1   0.2   0.5   1   2   5   10

[*]The five RCTs that did not have events in either the treated or placebo study groups were excluded from the fixed-effects meta-analysis but were included in the Bayes analysis: Fluoxetine HCJE (0/109 [treated], 0/110 [placebo]); Nefazodone CN104-141 (0/95, 0/95); Nefazodone CN104-187 (0/184, 0/94); Mirtazapine 003-045 (0/170, 0/89); and Venlafaxine 382 (0/80, 0/85).
[**]95% credible interval.

FIGURE 7.1

Forest plot on the relative risk scale comparing the risk of suicidal behavior for treatment with SSRI alone versus No-treatment for Phases I–III. The solid vertical line at 1 indicates the value corresponding to no risk. Each row gives an estimate of the relative risk and 95% confidence interval for each study in the meta-analysis of the RCT data (Phase I). Studies without an estimate or confidence interval had no events. A Mantel–Haenszel pooled estimate of relative risk with a 95% confidence interval based on a fixed-effects model is presented, as well as a Bayes estimate of risk with a 95% credible interval. The estimate of risk and confidence interval for the Restricted cohort (Phase III) is based on a propensity score analysis and a Poisson regression model. See the text for details. The triangle (▲) and dotted vertical line denote the calculated relative risk (RR = 2.7) in the unrestricted LifeLink cohort.

events, the relative risk is not calculable. We see that each study-wise risk is not statistically significant since the confidence interval contains 1. However, the fixed-effects, pooled estimate of the relative risk of suicidal behavior in children receiving antidepressants relative to placebo is 2.0 (95% confidence interval 1.01–3.95; p-value $= 0.046$) and is statistically significant. Finally, the Bayesian analysis yields an estimate of relative risk of 2.1 (95% credible interval 0.96–4.12), and the posterior probability that the relative risk is greater than 1 is 0.96. There was no significant between-study variability.

7.5.2 Phase II: IMS LifeLink Cohort

The IMS LifeLink cohort included 52,293 patients. After applying the trial exclusion criteria, 39,396 (75%) were eligible for our Restricted cohort (see Figure 7.2). Table 7.2 presents the sociodemographic characteristics for the

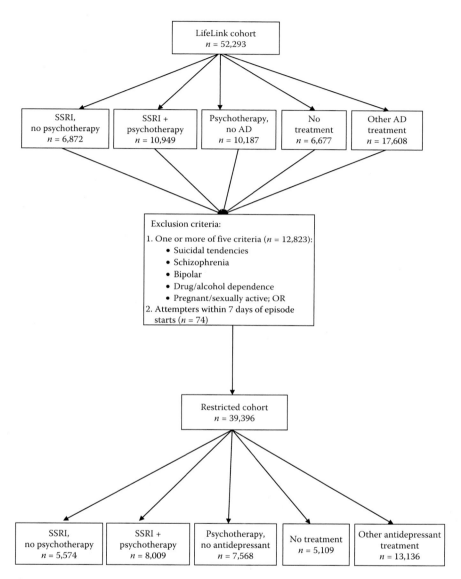

FIGURE 7.2

Consort flow chart. The flow chart depicts the creation of the *Restricted cohort* from the *Life-Link cohort* and the distribution of treatment modalities. The LifeLink cohort included 52,293 new episode depressed youths who were split into five mutually exclusive treatment groups. To create the Restricted cohort, youths were excluded from the LifeLink cohort based on having at least one of the RCT-identified exclusion criteria or had a suicide attempt within 7 days of episode start (see the text for details).

TABLE 7.2

Demographic Characteristics of Pediatric Cohorts

	LifeLink Cohort[a]	Restricted Cohort[b]	SSRI, No Psychotherapy	SSRI + Psychotherapy	Psychotherapy, No AD	No Treatment	Other Treatment
	52,293	39,396	5,574	8,009	7,568	5,109	13,136
Female (%)	30,765 (59%)	23,136 (59%)	3,537 (63%)	4,939 (62%)	4,185 (55%)	2,909 (57%)	7,566 (58%)
Mean age in years (SD)	14.5 (2.5)	14.3 (2.6)	14.8 (2.3)	14.4 (2.5)	13.8 (2.8)	14.3 (2.5)	14.3 (2.6)
Region							
East (%)	8,154 (16%)	5,739 (15%)	540 (10%)	1,227 (15%)	1,479 (19%)	693 (14%)	1,800 (14%)
Midwest (%)	31,778 (61%)	24,172 (61%)	3,108 (56%)	5,079 (63%)	4,577 (60%)	3,151 (62%)	8,257 (63%)
South (%)	5,628 (11%)	4,286 (11%)	796 (14%)	906 (11%)	632 (8%)	510 (10%)	1,442 (11%)
West (%)	6,733 (13%)	5,199 (13%)	1,130 (20%)	797 (10%)	880 (12%)	755 (15%)	1,637 (12%)
Medicaid claim (%)	2,370 (4%)	1,728 (4%)	318 (6%)	224 (3%)	308 (4%)	275 (5%)	603 (5%)

a LifeLink cohort includes attempters within 7 days of episode start.
b Restricted cohort excludes attempters within 7 days of episode start.

IMS LifeLink cohort and Restricted cohort, respectively, as well as by treatment group within the Restricted cohort. There are no statistically significant differences between the sociodemographic variables in the Restricted cohort and the IMS LifeLink cohort. This suggests that the Restricted cohort is statistically representative of the unrestricted cohort. The mean age of the Restricted cohort was 14.3 years, and more than half were girls (59%), quite similar to the gender and age distributions of the subjects in the pediatric SSRI trials found in the FDA's meta-analysis (Bridge et al. 2007). Because patients were not randomly assigned to treatments, it is not surprising that the distributions of sociodemographic characteristics varied significantly across the different treatment groups, indicating the need to statistically adjust for these confounders. We implemented these adjustments using propensity scores and regression models.

7.5.3 Phase III: Restricted Cohort

Our propensity score models fit the data well (e.g., Hosmer–Lemeshow test, $p = 0.72$) and successfully balanced treatment group assignments as assessed by propensity score stratification. Table 7.3 presents the results of our primary analysis comparing the "SSRI, No-psychotherapy" group to "No-treatment," the comparison most similar to the trial meta-analysis. Since the FDA black box warning included all antidepressants, we also present the comparison of the "Other-antidepressant" to the "No-treatment group." As noted earlier, the results for the IMS LifeLink cohort included all patients starting from day of diagnosis whereas the Restricted cohort excluded attempters within the first 7 days of diagnosis. The crude relative risk in the IMS

TABLE 7.3

Antidepressant Monotherapy: Crude and Adjusted Risk of Suicide Attempt

Group	n	Total Number of Events	Number of Events per 10,000 Subjects	Crude Relative Risk	Adjusted Rate Ratio[c] (95% CI)
LifeLink cohort[a]					
SSRI, no psychotherapy	6,872	63	91.7	2.7	
Other AD treatment	17,608	305	173.2	5.0	
No treatment (referent group)	6,677	23	34.4	1.0	
Restricted cohort[b]					
SSRI, no psychotherapy	5,574	25	44.9	2.5	2.3 (1.1, 5.1)
Other AD treatment	13,136	107	81.5	4.6	4.5 (2.3, 8.9)
No treatment (referent group)	5,109	9	17.6	1.0	1.0

[a] LifeLink cohort includes attempters within 7 days of episode start.
[b] Restricted cohort excludes attempters within 7 days of episode start.
[c] Restricted cohort estimates adjusted for propensity score, age, gender, region, and Medicaid status.

LifeLink cohort is 2.7 for the "SSRI, No-psychotherapy" group and 5.0 for the "Other-antidepressant" group, indicating that youths in the unrestricted cohort receiving any antidepressant monotherapy were at increased risk of suicide attempts. In the Restricted cohort, the adjusted rate ratio for suicide attempts for children and adolescents who received SSRI alone was 2.3 times greater than in the "No-treatment" group (95% confidence interval 1.1–5.1), a result remarkably close to

1. The estimate of risk from our meta-analysis of the trial data
2. The "population" risk in the IMS LifeLink cohort (see Figure 7.1)
3. The estimates in Hammad et al. (2006) and Valuck et al. (2004)

The adjusted relative risk in the Restricted cohort for the "Other-antidepressant" group is 4.5 (95% confidence interval 2.3–8.9), which is highly statistically significant. We note that the relative risk confidence intervals for the "SSRI-alone" group and the "Other-antidepressant" group overlap suggesting that the risk of suicidal behavior between these classes of antidepressants is not statistically significant (see also Schneeweiss et al. 2010; Cooper et al. 2014). Finally, we note that analyses of the Restricted cohort that *included* patients with suicide attempts within 7 days of diagnosis yielded nearly identical results.

7.6 Discussion

7.6.1 Case Study

We examined the risk of suicidal behavior with the initiation of antidepressant treatments in children and adolescents with major depressive disorder using two complementary data sources: randomized placebo-controlled trials where suicidal behavior was reported as an adverse effect and a large commercial database of longitudinal health claims. In our cross-design synthesis, we found at least a twofold increase in risk of suicidal behavior among antidepressant users. These results are similar to the results from the FDA's meta-analysis that was the basis for the black box warning. Our findings, however, differ from the FDA's in two important ways: our primary outcome was suicidal behavior not suicidality, and our results are generalizable to youths who would ordinarily be excluded from participation in randomized trials.

Our findings were robust across a variety of scenarios. For example, in the unrestricted IMS LifeLink cohort, we found a consistent increased risk of suicide attempts of at least 2.7 across all antidepressant treatment modalities. We also investigated the effect of selection due to excluding high-risk patients. There was little difference between the risks in the unrestricted and the restricted cohorts for the two antidepressant monotherapy groups, suggesting that the exclusion of patients based on the RCT exclusion criteria did not bias these estimates of risk. Thus, using multiple data sources, we find the weight of evidence compelling that a subset of youths initiating treatment with antidepressants are at increased risk of suicidal behaviors.

We have previously noted the limitations of using meta-analysis of randomized trials alone for these purposes, especially when outcomes are rare or treatment response or implementation is heterogeneous (Greenhouse and Kelleher 2005). Similarly, the limitations of large observational databases are also well known (Rubin 2010). The major concern for the latter is that alternative explanations, such as pretreatment differences between groups, could account for the observed increase in risk. In part, the convergence of evidence from multiple data sources, including randomized trial data, is reassuring that this is not the case. Finally, our use of sensitivity analyses also contributes to the robustness of our results.

In summary, the results of our cross-design synthesis show a convergence of evidence regarding the initiation of antidepressant treatment and an increased risk of suicidal behavior in a subset of youth with major depression. These results do not mean that antidepressant treatment is ineffective in relieving symptoms in a majority of depressed youths. These results, however, do identify a gap in our understanding about who is at risk and imply the need for further research to identify additional risk factors for this vulnerable subgroup to insure that children and adolescents with depression receive optimal treatment.

7.6.2 Cross-Design Synthesis

The use of cross-design synthesis in comparative effectiveness research is motivated in part by the recognition that evidence about patient outcomes is available from both RCTs and observational studies, and that neither data source is perfect, in the sense that RCTs may be rigorous but restricted, and observational studies more general but may be biased. Cross-design synthesis uses evidence from complementary studies to help answer questions about whether a treatment works across the full range of patients, providers, and settings. The challenge of this approach is to extract information from different kinds of research by capturing the strengths and minimizing the weaknesses of the different designs. Using state-of-the-art statistical and computational methods, such as hierarchical Bayesian models and propensity score matching, we believe cross-design synthesis is a valuable methodological approach that will help advance comparative effectiveness and patient-centered outcomes research, especially when there is concern about generalizability, treatment heterogeneity, and/or rare adverse effects.

Demonstrating a cause-and-effect relationship continues to be a challenging problem in the biomedical and public health sciences in general, and for comparative effectiveness research in particular. Nevertheless, public health agencies, such as the FDA, must make such determinations using the best available evidence (Hamburg and Sharfstein 2009). In our opinion, an underlying component of the controversy around the FDA's original finding of an increased risk of suicidality in pediatric antidepressant users was, in part, one of advocacy that pitted a belief in the value of evidence from randomized studies against the value of evidence from observational studies, sadly, a debate that continues even 10 years after the black box warning (see Stone 2014; Friedman 2014). Since a single study is rarely sufficient to show causation, especially for questions concerning the efficacy and/or safety of drugs, it is necessary to use methods that synthesize evidence from multiple sources. Our analysis demonstrates that evidence from both types of studies is valuable. Cross-design synthesis provides a methods template for the synthesis of evidence across complementary study designs. The strengths of cross-design synthesis include the ability to investigate the generalizability of trial results, the ability to synthesize evidence from multiple data sources, including experimental and observational studies, and the ability to generate new evidence. To answer important and similarly challenging healthcare questions when randomized trials are not adequate or not feasible, it will be necessary to use evidence from multiple data sources. We believe that the careful use of cross-design synthesis provides a foundation for generating and synthesizing evidence that is vital for advancing comparative effectiveness research.

Acknowledgments

The authors acknowledge Professor Howard Seltman, Department of Statistics, Carnegie Mellon University, for his contributions to the implementation of the Bayesian meta-analysis. This work was supported in part from grant number MH7862 (Greenhouse, Kelleher) and MH (Bridge) from the National Institute of Mental Health, and K12HS019464 from the Agency for Healthcare Research and Quality (Anderson, Libby, Valuck). The content is solely the responsibility of the authors and does not necessarily represent the official views of either funding agency.

References

Baldessarini R.J., Pompili M., Tondo L. 2006. Suicidal risk in antidepressant drug trials. *Archives of General Psychiatry*, 63(3):246–8.

Barbui C., Esposito E., Cipriani A. 2009. Selective serotonin reuptake inhibitors and risk of suicide: A systematic review of observational studies. *Canadian Medical Association Journal*, 180(3):291–7.

Bridge J.A., Iyengar S., Salary C.B., Barbe R.P., Birmaher B., Pincus H.A. et al. 2007. Clinical response and risk for reported suicidal ideation and suicide attempts in pediatric antidepressant treatment: A meta-analysis of randomized controlled trials. *JAMA*, 297:1683–96.

Centers for Disease Control and Prevention. Proposed Matrix of E-Code Groupings. Available at: www.cdc.gov/injury/wisqars/ecode_matrix.html, Last accessed November 2, 2011.

Cooper W.O., Callahan S.T., Shintani A., Fuchs D.C., Shelton R.C., Dudley J.A., Graves A.J., Ray W.A. 2014. Antidepressants and suicide attempts in children. *Pediatrics*, 133(2):1–7.

D'Agostino R.B., Jr. 1998. Propensity score methods for bias reduction in the comparison of a treatment to a non-randomized control group. *Statistics in Medicine*, 17(19):2265–81.

Droitcour J., Silberman G., Chelimsky E. 1993. A new form of meta-analysis for combining results from randomized clinical trials and medical-practice databases. *International Journal of Technology Assessment in Health Care*, 9(3): 440–9.

FDA Report. 2004. Hammad TA. Review and Evaluation of Clinical Data. Available at: http://www.fda.gov/ohrms/dockets/ac/04/briefing/2004-4065b1-10-TAB08-Hammads-Review.pdf and http://www.fda.gov/ohrms/dockets/ac/04/briefing/2004-4065B1_28_Handout-Events-by-trial-table-Corrected.pdf; Last accessed October 1, 2010.

Friedman R.A. 2014. Antidepressants' black-box warning—10 years later. *New England Journal of Medicine*, 371:1666–8, October 30, 2014, DOI: 10.1056/NEJMp1408480. http://www.nejm.org/doi/full/10.1056/NEJMp1408480

GAO. 1992. *Cross-Design Synthesis: A New Strategy for Medical Effectiveness Research, (GAO/PEMD-92-18)*. U.S. General Accounting Office, Washington, DC.

GAO. 1994. *Breast Conservation versus Mastectomy: Patient Survival in Day-to-Day Medical Practice and in Randomized Studies (GAO/PEMD-95-9)*. U.S. General Accounting Office, Washington, DC.

Gibbons R.D., Brown C.H., Hur K., Marcus S.M., Bhaumik D.K., Mann J.J. 2007. Relationship between antidepressants and suicide attempts: An analysis of the Veterans Health Administration data sets. *American Journal of Psychiatry*, 164(7):1044–9.

Greenhouse J., Iyengar S. 2009. Sensitivity analysis and diagnostics in *The Handbook of Research Synthesis*, 2nd ed., H.M. Cooper, L. Hedges and J. Valentine, eds. Russell Sage Foundation, New York, pp. 417–433.

Greenhouse J.B., Kaizar E.E., Kelleher K., Seltman H., Gardner W. 2008. Generalizing from clinical trial data: A case study. The risk of suicidality among pediatric antidepressant users. *Statistics in Medicine*, 27(11):1801–13.

Greenhouse J.B., Kelleher K. 2005. Thinking outside the (black) box: Antidepressants, suicidality, and research synthesis. *Pediatrics*, 116:231–3.

Hamburg M.A., Sharfstein J.M. 2009. The FDA as a public health agency. *New England Journal of Medicine*, 360(24):2493–5.

Hammad T.A., Laughren T., Racoosin J. 2006. Suicidality in pediatric patients treated with antidepressant drugs. *Archives of General Psychiatry*, 63:332–9.

Hammad T.A., Pinheiro S.P., Neyarapally G.A. 2011. Secondary use of randomized controlled trials to evaluate drug safety: A review of methodological considerations. *Clinical Trials*, 8(5):559–70.

Hernán M.A., Alonso A., Logan R., Grodstein F., Michels K.B., Willett W.C., Manson J.E., Robins J.M. 2008. Observational studies analyzed like randomized experiments: An application to postmenopausal hormone therapy and coronary heart disease (with discussion). *Epidemiology*, 19:766–79.

Horwitz R.I., Viscoli C.M., Clemens J.D., Sadock R.T. 1990. Developing improved observational methods for evaluating therapeutic effectiveness. *American Journal of Medicine*, 89(5):630–8.

IMS LifeLink®. 2009. *Health Plan Claims Database*, Pharmetrics, Inc., A unit of IMS Health, Watertown, WA.

Kaizar E.E., Greenhouse J.B., Seltman H., Kelleher K. 2006. Do antidepressants cause suicidality in children? A Bayesian meta-analysis (with discussion). *Clinical Trials*, 3:73–98.

Klein D.F. 2006. The flawed basis for FDA post-marketing safety decisions: The example of anti-depressants and children. *Neuropsychopharmacology*, 31(4):689–99.

Leslie L.K., Newman T.B., Chesney P.J., Perrin J.M. 2005. The Food and Drug Administration's deliberations on antidepressant use in pediatric patients. *Pediatrics*, 116(1):195–204.

Libby A.M., Brent D.A., Morrato E.H., Orton H.D., Allen R., Valuck R.J. 2007. Decline in treatment of pediatric depression after FDA advisory on risk of suicidality with SSRIs. *American Journal of Psychiatry*, 164:884–91.

Longford N.T. 1999. Selection bias and treatment heterogeneity in clinical trials. *Statistics in Medicine*, 18(12):1467–74.

Olfson M., Marcus S.C., Shaffer D. 2006. Antidepressant drug therapy and suicide in severely depressed children and adults: A case-control study. *Archives of General Psychiatry*, 63:865–72.

Posner K., Oquendo M.A., Gould M., Stanley B., Davies M. 2007. Columbia Classification Algorithm of Suicide Assessment (C-CASA): Classification of suicidal events in the FDA's pediatric suicidal risk analysis of antidepressants. *American Journal of Psychiatry*, 164(7):1035–43.

Rothwell P.M. 2005. Treating individuals 1: External validity of randomised controlled trials: "To whom do the results of this trial apply?" *Lancet*, 365:82–93.

Rubin D.B. 1990. A new perspective. Chapter 14 in *The Future of Meta-Analysis*, K. Wachter and M. Straf, eds. Russell Sage Foundation, New York, pp. 155–165.

Rubin D.B. 1992. Meta-Analysis: Literature synthesis or effect-size surface estimation? *Journal of Educational Statistics*, 17:363–74.

Rubin D.B. 1997. Estimating causal effects from large data sets using propensity scores. *Annals of Internal Medicine*, 127(8 Pt 2):757–63.

Rubin D.B. 2010. On the limitations of comparative effectiveness research. *Statistics in Medicine*, 29(19):96–7.

SAS Institute Inc. 2002–2008. *SAS Language*, Version 9.2. SAS Institute, Cary, NC.

Schneeweiss S., Patrick A.R., Solomon D.H., Dormuth C.R., Miller M., Mehta J., Lee J.C., Wang P.S. 2010. Comparative safety of antidepressant agents for children and adolescents regarding suicidal acts. *Pediatrics*, 125(5):876–88.

Scholle S.H. 2005. NCQA behavioral health measurement efforts. *Journal of Managed Care Pharmacy*, 11(3 Suppl):S9–11.

Simon G.E., Savarino J. 2007. Suicide attempts among patients starting depression treatment with medications or psychotherapy. *American Journal of Psychiatry*, 164(7):1029–34.

Simon G.E., Savarino J., Operskalski B., Wang P.S. 2006. Suicide risk during antide-pressant treatment. *American Journal of Psychiatry*, 163(1):41–7.

Sox H.C., Greenfield S (chairs) Committee on Comparative Effectiveness Research Prioritization. 2009. *Initial National Priorities for Comparative Effectiveness Research, Institute of Medicine*, National Academy of Sciences Press, Washington, DC.

Stone M.B. 2014. The FDA warning on antidepressants and suicidality—Why the controversy. *New England Journal of Medicine*, 371:1668–71; October 30, 2014. DOI: 10.1056/NEJMp1411138. http://www.nejm.org/doi/full/10.1056/NEJMp1411138

Valuck R.J., Libby A.M., Sills M.R., Giese A.A., Allen R.R. 2004. Antidepressant treat-ment and risk of suicide attempt by adolescents with major depressive disorder: A propensity-adjusted retrospective cohort study. *CNS Drugs*, 18(15):1119–32.

Weisberg H.I., Hayden V.C., Pontes V.P. 2009. Selection criteria and generalizability within the counterfactual framework: Explaining the paradox of antidepressant-induced suicidality? *Clinical Trials*, 6(2):109–18.

Woodward M. 2005. *Epidemiology: Study Design and Data Analysis*, 2nd ed., Chapman & Hall/CRC Press, Boca Raton.

8

Heterogeneity of Treatment Effects

Issa J. Dahabreh, Thomas A. Trikalinos, David M. Kent,
and Christopher H. Schmid

CONTENTS

ABSTRACT   We survey concepts of heterogeneity of treatment effects (HTE) in the context of comparative effectiveness research and address variability of individual causal effects (person-level HTE) and variability of conditional average causal effects (group-level HTE or effect measure modification). We provide an overview of statistical methods for quantifying and testing HTE in randomized trials and observational studies and address the reporting and interpretation of such analyses in the biomedical literature. Using data from a clinical trial of diabetes prevention, we illustrate the concepts and methods discussed in the chapter. Finally, we touch upon the role of HTE assessment in meta-analyses and decision analyses.

8.1 Background

The core questions of comparative effectiveness research (CER)—which treatment works best, for whom, and under what circumstances—revolve around the idea that treatment effects vary among patients and settings [1]; this variability is termed *heterogeneity of treatment effects* (HTE). The careful assessment of HTE is an important CER activity because the presence of identifiable heterogeneity has practical implications for patient-centered care: HTE across measurable factors can be used to tailor treatment strategies to the needs of individuals (*personalized medicine*) and to identify whether particular subgroups of patients receive benefit or harm from treatment [2,3,142]. In addition, HTE is a key consideration when assessing the applicability and generalizability of study findings to a target population (see, e.g., Chapters 6 and 7 of this book).

Clinicians intuitively understand that no two patients are identical because the mechanisms of disease are diverse and because patients have biological differences in drug metabolism, live in different environments, and adhere variably to treatment. Thus, most clinicians believe that HTE is pervasive in their practice. However, statistical analyses, even when based on large randomized trials, rarely identify factors that reliably predict differential treatment effectiveness. This leaves clinicians with an evidence base composed principally of average trial results, which is often incongruent with their intuition derived from treating patients who appear to vary in their treatment responses. Furthermore, clinical practice guidelines rarely make targeted treatment recommendations [4,5].

In this chapter, we provide a causal definition of HTE and draw distinctions between effect heterogeneity and various concepts of interaction. We illustrate the relationship between effect modification and deviation from additivity in regression models and discuss issues that arise in analyses that aim to identify HTE using data from randomized trials and observational studies. We also briefly discuss the role of HTE in meta-analyses, and decision and cost-effectiveness analyses.

8.2 Concepts of HTE

We examine concepts of HTE in the Neyman–Rubin potential outcomes (counterfactual) causal framework already discussed in Chapters 1, 2, and 6 of this book [6,7]. We adopt the counterfactual perspective [8] because it is applicable to both observational and randomized studies of interventions [9]. The topics developed in this chapter have close connections to concepts of variation of causal effects under alternative accounts of causality, including Pearl's nonparametric structural equation modeling approach using directed acyclic graphs [10,11] and Rothman's sufficient-component cause theory [12,13]. A detailed exploration of these alternative frameworks is beyond the scope of this chapter and interested readers should consult other sources [14].

Throughout, we assume that study participants are sampled from an infinite population and that we are interested in estimating causal effects in that population. We adopt a deterministic counterfactual model; extension to the stochastic case is possible [15] but not pursued here. To introduce some notation, the potential outcome under treatment $A = a$ is a random variable Y^a. A study collects data on n individuals; for the ith individual, with $i = 1, \ldots, n$, the *potential outcome* under treatment $A = a$ is Y_i^a. This outcome is called "potential" because it is only realized if the individual actually receives treatment $A = a$. We observe independent copies of (Y, X, A), where Y is the observed outcome, X is a vector of covariates (measured at baseline and possibly high-dimensional), and A is the treatment. We adopt the convention of using capital letters for random variables and lowercase letters for realizations. To simplify exposition, we focus on a case with only two possible treatments; extensions to the case of multiple treatments are fairly straightforward. We sometimes refer to the two treatments as the "treatment" and "control" exposures and the corresponding participant groups as the "treatment" and "control" groups; however, both groups may receive active care. We assume consistency (i.e., that the observed outcome Y equals the counterfactual outcome Y^a for those receiving $A = \alpha$), no interference (i.e., that treatment of any one individual does not influence the potential outcomes of other individuals in the population), no "hidden versions" of treatment, no measurement error, and no dropouts [16–18]. Chapters 1 through 3 of this book provide additional background on causal assumptions. We only consider point exposures because this is adequate for conceptualizing analyses in simple parallel randomized trials that aim to assess HTE for being assigned to the treatments under study. The more general longitudinal causality theory of Robins can be used to address effect heterogeneity when the exposure is time-varying [19,20].

We define *person-level treatment effects* as contrasts between *potential outcomes*, under the different treatments being compared. Thus, when comparing treatments $A = 1$ and $A = 0$, the treatment effect for the ith individual is

$$\Delta_i = Y_i^1 - Y_i^0.$$

Although the definition of person-level treatment effects as contrasts of potential outcomes is conceptually appealing, for each person at a given time point, we can only observe one of the potential outcomes (the "factual" outcome), while the other potential outcome is not observed (it remains counterfactual). Under our causal assumptions, the relationship between the observed (Y) and potential outcome random variables is

$$Y = AY^1 + (1 - A)Y^0.$$

It follows that the person-level treatment effects are in general not identifiable; this is known as the *fundamental problem of causal inference* [21]. Nevertheless, counterfactuals provide a powerful means for modeling causal effects [22]. For example, we can now use them to define person-level HTE:

Definition 8.1 (Person-level HTE)

Heterogeneity of person-level treatment effects exists when, for at least two individuals, i and j, we have that $\Delta_i \neq \Delta_j$ or, equivalently, $Y_i^1 - Y_i^0 \neq Y_j^1 - Y_j^0$.

The average treatment effect, ψ, is the expectation of the person-level effects: $\psi = \mathbb{E}[\Delta_i] = \mathbb{E}[Y_i^1 - Y_i^0] = \mathbb{E}[Y_i^1] - \mathbb{E}[Y_i^0]$. Clearly, the existence of person-level HTE implies that the variance of the person-level treatment effects,

$$\text{Var}[\Delta_i] = \text{Var}[Y_i^1 - Y_i^0] = \text{Var}[Y_i^1] + \text{Var}[Y_i^0] - 2\text{Cov}[Y_i^1, Y_i^0],$$

is not zero. The fundamental problem of causal inference means that the data provide no information on the covariance of the two potential outcomes and the variance of the treatment effects cannot be estimated (even though the marginal variances, $\text{Var}[Y_i^1]$ and $\text{Var}[Y_i^0]$, can be estimated).

One approach for assessing HTE is to obtain bounds for the variance of the person-level treatment effects without making assumptions about the joint distribution of the potential outcomes [23]; such bounding methods are most useful for HTE analyses of continuous outcomes. One can also explore what different (parametric) distributional assumptions imply for the magnitude of HTE. For example, for continuous outcomes, strong assumptions about the distribution of the outcome under treatment and control, conditional on a baseline covariate, can be used to bound the variance of causal effects or the correlation between treatment and outcome (given the estimated correlation of the covariate–treatment and covariate–outcome associations) [24]. In a similar spirit, beliefs about the joint distribution of potential outcomes can be expressed as prior distributions in a Bayesian analysis, in which case posterior-based inference about the (unidentifiable) proportions of the response types is possible [25]. Because assumptions about the joint distribution of potential outcomes have no empirical content, we view these analyses simply as sensitivity analyses based on rather implausible assumptions.

To see that person-level HTE is likely to be pervasive, consider a study evaluating the effect of treatment ($A = 1$) versus control ($A = 0$) for a binary outcome. From here on, and without loss of generality, we assume that the outcome is undesirable, for example, death, progression or recurrence of disease, or the development of an adverse drug reaction. As shown in Table 8.1, in such a study, there are four possible *response types* [26]: individuals who would experience the outcome regardless of exposure (doomed); those who would experience the outcome under treatment but not under control (harmed); those who would experience the outcome under control but not under treatment (responders); and those who would not experience the outcome regardless of treatment (immune).

As long as the study includes individuals from rows in the table with different values of Δ_i (i.e., as long as response types with different treatment effects are represented in the study), we would say that individual causal effects are heterogeneous, or that there exists HTE at the person level. We argue—on the basis of the complexity of disease biology, interindividual differences in drug metabolism, and variability in compliance—that person-level HTE is the norm in clinical studies. Unfortunately, even in very large and well-conducted randomized trials, the proportion of each response type

TABLE 8.1

Response Types with Respect to Potential Outcomes under Two Different Treatments

Response Type	Y^1	Y^0	Δ	Proportion of Response Type in the Population
Doomed	1	1	0	π_{11}
Harmed	1	0	1	π_{10}
Responder	0	1	-1	π_{01}
Immune	0	0	0	π_{00}

is not identifiable because among treated patients there is no way to distinguish doomed from treatment-harmed individuals, or treatment responders from immune individuals. Similarly, among untreated patients, there is no way to distinguish doomed individuals from treatment responders, or treatment-harmed from immune individuals.

Even though person-level treatment effects and the proportion of each response type are not identifiable, information can be obtained about the average treatment effect in the population [27]. Using the causal risk difference in the population RD_{causal} as the effect measure,

$$RD_{causal} = \mathbb{E}[Y^1 - Y^0] = Pr[Y^1 = 1] - Pr[Y^0 = 1] = (\pi_{11} + \pi_{10})$$
$$- (\pi_{11} + \pi_{01}).$$

The above equation shows that RD_{causal} is determined by the difference between the proportion of harmed and responder types, $\pi_{10} - \pi_{01}$. In other words, studies will tend to find large treatment effects if they enroll individuals with response types for which different treatments lead to discrepant outcomes. Under our causal assumptions, the term $(\pi_{11} + \pi_{10})$ is equal to $Pr[Y = 1 | A = 1]$ and the term $(\pi_{11} + \pi_{01})$ is equal to $Pr[Y = 1 | A = 0]$; both these probabilities can be estimated from the observed data. For example, in a randomized trial, these probabilities can be consistently estimated as

$$\widehat{Pr}[Y = 1 | A = 1] = \frac{\sum_{k=1}^{n} A_k Y_k}{\sum_{k=1}^{n} A_k} \text{ and } \widehat{Pr}[Y = 1 | A = 0] = \frac{\sum_{k=1}^{n} (1 - A_k) Y_k}{\sum_{k=1}^{n} (1 - A_k)}.$$

In a similar manner, using potential outcomes, we can define two other common measures of effect, the causal relative risk and the causal odds ratio, respectively, as

$$RR_{causal} = \frac{Pr[Y^1 = 1]}{Pr[Y^0 = 1]} \quad \text{and} \quad OR_{causal} = \frac{Pr[Y^1 = 1]/(1 - Pr[Y^1 = 1])}{Pr[Y^0 = 1]/(1 - Pr[Y^0 = 1])}.$$

In the remainder of this chapter, we mainly consider causal effects on the difference scale both for parsimony, and because the risk difference scale is the scale most pertinent to individual, and policy decision making [28] (we briefly revisit this issue in Section 8.7.2). When the outcome is continuous, of course, the difference is taken between the means of the two treatment groups, but this introduces nothing new conceptually. For simplicity, when the particular choice of effect measure is not important, we represent measures generically as functions of the expectations of potential outcomes under the two alternative treatments, $m(\mathbb{E}[Y^1], \mathbb{E}[Y^0])$ [29].

To recap, by focusing on populations instead of individuals, we can estimate average treatment effects. Yet, it should be clear that our attempt to circumvent the fundamental problem of causal inference has shifted our focus to the mean of the person-level treatment effects rather than their variability (heterogeneity). To some extent, we can assess heterogeneity by examining not individuals, but groups of individuals with similar characteristics. This is done by examining average treatment effects *conditional* on specific covariates and estimating causal effects within subgroups: $m\left(\mathbb{E}[Y^1|X = x], \mathbb{E}[Y^0|X = x]\right)$, where X can be a single characteristic or a vector of characteristics, such as age, sex, disease severity, genetic background, medical care environment, and so on.

8.2.1 Group-Level HTE as Effect Measure Modification

We identify HTE across groups with the epidemiological concept of effect (measure) modification [28–30]:

Definition 8.2 (Group-level HTE)

Heterogeneity of treatment effects exists when the effect measure $m\left(\mathbb{E}[Y^1|X = x], \mathbb{E}[Y^0|X = x]\right)$ varies over levels of covariate X, which is not affected by treatment.

We restrict our attention to covariates not affected by treatment to avoid conditioning on effects of the exposure. Standard regression methods can be biased when effects of exposures are used as covariates [31]. Causal methods that can estimate effects of treatments conditional on postexposure outcomes are available [32,33], but their discussion is beyond the scope of this chapter.

To make the definition of HTE more concrete, consider the case where the treatment, effect modifier, and outcome are binary. If our measure of choice is the risk difference, we can define HTE on the risk difference scale as follows:

Definition 8.3 (HTE on the risk difference scale over a binary modifier)

Heterogeneity of treatment effects exists on the risk difference scale when the causal risk difference varies over levels of the binary covariate X that is not affected by treatment:

$$Pr[Y^1 = 1|X = 1] - Pr[Y^0 = 1|X = 1] \neq Pr[Y^1 = 1|X = 0]$$
$$- Pr[Y^0 = 1|X = 0]. \tag{8.1}$$

Under exchangeability of treated and untreated individuals (see Chapter 3) and consistency the expression in the definition above can be written as

$$Pr[Y = 1|A = 1, X = 1] - Pr[Y = 1|A = 0, X = 1] \neq$$
$$Pr[Y = 1|A = 1, X = 0] - Pr[Y = 1|A = 0, X = 0]. \tag{8.2}$$

Thus, in a well-conduced randomized trial, HTE over a covariate can be assessed using the observed data on the outcome, covariate, and treatment assignment, by examining the risk differences in each stratum defined by the variable X. When the two risk differences are not equal, we say that there exists evidence of HTE on the risk difference scale. Section 8.5 discusses how standard regression models can be used to examine whether HTE is present, and to estimate stratum-specific causal effects.

8.2.2 Distinction between HTE and Causal Interaction

The concept of *interaction*, viewed heuristically as the interdependence of the effects of two or more causes, has a long history in statistics and epidemiology [28,34–36]. To define causal interaction and distinguish it from effect modification, we need to expand our consideration to more than one treatment; so, in addition to treatment A, we also consider treatment B (also binary). The potential outcome random variables for each individual have the form $Y_i^{a,b}$ and there are 4 (2×2) potential outcomes (i.e., $Y_i^{1,1}$, $Y_i^{1,0}$, $Y_i^{0,1}$, and $Y_i^{0,0}$) and 16 (2^4) response types to consider. We begin by defining counterfactual interaction on the risk difference scale, using this expanded framework for two binary treatments:

Definition 8.4 (Additive counterfactual causal interaction)

A causal interaction on the additive scale between binary treatments A and B exists when

$$Pr[Y^{1,1} = 1] - Pr[Y^{0,1} = 1] \neq Pr[Y^{1,0} = 1] - Pr[Y^{0,0} = 1]. \tag{8.3}$$

By subtracting $Pr[Y^{0,0} = 1]$ from both sides of the equation above and rearranging terms, we obtain the following expression:

$$Pr[Y^{1,1} = 1] - Pr[Y^{0,0} = 1] \neq (Pr[Y^{0,1} = 1] - Pr[Y^{0,0} = 1])$$
$$+ (Pr[Y^{1,0} = 1] - Pr[Y^{0,0} = 1]),$$

which serves to illustrate the meaning of counterfactual causal interactions: compared to no exposure at all, the presence of both exposures (left-hand side) has an effect on the outcome that is different from the sum of the effect of each exposure separately (bracketed terms on the right-hand side). The definition of additive counterfactual interactions can be used to motivate an index that is sometimes called the "interaction contrast":

$$IC = Pr[Y^{1,1} = 1] - Pr[Y^{0,1} = 1] - Pr[Y^{1,0} = 1] + Pr[Y^{0,0} = 1].$$

Nonzero values of the *IC* denote the presence of interaction; $IC > 0$ denotes "super-additive" interaction and $IC < 0$ denotes "sub-additive" interaction.

Miettinen [34] was the first to provide a description of causal interdependence along these lines, using the terms "causal" and "preventive synergism." Greenland and Poole [37] proposed a grouping of the 16 counterfactual response types induced by two treatments into seven mutually exclusive and exhaustive classes (shown in Table 8.2): doomed (C_{doomed}); treatment *A* causes the outcome but *B* does not (C_A); *B* causes the outcome but *A* does not (C_B); mutual antagonism (C_{ma}); disease occurs for only a single treatment combination (C_{single}); disease occurs for three treatment combinations (C_{three}); and immune (C_{immune}). This grouping is invariant to recoding of the treatments (i.e., replacing 0 with 1 and 1 with 0 in the potential outcomes).

As in the case of a single treatment, the proportion of individuals in the population belonging to each response type is not identifiable when examining interactions between two (or more) treatments. Nevertheless, if the population consists only of a combination of individuals with response types from classes C_{doomed}, C_A, C_B, or C_{immune}, we could say that there exists no causal interaction (and $IC = 0$). The converse is not true: we could have

TABLE 8.2

Response Types for Two Exposures

Response Type	$Y^{1,1}$	$Y^{0,1}$	$Y^{1,0}$	$Y^{0,0}$	IC	Proportion of Response Type in the Population
Doomed (C_{doomed})	1	1	1	1	0	π_{1111}
Single plus joint causation (C_{three})	1	1	1	0	−1	π_{1110}
Preventive antagonism (C_{three})	1	1	0	1	1	π_{1101}
B is causal, A has no effect (C_B)	1	1	0	0	0	π_{1100}
Preventive antagonism (C_{three})	1	0	1	1	1	π_{1011}
A is causal, B has no effect (C_A)	1	0	1	0	0	π_{1010}
Mutual blockage (C_{ma})	1	0	0	1	2	π_{1001}
Causal synergism (C_{single})	1	0	0	0	1	π_{1000}
Preventive synergism (C_{three})	0	1	1	1	−1	π_{0111}
Mutual blockage (C_{ma})	0	1	1	0	−2	π_{0110}
A is preventive, B has no effect (C_A)	0	1	0	1	0	π_{0101}
Causal antagonism (C_{single})	0	1	0	0	−1	π_{0100}
B is preventive, A has no effect (C_B)	0	0	1	1	0	π_{0011}
Causal antagonism (C_{single})	0	0	1	0	−1	π_{0010}
Single plus joint prevention (C_{single})	0	0	0	1	1	π_{0001}
Immune (C_{immune})	0	0	0	0	0	π_{0000}

Note: Terminology from Modern Epidemiology. 2008. K. J. Rothman, S. Greenland, and T. L. Lash. LWW (publisher), p. 76. Notation in parentheses is used in the text to refer to invariant groupings of response types.

$IC = 0$ while the population included at least some individuals from response types other than C_{doomed}, C_A, C_B, and C_{immune}, provided their proportions "balanced out."

A comparison of the definition of additive counterfactual interaction in Equation 8.3 against the definition of HTE on the additive scale in Equation 8.1 helps clarify the distinction between HTE (i.e., effect modification) and interaction [38,39]. HTE is defined with respect to a single cause of the outcome and an effect modifier, which does not necessarily have to be a cause of the outcome (e.g., it does not have to be manipulable, or it may be a proxy for a cause of the outcome with no direct effect on the outcome). In contrast, interaction is defined with respect to two causes of the outcome. This is reflected in the "asymmetry" inherent in the definition of HTE: the role of the treatment (A) and the effect modifier (X) is not the same; in contrast, in the definition of causal interaction, the two treatments (A and B) are treated symmetrically. If we can only intervene on a single cause, then HTE is the natural focus of investigation; if we can intervene on both causes, interaction may be a more natural focus.

Nevertheless, there is an obvious connection between interaction and effect modification in our example: if we have exchangeability for both treatments, then the comparison needed to assess the presence of interaction on the additive scale can be performed using empirical data; the two treatments would be said to interact on the additive scale if

$$Pr[Y = 1 | A = 1, B = 1] - Pr[Y = 1 | A = 0, B = 1] \neq$$
$$Pr[Y = 1 | A = 1, B = 0] - Pr[Y = 1 | A = 0, B = 0]. \quad (8.4)$$

Expression (8.4) is identical to expression (8.2) if in the latter we replace the effect modifier X with the treatment B. However, we caution that the assumptions required for obtaining the two expressions are not the same: we obtained expression (8.2) based on an assumption of exchangeability of A-treated and A-untreated patients. In contrast, we obtained expression (8.4) by assuming exchangeability for both treatments A and B. While expression (8.4) is written in a way that emphasizes the effect of A given B, it can be rearranged with the roles of A and B reversed. However, it is less meaningful, in a causal sense, to reverse the roles of A and X in expression (8.2). This is a reminder that the interpretation of data analysis results (i.e., estimates of the quantities in expressions (8.4) and (8.2)) depends on study design and background knowledge. The assumption that both treatments are unconfounded is fairly strong; it is realistic, for example, if assignment to both treatments is randomized. In such a trial (e.g., in a 2×2 factorial trial), the assessment of causal interaction between the two treatments would be equivalent to the assessment of effect modification.

We should also clarify that HTE and counterfactual causal interactions are not necessarily tied to biologic interactions [40,41]. To see why this is the case, consider a 2 × 2 factorial trial examining the use of a lipid-lowering agent (vs. none), and the use of an anticoagulant agent (vs. none). We may well find an interaction, say a larger decrease in the risk of cardiovascular adverse outcomes when comparing patients who receive both treatments (vs. none), as compared to the sum of the reductions in risk in the groups receiving only one of the agents. Even though such a finding would be indicative of a counterfactual causal interaction on the additive scale, it does not (necessarily) require the drugs to have the same biological targets (e.g., the antihypertensive agent may act by reducing the formation and growth of atherosclerotic plaques, while the antithrombotic agent may act by reducing clot formation on already-formed and ruptured plaques) or to physically come in contact. More generally, the results of epidemiological data analyses cannot identify the "true" biological model without strong additional assumptions [40,42,43].

8.2.3 A Note on Terminology

In the statistical and epidemiological literature, the terms "interaction," "effect modification," and "heterogeneity of treatment effect" are often used interchangeably [41,44]. To make matters worse, the term "interaction" is used to describe "statistical interactions" (i.e., deviations from additivity of effects in a particular statistical model), counterfactual causal interactions, and even biologic interactions. The important differences between these concepts, together with the degree to which different concepts have been associated with the same term in different literatures, suggest that the adoption of a common set of terms and definitions is unlikely. Some authors have proposed that use of the term "interaction" (or, more narrowly, "biologic interaction") should be discouraged in specific contexts to avoid confusion [41,45–47]. Here, we simply suggest that the term "heterogeneity of treatment effects" should be identified with the epidemiological concept of effect measure modification; we find that this term resonates with patients, researchers, and policy makers and directly conveys the key idea of variability of causal effects across well-defined groups of patients. As an added benefit, the term "heterogeneity of treatment effects" avoids any connotations of biologic interactions, which are in general not identifiable using empirical data [40].

In the remainder of this chapter, we limit ourselves to cases where exchangeability is achieved by design (in randomized trials) or assumed to hold conditional on covariates (e.g., in observational studies with rich covariate data) between patients receiving or not receiving a single treatment. We do not consider causal interactions further, and instead refer readers to a recent well-referenced tutorial [48] and some selected papers from the vast literature on this topic [38,43–47,49–51].

8.3 Potential Effect Modifiers, the Reference Class Problem, and the Curse of Dimensionality

8.3.1 Reference Class Problem

The discussion in Section 8.2 suggests that the number of potential effect modifiers in clinical research is very large, which means that HTE may be present over any of a myriad factors. Practically, any baseline covariate that is directly or indirectly associated with the outcome of interest might be an effect modifier. Characteristics of the patient (e.g., age, sex, race/ethnicity), the disease (severity, duration of symptoms, pathological subtype), the physician (specialty, years of training), and the setting of care (e.g., across centers in a multicenter trial; the volume of cases of a particular disease addressed by different hospitals) can all take the place of X in Definition 8.2.

The very large number of potential effect modifiers means that one-variable-at-a-time examination of potential modifiers does not produce results that can be applied in clinical practice. Patients simultaneously differ on multiple characteristics and the number of possible subgroups is enormous. Because each subgroup may be associated with a different magnitude of the treatment effect, it is not clear which estimate should be used to inform decision making for the particular patient—this is a version of the *reference class problem* [52–54]. To see why one-variable-at-a-time HTE analyses are inadequate for guiding practice, consider the following extreme scenario: two separate subgroup analyses conducted in the same trial reveal that women benefit from treatment whereas men are harmed by it and patients younger than 65 years old benefit from treatment whereas older patients are harmed. In view of such findings, the preferred treatment for a young male patient or for an old female patient would require analyzing HTE over subgroups defined by considering age and sex jointly. In addition to not producing clinically applicable results, one-variable-at-a-time analyses produce many false-positive results when a large number of effect modifiers are explored [55,56] (we further discuss the issue of multiplicity in Section 8.5.3). The risk of false-positive errors can be controlled by using appropriate procedures that control the family-wise error rate for *a priori* specified statistical comparisons, but such methods do not address the complex covariate–treatment–outcome relationships that are typical of chronic diseases (when they emphasize the examination of one-variable-at-a-time).

8.3.2 Curse of Dimensionality

Clinically meaningful HTE analyses need to examine multiple potential effect modifiers jointly. Unfortunately, the number of subgroups of interest can very quickly become intractable as the number of covariates increases, even in very large datasets (e.g., megatrials with tens of thousands of randomized participants), the number of covariates of interest can very quickly become intractable as the dimensionality of the problem becomes very high. For example, in addition to age, sex, and race, the set of covariates can include a large number of comorbidities, as well as "omic" information (genomic, proteomic, and metabolomic markers). For a single individual, it is now possible to measure millions of variables at a single point in time. To see the magnitude of the problem, for just 20 binary covariates the number of possible combinations is $2^{20} = 1,048,576$, a number large enough to suggest that estimating treatment effects for each combination of covariates is nearly impossible even in very large datasets (and the situation is worse when the prevalence of the covariates is small or when the outcome rate is low). This means that we need to reduce the dimension of the covariate space by leveraging background knowledge and by using models to extract information from data. We discuss some strategies for doing this in Section 8.5.

8.4 Study Design Considerations

Heterogeneity can arise in both randomized trials and in observational studies. While some differences in analysis will be discussed below, a primary distinction between the two types of studies is that trials can be planned to consistently estimate HTE over factors of interest, whereas observational studies may suffer from non-exchangeability of the compared groups and may lack information on key variables necessary to discover HTE. Prospective cohort studies can, however, control enrollment to focus on subgroups of interest.

8.4.1 Issues with Specific Study Types

8.4.1.1 Randomized Trials

Clinical trials for CER randomize participants to two or more interventions in order to eliminate confounding of treatment effects by other factors. Trials can also randomize participants in blocks or subgroups to address potential heterogeneity. A multisite trial is a simple example. Participants are separately randomized by site, to control for between-site variation. One common strategy for exploring heterogeneity uses factorial or fractional factorial designs to randomize participants to a set of predetermined treatments and conditions that are believed to affect outcomes. Comparison of results among these participants enables assessment of both the main effects of all the treatments and subgroups, as well as interactions among them [57]. Such designs can be embedded within an adaptive strategy that learns from the effects discovered to plan a new study focusing on the most effective treatment strategies and on those that exhibit the most heterogeneity.

Blocking of participants within subgroups that have similar outcomes also increases the precision with which treatment effects may be estimated. The increased precision is particularly important when assessing heterogeneity because interactions are typically estimated with considerably less precision than main effects. Studies designed to have sufficient power to test the main effects typically have insufficient sample sizes to test for effect modification. Thus, exploring heterogeneity requires either larger sample sizes or carefully constructed designs that minimize sources of variability. In particular, it is crucial that study designs explicitly address heterogeneity so that sufficient numbers of participants will be available for accurately assessing the heterogeneity.

Designs set up to adapt as data accrue may also aid the detection of heterogeneity. Such designs require analysis at interim times to assess results and make appropriate changes. One simple adaptive design changes the allocation proportions of participants among treatment groups to favor those treatments that appear to be the most effective. This strategy also promotes the detection of heterogeneity within the optimal treatment groups because it increases the numbers of participants assigned to those groups. For instance, in a cancer treatment trial, it may be found that some treatments are working more effectively than others on average. By allocating more participants to the more effective arms, a larger sample will be available to investigate differences in efficacy of that treatment within subgroups of participants.

8.4.1.2 N-of-1 Studies

The N-of-1 design is particularly strong for extending the exploration of HTE from the subgroup level all the way to the individual [58]. An N-of-1 study is a multiple crossover design in which a single participant receives a (randomized) sequence of two or more treatments three or more times. The outcomes on each treatment are averaged across each instance and compared to determine efficacy on that individual. Because of the single-subject design, replication is provided by the repeated crossovers and power derives from repeatability of the effect. If data are sufficient, one can determine the best treatment for each individual. Assuming that the individual's treatment effect remains stable over the course of the N-of-1 study, this design can directly estimate person-level treatment effects. But because the number of crossovers is usually small, randomization may fail to eliminate all confounding so that the person-specific effect does not provide an unbiased estimate of the person-level treatment effect. In any case, a proper analysis needs to account for the correlation among observations taken within a participant and for potential carryover and time trends. Analysis of multiple N-of-1 trials together in a multilevel framework permits estimating both person-level effects as well as the average treatment effect and conditional average effects across subgroups [59–61]. The person-level effects may actually be estimated more precisely in the multilevel framework because the borrowing of strength across individuals adds information.

8.4.1.3 Observational Studies

Observational studies of treatment effectiveness are used when randomized trials are infeasible to conduct for ethical or logistical issues, when information from RCTs cannot be obtained in a timely manner, or when information about treatment effectiveness in routine practice is needed. Because of their large sample sizes, observational studies can offer opportunities to assess HTE over factors that are impossible to explore in randomized trials. The main concern in observational studies is lack of exchangeability between treatment groups, primarily because treatment choice is influenced by characteristics that are also causes of the outcome (confounding). Because of the lack of randomization, marginal exchangeability of treated and untreated individuals is implausible in observational studies and we can only hope that exchangeability can be achieved conditional on covariates, some of which may also be effect modifiers. Meaningful HTE analysis over baseline variables (X) can only be performed if we "control" condition on confounding varibales [62], which we denote by L (note that X and L can have common elements):

Definition 8.5 (HTE for conditional average causal effects)

Heterogeneity of treatment effects over variable X exists when the effect measure $m\left(\mathbb{E}[Y^1|X=x, L=l], \mathbb{E}[Y^0|X=x, L=l]\right)$ varies over levels of X, conditional on L.

Often, interest centers on heterogeneity of conditional average causal effects marginalized over other pretreatment variables (e.g., confounders that are not of interest as possible effect modifiers). This idea is captured by the following definition:

Definition 8.6 (HTE for conditional average causal effects marginalized over covariates)

Heterogeneity of treatment effects over variable X exists when the effect measure

$$m\left(\sum_l \mathbb{E}[Y^1|X=x, L=l]Pr[L=l|X=x], \sum_l \mathbb{E}[Y^0|X=x, L=l]\right)$$

$$Pr[L=l|X=x]\right)$$

varies over levels of X.

In the presence of confounding, investigators can attempt to achieve exchangeability using design-based approaches other than randomization (e.g., by restricting the sample to patients with a particular value of the confounder, matching, or stratification) or using appropriate statistical analysis methods (e.g., outcome regression, inverse probability weighting). The adequacy of these techniques for drawing causal inferences about treatment effects and effect modification relies on the assumption that treatment is randomized within strata defined by the covariates; this assumption is generally never exactly true and cannot be verified using data from the study [63]. As such, in observational studies, exchangeability is a judgment made by researchers based on background knowledge [64]. Sensitivity and bias analyses have received considerable attention for assessing the robustness of observational study results to residual confounding [65,66], though these methods have rarely been examined in settings with heterogeneous treatment effects [67,68].

8.4.2 Power, Precision, and Sample Size

Typically, studies are designed with the goal of estimating the average treatment effect or testing hypotheses about it. Analyses that aim to identify HTE generally need much larger sample sizes than analyses focused on average effects to attain the same level of statistical power. Numerous studies have assessed the performance of statistical testing for effect modification using permutation methods, stratified analyses, or a regression framework [56,69–78]; as usual, no single testing procedure is universally better. However, two rules of thumb are often useful. First, for a given sample size, the power to detect effect measure modification is typically an order of magnitude lower than the power to detect main effects. Second, the variance of the statistical interaction term is an order of magnitude greater than the variance of the main effects estimate under a no-interaction model [44,74]. This suggests that, in general, HTE analyses using data from studies designed for inference about average effects (e.g., re-analyses of phase III randomized trials) will often be underpowered to detect effect modification. This is important for the interpretation of unplanned subgroup analyses: nonstatistically significant results should not be taken to imply lack of heterogeneity, because the probability of false-negative tests is fairly high in that setting. Thus, nonstatistically significant results should not be taken to imply that treatment benefits (or harms) all patients equally.

8.5 Statistical Analysis to Detect and Quantify HTE

HTE implies that treatment effects differ across subgroups of patients. Detecting HTE empirically requires comparing the treatment effects in each subgroup by a statistical analysis. This requires estimating and comparing $m\left(\mathbb{E}[Y^1|X=x_1], \mathbb{E}[Y^0|X=x_1]\right)$ and $m\left(\mathbb{E}[Y^1|X=x_2], \mathbb{E}[Y^0|X=x_2]\right)$, where X is the covariate defining the subgroups that take values x_1 and x_2. These subgroup-specific effects may be estimated by separately analyzing each subgroup; the magnitude of effect modification can be assessed by taking the difference of these separate treatment effects and estimating the standard error of the difference. It is incorrect, although lamentably common, to heuristically compare the treatment effects by examining the overlap of their confidence intervals or comparing p-values for the null hypothesis of no treatment effect obtained separately in each subgroup (these problems are common in medical publications, despite repeated cautionary notes [55,79–83]).

The following sections touch upon several issues that arise in statistical analyses for HTE. The relevant literature is vast and rapidly expanding, so our goal here is to identify key themes and point readers to selected references.

8.5.1 Regression Models for HTE Assessment

In our running clinical trial example where the treatment and covariate are both binary, treatment effects in the two subgroups can be easily assessed by constructing a statistical model that includes the treatment, the covariate, and their product as regressors. A fully saturated model for the expectation of the response has the form

$$\mathbb{E}[Y|A, X] = g^{-1}(\beta_0 + \beta_1 A + \beta_2 X + \beta_3 AX). \tag{8.5}$$

Here, g is the link function, which for binary outcomes is often taken to be the identity, log, or logistic function. For example, assume that we want to determine if treatment effects differ between men and women. Representing the treatment as $A=1$ for those treated and $A=0$ for controls and gender as $X=1$ if female and $X=0$ if male, the interaction term is $A \times X = 1$ for treated females and 0 for others. On the risk difference scale (i.e., using the identity link function), the probability of the outcome can be modeled as a function of treatment and gender, using the following linear probability model:

$$Pr[Y = 1|A, X] = \beta_0 + \beta_1 A + \beta_2 X + \beta_3 AX. \tag{8.6}$$

The parameters β_1 and β_2 are called the main effects of treatment and gender, β_3 is the statistical interaction, and β_0 is the intercept that describes the expected response when $A=0$ and $X=0$ (i.e., for untreated males). The interpretation of these coefficients is easily seen by laying out the expected responses under the four conditions as in Table 8.3. The treatment effect in males, the difference between the expected response in treated and control

TABLE 8.3

Subgroup Specific Effects from the
Model in Equation 8.6

	Male	Female
Control	β_0	$\beta_0 + \beta_2$
Treated	$\beta_0 + \beta_1$	$\beta_0 + \beta_1 + \beta_2 + \beta_3$

males, is β_1. Likewise, the treatment effect in females is $\beta_1 + \beta_3$. The difference between the treatment effects in male and female individuals is β_3, which is the coefficient of the product term in the regression model. To determine whether this difference is statistically significant, we can simply test the null hypothesis that $\beta_3 = 0$. The model thus gives us both subgroup-specific treatment effects as well as their difference and allows us to make valid statistical tests of key hypotheses. To test whether the effect in males is nonzero, we would test $\beta_1 = 0$, and to test whether the effect in females is nonzero, we test $\beta_1 + \beta_3 = 0$. Of course, in the absence of HTE, that is, when $\beta_3 = 0$, the main effects β_1 and β_2 have their usual interpretations as the average effects of treatment and gender.

These results can be obtained by separate analyses of the treatment effect in males and females, but the single model is simpler to fit with standard software. Moreover, it conveniently generalizes to multiple regression when one wants to control for other factors or simultaneously test for multiple interactions. A further advantage of the regression framework is that it easily generalizes to link functions other than the identity using the generalized linear model framework [84]. When Y is a binary outcome, logistic regression using the logit($\cdot$) link function estimates the log odds ratio as the treatment effect and separate log odds ratios for each subgroup. In that case, the regression coefficients on the right-hand side of Equation 8.5 are differences in logits of the probabilities and represent log odds ratios. For instance, β_3 is the difference in the log odds ratios of the treatment effect for males and females. Similarly, log-linear regression using the ln($\cdot$) link function estimates the log relative risk as the treatment effect and separate log relative risks for each subgroup.

8.5.2 Scale Dependence of HTE

It is quite easy to see that a factor that induces HTE on one scale may show no HTE on another [85]. A numerical example illustrates the effect. If the event probability in the control group is 0.05 and the relative risk is 0.5, the probability in the treatment group is 0.025, so the risk difference is -0.025. However, if the event probability in the control group is 0.5, with the same relative risk of 0.5, the probability in the control group is 0.25 and the risk difference is -0.25. In this case, substantial HTE is present on the risk difference scale, but not on the relative risk scale. One can show that there is also HTE on the odds ratio scale. In the example, when the event probability in the control group is 0.05, the odds ratio is 0.49, but when the probability in the control group is 0.5, the odds ratio is 0.33.

In fact, for binary treatment, outcome, and effect modifier, it can be shown in general that if effects are homogeneous on both the risk difference and relative risk scales, then either the treatment has no effect or the effect modifier is not associated with the probability of the outcome. To see this, let $p_{ij} = Pr[Y = 1 | A = i, X = j], i = 0, 1, j = 0, 1$, and consider that effect homogeneity on the risk difference scale can be expressed as $p_{11} - p_{01} = p_{10} - p_{00}$, or equivalently, as

$$\frac{p_{11}}{p_{00}} = \frac{p_{10}}{p_{00}} + \frac{p_{01}}{p_{00}} - 1. \tag{8.7}$$

Effect homogeneity on the relative risk scale can be expressed as $\frac{p_{11}}{p_{01}} = \frac{p_{10}}{p_{00}}$, or equivalently as

$$\frac{p_{11}}{p_{00}} = \frac{p_{01}}{p_{00}} \frac{p_{10}}{p_{00}}. \tag{8.8}$$

Equating the right-hand sides of Equations 8.7 and 8.8 and rearranging, we obtain

$$\left(\frac{p_{01}}{p_{00}} - 1\right)\left(\frac{p_{10}}{p_{00}} - 1\right) = 0,$$

which, together with the homogeneity assumptions, implies that either the effect modifier or the treatment does not affect the outcome probability. Furthermore, if treatment and the modifier are associated with the outcome, then homogeneity on the risk difference scale implies heterogeneity on the relative risk scale, and vice versa. The relationships between the presence or absence of heterogeneity on various scales become rather complex when one considers what the relationships between estimates of effect in a particular scale imply for the magnitude of effect modification in other scales. Two simulation-based studies have explored these relationships in depth [86,87]. Figure 8.1 depicts how each of the two measures of effect behaves when the other is held constant (over baseline risk).

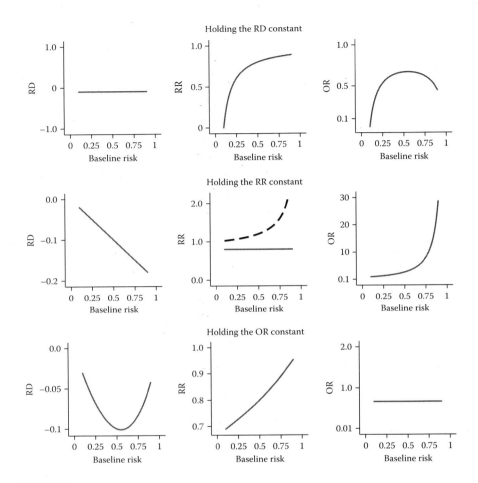

FIGURE 8.1

Scale dependence of HTE. When the treatment effect is nonnull and the baseline risk varies, HTE is inevitable on the other commonly used scales for treatment effect. The graphs show that when one measure of treatment effect is held constant, the other two will vary substantially as the baseline risk changes. The center panel also demonstrates that when the treatment effect is nonnull and the baseline risk varies, when the RR is held constant for "event occurrence," then there will exist HTE for the complementary outcome (i.e., "no event occurrence," shown by the dotted line). HTE = heterogeneity of treatment effects; OR = odds ratio; RD = risk difference; RR = relative risk. When held constant, RD = −0.1, RR = 0.8, and OR = 0.66. Results are shown over baseline outcome risks ranging from 0.1 to 0.9. (Reproduced from I. J. Dahabreh et al. *International Journal of Epidemiology*, November 17, 2016. pii: dyw125. [Epub ahead of print] Review.)

To connect these ideas to modeling, consider again the model in Equation 8.5; when the treatment effect does not vary by subgroup, β_1 is the common treatment effect and $\beta_3 = 0$. However, the presence (or absence) of HTE depends on the scale of the response in the model. Assume that no

HTE is present on the relative risk scale. This means that the generalized linear model with a log-link function and no product term would be correctly specified:

$$\log Pr[Y = 1|A, X] = \beta_0 + \beta_1 A + \beta_2 X.$$

This model implies that the event probability is $\exp(\beta_0 + \beta_1)$ for treated men, $\exp(\beta_0)$ for untreated men, $\exp(\beta_0 + \beta_1 + \beta_2)$ for treated women, and $\exp(\beta_0 + \beta_2)$ for untreated women. There is no HTE on the relative risk scale because the treatment effect in men is equal to the treatment effect in women:

$$\frac{\exp(\beta_0 + \beta_1)}{\exp(\beta_0)} = \frac{\exp(\beta_0 + \beta_1 + \beta_2)}{\exp(\beta_0 + \beta_2)} = \exp(\beta_1).$$

However, because of the nonlinear link function, the subgroup-specific risk differences are in general not equal (except when the treatment effect is null or when the event rate under no treatment is the same in both subgroups), which implies the presence of HTE on the risk difference scale:

$$\exp(\beta_0 + \beta_1) - \exp(\beta_0) \neq \exp(\beta_0 + \beta_1 + \beta_2) - \exp(\beta_0 + \beta_2).$$

So what is the responsible analyst to do in light of such discrepancies? It is important to keep two principles in mind: use simple (parsimonious), valid models and interpret on the most relevant scale. These principles may lead to analyzing on a scale different from that which is finally reported. Generally, the simplest model is the one on which effects are additive (i.e., on which there is no interaction).

In simple problems, like those discussed above, one could do the analysis on either scale without any difficulty. In more complex problems, with additional variables to adjust for and other nonlinear or nonadditive effects, model specification becomes more challenging. Consider, treatment effects for continuous outcomes, such as change in CD4 count for patients with HIV. Outcomes such as these that are biochemical concentrations often change by proportional amounts and are more normally distributed on a logarithmic scale. Modeling on the logarithmic scale will more likely satisfy assumptions of the linear model such as additivity, homoskedasticity, and normality. If interpretation is needed on the original scale, one simply transforms back with the antilogarithm. This, of course, implies that the treatment effects will vary with the base CD4 count. More generally, model selection with multivariable models is complicated because model parsimony is typically incompatible with correct specification. In most cases, a complex and approximately correctly specified model is preferable to a simple but grossly misspecified one; appropriate numerical summaries (e.g., standardized probabilities or risk differences) and graphical methods can be used to ease interpretation of complex models.

8.5.3 Multiplicity

As noted in Section 8.3, the number of potential effect modifiers is often very large. Examining all of these potential modifiers in a series of statistical models using a constant type I error rate raises the danger of multiplicity of testing and inflated error rates across the family of tests. This can lead to false-positive findings of HTE where it does not really exist. Section 8.5.4 discusses low summary variables can be used to the number of modifiers being considered and capture the joint and overlapping effects of multiple modifiers. However, it is also important to note that all effect modifiers are not created equal.

Very often, prior studies or biological insight suggest that some variables are more likely to be effect modifiers than others. In many trials and prospective studies, protocols identify certain variables to be tested explicitly as effect modifiers as primary or secondary aims. When based on prior findings supporting these hypotheses, the resulting tests are often labeled confirmatory and the clinical trials aim to test both an average treatment effect and the average effect in one or more particular subgroups identified in advance. Because the tests are defined in advance, confirmation of the hypothesis in the study leads to a more credible finding that policy makers can trust. An example in which one of the authors is involved concerns the confirmation of a small study that suggested tai chi substantially reduced pain among patients with knee osteoarthritis [88]. A larger confirmatory trial has been designed to replicate this result but also to test whether the effect can be generalized to different tai chi instructors, as the intervention in the first study was led by an experienced instructor who had customized the treatment for patients with difficulty in bending and moving. In the follow-up study, the instructor's protocol has been taught to two other instructors and it is of interest to determine whether results can be maintained consistently in each class [89].

On the other hand, analysts may still wish to test for effect modification by factors that have not been prespecified. Such analyses are exploratory; the results will need later explicit confirmation from another study. Nevertheless, exploratory tests of heterogeneity are useful in suggesting new avenues for research and can be quite informative for comparative effectiveness studies and for individualized patient decision making because they can point to subgroups and individuals in whom treatment may be either more or less effective than the average. It is important that reports of exploratory tests of heterogeneity qualify their results for the variables examined and tests run, perhaps carrying out a rough statistical adjustment if p-values are reported.

Several methods for adjusting for multiple tests are commonly employed. The most stringent employs the Bonferroni adjustment which carries out the significance test at the nominal level (often $\alpha = 0.05$) divided by the number of tests done. This approach, while appropriate if all tests are independent, is extremely conservative when they are related which they will be when effect modification is assesses over subgroups that overlap. Nevertheless, for a small number of tests, the Bonferroni adjustment may be adequate. A second related approach creates a more stringent significance level for all interactions tests that is set at some round number such as $\alpha = 0.01$ or $\alpha = 0.001$. This is quite common for genetic tests where the subgroups may be defined using large group of genetic markers. With microarrays that have an extremely large number of potential markers, the significance level is often orders of magnitude lower. A third approach is to use a permutation test in which the outcome and treatment variables are fixed, but the covariate values of the effect modifier are randomly permuted so that they are matched with different outcome–treatment combinations. The permutation p-value is determined by the location of the original p-value from the interaction test within the distribution generated by the permutations. Observed interactions that are unusual relative to the permutations are more likely to be real. With multiple covariates, the same procedure can be employed, but the observed p-values are compared as order statistics. For instance, the second smallest observed p-value would be compared to the distribution of the second smallest p-values from the permutations. This will, of course, not always correspond to the same variable.

An alternative approach that combines the goals of separating effect modifies by their plausibility and holding some to a higher standard than others without requiring arbitrary standards that are hard to defend beyond custom is to use Bayesian inference. The Bayesian approach assigns a prior probability to the chance that an interaction is present [90]. This explicitly quantifies the uncertainty that the analyst attaches to the interaction effect and allows for attaching different levels of prior uncertainty to different interactions. This seems to be a more principled approach than one that arbitrarily assigns one or more significance level bars that interactions must pass. Assessments of effect modifier with previous supporting evidence, which are perhaps being treated as confirmatory tests, can use prior distributions that assign more probability to the presence of effect modification. Such priors have been termed enthusiastic [91]. Other modifiers with little prior support, but scientifically plausible, may be given neutral priors centered on zero with more chance of the magnitude of effect modification being small. Finally, modifiers assessed in an exploratory fashion may be given skeptical priors centered strongly on zero so that the data must be quite strong to counteract them. The resulting posterior distributions will then reflect the relative weight of the priors and the likelihood so that modifiers with higher prior probabilities of nonzero effects will be more likely to have posterior probabilities of nonzero effects. Conversely, unlikely modifiers will be much less likely to have posteriors that suggest true effect modification. It is, of course, crucial that the prior distributions reasonably represent the prior beliefs. The common objection to priors as being subjective can be countered by noting that different scientists may reasonably have different beliefs about both before and after analyzing the data. The Bayesian formulation simply quantifies these beliefs so that they can be concretely discussed.

8.5.4 HTE Analyses Using Summary Variables

One strategy for addressing to some extent the problems engendered by the large number of potential effect modifiers is to perform HTE analyses over variables that summarize information from multiple covariates [92,93]. Analysts often use modeling to reduce a person's (column) vector of covariates, $\mathbf{X}$, into a lower-dimensional object, $h(\mathbf{X})$, so that HTE is assessed over its levels; for example, by examining

$$\mathbb{E}[Y^1 - Y^0 | h(x)] = \mathbb{E}[Y | A = 1, h(x)] - \mathbb{E}[Y | A = 0, h(x)]$$

over levels of $\mathbf{X}$.

One approach that has been recommended on the grounds that outcome risk in the control group is an important determinant of the treatment effect [92,94,95] is to use a regression model for the outcome without treatment to estimate a *risk score*,

$$\mathbb{E}[Y | A = 0, \mathbf{X}] = g^{-1}(\mathbf{X}^{\mathsf{T}} \beta), \tag{8.9}$$

where g is a link function and β is a vector of regression coefficients. By estimating the parameters of this model, we can obtain the predicted outcome risk for each patient under no treatment and use that to stratify the patient population, using the risk score (a scalar) instead of the possibly very high-dimensional $\mathbf{X}$ as the effect modifier. In general, it is dangerous to use data from the control group when developing the risk score model and then apply the risk score to the entire trial; such an approach risks overfitting the risk model to the control group (especially when the number of covariates is large, the trial sample size is small, or model selection is aggressive), which can lead to serious distortion of estimates and tests for HTE [95]; such problems can be overcome with appropriate statistical methods (e.g., leave-on-out or split-sample estimation [95]) or the use of externally developed models. Obviously, analyses based on predicted outcome risk in the absence of treatment can take advantage of the fairly large number of available (previously developed) predictive models for various index conditions and outcomes and the extensive background knowledge on risk factors for various outcomes.

An obvious alternative is to use an *effect score* [93,96–99]. One begins by modeling outcomes conditional on treatment as a function of covariates separately for each treatment group,

$$\mathbb{E}[Y^a | \mathbf{X}] = \mathbb{E}[Y | A = a, \mathbf{X}] = g_a^{-1}(\mathbf{X}^{\mathsf{T}} \beta_a), \tag{8.10}$$

where g_a is a link function (possibly different for each treatment group) and β_a is a vector of coefficients to be estimated separately for each treatment. The effect score for individuals with $\mathbf{X} = \mathbf{x}$ is then obtained as

$$\hat{\delta}(\mathbf{x}) = g_1(\mathbf{x}^\mathsf{T}\hat{\beta}_1) - g_0(\mathbf{x}^\mathsf{T}\hat{\beta}_0).$$

In a sense, assessing effect heterogeneity over the predicted treatment effect is the most "informative" analysis possible, given that interest typically centers on identifying predictors of differential treatment magnitude. However, developing predictive outcome models separately within each arm of a randomized trial may lead to substantial overfitting. When the number of predictors is modest and the sample size is moderate to large, the use of resampling methods and cross-validation can address these issues. As always, model evaluation is best performed using data that were not used in model development. Also, even though the exposition in this section adopts a generalized linear model framework, the risk or effect score strategies can also be used with time-to-event where the primary additional challenge is accounting for censoring (e.g., [99–102]).

Another issue is that, for the effect score to consistently estimate the conditional average treatment effect, the outcome model for each treatment group needs to be correctly specified. This will generally not be possible (because determinants of the outcome are unmeasured or the functional form of the regression is misspecified) and it is more productive to view the models used to estimate the effect score as *working models*. Yet, the use of the summary variables for examining estimated treatment effects within "bins" of risk or effect score values does not require correct model specification (e.g., modifiers may be omitted or the functional form of their relationships with the outcome may be incorrectly modeled). Even when the working models are misspecified (which will almost always be the case), within groups of individuals with similar summary variable values, conditional average treatment effects are estimated consistently (in simple randomized trials). In other words, the treatment effect conditional on the risk and effect score can be consistently estimated (even when the models are misspecified) by virtue of randomization, and valid inference on the relationship between the score and the treatment effect is possible using held-out data or external data from a second trial of the same treatments (the availability of data from a second trial is not uncommon in drug development programs under the current regulatory framework).

Finally, we note that summary variables can only offer a partial solution to the problems engendered by the high dimensionality of the covariate space. With datasets of modest sample size (as are typical in applied CER), there will always be restrictions on the complexity of the models that can be fit (e.g., to develop risk or effect scores), the ability to explore heterogeneity will always be limited, and background knowledge will be needed for model building.

8.5.5 Assessing HTE in Observational Studies

Under the assumption of conditional exchangeability, the approach for quantifying HTE in observational studies is similar to that in RCTs. For example, exploration of HTE conditional on covariates via outcome regression involves the expansion of model (8.5) to include additional covariates. The correctness of inferences based on outcome regression generally depends on correctly specifying the outcome model (i.e., no omitted variables and correct specification of the functional form of the relationship between covariates and the outcome). Subgroup-specific average treatment effects adjusted for multiple covariates can be obtained by estimating effects conditional on all covariates and then marginalizing over the covariate distribution in each subgroup (a process referred to as "standardization").

In realistic problems, investigators will often adjust for a large number of covariates many of which may be effect modifiers. Standard outcome regression methods cannot easily handle large sets of covariates and interactions of these covariates with the treatment variable. One approach is to use methods with different sparsity constraints over the main effects and interaction terms in the regression model; for example, one recent study used support vector machine classifiers with separate LASSO (least absolute shrinkage and selection operator) penalty parameters for interactions between the treatment and covariates, and other adjustment variables [3]. Even though this approach is promising, it still relies on correct specification of the outcome model for valid causal inference.

Exposure modeling methods [103] to control confounding are available when investigators have some knowledge of the treatment assignment mechanism (e.g., various methods based on modeling the propensity score for fixed exposures). For the examination of HTE over a nominal effect modifier, one can use propensity scores derived separately for each stratum of the modifier and then use the scores to estimate treatment effects within each stratum of the modifier; though this strategy has been recommended [105], its performance has not been thoroughly evaluated. We would expect this strategy to be the most appealing when the subgroups are fairly large and when background knowledge suggests that confounding may behave differentially within each subgroup. A simulation study of propensity score matching in the presence of effect modification and confounding showed that matching within subgroup using a propensity score developed in the entire study is adequate to eliminate confounding, provided that the propensity score is correctly specified [104].

The exploration of HTE using marginal structural models (both for fixed and time-varying exposures) is also fairly straightforward: inverse probability of treatment weights is used to control for confounding and the outcome model is expanded to include potential effect modifiers of substantive interest [106]. That said, information on the relative performance of alternative analytical methods of detecting HTE in observational data, particularly using methods that rely on exposure modeling (e.g., propensity score matching or marginal structural models), is limited and further research is needed.

Model specification is important when analyzing observational data and misspecification can lead to serious bias in the estimation of causal effects [107].

Chapter 1 discusses alternative estimation approaches for observational studies; the importance of heterogeneity of effects in interpreting instrumental variable analyses is addressed in Chapter 2.

8.5.6 Policy Search Methods

The preceding sections have focused on methods that rely heavily on regression models for the outcome conditional on covariates; these are sometimes referred to as *regression-based methods* and are by far the most commonly used and easily implemented in standard software. There is growing interest in methods that search for and evaluate the performance of the best treatment rule (a function that maps patient characteristics into recommended treatments) within a prespecified class [108–110]. These methods are sometimes referred to as *policy search methods*, but the distinction between policy search and regression-based methods can be subtle [110–112]. Policy search methods involve the construction of an estimator for the *value of the treatment rule*, that is, an estimator of the expected outcome if all patients were to be treated according to a particular rule. The choice among rules is then made by searching among a prespecified class of rules for the *optimal regime* (i.e., the one that maximizes value). One appealing characteristic of policy search methods is that one can use estimators of value that are less reliant on the correct specification of the outcome model [109]. A second appealing feature is that maximization can be performed over a restricted class of rules (e.g., chosen to be feasible or have manageable costs) [111]. The development of policy search methods is an active area of research and the choice among methods (regression-based and policy search) requires careful consideration of the specifics of the research problem being considered.

8.6 Reporting of HTE Analyses

In general, the choice of effect modifiers to be considered in any given study should depend on substantive considerations about factors that can plausibly be thought to influence the magnitude of the treatment effect. In addition, in some cases, analyses of HTE can be conducted with the explicit goal to demonstrate that large variability in treatment effects is unlikely, in order to support uniform treatment recommendations among patients with the same index condition. Some "default" subgroup and model-based HTE analyses over key demographic characteristics (e.g., age, sex, race) often make sense, provided that subgroups defined by these variables are sufficiently represented in the study population. These analyses can facilitate future attempts to synthesize data (and thus are justified even when the subgroup analysis was not prespecified in the study protocol [113]). Such analyses may also be mandated legally or required as a condition for the provision of research funding. In any case, all analyses actually performed should be fully reported to avoid selective reporting bias and address issues related to multiplicity.

The reporting of HTE analyses varies across published medical studies [114,115], leading at least one major medical journal to issue reporting guidelines [116]. Recommendations are also available for the reporting of subgroup analyses in clinical trials [117] and effect modification and interaction analyses in epidemiologic studies [118]. Some special issues arise when reporting results from multivariable regression models [119].

When reporting analyses of HTE over levels of a binary, nominal, or ordinal effect modifier, it is helpful to provide sufficient information to allow the calculation of the treatment effect (and its associated standard error) within the strata of the modifier. For example, in a head-to-head randomized trial of two treatments with a binary outcome assessing HTE between men and women, the number of events and number of participants should be presented, cross-tabulated by treatment group and sex. In randomized trials, this level of reporting is adequate to "recreate" a person-level dataset with three variables (treatment, sex, and the outcome). When considering two exposures, it makes sense to present data adequate for calculating treatment effects within levels of each treatment using different measures of association (i.e., the effect of A within strata defined by B, as well as the effect of B within strata of A) and also to estimate treatment effects using a common baseline group (i.e., the effects of A alone, B alone, and A plus B, using no treatment as a common baseline category). Both analyses of HTE and causal counterfactual interaction should be accompanied by appropriate statistical indexes such as tests for statistical interaction (e.g., tests for nonadditivity on the risk difference and nonproportionality on the relative risk scale). If any analyses are adjusted for other variables (as would be expected in observational studies and some trial analyses where covariate adjustment is deemed useful), details about the modeling strategy, the variables considered, and their functional form should also be provided.

Detailed reporting allows readers to examine HTE on different scales (risk difference, relative risk) and also gives a better sense of the outcome rate within subgroups. Another reason to favor such detailed reporting is to facilitate future meta-analyses that will need to explore HTE using published (aggregate data). When detailed data are available, meta-analysts can select a meta-analysis model without being constrained by the unavailability of appropriate data from some studies under a particular model. In many cases, individual studies are not powered to detect HTE, so meta-analysis may be the only way to explore potential effect modification by binary covariates.

The above recommendations are not very practical when considering multivalued or continuous potential effect modifiers, survival analyses with censoring, or when—as in most cases—one wants to examine multiple modifiers jointly. In such cases, access to the individual patient data may be the only way to reproduce study findings or perform detailed HTE analyses across studies. However, graphical approaches can be used to convey findings of HTE analyses over continuous covariates (e.g., [120]).

8.7 Interpreting the Results of HTE Analyses

The interpretation of HTE analyses has long been a source of debate in medicine and epidemiology [117,121,122]. Proper interpretation of findings from analyses that quantify HTE depends on the design of the study and the inferential goals, planning, and conduct of the analysis. As mentioned in Section 8.5.3, a commonly drawn distinction is between "hypothesis generating/exploratory" and "hypothesis testing/confirmatory" analyses. Hypothesis testing analyses need to be prespecified in the study protocol, typically assess a small number of effect modifiers, and are motivated by prior empirical research or background knowledge about the disease and treatments of interest. Statistical testing in such analyses is often combined with attempts to control the false-positive rate and in some cases, the study is designed with the goal of testing HTE (e.g., the sample size is chosen to attain adequate power for assessing effect modification). In contrast, exploratory analyses are not always fully specified in the study protocol, are done even if the study was not designed to have adequate power for exploring HTE, usually examine a moderate to large number of candidate modifiers, may be data driven, and are almost never combined with efforts to control the false-positive rate. A more refined classification of HTE analyses as confirmatory, descriptive, exploratory, or predictive has recently been proposed, based on the distinct analytic goals that can be pursued when examining HTE [113,123]. More generally, when interpreting the results of HTE analyses, the following aspects should be considered: the number of effect modifiers, how the modifiers were selected, whether the study was specifically designed and powered to assess HTE, the degree to which the analyses were prespecified (e.g., variables to be considered, their functional form, any cut-offs, and details of the modeling strategy), and whether an attempt to control the false-positive error rate was made. In any cases, all HTE analyses performed (whether planned or not) and the methods used to conduct them should be fully reported, regardless of what the findings were (e.g., regardless of statistical significance or agreement with prior beliefs about the magnitude and direction of HTE).

8.7.1 Credibility of HTE Analyses Using Subgroups

Especially when HTE analyses are considered to guide treatment recommendations, the considerations listed above have a bearing on the credibility of HTE analyses, an issue that has been discussed extensively in the clinical trials literature. In 1992, Oxman and Guyatt proposed a set of items for assessing the plausibility of subgroup analyses in randomized-controlled studies [124]. They suggested considering the following questions:

1. Is the magnitude of the difference clinically important?
2. Was the difference statistically significant?
3. Did the hypothesis precede rather than follow the analysis?
4. Was the subgroup analysis one of a small number of hypotheses tested?
5. Was the difference suggested by comparisons within rather than between studies?
6. Was the difference consistent across studies?
7. Is there indirect evidence that supports the hypothesized difference?

This list was expanded in 2010 [125] to include a total of 11 prompting questions:

8. Is the subgroup variable a characteristic measured at baseline or after randomization?
9. Was the direction of the subgroup effect specified *a priori*?
10. Is the significant subgroup effect independent? (This question asks whether an interaction term in a model remains statistically significant after adjusting for another potential effect modifier.)
11. Is the interaction consistent across closely related outcomes within the study?

Using criteria very similar to these, a review of 207 trials reporting subgroup analyses concluded that "the credibility of subgroup effects, even when claims are strong, is usually low" [126].

In view of the concepts discussed earlier in this chapter, most of these items appear to have face validity and may be useful as reminders of *issues to consider* when interpreting claims about effect modification. However, some caveats need to be mentioned. First, the questions are impossible to apply on continuous effect modifiers (without dichotomizing them) and seem to place too much emphasis on hypothesis-testing procedures. Second, operationalizing the questions for application to a specific analysis (e.g., what is a "clinically important effect," what exactly counts as "indirect evidence," and how is the strength of that evidence to be assessed?) appears challenging.

Third, a practical method for jointly assessing all 11 questions to determine the "likelihood that a subgroup effect is real" may be hard to defend (e.g., how many questions need to be answered in the affirmative? How are matters of degree to be resolved?). Fourth, the authors proposed that the plausibility of subgroup effects should be *exclusively* assessed using relative measures of effect (e.g., relative risks). As we discuss in Section 8.7.2, HTE on the risk difference scale is usually of greater interest for decision making, both for individual-level and public policy decisions. More generally, although heuristics can be useful, they may encourage formulaic application and discourage in-depth examination of HTE findings.

A more comprehensive examination of HTE would involve case-by-case deliberation using background knowledge, intimate knowledge of the study design and conduct, and statistical principles to interpret study data [127]. This form of assessment cannot be easily reduced to a checklist of items and usually requires the involvement of topic-area and methods experts. Case-by-case deliberation is necessary when facing complex questions (treatments with many possible modifiers) and difficult decisions (e.g., approval of a drug only for a subgroup of patients).

8.7.2 Decoupling the Analysis Scale from the Interpretation Scale

In the context of CER, what is ultimately most germane is detecting, quantifying, and reporting in a clear and usable manner clinically relevant HTE. For person-level and policy decisions, HTE is best assessed on an additive scale. However, because model building on a multiplicative risk scale (e.g., log-linear or logistic regression models) is often believed to produce more parsimonious models and because logistic and Cox regression models are computationally convenient (and numerically more stable) than models on the additive scale, the vast majority of published analyses in biomedical journals analyze and interpret HTE on multiplicative scales (this relates to the general preference for quantifying effects using relative risks in epidemiology [128,129]). The choice of scale, together with the preference for parsimonious models, may have unintended effects: insisting on parsimony when modeling on a relative risk scale can lead to highly nonlinear models for the effect of the exposure; in contrast, insisting on parsimony when modeling on the risk difference will lead to linear models [130]. In both cases, models will have few product terms between the exposure and effect modifiers (a consequence of insisting on parsimony). As such, models on different scales can produce very different predictions for the effect of exposure, even when they have comparable fit. We argue that in many cases (and when justified by the study design), the analysis and interpretation of HTE should be decoupled: analyses should aim to reflect as closely as possible the relationship between treatment, covariates, and the outcome of interest, using background knowledge about the condition of interest and the treatment, making use of advances in statistical modeling, and using a computation-ally convenient approach for estimation [42,130]. However, when using the analysis results to make decisions, it is important to present results in a way that is intuitively accessible to decision makers; in most cases, this means "back-transforming" the results to the risk difference scale.

8.8 HTE Assessment in Practice: The Diabetes Prevention Program

To illustrate the concepts and methods discussed in the previous sections, we use a dataset derived from the Diabetes Prevention Program (DPP), a three-arm randomized trial of interventions for preventing the development of diabetes among high-risk individuals [131]. Briefly, the DPP enrolled patients with a body mass index of 24 or higher (22 or higher in Asians), impaired fasting glucose (plasma concentration of 95–125 mg/dL), and impaired glu-cose tolerance (plasma concentration of 140–199 mg/dL 2 h after a 75 g oral glucose load). Participants were randomly assigned into three groups: (1) standard lifestyle recommendations (written information and an annual individual session that emphasized the importance of a healthy lifestyle, fol-lowing dietary guidelines, weight reduction, and increased physical activity) plus metformin, an antidiabetic medication; (2) standard lifestyle recommen-dations plus placebo; and (3) an intensive program of lifestyle modification (a 16-lesson individualized curriculum on diet, exercise, and behavior modifi-cation followed by individual sessions and group sessions aiming to achieve and maintain a weight reduction of at least 7% of initial weight through healthy diet and to engage in moderate-intensity physical activity for ≥ 150 min per week). The outcome of interest was diabetes, diagnosed on the basis of annual oral glucose tolerance tests or biannual fasting plasma glucose tests, according to the 1997 criteria of the American Diabetes Association. Data for the analyses presented here were available from 3,081 individual patients (of 3,234 DDP participants, 95%; local institutional review boards decided not to make data available for the remaining participants). Read-ers should consult Reference 132 for a clinically oriented discussion of the findings.

In the overall trial population, both metformin (plus standard lifestyle recommendations) and aggressive lifestyle intervention were more effec-tive than standard lifestyle recommendations (plus placebo). After a median follow-up period of 2.8 years, progression to diabetes was reduced by 58% in the lifestyle modification group and by 31% in the metformin group, both compared with the standard recommendations plus placebo group. Many factors measurable at baseline (e.g., fasting blood sugar, blood lipids, and BMI) are predictive of progression to diabetes and are candidate treatment effect modifiers on the multiplicative or additive scale. In addition, the implementation of the interventions in practice has proven difficult because of concern about side effects (for metformin) and logistical challenges (for aggressive lifestyle modification). Thus, there is interest in targeting these effective treatments to subsets of the population that are likely to benefit most from intervention.

We used an "external" risk model developed in the Framingham Offspring Study [133] to obtain the predicted outcome risk for trial participants. The model is based on the following covariates: age, sex, parental history of diabetes, BMI, systolic blood pressure, HDL-C levels, triglyceride levels, waist circumference, and fasting glucose. We stratified patients into quartiles of predicted risk obtained from the Framingham model, calculated treatment effects in each quartile, and tested the null hypothesis of no effect heterogeneity across quartiles.

It is worth noting that many other determinants of risk for diabetes can be considered. For example, a systematic review [134] of studies on models predicting diabetes risk identified 17 factors that were found to be predictive of diabetes development in at least three previously developed models: fasting blood sugar, hemoglobin A1c, age, body mass index (in kilograms per meter of height squared), waist-to-hip ratio, waist circumference, height, triglycerides, high-density lipoprotein cholesterol, systolic blood pressure, physical activity metabolic equivalent, sex, race/ethnicity, family history of diabetes, self-reported history of hypertension, self-reported history of high blood glucose (including "borderline" high glucose or only during pregnancy), and smoking status. These variables were combined in a predictive model for the outcome that was fit to the trial data without using information on the trial arm in which participants were assigned. This strategy is sometimes used to avoid issues induced by overfitting when using only the control arm to estimate the parameters of the risk model, while using all available data. Though increasingly popular and supported by a small simulation study [135], the strategy is not fully satisfactory (e.g., it is clear that, when the treatment has an effect on the outcome, the outcome model is "intentionally" misspecified). For comparison with the results obtained using the Framingham model, we also examined effect heterogeneity over quartiles of predicted risk defined on the basis of the internally developed risk model.

We summarize the results from all analyses in Figure 8.2 by plotting effect estimates both on the hazard ratio scale (assuming proportional hazards and using the Cox model) and on the risk difference scale (at median follow-up, with risk calculations based on estimates from the Cox model). For the comparison of intensive lifestyle modification versus standard lifestyle recommendations and placebo, there was little evidence of HTE on the multiplicative scale but there was statistically significant evidence of strong heterogeneity on the absolute risk difference scale. For the comparison of metformin plus standard lifestyle recommendations versus standard lifestyle recommendations plus placebo, there was statistically significant evidence of

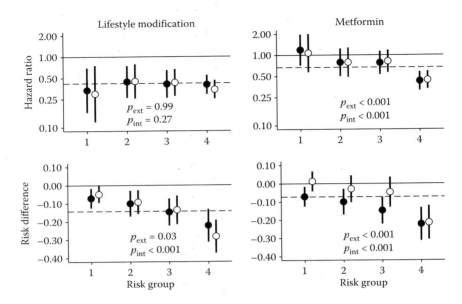

FIGURE 8.2
HTE analyses in the Diabetes Prevention Program. Panels on the left present results from the comparison of lifestyle modification against standard lifestyle recommendations plus placebo; panels on the right present results from the comparisons of metformin plus standard lifestyle recommendations versus standard lifestyle recommendations plus placebo. Top panels present results for treatment effects on the multiplicative (hazard ratio) scale and bottom panels present results on the risk difference scale. Risk groups correspond to quartiles of predicted risk based on an externally developed model (black markers) or an internally developed model (white markers). Extending vertical lines denote 95% confidence intervals. *p*-values are based on tests of the null hypothesis of no effect modification (separately for the externally and internally developed risk models). Horizontal dashed lines denote the estimate of the merge effect for each comparison.

HTE on both the multiplicative and additive scale. Results were qualitatively similar when heterogeneity was assessed over quartiles of risk predicted using the Framingham model and using the internally developed model.

8.9 HTE in Meta-Analysis

When heterogeneity manifests itself across a set of comparative effectiveness studies in such a way that some studies favor one treatment and others either favor another or find no significant difference between them, it may be possible to use meta-analysis to assess the sources of the heterogeneity (see Chapter 10, [136]). While some of these differences may simply reflect random variation, others reflect systematic differences in study populations, designs, and quality of execution. Meta-regression can be used if only study summaries like averages are available or multilevel modeling if individual participant data from each of the studies can be obtained. Analysis of across-study heterogeneity extends the methods for analyzing heterogeneity in a single study discussed so far in this chapter to incorporate between-study differences. Some of these differences could just as easily be present in a single study (e.g., different types of individuals), but others related to study design and execution are fundamentally differences that only appear across studies. For instance, estimated treatment effects in a well-conducted randomized trial are often quite different from those found in an observational study that has not properly controlled for baseline differences between the treatment groups.

Evaluation of heterogeneity depends crucially on the type of data available. When data from each participant in each study are available, one can assess heterogeneity over person-level characteristics (e.g., age, gender, or disease severity) [137,138]. Such assessment is also possible when individual studies consistently report results stratified by person-level characteristics (e.g., subgroup analyses) or when studies report the results of HTE analyses (estimates of product terms between treatment and the effect modifier of interest in regression models). If only aggregate data such as the average age of participants in the study are available, it is only possible to get a sense of heterogeneity by examining the association of these characteristics with the estimated treatment effect. Associations of treatment effects with study-level covariates may not reflect HTE over patient-level characteristics, even when effects are truly variable at the patient level [139,140]. As an example, consider a treatment such as flu vaccine that is particularly effective among older individuals. Two studies of flu vaccine may find different treatment effects because of different distributions of elderly individuals in the studies even if the average age of the participants varies little. The presence of a small group of elderly individuals at risk in one study may be enough to impact the overall treatment effect estimate without substantially changing the mean age. Study-level characteristics, such as the year when the study was conducted, that apply to every individual in the treatment group or in the entire study do not require such individual data, but require information from different studies to properly assess heterogeneity. Unfortunately, because the studies may differ in other aspects as well, the influence of different study characteristics on results cannot be can be difficult to disentangle.

8.10 HTE and Clinical Decision Making

Clinicians choose how to treat a patient by considering the anticipated effects of treatments and their understanding of their patient's values (preferences). For example, most clinicians would not prescribe statins to a 50-year-old man at very low risk of cardiac disease. The minor anticipated benefit does not offset the inconvenience of daily pill-taking, the risk of experiencing a rare but serious adverse event (rhabdomyolysis), or the associated cost. By contrast, most clinicians would prescribe statins to a woman with high low-density cholesterol uncontrolled by lifestyle modifications, because they would perceive that the balance of benefits and risks favors treatment [141]. This "heterogeneity" in decision making across different patient subgroups is pervasive in clinical practice and is intuitively clear to practitioners. It is conceptually related to HTE as examined in this chapter, but additional considerations apply.

First, decisions are rarely determined by a single outcome. In the examples above, the optimal action is chosen based on the valuation and aggregation of several dimensions, namely, benefits, harms, preferences for different outcomes, and costs. Each dimension can have different treatment effect modifiers, and more generally, a different instantiation of group-level HTE (Definition 8.2). Even if HTE in each dimension is satisfactorily modeled using regression methods, the relationship of effect modifiers with the evaluated and aggregated decision-relevant quantity can be complex.

Second, as discussed in Section 8.5.2, the scale on which decisions are made can differ from (be a nonlinear transformation of) the scale on which HTE is modeled. Thus, even if the model used to assess HTE using Definition 8.2 includes no product terms ("statistical interactions") of treatment with other variables on the logit scale, the risk difference between treatment and control will change across levels of the variables in the model. When relative treatment effects are constant for all outcomes of interest, difference in the decision-relevant quantity in the risk difference scale can be large or small depending on the baseline risk of each outcome in various populations.

Third, decisions correspond to a discretization of an underlying decision-relevant quantity (equivalently, a loss function) according to some decision criterion (e.g., to minimize expected loss). The decision may therefore depend on factors in addition to HTE and so the optimal choice may either be the same across subgroups despite HTE or different despite a lack of HTE. For example, one may still decide to treat both men and women, even if the treatment is moderately beneficial in men and very beneficial in women. Conversely, a treatment with a moderate cost and a constant relative treatment effect with respect to a key health outcome will have a different benefit on the risk difference scale for individuals with different baseline risks. Consideration of the unit cost per percentage change in risk may lead to different decision thresholds so that treatment is reserved for the higher-risk patients.

8.11 Concluding Remarks

The exploration of HTE is now widely recognized as a key activity in patient-centered CER and a prerequisite for personalized care. This chapter reviewed concepts of HTE at the individual level (as heterogeneity of person-level causal effects) and at the group level (as heterogeneity of conditional average treatment effects or effect measure modification). We discussed the relationship between HTE, causal interactions, and statistical interactions (deviations from additivity) and their implications for the interpretation of statistical analyses. The very large number of potential effect modifiers means that analyses must consider multiple modifiers jointly, in order to address the reference class problem. However, advances in measurement and data storage mean that the number of potential effect modifiers covariate space to explore far exceeds the sample size of our clinical studies. Consequently, even as routine data collection of observational data (e.g., availability of electronic health record information) leads to increases in the number of available observations, a lot of methodological research remains to be done. Our ability to understand HTE can be improved by developing methods to design randomized trials to optimally address HTE questions, by finding ways to leverage background knowledge, observational data, and randomized trials to address clinically meaningful questions, and by developing analytical methods that can better cope with the complex questions we need answered.

Acknowledgments

This work was supported by a Patient-Centered Outcomes Research Institute Methods Research Award (PCORI, ME-1306-03758) and an Agency for Health Care Research and Quality training grant (AHRQ, R25HS023299). All statements in this chapter are solely those of the authors and do not necessarily represent the views of PCORI, its board of governors, the PCORI Methodology Committee, AHRQ, or the Department of Health and Human Services.

References

1. S. R. Tunis, J. Benner, and M. McClellan, Comparative effectiveness research: Policy context, methods development and research infrastructure, *Statistics in Medicine*, vol. 29, no. 19, pp. 1963–1976, 2010.
2. R. L. Kravitz, N. Duan, and J. Braslow, Evidence-based medicine, heterogeneity of treatment effects, and the trouble with averages, *Milbank Quarterly*, vol. 82, no. 4, pp. 661–687, 2004.
3. K. Imai et al., Estimating treatment effect heterogeneity in randomized program evaluation, *The Annals of Applied Statistics*, vol. 7, no. 1, pp. 443–470, 2013.

4. J. J. Goldberger and A. E. Buxton, Personalized medicine vs guideline-based medicine, *JAMA*, vol. 309, no. 24, pp. 2559–2560, 2013.
5. D. M. Eddy, J. Adler, B. Patterson, D. Lucas, K. A. Smith, and M. Morris, Individualized guidelines: The potential for increasing quality and reducing costs, *Annals of Internal Medicine*, vol. 154, no. 9, pp. 627–634, 2011.
6. J. Splawa-Neyman et al., On the application of probability theory to agricultural experiments. Essay on principles. Section 9, *Statistical Science*, vol. 5, no. 4, pp. 465–472, 1990.
7. D. B. Rubin, Estimating causal effects of treatments in randomized and non-randomized studies, *Journal of Educational Psychology*, vol. 66, no. 5, p. 688, 1974.
8. D. Lewis, Causation, *Journal of Philosophy*, vol. 70, no. 17, pp. 556–567, 1973.
9. J. M. Robins and S. Greenland, Causal inference without counterfactuals: Comment, *Journal of the American Statistical Association*, vol. 95, no. 450, pp. 431–435, 2000.
10. J. Pearl, *Causality: Models, Reasoning and Inference*, vol. 29. Cambridge University Press, New York, 2000.
11. T. J. VanderWeele and J. M. Robins, Four types of effect modification: A classification based on directed acyclic graphs, *Epidemiology*, vol. 18, no. 5, pp. 561–568, 2007.
12. K. J. Rothman, Causes, *American Journal of Epidemiology*, vol. 104, no. 6, pp. 587–592, 1976.
13. W. D. Flanders, On the relationship of sufficient component cause models with potential outcome (counterfactual) models, *European Journal of Epidemiology*, vol. 21, no. 12, pp. 847–853, 2006.
14. S. Greenland and B. Brumback, An overview of relations among causal modelling methods, *International Journal of Epidemiology*, vol. 31, no. 5, pp. 1030–1037, 2002.
15. J. M. Robins and S. Greenland, The probability of causation under a stochastic model for individual risk, *Biometrics*, vol. 45, pp. 1125–1138, 1989.
16. D. B. Rubin, Statistics and causal inference: Comment: Which ifs have causal answers, *Journal of the American Statistical Association*, vol. 81, no. 396, pp. 961–962, 1986.
17. D. B. Rubin, Reflections stimulated by the comments of Shadish (2010) and West and Thoemmes (2010). *Psychological Methods*, vol. 15, no. 1, pp. 38–46, 2010.
18. T. J. VanderWeele, Concerning the consistency assumption in causal inference, *Epidemiology*, vol. 20, no. 6, pp. 880–883, 2009.
19. J. M. Robins, A new approach to causal inference in mortality studies with a sustained exposure period—Application to control of the healthy worker survivor effect, *Mathematical Modelling*, vol. 7, no. 9, pp. 1393–1512, 1986.
20. J. M. Robins, Addendum to "A new approach to causal inference in mortality studies with a sustained exposure period—Application to control of the healthy worker survivor effect", *Computers & Mathematics with Applications*, vol. 14, no. 9, pp. 923–945, 1987.
21. P. W. Holland, Statistics and causal inference, *Journal of the American Statistical Association*, vol. 81, no. 396, pp. 945–960, 1986.
22. S. Greenland, J. M. Robins, and J. Pearl, Confounding and collapsibility in causal inference, *Statistical Science*, vol. 14, no. 1, pp. 29–46, 1999.

23. A. S. Gerber and D. P. Green, *Field Experiments: Design, Analysis, and Interpretation*. WW Norton, New York, 2012.

24. G. L. Gadbury and H. K. Iyer, Unit–treatment interaction and its practical consequences, *Biometrics*, vol. 56, no. 3, pp. 882–885, 2000.

25. E. J. Mascha and J. M. Albert, Estimating treatment effect heterogeneity for binary outcomes via Dirichlet multinomial constraints, *Biometrical Journal*, vol. 49, no. 3, pp. 378–393, 2007.

26. J. Copas, Randomization models for the matched and unmatched 2×2 tables, *Biometrika*, vol. 60, no. 3, pp. 467–476, 1973.

27. M. Hernan, A definition of causal effect for epidemiological research, *Journal of Epidemiology and Community Health*, vol. 58, no. 4, pp. 265–271, 2004.

28. K. J. Rothman, S. Greenland, and A. M. Walker, Concepts of interaction, *American Journal of Epidemiology*, vol. 112, no. 4, pp. 467–470, 1980.

29. T. J. VanderWeele, Confounding and effect modification: Distribution and measure, *Epidemiologic Methods*, vol. 1, no. 1, pp. 55–82, 2012.

30. O. Miettinen, Confounding and effect-modification, *American Journal of Epidemiology*, vol. 100, no. 5, pp. 350–353, 1974.

31. P. R. Rosenbaum, The consequences of adjustment for a concomitant variable that has been affected by the treatment, *Journal of the Royal Statistical Society. Series A (General)*, vol. 147, no. 5, pp. 656–666, 1984.

32. J. M. Robins and S. Greenland, Adjusting for differential rates of prophylaxis therapy for PCP in high-versus low-dose AZT treatment arms in an AIDS randomized trial, *Journal of the American Statistical Association*, vol. 89, no. 427, pp. 737–749, 1994.

33. C. E. Frangakis and D. B. Rubin, Principal stratification in causal inference, *Biometrics*, vol. 58, no. 1, pp. 21–29, 2002.

34. O. S. Miettinen, Causal and preventive interdependence: Elementary principles, *Scandinavian Journal of Work, Environment & Health*, vol. 8, no. 3, pp. 159–168, 1982.

35. D. L. Weed, M. Selmon, and T. Sinks, Links between categories of interaction, *American Journal of Epidemiology*, vol. 127, no. 1, pp. 17–27, 1988.

36. D. R. Cox, Interaction, *International Statistical Review/Revue Internationale de Statistique*, vol. 52, no. 1, pp. 1–24, 1984.

37. S. Greenland and C. Poole, Invariants and noninvariants in the concept of interdependent effects, *Scandinavian Journal of Work, Environment & Health*, vol. 14, no. 2, pp. 125–129, 1988.

38. T. J. VanderWeele, On the distinction between interaction and effect modification, *Epidemiology*, vol. 20, no. 6, pp. 863–871, 2009.

39. T. J. VanderWeele and M. J. Knol, Interpretation of subgroup analyses in randomized trials: Heterogeneity versus secondary interventions, *Annals of Internal Medicine*, vol. 154, no. 10, pp. 680–683, 2011.

40. W. D. Thompson, Effect modification and the limits of biological inference from epidemiologic data, *Journal of Clinical Epidemiology*, vol. 44, no. 3, pp. 221–232, 1991.

41. S. Greenland, Interactions in epidemiology: Relevance, identification, and estimation, *Epidemiology*, vol. 20, no. 1, pp. 14–17, 2009.

42. S. Greenland, Modeling and variable selection in epidemiologic analysis, *American Journal of Public Health*, vol. 79, no. 3, pp. 340–349, 1989.

43. J. Siemiatycki and D. C. Thomas, Biological models and statistical interactions: An example from multistage carcinogenesis, *International Journal of Epidemiology*, vol. 10, no. 4, pp. 383–387, 1981.

44. S. Greenland, Basic problems in interaction assessment, *Environmental Health Perspectives*, vol. 101, no. Suppl 4, p. 59, 1993.

45. J. S. Kaufman, Interaction reaction, *Epidemiology*, vol. 20, no. 2, pp. 159–160, 2009.

46. D. A. Lawlor, Biological interaction: Time to drop the term? *Epidemiology*, vol. 22, no. 2, pp. 148–150, 2011.

47. T. J. VanderWeele, A word and that to which it once referred: Assessing biologic interaction, *Epidemiology*, vol. 22, no. 4, pp. 612–613, 2011.

48. T. J. VanderWeele and M. J. Knol, A tutorial on interaction, *Epidemiologic Methods*, vol. 3, no. 1, pp. 33–72, 2014.

49. N. Pearce, Analytical implications of epidemiological concepts of interaction, *International Journal of Epidemiology*, vol. 18, no. 4, pp. 976–980, 1989.

50. T. J. VanderWeele and J. M. Robins, The identification of synergism in the sufficient-component-cause framework, *Epidemiology*, vol. 18, no. 3, pp. 329–339, 2007.

51. T. J. VanderWeele, A unification of mediation and interaction: A 4-way decomposition, *Epidemiology*, vol. 25, no. 5, pp. 749–761, 2014.

52. J. Venn, *The Logic of Chance: An Essay on the Foundations and Province of the Theory of Probability, with Especial Reference to Its Application to Moral and Social Science.* Macmillan, London, 1866.

53. H. Reichenbach, *The Theory of Probability.* University of California Press, Berkeley, 1949.

54. A. Hájek, The reference class problem is your problem too, *Synthese*, vol. 156, no. 3, pp. 563–585, 2007.

55. S. W. Lagakos, The challenge of subgroup analyses-reporting without distorting, *New England Journal of Medicine*, vol. 354, no. 16, p. 1667, 2006.

56. S. T. Brookes, E. Whitley, T. J. Peters, P. A. Mulheran, M. Egger, and G. Davey Smith, Subgroup analyses in randomised controlled trials: Quantifying the risks of false-positives and false-negatives, *Health Technology Assessment*, vol. 5, no. 33, pp. 1–56, 2001.

57. G. E. Box et al., *Statistics for Experimenters*, Wiley, New York, 1978.

58. R. L. Kravitz, N. Duan, and the DEcIDE Methods Center N-of-1 Guidance Panel, eds., *Design and Implementation of N-of-1 Trials: A User's Guide*. Agency for Healthcare Research and Quality, Rockville, MD, 2014.

59. D. Zucker, C. Schmid, M. McIntosh, R. D'Agostino, H. Selker, and J. Lau, Combining single patient (n-of-1) trials to estimate population treatment effects and to evaluate individual patient responses to treatment, *Journal of Clinical Epidemiology*, vol. 50, no. 4, pp. 401–410, 1997.

60. D. R. Zucker et al., Lessons learned combining n-of-1 trials to assess fibromyalgia therapies, *Journal of Rheumatology*, vol. 33, no. 10, pp. 2069–2077, 2006.

61. D. R. Zucker, R. Ruthazer, and C. H. Schmid, Individual (n-of-1) trials can be combined to give population comparative treatment effect estimates: Methodologic considerations, *Journal of Clinical Epidemiology*, vol. 63, no. 12, pp. 1312–1323, 2010.

62. T. Kurth, A. M. Walker, R. J. Glynn, K. A. Chan, J. M. Gaziano, K. Berger, and J. M. Robins, Results of multivariable logistic regression, propensity matching,

propensity adjustment, and propensity-based weighting under conditions of nonuniform effect, *American Journal of Epidemiology*, vol. 163, no. 3, pp. 262–270, 2006.

63. J. M. Robins and L. Wasserman, On the impossibility of inferring causation from association without background knowledge, *Computation, Causation, and Discovery*, MIT Press, Cambridge, MA, pp. 305–321, 1999.

64. J. M. Robins, Data, design, and background knowledge in etiologic inference, *Epidemiology*, vol. 12, no. 3, pp. 313–320, 2001.

65. J. M. Robins, A. Rotnitzky, and D. O. Scharfstein, Sensitivity analysis for selection bias and unmeasured confounding in missing data and causal inference models, in *Statistical Models in Epidemiology, The Environment, and Clinical Trials*, pp. 1–94, Springer, New York, 2000.

66. T. L. Lash, M. P. Fox, R. F. MacLehose, G. Maldonado, L. C. McCandless, and S. Greenland, Good practices for quantitative bias analysis, *International Journal of Epidemiology*, p. dyu149, vol. 43, no. 6, pp. 1969–1985, http://ije.oxfordjournals.org/content/early/2014/07/30/ije.dyu149.short, 2014.

67. T. J. VanderWeele, B. Mukherjee, and J. Chen, Sensitivity analysis for interactions under unmeasured confounding, *Statistics in Medicine*, vol. 31, no. 22, pp. 2552–2564, 2012.

68. E. J. Tchetgen Tchetgen and T. J. VanderWeele, Robustness of measures of interaction to unmeasured confounding, COBRA Preprint Series. Working Paper 89. http://biostats.bepress.com/cobra/art89, 2012.

69. M. Gail and R. Simon, Testing for qualitative interactions between treatment effects and patient subsets, *Biometrics*, vol. 41, no. 2, pp. 361–372, 1985.

70. M. Schemper, Non-parametric analysis of treatment—Covariate interaction in the presence of censoring, *Statistics in Medicine*, vol. 7, no. 12, pp. 1257–1266, 1988.

71. E. Edgington and P. Onghena, *Randomization Tests*. CRC Press, Boca Raton, 2007.

72. R. F. Potthoff, B. L. Peterson, and S. L. George, Detecting treatment-by-centre interaction in multi-centre clinical trials, *Statistics in Medicine*, vol. 20, no. 2, pp. 193–213, 2001.

73. R. Wang, D. A. Schoenfeld, B. Hoeppner, and A. E. Evins, Detecting treatment-covariate interactions using permutation methods, *Statistics in Medicine*, vol. 34, no. 12, pp. 2035–2047, 2015.

74. S. Greenland, Tests for interaction in epidemiologic studies: A review and a study of power, *Statistics in Medicine*, vol. 2, no. 2, pp. 243–251, 1983.

75. D. A. Follmann and M. A. Proschan, A multivariate test of interaction for use in clinical trials, *Biometrics*, vol. 55, no. 4, pp. 1151–1155, 1999.

76. S. A. Kovalchik, R. Varadhan, and C. O. Weiss, Assessing heterogeneity of treatment effect in a clinical trial with the proportional interactions model, *Statistics in Medicine*, vol. 32, no. 28, pp. 4906–4923, 2013.

77. P. Royston and W. Sauerbrei, Interaction of treatment with a continuous variable: Simulation study of significance level for several methods of analysis, *Statistics in Medicine*, vol. 32, no. 22, pp. 3788–3803, 2013.

78. P. Royston and W. Sauerbrei, Interaction of treatment with a continuous variable: Simulation study of power for several methods of analysis, *Statistics in Medicine*, vol. 33, no. 27, pp. 4695–4708, 2014.

79. S. J. Pocock, M. D. Hughes, and R. J. Lee, Statistical problems in the reporting of clinical trials, *New England Journal of Medicine*, vol. 317, no. 7, pp. 426–432, 1987.

80. J. N. Matthews and D. G. Altman, Statistics notes: Interaction 2: Compare effect sizes not p values, *BMJ*, vol. 313, no. 7060, p. 808, 1996.
81. S. F. Assmann, S. J. Pocock, L. E. Enos, and L. E. Kasten, Subgroup analysis and other (mis) uses of baseline data in clinical trials, *Lancet*, vol. 355, no. 9209, pp. 1064–1069, 2000.
82. S. J. Pocock, S. E. Assmann, L. E. Enos, and L. E. Kasten, Subgroup analysis, covariate adjustment and baseline comparisons in clinical trial reporting: Current practice and problems, *Statistics in Medicine*, vol. 21, no. 19, pp. 2917–2930, 2002.
83. A. V. Hernández, E. Boersma, G. D. Murray, J. D. F. Habbema, and E. W. Steyerberg, Subgroup analyses in therapeutic cardiovascular clinical trials: Are most of them misleading? *American Heart Journal*, vol. 151, no. 2, pp. 257–264, 2006.
84. P. McCullagh, J. A. Nelder, and P. McCullagh, *Generalized Linear Models*, vol. 2. Chapman & Hall, London, 1989.
85. N. Mantel, C. Brown, and D. P. Byar, Tests for homogeneity of effect in an epidemiologic investigation, *American Journal of Epidemiology*, vol. 106, no. 2, pp. 125–129, 1977.
86. B. Brumback and A. Berg, On effect-measure modification: Relationships among changes in the relative risk, odds ratio, and risk difference, *Statistics in Medicine*, vol. 27, no. 18, pp. 3453–3465, 2008.
87. A. Morabia, T. Ten Have, and J. R. Landis, Interaction fallacy, *Journal of Clinical Epidemiology*, vol. 50, no. 7, pp. 809–812, 1997.
88. C. Wang, C. H. Schmid, P. L. Hibberd, R. Kalish, R. Roubenoff, R. Rones, and T. McAlindon, Tai chi is effective in treating knee osteoarthritis: A randomized controlled trial, *Arthritis Care & Research*, vol. 61, no. 11, pp. 1545–1553, 2009.
89. C. Wang et al., Assessing the comparative effectiveness of tai chi versus physical therapy for knee osteoarthritis: Design and rationale for a randomized trial, *BMC Complementary and Alternative Medicine*, vol. 14, no. 1, p. 333, 2014.
90. D. O. Dixon and R. Simon, Bayesian subset analysis, *Biometrics*, vol. 47, no. 3, pp. 871–881, 1991.
91. D. J. Spiegelhalter, L. S. Freedman, and M. K. Parmar, Bayesian approaches to randomized trials, *Journal of the Royal Statistical Society. Series A (Statistics in Society)*, vol. 157, pp. 357–416, 1994.
92. P. John and J. Lau, Heterogeneity of the baseline risk within patient populations of clinical trials. A proposed evaluation algorithm, *American Journal of Epidemiology*, vol. 148, no. 11, pp. 1117–1126, 1998.
93. T. Cai, L. Tian, P. H. Wong, and L. Wei, Analysis of randomized comparative clinical trial data for personalized treatment selections, *Biostatistics*, vol. 12, no. 2, pp. 270–282, 2011.
94. D. M. Kent, P. M. Rothwell, J. P. Ioannidis, D. G. Altman, and R. A. Hayward, Assessing and reporting heterogeneity in treatment effects in clinical trials: A proposal, *Trials*, vol. 11, no. 1, p. 85, 2010.
95. A. Abadie, M. M. Chingos, and M. R. West, Endogenous stratification in randomized experiments, Tech. Rep., National Bureau of Economic Research, 2013.
96. J. A. Dorresteijn, F. L. Visseren, P. M. Ridker, A. M. Wassink, N. P. Paynter, E. W. Steyerberg, Y. van der Graaf, and N. R. Cook, Estimating treatment effects for individual patients based on the results of randomised clinical trials, *BMJ*, vol. 343, p. d5888, 2011.

97. L. Zhao, L. Tian, T. Cai, B. Claggett, and L.-J. Wei, Effectively selecting a target population for a future comparative study, *Journal of the American Statistical Association*, vol. 108, no. 502, pp. 527–539, 2013.

98. B. Claggett, L. Tian, D. Castagno, and L.-J. Wei, Treatment selections using risk–benefit profiles based on data from comparative randomized clinical trials with multiple endpoints, *Biostatistics*, vol. 16, no. 1, pp. 60–72, 2015.

99. L. Tian and X. Zhao, *Statistical Methods for Personalized Medicine*, p. 79, World Scientific Publishing Co, Singapore, 2015.

100. R. Li and L. Chambless, Test for additive interaction in proportional hazards models, *Annals of Epidemiology*, vol. 17, no. 3, pp. 227–236, 2007.

101. T. J. VanderWeele, Causal interactions in the proportional hazards model, *Epidemiology*, vol. 22, no. 5, p. 713, 2011.

102. N. H. Rod, T. Lange, I. Andersen, J. L. Marott, and F. Diderichsen, Additive interaction in survival analysis: Use of the additive hazards model, *Epidemiology*, vol. 23, no. 5, pp. 733–737, 2012.

103. S. Greenland, Invited commentary: Variable selection versus shrinkage in the control of multiple confounders, *American Journal of Epidemiology*, vol. 167, no. 5, pp. 523–529, 2008.

104. J. A. Rassen, R. J. Glynn, K. J. Rothman, S. Setoguchi, and S. Schneeweiss, Applying propensity scores estimated in a full cohort to adjust for confounding in subgroup analyses, *Pharmacoepidemiology and Drug Safety*, vol. 21, no. 7, pp. 697–709, 2012.

105. K. M. Green and E. A. Stuart, Examining moderation analyses in propensity score methods: Application to depression and substance use, *Journal of Consulting and Clinical Psychology*, vol. 82, no. 5, p. 773, 2014.

106. M. A. Hernan and J. M. Robins, *Causal Inference*. CRC Press, Boca Raton, 2010.

107. S. Vansteelandt, M. Bekaert, and G. Claeskens, On model selection and model misspecification in causal inference, *Statistical Methods in Medical Research*, vol. 21, no. 1, pp. 7–30, 2012.

108. D. B. Rubin and M. J. van der Laan, Statistical issues and limitations in personalized medicine research with clinical trials, *International Journal of Biostatistics*, vol. 8, no. 1, 2012.

109. B. Zhang, A. A. Tsiatis, E. B. Laber, and M. Davidian, A robust method for estimating optimal treatment regimes, *Biometrics*, vol. 68, no. 4, pp. 1010–1018, 2012.

110. C. Kang, H. Janes, and Y. Huang, Combining biomarkers to optimize patient treatment recommendations, *Biometrics*, vol. 70, no. 3, pp. 695–707, 2014.

111. E. B. Laber, A. A. Tsiatis, M. Davidian, and S. T. Holloway, Discussion of combining biomarkers to optimize patient treatment recommendations, *Biometrics*, vol. 70, no. 3, pp. 707–710, 2014.

112. C. Kang, H. Janes, and Y. Huang, Rejoinder: Combining biomarkers to optimize patient treatment recommendations, *Biometrics*, vol. 70, no. 3, p. 719, 2014.

113. R. Varadhan, J. B. Segal, C. M. Boyd, A. W. Wu, and C. O. Weiss, A framework for the analysis of heterogeneity of treatment effect in patient-centered outcomes research, *Journal of Clinical Epidemiology*, vol. 66, no. 8, pp. 818–825, 2013.

114. N. B. Gabler, N. Duan, D. Liao, J. G. Elmore, T. G. Ganiats, and R. L. Kravitz, Dealing with heterogeneity of treatment effects: Is the literature up to the challenge, *Trials*, vol. 10, no. 1, pp. 43–55, 2009.

115. M. J. Knol, M. Egger, P. Scott, M. I. Geerlings, and J. P. Vandenbroucke, When one depends on the other: Reporting of interaction in case-control and cohort studies, *Epidemiology*, vol. 20, no. 2, pp. 161–166, 2009.

116. R. Wang, S. W. Lagakos, J. H. Ware, D. J. Hunter, and J. M. Drazen, Statistics in medicine—Reporting of subgroup analyses in clinical trials, *New England Journal of Medicine*, vol. 357, no. 21, pp. 2189–2194, 2007.

117. P. M. Rothwell, Subgroup analysis in randomised controlled trials: Importance, indications, and interpretation, *Lancet*, vol. 365, no. 9454, pp. 176–186, 2005.

118. M. J. Knol and T. J. VanderWeele, Recommendations for presenting analyses of effect modification and interaction, *International Journal of Epidemiology*, vol. 41, no. 2, pp. 514–520, 2012.

119. D. Westreich and S. Greenland, The table 2 fallacy: Presenting and interpreting confounder and modifier coefficients, *American Journal of Epidemiology*, vol. 177, no. 4, pp. 292–298, 2013.

120. C. Lamina, G. Sturm, B. Kollerits, and F. Kronenberg, Visualizing interaction effects: A proposal for presentation and interpretation, *Journal of Clinical Epidemiology*, vol. 65, no. 8, pp. 855–862, 2012.

121. A. R. Feinstein, The problem of cogent subgroups: A clinicostatistical tragedy, *Journal of Clinical Epidemiology*, vol. 51, no. 4, pp. 297–299, 1998.

122. D. A. Berry, Subgroup analyses, *Biometrics*, vol. 46, no. 4, pp. 1227–30, 1990.

123. R. Varadhan, E. A. Stuart, T. A. Louis, J. B. Segal, and C. O. Weiss, Review of guidance documents for selected methods in patient centered outcomes research: Standards in addressing heterogeneity of treatment effectiveness in observational and experimental patient centered outcomes research, A Report to the PCORI Methodology Committee Research Methods Working Group, 2012.

124. A. D. Oxman and G. H. Guyatt, A consumer's guide to subgroup analyses, *Annals of Internal Medicine*, vol. 116, no. 1, pp. 78–84, 1992.

125. X. Sun et al., Is a subgroup effect believable? Updating criteria to evaluate the credibility of subgroup analyses, *BMJ*, vol. 340, p. c117, 2010.

126. X. Sun et al., Credibility of claims of subgroup effects in randomised controlled trials: Systematic review, *BMJ*, vol. 344, p. e1553, 2012.

127. A. B. de González et al., Interpretation of interaction: A review, *Annals of Applied Statistics*, vol. 1, no. 2, pp. 371–385, 2007.

128. C. Poole, On the origin of risk relativism, *Epidemiology*, vol. 21, no. 1, pp. 3–9, 2010.

129. T. Gordon, Hazards in the use of the logistic function with special reference to data from prospective cardiovascular studies, *Journal of Chronic Diseases*, vol. 27, no. 3, pp. 97–102, 1974.

130. S. Greenland, Limitations of the logistic analysis of epidemiologic data, *American Journal of Epidemiology*, vol. 110, no. 6, pp. 693–698, 1979.

131. Diabetes Prevention Program Research Group et al., Reduction in the incidence of type 2 diabetes with lifestyle intervention or metformin, *New England Journal of Medicine*, vol. 346, no. 6, p. 393, 2002.

132. J. B. Sussman, D. M. Kent, J. P. Nelson, and R. A. Hayward, Improving diabetes prevention with benefit based tailored treatment: Risk based reanalysis of diabetes prevention program, *BMJ*, vol. 350, p. h454, 2015.

133. P. W. Wilson, J. B. Meigs, L. Sullivan, C. S. Fox, D. M. Nathan, and R. B. D'Agostino, Prediction of incident diabetes mellitus in middle-aged adults:

The Framingham offspring study, *Archives of Internal Medicine*, vol. 167, no. 10, pp. 1068–1074, 2007.

134. G. S. Collins, S. Mallett, O. Omar, and L.-M. Yu, Developing risk prediction models for type 2 diabetes: A systematic review of methodology and reporting, *BMC Medicine*, vol. 9, no. 1, p. 103, 2011.

135. J. F. Burke, R. A. Hayward, J. P. Nelson, and D. M. Kent, Using internally developed risk models to assess heterogeneity in treatment effects in clinical trials, *Circulation: Cardiovascular Quality and Outcomes*, vol. 7, no. 1, pp. 163–169, 2014.

136. J. Lau, J. P. Ioannidis, and C. H. Schmid, Quantitative synthesis in systematic reviews, *Annals of Internal Medicine*, vol. 127, no. 9, pp. 820–826, 1997.

137. L. Koopman, G. J. van der Heijden, P. P. Glasziou, D. E. Grobbee, and M. M. Rovers, A systematic review of analytical methods used to study subgroups in (individual patient data) meta-analyses, *Journal of Clinical Epidemiology*, vol. 60, no. 10, pp. 1002–1009, 2007.

138. D. Fisher, A. Copas, J. Tierney, and M. Parmar, A critical review of methods for the assessment of patient-level interactions in individual participant data meta-analysis of randomized trials, and guidance for practitioners, *Journal of Clinical Epidemiology*, vol. 64, no. 9, pp. 949–967, 2011.

139. J. A. Berlin, J. Santanna, C. H. Schmid, L. A. Szczech, and H. I. Feldman, Individual patient-versus group-level data meta-regressions for the investigation of treatment effect modifiers: Ecological bias rears its ugly head, *Statistics in Medicine*, vol. 21, no. 3, pp. 371–387, 2002.

140. C. H. Schmid, P. C. Stark, J. A. Berlin, P. Landais, and J. Lau, Meta-regression detected associations between heterogeneous treatment effects and study-level, but not patient-level, factors, *Journal of Clinical Epidemiology*, vol. 57, no. 7, pp. 683–697, 2004.

141. Ž. Reiner et al., ESC/EAS guidelines for the management of dyslipidaemias. The Task Force for the management of dyslipidaemias of the European Society of Cardiology (ESC) and the European Atherosclerosis Society (EAS), *European Heart Journal*, vol. 32, no. 14, pp. 1769–1818, 2011.

142. I. J. Dahabreh, R. Hayward, D. M. Kent. Using group data to treat individuals: Understanding heterogeneous treatment effects in the age of precision medicine and patient-centred evidence. *International Journal of Epidemiology*, November 17, 2016. pii: dyw125. [Epub ahead of print] Review.

9

Challenges in Establishing a Hierarchy of Evidence*

Robert T. O'Neill

CONTENTS

ABSTRACT   This chapter discusses a range of issues that might help frame how evidence of comparative effectiveness (CE) is judged in the regulatory setting, taking into account the experiences gained from evaluating the efficacy of medical products, especially pharmaceuticals. We propose a

---

* The opinions reflected in this chapter are those of the author and do not reflect the FDA policies
   or positions.

hierarchy of standards of evidence that are aligned with the questions and issues of importance to each constituency that will use the evidence. The Food and Drug Administration regulatory experience for pharmaceuticals is based upon the evaluation of substantial evidence of the efficacy and safety of pharmaceutical products. The regulatory standard is derived from randomized-controlled clinical trials and can inform about the types of studies, including randomized studies and observational studies that could be conducted to support CE conclusions. There are several government bodies that have sponsored work on guidances and methodologies relevant to comparative effectiveness research and some of this material will be briefly covered.

9.1 Introduction and Goal of the Chapter

Comparative effectiveness research (CER) may mean different things to different constituencies. In one of its forms, as defined by the Institute of Medicine (IOM) [1], it is research that is used to provide evidence for decision makers to make informed choices. More specifically, the IOM defines CER as "the generation and synthesis of evidence that compares the benefits and harms of alternative methods to prevent, diagnose, treat, and monitor a clinical condition or to improve the delivery of care. The purpose of CER is to assist consumers, clinicians, payers, and policy makers to make informed decisions that will improve health care at both the individual and population level." In order to make any substantive statistical contributions in this area, it is important to consider who those decision makers are; what are the consequences of those decisions for an individual, a population, a health plan, or a payer, or for marketing approval; and what types of evidence are necessary for the particular situation. Essentially, what is needed is a hierarchy of standards of evidence that are aligned with the questions and issues of importance to each constituency that will use the evidence.

The goal of this chapter is to propose a framework for how evidence of CER might be judged taking into account the experience gained from evaluating the efficacy of medical products, especially pharmaceuticals, in the regulatory setting. The Food and Drug Administration (FDA) regulatory experience for pharmaceuticals is based upon the evaluation of substantial evidence of the efficacy and safety of these products, the regulatory standard, which is derived from randomized-controlled clinical trials, and this experience is relevant to inform about the types of studies, including randomized studies that could be conducted to support CER conclusions.

With regard to observational studies and research, FDA supported the Sentinel initiative (Mini-Sentinel, Observational Medical Outcome Partnership [OMOP]) [3,21] to evaluate the performance of study designs for observational data used for active safety surveillance, focused on detecting signals of safety risk associated with regulated medical products. The Mini-Sentinel and OMOP experience might contribute to framing the role of observational studies in a CER hierarchy of evidence. Establishing a hierarchy of evidence aligned with the objectives, data sources, study designs, methods of analysis, and the consequences of the conclusions and actions based on studies seems a relevant goal given the current discussions and controversies surrounding CER. While it is challenging to do so, it is important to balance the strength of evidence needed to support the actions for different decision makers against the consequences of an incorrect decision.

It is argued that studies that provide evidence for regulatory decisions are often too narrowly focused and conducted under controlled conditions and therefore are not likely to apply in the actual practice of medicine or health-care delivery. CER promotes the concept that studies conducted in a more uncontrolled real-world setting, including what are called pragmatic trials, are more relevant. While this may be the case, these pragmatic-type designs face challenges to their interpretation and evidentiary role. Thus, studies that provide evidence in more "real-world settings" should be judged in the context of what decisions will be made on the basis of their conclusions, and what are the risks to the use of flexible standards that attempt to balance real-world studies with the validity of their conclusions.

At the core of the CER initiative are three important areas: the measurement and assessment of real-world outcomes in actual practice and conditions of use; the increasing availability of health claims data and electronic health records that can serve as the basic data source for studies; and the proposed use of observational studies based upon electronic records or pragmatic randomized clinical trials. With regard to the interest in real-world outcomes in the current practice of medical care delivery, that need is driven by the many unanswered questions of importance that pertain to informing patient or provider decisions for which treatments to choose from when alternatives exist. It is the hope that the Affordable Care Act [4] with its expanded health insurance coverage and the emerging availability of electronic health records will facilitate the ability to address these questions with studies that use real-world data collected as part of the real-world delivery of health care. This of course is a tall order if scientific rigor is to be addressed at the same time since there will be a need for a balance between scientific rigor, practicality and cost of obtaining answers, and the consequence of the wrong conclusions drawn from inadequate CER studies.

That is why a consensus is needed on some form of evidentiary standards because all situations requiring information for decision making should not be held to the same standards. These standards are set very high for medical products that are regulated and which must demonstrate their efficacy and safety before entering the market place. Much can be learned from how these standards of evidence and the principles of research derived from them have served the public health and improved the evidentiary database of comparative trials. The clinical study designs that rely on randomization and other design principles to minimize bias and afford high degree of certainty to study conclusions have matured over the last 50 years or so since the efficacy standards for new drugs were placed into law by Congress [5]. There are many lessons learned from this regulatory experience with evaluating the efficacy of new drugs and monitoring their safety. Some of this experience relates to comparing two or more alternative therapies, one of which is investigational and the other of which is an approved effective therapy, in what are called noninferiority (NI) trials. The NI design is one design that is used to infer efficacy for an investigational treatment based on a comparison with an already-approved and marketed effective treatment. The objective of an NI design is to show that the response to an investigational drug is not materially different from that of an approved on-the-market therapy by an empirically based predetermined effect size margin that is carefully chosen to be a medically acceptable zone of difference in efficacy with regard to an outcome supporting the claim. Very few proven effective therapies have gone head to head in a trial where one is demonstrated to be superior to the other, and when that does occur, the relative treatment differences in effects are usually modest. The regulatory experience with active controlled NI trials is relevant to the design and interpretation of CER studies intended to compare two or more treatment strategies that are used in actual practice.

This chapter will touch upon some of the regulatory experience that might be useful for setting a hierarchy of evidence for interventions, treatments, and medical products, especially those that do not require regulatory approval but that do require sound scientific approaches and rigor to minimize false conclusions. We will discuss some challenges to arriving at a hierarchy for evidence.

9.2 Challenges in Developing a Hierarchy of Evidence

9.2.1 Aligning the Type of Evidence with the Decision Maker's Use of It

Goodman [6] addressed the issue cited in Challenge 1 in the context of what type of clinical trial may be sufficient for different decision makers in the CER space based on the type of evidence the study provides and the questions that the study addresses. The study designs themselves are likely to be different depending upon the decision maker's objectives. A clinical trial for regulatory purposes may be different than one conducted for a payer. For example, the FDA may accept certain outcomes, or certain study designs, or certain comparators to support a label claim, and require blinded adjudication of an investigator's ascertainment of patient outcomes where documentation can be audited for confirmation. But the outcomes or the questions addressed by the regulatory trial may not be as relevant to a decision maker whose decisions affect coverage policies for their subscribers, such as health insurance plans. Thus, a payer may need different answers to comparative questions for which the certainty of the conclusion is just as important, perhaps as the regulatory approval decision in terms of the impact on populations.

Goodman [6] argues for aligning the questions addressed by the trial with the needs of the decision maker. As he notes, even randomized trials that are well conducted may not be useful for some purposes—in other words, the objectives need to be aligned with the need. The generalization of the randomized clinical trial and the comparators used in the trial is important to the decision makers because of their population of interest. A pragmatic trial (discussed in Challenges 4 and 5) conducted within a health plan population, in contrast to an explanatory trial conducted under more controlled conditions in a selected population, may be more relevant to these payer decision makers. The choice of such a design however must take into account that a pragmatic trial faces challenges to its interpretation, as we will discuss in more detail later.

Woodcock [7] commented on the potential promise of electronic medical records as the data capture source in a randomized pragmatic trial within a healthcare system, and how such a study could be useful for regulatory decisions on pharmaceuticals or other medical products. Woodcock [7] notes that such trials could provide relevant data on longer-term safety of drugs, their use in heterogeneous populations, or the optimal durations of use. She further suggests that such randomized outcome studies could be robust enough for regulatory use and fill gaps left by the current product development process. However, a lot needs to be done to align the practice of healthcare delivery with the research agenda, and it seems this is a very fruitful area for methodological research and collaboration. It is unlikely that, at this time, the use of pragmatic trials that would use medical records for data capture would or could be conducted preapproval or prior to marketing authorization, a point that has been made by both FDA and European Medicines Agency (EMA) officials [8].

The type of data needed may depend on the decision maker and the consequences of the decision. For example, if the decision maker is a medical practitioner, or a patient, the choices they make impact that individual alone so the consequences and the types of data that are relevant to them may be different from a payer setting policy or a regulator approving an efficacious drug. Information on hip replacement surgeries is of interest to many constituencies, including patients who need to make choices about surgeons, hospitals, techniques, and/or devices. Information for an individual choice, for example, is provided in a report prepared by the Vermont Program for Quality in Health Care, which collected data on infections following hip replacements for Vermont hospitals from October 1, 2009 through September 30, 2010 [9]. A standardized infection ratio was created to compare the number of infections following hip replacement surgeries in Vermont to national data for people having the same surgery. The ratio takes into account patient and medical characteristics such as age, gender, length of surgery, and overall assessment of physical health that may increase or decrease the patient's risk of infection. This adjustment is a typical epidemiological approach to standardization. This type of data, while not a randomized study, is useful for comparative purposes and may be all that is available to make decisions. The data are descriptive yet potentially useful for the use to which they are being put. This leads to the next challenge.

9.2.2 Descriptive Assessments versus Causal Conclusions

With the availability of electronic claims data and electronic medical records, registries, and the like, the opportunity exists to evaluate, analyze, summarize, and describe massive amounts of information that are collected but not currently used systematically to inform decision making. Some databases, such as Medicare and Medicaid claims data, and longitudinal linked electronic records maintained by health insurance plans can inform on many questions of interest to an individual as well as to policy makers. For this purpose, there are many descriptive analyses of already-collected data that could inform about patterns of use, exposure, access, geographic patterns, practice patterns, provider choice differences, relative frequency of choosing one versus an alternative approach, and so on.

The descriptive statements about these data should be recognized as such, and should not be overinterpreted or compared to other descriptive summaries. Generally, two or more descriptive summaries when compared likely will not provide an unbiased comparison or a fair one, without an assurance that competing therapies are each being used optimally under their proposed conditions of use, and the populations are similar. There are many examples of how descriptive data might be useful. Simply summarizing usage or exposures or prescriptions for different states, geographic regions, clinical practice types, Medicare plans, age and gender groups, and so on provides information on variation of practice without making any causal conclusions as to the reasons why such variation occurs. Prevalence of different types of surgery in different geographic regions or different health plans, stratified by relevant categories, is informative. Incidence of certain codes used to capture outcomes associated with different patient treatment or response patterns can be informative, even as a prelude to understanding factors that inform about the propensity to prescribe or use a treatment.

Thus, descriptive statements that are factual about how medical interventions are assigned, used, tolerated, used in conjunction with other therapies, and switched to alternatives may be useful to an individual patient, an individual medical practitioner, a health plan analyst, or a payer.

On the other hand, causal conclusions about comparative benefits, risks, or trade-offs rise to a different level of evidentiary standard. Inferential conclusions are usually associated with causal conclusions backed by tests of hypotheses that are prespecified and whose uncertainties of conclusions can be quantified. This is where randomized studies shine and such studies are needed for most causal conclusions, but in some situations, observational research may serve the causal conclusion role if factors, that can be controlled for by design or analysis, can overcome unobserved confounding and other sources of bias inherent in observational research. Usually, drawing causal conclusions from observational research should be reserved for large treatment effect sizes, which may not be the situation for most alternative treatments that are compared. It has been suggested that knowledge of database features and outcomes to be assessed should be evaluated in advance of planning a CER study as a basis for deciding whether it is feasible to study the anticipated treatment differences [39]. The regulatory experience in this area is very important to understand and that will be discussed next.

9.2.3 Building on the Regulatory Experience in Evaluating Evidence of Efficacy and Treatment Effects in Noninferiority Studies—A Form of Comparative Efficacy

There are lessons to be learned from the regulatory experience of evaluating clinical research and clinical trials conducted to support the efficacy and safety of medical products. As Woodcock [7] noted, these lessons range from moving beyond the era of anecdotal clinician statements about the alleged efficacy of a medical product or intervention, to the era of conduct of poorly designed or conducted studies whose conclusions were suspect and could not support evidentiary conclusions, to a modern evidentiary standard where the drug development and regulatory review process requires statistical study design and analysis methods developed to control or minimize incorrect conclusions and where study designs and procedures are employed to assure the use of appropriate control groups, comparisons that are unbiased or account for various biases to reach valid causal conclusions.

The most important milestone in establishing the evidentiary standard for drug efficacy and safety came about with the Harris Kefauver amendments of 1962 [5] outlining the need for substantial evidence derived from adequate and well-controlled trials. Subsequently in 1970, the features of an adequate and well-controlled trial were defined including a focus on study design, choice of control group, randomization, outcome ascertainment, minimizing bias, and appropriate analysis methods. Historical controls is one of the acceptable controls when appropriate. This could be a nonrandomized comparison that involves comparing a concurrently treated cohort with past historical cohorts for which valid comparisons is achievable. But that study design is not the norm, and it is usually limited to situations where large treatment effects over and above historical response are demonstrable.

The comparison of an investigational treatment to a control group to support evidence of treatment efficacy and the other principles for experimental evidence such as randomization and blinding, minimizing observer bias, and assuring comparability of treatment groups is the basic framework of current product development and regulatory review. In particular, the choice of control groups is one of the considerations in the regulations as is the choice of a study design to establish whether a drug is effective or not. As Temple [11] has noted in an extensive discussion about regulatory experience in comparative evaluations, the randomized NI study design contains many lessons learned that are applicable to CER studies that might use the observational approach. The key point here is that an observational study conducted as if it were an NI study would likely lack assay sensitivity, a critical design requirement for a randomized NI study, as explained below.

Temple [11] and Woodcock [7] summarized different aspects of the regulatory experience and these references are worth reading in order to obtain a deeper understanding of the relevance of that regulatory experience to CER evaluation. We will only summarize a few points from those articles.

When one cannot ethically conduct a placebo-controlled comparative clinical trial to evaluate an investigational agent, there are several alternative designs that might be used, one of which is known as the NI design. This design is a direct randomized comparison of a marketed effective treatment to one that is still in its investigational stage and unproven as effective. The marketed treatment is a drug that has demonstrated its efficacy, usually in one or more randomized placebo-controlled trials, and the magnitude of the treatment effect is known (estimated) based upon those trials with a placebo comparator. Knowledge of the magnitude of effect for the marketed product allows an empirically established margin of treatment effect to be chosen for the NI study, whose objective is to show that the investigational drug is not materially inferior in effect to the market product. The NI design does not require that one show a difference in effects or superiority of one treatment to the other. While this is a direct randomized comparison to demonstrate the investigational drug does not differ by more than a prespecified amount based upon the empirically demonstrated effect of the marketed approved product, the NI design also provides an indirect inference that the investigational product is effective in that it would have been superior to a placebo or perhaps a standard of care, were one included in the NI design.

However, that conclusion from an NI design requires an additional condition that needs to be satisfied to make a valid inference. The prespecification of the margin for how different the two treatments in the NI design can be in order to make a valid conclusion is a challenging task. It is not always possible to determine that margin in order to demonstrate the efficacy of the investigational drug. In the regulatory setting, this NI design and choice of margin is critical for demonstrating evidence that the investigational treatment (not yet approved for that claim) meets legal standards to prove it is effective based upon the size of the treatment effect of the active comparator and how much of it the investigational comparator should preserve. The additional assumption is that the approved and marketed effective comparator will, in this NI study, have the same effect it has demonstrated in prior studies. Whether the approved comparator will have that effect in the current

NI study under its conditions of use is something that is often not the case for treatments that produce variable symptomatic response, and something that may be challenging to support for real-world NI study under less controlled conditions. There are many examples where an effective treatment may not be replicable in any particular study. For example, treatments for symptomatic disease like depression and anxiety are difficult to repetitively demonstrate effects for known effective treatments, that is why a placebo is usually needed and NI studies are seldom used in that setting.

Consider how the study of a subjective outcome like patient-reported outcomes or quality of life measures might be addressed in CER. The regulatory experience illustrates the difficulty in interpreting the results of a direct comparison of two treatments, particularly when there is no discernible difference in effect size between them, as there might be with CER comparisons of competing or alternative therapies. For a randomized study, the interpretation of superiority (i.e., a real difference) of one treatment relative to another is easier than the interpretation of similarity or no observed difference between alternative therapies. A CER study comparing two alternative therapies that results in no material observed difference between them might be uninterpretable for many of the reasons well known to the NI design and articulated in numerous literature articles, and regulatory guidances [12,13]. Without a no-treatment or a standard-of-care control group (like a placebo) incorporated into a planned comparison to distinguish if true effects are detectable, two treatments whose effects are observed to be similar can either both be comparably effective or both be ineffective under the circumstances of study but one cannot distinguish which is true. However, if a treatment was compared to a standard of care, using an appropriate population, and found not to be different, that is probably an interpretable conclusion.

The comparative study becomes more complex when three or more alternative therapies are compared among each other, as the certainty of the conclusions for each pairwise comparison, or all possible comparisons, is subject to statistical multiplicity concerns, which are well known to the clinical trial community and discussed in international guidelines for statistical principles for clinical trials [32]. One solution is to plan the study for strong control of the type 1 error (false-positive conclusion) whenever there is more than one comparison of interest.

9.2.4 Introducing Randomization into Comparative Evaluations in Healthcare Systems Where Equipoise Exists

A pragmatic clinical trial is a naturalistic experiment defined as a prospective randomized study where, following randomization of patients to an intervention, patient care is left to the practitioner according to his/her typical practice. The pragmatic trial is intended to maintain the advantages of randomization while examining outcomes in routine care setting. This is in contrast to an explanatory trial that is conducted in more controlled circumstances and selective patient populations, and this type of study is usually the basis for regulatory decision making. The idea of using randomization for comparative studies within the healthcare system and making use of the electronic health record for data capture and collection is receiving increasing attention [14,15,35,37,38]. A pragmatic trial is not the same as a large simple trial, but it may appear to be so when the large simple trial is conducted in the routine delivery of care. Sample size of the trial is usually not the distinguishing feature between the large simple trial and a pragmatic trial conducted in a real-world unblinded setting. A large simple trial, such as those conducted for postapproval safety assessment, often involves considerable resources for event ascertainment, adjudication, and data cleaning and monitoring. For a pragmatic trial that may be conducted within a healthcare plan, it is likely that the healthcare record will be the source of data capture so there is a need to assess the quality of the data in medical record databases. Classical large simple trials evaluate a hard endpoint that is usually not misclassifiable, such as mortality. The large simple trial is designed to capture a limited number of outcomes and patient characteristics so that there is some protocol-induced uniformity and structure to the information collected. Sometimes, the endpoints may be adjudicated blindly by an independent committee if cause-specific events are the objective of the study. When that is needed to support the credibility of conclusions, the large simple trial is not so simple, although it may be called so. Large simple trials of this type may not be synonymous with a pragmatic trial considered within a healthcare system when no additional adjudication of outcomes or patient electronic records is envisioned.

It is tempting to favor pragmatic clinical trials to address some of the real-world comparisons of interest to the CER community because these trials would be conducted within the practice of medicine and normal delivery of health care, using as source data the electronic medical record from which key outcome variables and other preexposure and/or exposure variables are extracted. However, there are challenges to the interpretability of pragmatic trials. Experience with pragmatic trials conducted within a healthcare system is relatively limited at this time, and methodological research is needed to help design and extract as much causally valid inference from these studies as feasible. Pragmatic trials are likely to be the major cost-effective way of addressing future CER questions, aside from observational studies that may fill another evidentiary gap, but we would rank order randomized pragmatic trials as a higher standard of evidence than observational cohort studies.

Because there is no control for how patients may be treated or managed once assigned to randomized interventions, pragmatic trials soon face the issues that the best observational study will face. Goodman [6] recognized this and gave as an example the difficulty in interpreting the Spine Patient Outcomes Research Trial (SPORT), which looked at surgical treatment for back pain relative to a host of nonsurgical options, arguing that the results may not be very convincing to the orthopedic community. Goodman suggests that in the future, randomized pragmatic trials will be a rich ground for applying observational research methods to them for making valid subgroup inferences, where observational research methods might address sources of noise that will occur in the real-world situation.

Ware and Hamel [17] have also provided some insight into the difficulties in interpreting pragmatic trials when conducted in real-world settings. They discuss challenges with interpretation resulting from potential biases and uncontrolled factors. In commenting on two pragmatic trials published in the *New England Journal of Medicine*, they provide a very useful discussion for how difficult the interpretation of causal conclusions can be because of very fundamental issues that pragmatic trials face. Ware and Hamel acknowledge the strengths of these trials, such as the full assessment of outcomes on all randomized subjects, full follow-up during the 2-year treatment to capture longer-term effects, as was done in the studies commented on. Full follow-up and outcome ascertainment is always a good feature for any study but is a challenge for an explanatory randomized trial in the face of switching of therapies. The retention of subjects for a defined period of time with little to no loss to follow-up may be a strength of a pragmatic trial but this strength may be counterbalanced by informative censoring of exposure and outcomes as a result of switching of therapies for causal reasons not allowing an otherwise observable outcome to be counted against a prior exposure.

Ware and Hamel [17] point out a number of challenges to the causal interpretation of findings of a comparison in these pragmatic trials. For example, if patients change or discontinue treatment, this is not a nonadherence problem but rather nonadherence is an outcome in itself and can inform about the usefulness of two or more treatments that are compared. If adherence is differential, any comparative outcomes are likely to be difficult to interpret particularly for time-dependent outcomes. Nonadherence will impact any intent to treat analysis, and has different consequences for a trial designed to demonstrate superiority versus a trial to demonstrate noninferiority, or in this instance, sameness. As noted above, NI trials are used when placebos cannot ethically be used, and are intended to show that one treatment is not materially worse than another. CER studies will face the same issues in some form or the other.

Related to nonadherence is the switching from one treatment to another, especially for long-term treatment with extended follow-up of longer-term outcomes. Such switching of treatments, the timing of such switches, and the multiple outcome events leading up to that switch will be challenging to address in analysis. It is unclear if any analysis may be able to overcome this obstacle to produce valid, interpretable causal conclusions. Ware and Hamel [17] go on to point out that most pragmatic trials conducted in real-world setting are unblinded so that patient-reported outcomes and clinician assessment of events and outcomes, and behavioral choices may also be potentially biasing to the comparative evaluation. They also point out that there are few strategies available to assess bias or its impact associated with differential patient behavior, or provider choices subsequent to randomization. One solution they propose is to include both objective and subjective outcome measures that may be compared for consistency.

Ware and Hamel [17] conclude that pragmatic trials are designed to study real-world practice and represent a less than perfect experiment than pure efficacy trials because they sacrifice internal validity for generalizability. The challenge is to keep the balance right so that the findings are likely to be both correct and applicable to the clinical practice or healthcare delivery system. This is also a challenge to the establishment of a hierarchy of evidence aligned with the questions needing to be addressed and the consequences of getting it wrong.

9.2.5 Tapping the Potential to Conduct Comparative Randomized Trials within the Healthcare System without Burdening the Data Collection Process

While discussions of how to conduct randomized trials within the current healthcare delivery systems have occurred, there are only a few examples to illustrate the challenges and obstacles to their interpretability. Goodman [6] has argued that any changes made to the process of care delivery to improve outcomes should be studied in a more systematic way because there is no way to assess the impact of small changes in the delivery of care without an experimental design. Measuring and quantifying the impact of planned changes on interesting outcomes generally cannot be accomplished in an observational setting if causal conclusions are needed. This is a very novel yet profound concept, and is consistent with the Deming philosophy [18] of identifying the factors that impact systematic differences and variability of outcomes, monitoring them, and evaluating whether changes impact outcomes. Goodman argued for more experimental control of the process of healthcare delivery in his article about randomized trials in CER [6]. Goodman is correct in arguing for the use of experimental designs with randomization within healthcare systems to help them deliver better outcomes to patients because concluding that some processes need small incremental changes or not can only be accomplished by introducing an experimental design into the delivery of health care.

Comparative treatment evaluations may require a change in our approach to the evaluation of systematic changes to the delivery of medical care and use of treatments or strategies within that process. Even for medical products that go through the regulatory evaluation process and are deemed effective, there are many open questions that remain as to whether the medical product or intervention works in certain situations relevant to the healthcare system, and when to use the product and on which patients. Addressing these issues has usually been a matter of judgment and not supported by measurement of outcomes. Essentially, the issue is about introducing the Deming philosophy [18] into evaluation of the healthcare delivery system. Utah's Intermountain Healthcare system [19] is an example where this philosophy seems to have been successfully introduced into continuous improvement goals in its system by using the electronic records system to track outcomes, adjust care accordingly, and quantify the impact of system changes on outcomes.

CER might be the driver of the use of rigorous experimental designs embedded in the system at point of care of healthcare delivery to evaluate the impact of two or more choices or process changes to facilitate the continuous improvement in healthcare delivery. In order to evaluate the impact of incremental changes in intervention/treatment strategies on outcomes, which are a form of CER, the factors of interest need to be controlled for, and this will not likely occur without some form of experimental design with randomization within the system of interest, perhaps embedded on a smaller scale, in larger pragmatic trials. As Goodman [6] proposes, some process variables should be measured and process changes evaluated in some form of an experimental design that can detect outcomes impacted by process changes. Essentially, Goodman is proposing to implement the Deming philosophy [18] of "plan, do, measure, act" for continuous improvement to evaluate the impact of process changes to healthcare delivery. This proposal has yet to be considered seriously in CER and is ripe for future research and piloting.

9.2.6 Interpreting Differential Treatment Effects in Subgroups and Assessing Predictors of Differential Treatment Effects

One of the goals of CER is to assess whether some patient subgroups respond better or worse to some treatments and to assess the relative benefits or risks of alternative treatments in different patient subgroups. This information would be of use to a patient, a provider, or a decision maker when choosing what is the best alternative for them. The task of identifying subgroup treatment effects that are truly different from other subgroups and are real and not due to chance is very challenging and difficult, even for randomized clinical trials that control or stratify on some of these potential predictors. Chapter 8 in this volume provides a detailed discussion of heterogeneity of treatment effects. The literature on the use and misuse of subgroup analysis in clinical trials is extensive [20] and it is not the intention of this chapter to discuss the issues in depth. Rather, the goal is to point out how the certainty of a conclusion is dealt with within a statistical framework for drawing inferential or causal conclusions from comparative studies, whether randomized or observational.

The literature on subgroup analysis primarily focuses on the false-positive rates of concluding there is a real treatment effect based upon an observed effect in a subgroup when in fact there is no true effect, or the effect does not truly differ from other subgroups, and thus drawing an inference that is erroneous. It is well known that, under the global null hypothesis of no treatment effects (no differences), the more subgroup comparisons within a clinical study, the higher the chance for a false-positive conclusion that treatment is effective in at least one of the subgroups. When an overall study conclusion is that there is no difference in the effects of two or more alternative therapies, and no prospective plan is in place with statistical adjustments, it is inappropriate to proceed to analyze subgroups and conclude that real treatment differences exist in some of the subgroups. This practice is discouraged for clinical trial inference, except if there is a prespecified plan to identify a subgroup(s) for which a conclusion is of interest and appropriate multiplicity adjustments made. CER practitioners should follow a similar philosophy as it would contribute to the hierarchy of evidence framework we are trying to build.

Of equal concern is the error in making a false conclusion that no treatment effect exists in a subgroup when there is one. For example, in a comparison of two alternative therapies, if an overall difference is observed that is statistically significant for the prespecified outcomes, the conclusion is that one treatment is superior to the other. To proceed to evaluate the subgroups for the purpose of choosing which has the largest or smallest treatment effect is a challenging task that can easily lead to false conclusions, especially without a proper prespecified analysis plan. This approach may sometimes be used inappropriately when seeking a treatment decision tailored to an individual's unique factors.

A reversal occurs when one treatment is observed to be superior in one subgroup and the other alternative treatment is observed to be superior in another subgroup. This observed reversal of observed treatment benefit among subgroups may occur simply by chance. Li et al. [2] consider this issue in discussing the probability of observing negative subgroup results when the treatment effect is positive and homogeneous across all subgroups. Recognizing the expected variability in treatment effects solely due to chance when all subgroups share no effect or all subgroups share the same effect is an important concept to understand. The lessons learned from the clinical trial experience regarding how cautious to be when interpreting observed subgroup differences in direction of effects or in magnitude of effects can be useful to CER study investigators.

9.2.7 Characterization of Performance of Observational Study Designs and Standards for Conduct and Analysis

As mentioned in the introduction, the focus of this chapter is on CER evidence development that would rely upon randomized studies, either of the explanatory, pragmatic, or hybrid type that are conducted in nontraditional settings, such as healthcare plans or community-based networks. But interest is high in the use of observational research to support CER. There is regulatory interest in using observational healthcare data for active surveillance of the safety of medical products once they enter the market place. Two recent efforts supported by the FDA, Mini-Sentinel [3], and OMOP [21] are devoted to methods development, and study design and database evaluation to determine how reliable such observational health outcomes data and studies are for early risk detection.

The OMOP [21–25] team studied the performance of the new user cohort design as a tool for risk identification in observational healthcare data. OMOP evaluated methods applied to 165 positive controls (considered true drug–outcome associations) and 234 negative controls (considered null drug–outcome associations) across four health outcomes of interest in five real observational databases (four administrative claims and one electronic health record) and in six simulated datasets with no effect and injected relative risks of 1.25, 1.5, 2, 4, and 10. The performance measures included the sensitivity, specificity, and positive predictive value of the methods to detect known positive and negative (neutral) signals of risk, and Area Under the Curve (AUC) metrics to compare performances of study designs. Using traditional levels of statistical significance of $p < 0.05$ for controlling for a false conclusion, OMOP empirically determined the false-positive and false-negative rates for different thresholds of relative risk for these different combinations of study designs, outcome pairs, and databases. The OMOP investigators found that the new incident user cohort design, which might be used in CER evaluation of two or more alternative treatments, has relatively high false-positive rates and that different databases in which such designs are conducted may themselves have different performance characteristics. There are limitations to OMOP's empirical assessment, including that short-term outcomes (e.g., event within 30 days of initial exposure) were evaluated, so that longer-term exposures and longer-term outcomes that might be evaluated in time to event studies were not addressed. However, the variability of the results across combinations was alerting.

The OMOP work illustrated how variable study findings can be and how lack of replication of a study finding, either in the same database, or different databases, is an issue. The OMOP experiment has important implications for setting a hierarchy of evidence for observational studies. It seems that a critical component of that hierarchy should be replication of any observational finding in at least two different databases, perhaps using different designs. The OMOP experiment empirically illustrated that with the databases and drug/disease pairs used, replication of a study finding may not be that easy, especially for treatments with modest effect sizes so that only comparative effect sizes of a rather large magnitude may be replicable in other studies. The OMOP team [25,27] claims that they replicated most of the findings from the U.S. databases, in six databases of the EU-ADR (Exploring and Understanding Adverse Drug Reactions) database network in Europe. The OMOP experiment also suggests that another component of the evidentiary hierarchy might be the provision of a prespecified lower bound on the magnitude of the comparative effect size that is detectable in the evaluation of effectiveness of two or more comparators if that result is to be believed and acted upon (i.e., a true-positive or a true-negative finding).

There are several relevant guidance documents that bear upon best practices for CER that have been published by agencies or professional societies. The Patient-Centered Outcomes Research Institute (PCORI) was authorized by the Affordable Health Care Act and it has as a mandate the promotion of CER mostly based upon "real-world" observational data. PCORI published a Methodology Standards Document [31] intended to lay the foundation for best practices. The table of contents in that document covers a wide variety of topics, including standards for formulating the research question, systematic reviews, heterogeneity of treatment effects, preventing and handling missing data, data networks, adaptive and Bayesian trial designs, data registries, studies of diagnostic tests, and for causal inference. In addition to its recommendations in these areas, the documents contain a discussion of general and cross-cutting methods for all patient-centered outcomes research.

Perhaps not as well emphasized in this document, but which this author takes a position on, is that any observational study is not a replacement for a randomized study even if such an observational study mimics the randomized study as best as it can. So, even if a randomized study is not possible or feasible to address a CER question within a healthcare system, the decision to conduct some other design to address a question of interest is not without its risks for interpretability and use by decision makers. Indeed, a similar point is made by Rubin [33] who argues that one should design an observational study as much to conform to what one would do for a randomized study of the same question, except for the introduction of randomization. Hernan [26] also argues for analyzing observational studies like randomized experiments, but criticizes the intent to treat philosophy as addressing the wrong questions of interest to others. The reader can consult the discussion in Chapter 3 of this volume. Prentice [30] on the other hand, while acknowledging the potential of modern data analysis methods for observational studies such as causal inference and inverse probability weighting strategies, to enhance the reliability and interpretation of epidemiological data, emphasizes the benefits of the intent to treat analysis and cautions that adherence-adjusted analyses depend directly on the ability to model the nonadherence process, which is analogous to modeling for control of confounding. Prentice suggests that the factors that determine adherence to each treatment in a study population must be accurately measured and correctly modeled, and our current knowledge in this area is limited.

The Agency for Healthcare Research and Quality (AHRQ) published a handbook [36] *Developing a Protocol for Observational Comparative Effectiveness Research: A User's Guide*. This guide provides information for designing CER protocols and minimal standards and best practices for designing CER studies. The guide reflects an extensive and broad participation by authors and contributors from government, academic, and private sectors. The topics considered in the guide include defining the study objectives and questions to be addressed by a study, study design issues, estimation and reporting of heterogeneity of treatment effects, exposure definitions and measurement, comparator selection, outcome definition and measurement, covariate selection, data source selection, study size planning, statistical analysis considerations, and proposal for sensitivity analysis.

The International Society for Pharmacoeconomics and Outcomes Research (ISPOR) issued a task force report [34,36] on good research practices focused on prospective observational studies to assess comparative effectiveness. The task force report emphasizes the need for precision and clarity in specifying the key policy questions that are addressed by research and recommends that studies should be designed with the goal of drawing causal inferences whenever possible. They state that "if a study is being performed to support a policy decision, then it should be designed as hypothesis testing which requires drafting a protocol as if subjects were to be randomized and that investigators clearly state the purpose or main hypotheses, define the treatment groups and outcomes, identify all measured and unmeasured confounders, and specify the primary analyses and required sample size." They go on to state that "similar to the concept of the importance of declaring a prespecified hypothesis, we believe that the credibility of many prospective observational studies would be enhanced by their registration on appropriate publicly available accessible sites (e.g. Clinicaltrials.gov and encepp.eu) in advance of their execution."

The ISPOR task force report covers many important topics and provides insight into how complex and difficult it will be to conduct interpretable research that is valid and actionable by decision makers who deal with questions of policy. While most of the report is about observational research and the complexities of designing and analyzing such studies to address switching of therapies, immortal time bias (see report for discussion), value of intent to treat analysis relative to as treated analysis, time-varying and time-invariant confounding, and bias control, there is mention of the use of the study design known as the pragmatic trial. This design, as mentioned earlier in this chapter, is a naturalistic experiment that is a prospective randomized clinical study in which, following randomization to an intervention, patient care is left to the practitioners according to their typical practice. The pragmatic trial is intended to maintain the advantages of randomization while examining outcomes in routine care setting. However, they do not address that this type of trial is not without its own challenges to interpretability as was discussed earlier.

Finally, the Center for Medicare and Medicaid Services (CMS) has broad authority regarding payment and coverage for many health-related interventions and treatments in the United States. CMS issued a Draft Guidance for the Public, Industry, and CMS Staff on "Coverage with Evidence Development in the context of coverage decisions" [26]. It is instructive to read the standards that are articulated in that document relative to evidence development.

CMS created coverage with evidence development (CED) to address coverage of items and services that were believed to be promising but whose ultimate impact on Medicare beneficiary health outcomes remained unconfirmed. The CED concept considers the item or service to be reasonable and necessary only while evidence is being developed pursuant to AHRQ's authority. AHRQ can conduct and support research on the outcomes, effectiveness, and appropriateness of healthcare services and procedures to identify the manner in which diseases, disorders, and other health conditions can be prevented, diagnosed, treated, and managed clinically. In addition, AHRQ can conduct or support evaluations of the comparative effects, on health and functional capacity, of alternative services and procedures utilized in preventing, diagnosing, treating, and clinically managing diseases, disorders, and other health conditions. It is important to note that no preference for study design is provided.

9.2.8 Improving the Quality of Data Collected in Real-World Settings

A false assumption in the use of electronic claims data and health records is that the data will be directly useable without some preprocessing or additional processing to standardize outcome definitions or exposure definitions. The quality of patient-level outcome data (i.e., occurrence of heart attack, fracture, cause-specific reason for hospitalization) either in claims data or electronic health records is a critical issue in any observational study. The cost of a study or its simplicity will be impacted, if there is a need to independently adjudicate, blindly or otherwise, key data elements from claims data or electronic medical records in order to conduct a credible study. Current medical event coding and health plan-specific payment and coding strategies impact the credibility, quality, and use of such data for CER. The hope is that electronically accessible health record data do not have to be extensively adjudicated to confirm the validity of procedures, exposures (drugs), or diagnoses (outcomes). It is probably an understatement to say that the quality of electronic data, its accuracy, interpretability, and utility for decision making will always be a challenge to the research community. It is likely to be an evolutionary process to make such data useful for research purposes [15,16,28,29].

Characterizing the occurrence of health outcomes of interest that have good sensitivity, specificity, and positive predictive value, and defining exposure periods so that the duration of exposure can be accounted for in the analysis, has been a goal of the Mini-Sentinel and OMOP experiments and much has been learned about the predictive value of different ways of defining events and exposures. Current approaches for the use of claims data and electronic medical records that rely on the coding of outcomes and exposures, and to deriving variables from raw recorded data so that the derived variables are reflective of true exposure durations and patterns and outcomes as defined by whatever study design is selected, remain a task that will impact the quality of CER research as well. Data that are collected for multiple purposes, whether administrative claims data or electronic medical health records, generally will not have the same level of oversight and quality control at a point of collection as a controlled clinical trial. It is interesting to examine the experiences of the Mini-Sentinel project and the OMOP project in terms of how they deal with the quality of the data and what limitations data quality may pose on the ability to address a comparative question. OMOP employed a common data model that standardizes data from multiple partners into a common format. Mini-Sentinel employed a distributed database model in which data partners kept their own data behind a firewall for confidentiality purposes but addressed common questions with the same algorithmic software. CER researchers may be able to build upon the experiences of these two projects [2,21].

Registries have been proposed as a source of efficient access to patients who can be randomized to comparative therapies, as carried out in the TASTE trial in Scandinavia [16]. Lauer and D'Agostino [16] discussed the challenges to the use of registries as the source for efficient and timely randomized effectiveness trials, at least in the electronic medical databases available in the U.S. healthcare system. Some of these challenges are missing data fields, addressing the privacy and informed consent process, the lack of blinding or whether blinding would ever be possible in an effectiveness trial, and the ability to actually capture long-term follow-up outcomes or composite outcomes. The randomized registry trial represents a potentially cost-effective, efficient, and disruptive technology that could transform some of the existing structures to carry out randomized trials, especially effectiveness trials in a real-world setting.

9.3 Reaching Consensus on a Hierarchy of Evidence for CER

A hierarchy of evidence is a function of the needs of the users, namely, the decision makers, the types of questions they ask, and the consequences of the decisions of users to the individual and to the public health. All these factors impact what types of CER studies and which types of databases are appropriate to address the question. Policy makers using CER studies for decisions impact public health in many ways, in contrast to individual patients and providers who may use information from studies to inform their own personal decisions that do not impact others. For untested medical products or for approved therapies never tested against each other, CER should not be considered a replacement for the regulatory process and standards of evidence for entry into the market place. The distinction between efficacy and effectiveness is more about use in uncontrolled conditions so the conditions of use may dominate the real efficacy of product, especially for treatment with modest effects.

Some consider that efficacy refers to the effects of treatment when used as directed and complied with. Effectiveness is generally considered as the effects of treatments when used in the real world and in less controlled environments—but comparison of effectiveness of two or more alternative therapies or interventions may still require a randomized experiment to validly interpret, but not the same type of randomized experiment. The principles of randomized clinical trials that are generally accepted internationally [32] recommend that the intent to treat principle be followed so that a causal conclusion can be drawn. This principle dictates that randomized trials should be analyzed in a manner that preserves the initial randomized treatment assignment of a patient or subject regardless of compliance to the assigned treatment. This is the only approach that preserves a causal conclusion. Conditioning on compliance or other behavioral choices is conditioning on postrandomization outcomes, as say in a per protocol analysis, and such an analysis can have problems of interpretation because the subset of randomized subjects complying is not a true randomized comparison but rather a subset of the randomized population for which the causal conclusions are less strong. It would seem that CER studies conducted in the real-world setting that are not analyzed according to the intention to treat principle and that rely on strong modeling assumptions will face these same challenges as do randomized studies, but the unblinding and selection bias in real-world setting is likely to further complicate any inferences.

It is the hope that randomized CER studies could supplement medical product development studies and be informative for evidence incorporated in product labels, if conducted under adequate conditions. When interest turns to comparing already-vetted products that have FDA-approved evidence of efficacy, under whatever conditions of use or outcomes assessed, the level of evidence to make decisions of relative benefit or safety should be high. This is because the consequences of those decisions by policy makers may impact patient access or the availability of competing interventions for which the conclusions about their relative benefits may be incorrect and therefore detrimental to public health. There are situations where real-world studies of already-marketed efficacious medical products may expand knowledge and claims in a valid manner, such as long-term outcomes, sequential use of multiple therapies, dosing strategies, and so on. Such studies should be held to regulatory standards of evidence currently employed for any investigational product, though flexibility in study design, outcomes, and conduct may be warranted.

There are many unregulated medical interventions, behaviors, and patterns of care that have never been systematically studied in any setting, and specifically in real-world settings. It will be challenging to conduct CER in an environment with many uncontrolled factors that also is intended to support robust conclusions but the research enterprise needs to proceed on how to best do so. Currently, there seem to be no best or new ideas that have not already been considered in publicly available documents discussed in Challenge 7 above.

The anticipated magnitude of the comparative benefits of alternative treatments or approaches should drive which study design choice is desired, as should the characteristics of the database in which the study is conducted. Because the regulatory history with the randomized trial that evaluates and compares two or more competing therapies indicates that relative differences among treatments are not likely very large, it would seem that only very large, and possibly unlikely large, differences among competing interventions will be reliably detected with observational studies. Despite the appeal to randomization designs for effectiveness evaluations, randomized studies conducted in real-world circumstances, such as pragmatic trials conducted in healthcare systems using the healthcare data collection system, may be difficult to interpret when the impact of adherence, compliance, open unblinded conditions of treatment use, and outcome reporting are assessed and analyzed with the intention to treat principle. Yet, the hope is that we can make them interpretable. It would seem that a minimum, the replication of any CER finding, not necessarily with the same study design or patient population, may be the only way to overcome the challenge of real-world unblinded studies, assuming the biases will not always be responsible for replicating similar findings in the same direction.

So, we end this chapter by suggesting possible steps forward for arriving at a hierarchy of evidence for nonrandomized CER observational studies. When this choice seems to be the most scientifically practical to address the question(s) of interest, investigators should follow best practices for observational studies as described in many recent guidances and documents referenced in the challenges above. In addition, the following advice is suggested to establish a hierarchy of evidence:

- The quality of the database to be used for a study should be adequately assessed and reported on with regard to its ability to capture important outcomes, to assess the positive predictive value of any coding schemes used to count the events, and to assess the types of missing data and misclassification of events. Generally, this should be considered prior to conducting a study [39].

- There should be independent replication of any conclusions (not necessarily the design) from more than one study and more than one database for which it is not likely that potential biases associated with observational research themselves are replicated and contributory to the replication.

- Conclusions of similarity of outcomes derived from the comparison of two or more alternative treatments or interventions should be judged differently than conclusions of superiority. A conclusion of similarity may result from sources of nondifferential bias like patient noncompliance, missing information on important confounders, or outcome misclassification, all of which tend to drive estimates or relative treatment differences toward the null of no difference. A definition of similarity for alternative treatments compared in observational research needs discussion and consensus on criteria for study assay sensitivity and how should a quantitative margin of acceptable similarity (not just no significant difference statistically) be determined. Further, the quantitative margin of "close enough" or NI should not be based on a judgment call but on evidence of the magnitude of effects from other independent empirical sources.

- Conclusions of superiority or differences in treatment effects between alternative interventions are more easily interpretable but may also be subject to or a result of biases inherent in observational studies, such as informative censoring, differential adherence, differential follow-up, or channeling bias that cannot be overcome by techniques such as propensity score matching, or causal analysis methods. The limits of detectability of the chosen study design, and the outcomes evaluated should be assessed before a study is conducted.

- Because treatment selections or strategies by patient or provider are unblinded in the real-world delivery of care, valid comparison of subjective outcomes among two or more groups may need a special control group or study design to address the subtle confounding impact of unblinded delivery of care.

- When more than two alternative competing interventions are compared, multiplicity adjustments in the statistically strong sense should be employed. That is, there should be strong control of type 1 error for studies with multiple interventions compared where the chances of making an erroneous false-positive conclusion for any one of the pairwise comparisons are of interest. Because, the goal of the study will generally be to identify and choose those therapies as best under the circumstances. Multiplicity considerations should be taken into account for subgroup analyses as well and where interest is in identifying factors predictive of differential treatment effects. This is particularly important as delivery of care that is individualized to a patient's covariates may be increasingly based upon causal interpretation of observational research.

- Descriptive statements about cohort exposures, outcomes, behaviors, risk factors, and variation in treatment patterns can be useful to patients and providers to inform practice and should not be confused with causal conclusions that rely on valid inferential approaches.

- To evaluate the impact on outcomes of incremental changes in intervention/treatment policy strategies in healthcare systems, the factors of interest need to be controlled for. Usually this will involve an experimental design stratified for the controlling factors, and most likely randomization to different intervention changes. That is, process variables should be measured and process changes evaluated in some form of an experimental design that can detect changes in outcomes impacted by process changes. The Deming philosophy should be applied to evaluating the impact of process changes to healthcare delivery. This can still be accomplished in an observational real-world delivery of care model, where randomization is introduced to control factors of interest.

- Some also argue for preregistration of the protocol for all CER studies, whether randomized or observational in a system such as Clinicaltrials.gov. This seems like a sensible idea.

References

1. Institute of Medicine. *Initial National Priorities for Comparative Effectiveness Research*. Washington, DC. The National Academies Press, 2009.
2. Li Z, Chuang-Stein C, Hoseyni C. The probability of observing negative subgroup results when the treatment effect is positive and homogeneous across all subgroups. *Drug Information Journal*, 2007; 41: 47–56.
3. Mini-Sentinel. www.minisentinel.org
4. Affordable Care Act, as amended May 1, 2010. http://housedocs. house.gov/energycommerce/ppacacon.pdf
5. The Federal Food, Drug, and Cosmetic Act of 1938 as amended by the Kefauver-Harris Amendments of 1962. http://www.fda.gov/Regulatory Information/Legislation/default.htm
6. Goodman SN. Quasi-random reflections on randomized controlled trials and comparative effectiveness research. *Clinical Trials*, 2012; 9: 22–26.
7. Woodcock J. Comparative effectiveness research and the regulation of drugs, biologics and devices. *Journal of Comparative Effectiveness Research*, 2013; 2(2): 95–97.
8. Temple and Eichler. Reported by Kelly for the Pink Sheet, June 11, 2012, Regarding an International Society for Pharmacoeconomics and Outcomes Research (ISPOR) Meeting, June 5, 2012.
9. The Vermont Program for Quality in Health Care. www.vpqhc.org
10. Walker AM, Patrick AR, Lauer MS. et al. A tool for assessing the feasibility of comparative effectiveness research. *Comparative Effectiveness Research*, 2013; 3: 11–20.

11. Temple R. A regulator's view of comparative effectiveness. *Clinical Trials*, 2012; 9: 56–65.
12. U.S. Food and Drug Administration. Guidance for Industry: ICH E-10, Choice of Control Group and Related Issues in Clinical Trials. Available at: http://www.fda.gov/RegulatoryInformation/Guidances/ucm125802.htm
13. U.S. Food and Drug Administration. Draft Guidance for Industry: Non-Inferiority and Clinical Trials. Available at: http://www.fda.gov/downloads/Drugs/GuidanceComplianceRegulatoryInformation/Guidances/UCM202140.pdf
14. Eapen ZJ, Lauer MS, Temple RJ. The imperative of overcoming barriers to the conduct of large simple trials. *JAMA*, 2014; 311(14): 1397–1398.
15. Frobert O, Lagerqvist B, Olivecrona GK et al. Thrombus aspiration during ST-segment elevation myocardial infarction. *The New England Journal of Medicine*, 2013, 369: 1587–1597. DOI: 10.0156/NEJMoa1308789.
16. Lauer MS, D'Agostino RB. The randomized registry trial—The next disruptive technology in clinical research. *The New England Journal of Medicine*, September 1, 2013; 389: 1–3.
17. Ware J, Hamel MB. Pragmatic trials—Guides to better patient care? *The New England Journal of Medicine*, 2011; 364(18): 1685–1687.
18. Deming WE. *Out of the Crisis*. Cambridge, US. MIT Press, 1986.
19. Caramenico A. Intermountain's Brent James: Patient-Centeredness Drives Quality, Savings, March 27, 2013. http://www.fiercehealthcare.com/story/intermountains-bret-james-patient-centeredness-drives-quality-savings/2013-03-27
20. Wang R, Lagakos SW, Ware JH, Hunter DJ, Drazen JM. Statistics in medicine—Reporting of subgroup analyses in clinical trials. *The New England Journal of Medicine*, 2007; 357: 2189–2194.
21. Observational Medical Outcomes Partnership. http://omop.fnih.org/
22. Ryan PB, Madigan D, Stang PE, Overhage JM, Racoosin JA, Hartzema AG. Empirical assessment of methods for risk identification in healthcare data: Results from the experiments of the Observational Medical Outcomes Partnership. *Statistics in Medicine*, 2012; 31: 4401–4415.
23. Madigan D, Ryan P. What can we really learn from observational studies? *Epidemiology*, 2011; 22(5): 629–631.
24. Ryan P. Statistical challenges in systematic evidence generation through analysis of observational healthcare data networks. *Statistical Methods in Medical Research*, 2011; 22(1): 3–6.
25. Ryan P, Schuemie M, Gruber S, Zorych I, Madigan D. Empirical performance of a new user cohort method: Lessons for developing a risk identification and analysis system. *Drug Safety*, 2013; 36(1 Suppl.); 59–72.
26. Hernan MA, Alons A, Logan R. et al. Observational studies analyzed like randomized experiments, an application to postmenopausal hormone therapy and coronary heart disease. *Epidemiology*, 2008; 19(6): 766–779.
27. Schuemie M, Gini R, Coloma PM, Straatman H. Replication of the OMOP experiment in Europe: Evaluating methods for risk identification in electronic health record databases. *Drug Safety*, 2013; 36(1 Suppl.); 171–180.
28. Rassen JA, Schneeweiss S. Newly marketed medications present unique challenges for nonrandomized comparative effectiveness analyses. Editorial. *Journal of Comparative Effectiveness Research*, 2012; 1(2): 109–111.

29. Schneeweiss S, Gagne JJ, Glynn RJ, Ruhl M, Rassen JA. Assessing the comparative effectiveness of newly marketed medications: Methodological challenges and implications for drug development. *Clinical Pharmacology & Therapeutics*, 2011; 90(6): 777–790.
30. Prentice RL. Data analysis methods and the reliability of analytic epidemiologic research. *Epidemiology*, 2008; 19(6): 785–787.
31. http://www.pcori.org/assets/2013/11/PCORI-Methodology-Report.pdf
32. U.S. Food and Drug Administration. Guidance for Industry: ICH E-9, Statistical Principles for Clinical Trials. Available at: http://www.fda.gov/ RegulatoryInformation/Guidances/ucm125802.htm
33. Rubin D. The design versus the analysis of observational studies for causal effects: Parallels with the design of randomized trials. *Statistics in Medicine*, 2007; 26: 20–36.
34. Berger ML, Dreyer N, Anderson F, Towse A, Sedrakyan A, Normand SL. Prospective observational studies to assess comparative effectiveness: The ISPOR good research practices task force report. *Value in Health*, 2012; 15: 217–230.
35. Thorpe KE, Zwarenstein M, Oxman AD et al. A pragmatic-explanatory continuum indicator summary (PRECIS): A tool to help trial designers. *Journal of Clinical Epidemiology*, 2009; 62: 464–475.
36. Draft Guidance for the Public, Industry, and CMS Staff. Coverage with Evidence Development in the Context of Coverage Decisions. Issued on November 29, 2012. Available at: http://www.cms.gov/medicare-coverage-database/details/medicare-coverage-document-details.aspx?MCDId=23
37. Curtis LH, Brown J, Platt R. Four health data networks illustrate the potential for a shared national multipurpose big-data network. *Health Affairs*, 2014; 33(7): 1178–1186.
38. Selker HP, Oye KA, Eichler H-G, Stockbridge NL, Mehta CR, Kaitin KI, McElwee NE, Honig PK, Erban JK, D'Agostino RB. A proposal for integrated efficacy to effectiveness (E2E) clinical trials. *Clinical Pharmacology & Therapeutics*, 2014; 95(2): 147–153.
39. Girman CJ, Faries D, Ryan P, Rotelli M, Belger M, Binkowitz B, O'Neill R. Pre-study feasibility and identifying sensitivity analyses for protocol pre-specification in comparative effectiveness research. *Journal of Comparative Effectiveness Research*, 2014; 3(3): 259–270.

Section III

Research Synthesis

10

Systematic Reviews with Study-Level and Individual Patient-Level Data

Joseph Lau, Sally C. Morton, Thomas A. Trikalinos,
and Christopher H. Schmid

CONTENTS

ABSTRACT   Systematic review and meta-analysis are the fundamental
tools of evidence-based healthcare. Combining information from multiple
studies can provide insights that individual studies cannot offer. In this chapter we explain these methods and show how they are applied by AHRQ
(a US-based healthcare agency) in its comparative effectiveness research program. We illustrate the challenges of conducting comparative effectiveness
reviews using study level data in three examples of reports produced by the
AHRQ evidence-based practice centers. In the second half of this chapter,
we provide a detailed discussion of the statistical methods used in individual patient data meta-analysis. The approach to combine patient level data
has the ability to answer questions that are directly applicable to individual patients, whereas study level meta-analysis can only offer conclusions
for a population. We anticipate that individual patient data will likely be
more readily available for future meta-analyses. The increasing demand for
comparative effectiveness reviews will need more efficient methods to produce them. We offer some suggestions to modernize systematic review and
meta-analyses methods.

10.1 Background

Individual studies, even those that are well designed, conducted, and
reported, typically do not answer all questions that pertain to healthcare
policy problems. Instead, a more complete picture can be had through combining information from multiple sources that address different aspects of a
policy problem, or several variations of a problem, including different populations, interventions, or settings. This is summarized in the basic maxim that
taking into account the totality of relevant evidence optimizes the likelihood
of high-quality decisions.

Informing decisions with the totality of relevant evidence requires a systematic, methodical approach to identifying, culling, synthesizing, and interpreting evidence, and most practitioners lack the time or skills to do these
tasks. The ever-growing volume of the biomedical literature magnifies these
challenges (Bastian et al., 2010).

10.1.1 The Need for Systematic Reviews of Healthcare Evidence

Systematic review and meta-analysis have developed and matured in response to the many shortcomings of the traditional approaches of finding and using healthcare evidence. Systematic reviews use an *a priori* formulated protocol and well-defined research questions to comprehensively identify, critically appraise, and carefully synthesize relevant data using rigorous methods that minimize bias. Meta-analysis is a quantitative synthesis of data across several studies addressing the same question, performed typically on summary data abstracted from primary studies during the conduct of a systematic review (Lau et al., 1997). These methods have become the foundation of the now widely promoted evidence-based approach to healthcare practices (Evidence-Based Medicine Working Group, 1992). They help to summarize evidence, increase the power of individual studies, and explore heterogeneity of treatment effects (Lau et al., 1998). Thousands of systematic reviews and meta-analyses have been published in recent years to inform healthcare practices, policies, and research. A study in 2010 found that 11 systematic reviews were being published each day (Bastian et al., 2010). As of October 2014, over 80,000 items have been indexed in Pubmed as meta-analyses or related articles. Institute of Medicine (IOM) reports on comparative effectiveness research, CER (Ratner et al., 2009), and evidence-based healthcare (Sox et al., 2008) have consistently included evidence synthesis as an essential component of healthcare decision making. The U.S. Congress affirmed this view in the 2010 Affordable Care Act in which it explicitly included the use of systematic reviews as part of the CER agenda in its legislation. Many funding agencies and journals worldwide now require systematic reviews to support the need for new studies and trials (Clarke et al., 2007).

10.1.2 Development of Comparative Effectiveness Reviews

Early meta-analyses generally were narrow in scope, partly due to the simpler nature of the questions asked, the types of evidence analyzed, and the synthesis methodologies available. They often addressed only one question and focused on randomized-controlled trials (RCTs) to assess the efficacy of a new intervention with an existing one (or with a placebo). The topics were selected primarily because of the authors' interest and the availability of a sufficient number of trials to merit synthesis and publication. In a 1998 analysis of 115 published meta-analyses of RCTs of interventions, the median number of included articles was found to be about 8 for Cochrane reviews and 11.5 for those published in journals (Schmid et al., 1998). An example of the early meta-analyses is one that compared the efficacy and adverse effects of single daily dosing with the traditional multiple daily dosing of aminoglycosides in the treatment of serious infections (Barza et al., 1996). This meta-analysis found that a once daily dosing regimen was at least as efficacious as multiple daily dosing regimens with likely less toxicity. Thus, the single daily dosing strategy was not only clinically better; it could potentially simplify treatment delivery and reduce cost.

As systematic reviews and meta-analyses gained acceptance, they began to take on broader and more complex questions that addressed the needs of healthcare practitioners and policy decision makers. Reviews compared the effectiveness and harms of multiple alternative interventions and often included different treatment modalities. They also included analyses to examine variation of treatment effects in different populations and settings. The lack of RCTs for many topics and the need to assess harms led to the inclusion of data from observational studies. Comprehensive systematic reviews that address multiple questions and evaluate several alternatives are now commonly referred to as comparative effectiveness reviews. In addition to evaluating treatments, comparative effectiveness reviews may also evaluate the accuracy of diagnostic tests in specific settings (meta-analysis of diagnostic tests performance is covered in Chapter 17). While comparative effectiveness reviews synthesize large bodies of evidence to inform research questions, the reviews by themselves do not make clinical or policy recommendations.

The need to compare multiple interventions has led to new synthesis methods in CER that combine direct and indirect comparisons of more than two interventions. The development of network meta-analysis in the last 15 years allows simultaneous comparison and ranking of multiple interventions from a set of studies, each of which directly compares only a subset (often two) of the interventions (covered in Chapters 11 and 12). Usually, in larger networks, some of the interventions are not directly compared at all; information about their relative performance comes about indirectly through common comparators.

New methods have also been developed to investigate and interpret discrepant results across trials and limitations of the primary literature (e.g., study quality, missing data, and biases). These investigations are much easier when individual participant data are available from the studies. Such data permit analyses that can answer questions which summary data from published studies cannot such as modeling heterogeneity of treatment effects (covered in Chapter 8) and performing time-to-event analyses. We discuss individual participant data meta-analysis (IPDMA) later in this chapter. In addition to providing assessments on effectiveness and harms, systematic reviews can also inform the design of future studies by identifying knowledge gaps and methodological deficiencies in the existing literature.

10.1.3 Producers and Users of Comparative Effectiveness Reviews

Comparative effectiveness reviews require significant amounts of time and resources to produce. While these reviews can be carried out by small teams of researchers without major funding, they are typically produced by established research units located either within academic centers or other large organizations. The reviews are sponsored by government agencies (e.g., Agency for Healthcare Research and Quality [AHRQ], Center for Disease Control and Prevention, National Institutes for Health, and the Department of Veterans Affairs; National Center for Clinical Excellence in the United Kingdom; World Health Organization) and major professional and international organizations (e.g., American Heart Association, Kidney Disease Improving Global Outcomes). AHRQ has been a leader in the United States conducting evidence reviews since 1997. The agency established the evidence-based practice center (EPC) program and contracts with research teams that have demonstrated to have the necessary expertise and infrastructure to carry out high-quality systematic reviews on a timely basis. Currently, 13 EPCs produce comparative effectiveness reviews under the AHRQ Effectiveness Health Care Program. The Cochrane Collaboration has been a global leader in producing and disseminating systematic reviews for over 20 years, and many of their current reviews could be considered as comparative effectiveness reviews. Many not-for-profit technology assessment organizations (e.g., Blue Cross Blue Shield Technology Evaluation Center, ECRI), and pharmaceutical and commercial companies (e.g., Doctor Evidence, LLC; Hayes Inc.; and Spectrum Research Inc.) also carry out comparative effectiveness reviews.

Comparative effectiveness reviews have been used by a wide range of stakeholders for many purposes including patients to understand healthcare options, clinicians to inform medical practices, professional societies to create clinical practice guidelines, healthcare payers to determine coverage decisions, government agencies to formulate public health policies, pharmaceutical companies and medical device manufacturers to identify marketing opportunities for their products, and funders of research to plan future studies. Results from comparative effectiveness reviews are also being used to inform calculations in pharmacoeconomic analyses. Under the Effective Health Care Program, research summaries about the benefits and risk of different treatments for different health conditions based on the comparative effectiveness review are also created for consumers, clinicians, and policymakers. However, these research summaries are not clinical recommendations or practice guidelines.

10.1.4 AHRQ Comparative Effectiveness Reviews

The 2003 Medicare Modernization Act authorized AHRQ to conduct and support research with a focus on "outcomes, comparative clinical effectiveness, and appropriateness of healthcare items and services" for Medicare and Medicaid populations. Over 170 comparative effectiveness reviews have been published by AHRQ since 2005 under the Effective Healthcare Program and many more are underway. In a sample of the 50 reviews published between 2013 and 2015, 33 assessed the comparative effectiveness of interventions, 14 dealt with comparative effectiveness of diagnostic/screening tests, two addressed both issues, and one assessed decision aids. Nineteen of the 50 topics are among those listed in the IOM report on *100 Initial Priority Comparative Effectiveness Research Topics*. The most common topics were cardiovascular conditions (11 reports), cancers (10), and mental health issues (7); there were also five reports on pediatric and adolescent topics. Six reports updated prior reviews. The number of key questions in these reviews ranged from 2 to 8 with a median of 4. The number of included articles ranged from 11 to 326 publications with a median of 61. In addition to the comparative effectiveness reviews, 30 technical briefs have also been published. Technical briefs are generally commissioned for topics that have limited research data to support definitive conclusions. Instead, they use systematic review methodologies to provide an overview of key issues related to a clinical intervention or healthcare service, to describe what is known and unknown about the technology, and how the technology fits within the CER framework. They also summarize the state of research and identify information needed to conduct meaningful comparative effectiveness reviews in the future.

In this section, we discuss two AHRQ comparative effectiveness reviews and a technical brief to illustrate their scope, methodological issues encountered, and some of the challenges in carrying them out. The first example we discuss below is on the *Management of Gastroesophageal Reflux Disease* (GERD). This 2005 report was the first comparative effectiveness review of the EPC program (Ip et al., 2005). The second example is a 2013 comparative effectiveness review of *Treatment Modalities* for *Chronic Venous Ulcers* (Zenilman et al., 2013). The third example is a technical brief on *Particle Beam Radiation Therapies for Cancer* (Trikalinos et al., 2009).

EXAMPLE 10.1: MANAGEMENT OF GERD

GERD is one of the most common health conditions affecting about 4% of people in the United States with estimated annual incremental health benefit costs (employers' perspective) of $23 billion (Brook et al., 2007). It ranked in the first quartile of 100 initial priority topics in the 2009 IOM report on *Initial National Priorities for Comparative Effectiveness Research*. The 2005 report on management options for adults asked three key questions: (1) What is the evidence of the comparative effectiveness of medical, surgical, and endoscopic treatments for improving objective and subjective outcomes in patients with chronic GERD? (2) Is there evidence that effectiveness of medical, surgical, and endoscopic treatments varies for specific patient subgroups? (3) What are the short- and long-term adverse effects associated with specific medical, surgical, and endoscopic therapies for GERD?

Management of GERD brings out many comparative effectiveness review and patient-centered outcomes issues. GERD is a chronic disease that has diverse clinical and symptomatic manifestations. Multiple-treatment modalities (i.e., drugs, surgery, and endoscopic procedures) and alternatives within a modality (i.e., several classes of drugs and multiple drugs within a class) are available to manage this condition. Subjective (e.g., symptoms, lifestyle modifications) and objective outcomes (e.g., development of cancers, mortality) are important patient-centered outcomes to consider, in addition to other relevant outcomes such as endoscopic findings. To identify effective and appropriate management, all of the treatment modalities, types of outcomes, and harmful effects of the interventions must be assessed and taken into consideration in different patient subgroups. The need to use observational data to assess harms, and the availability of many trials and existing systematic reviews present challenges and opportunities of synthesizing a large and diverse body of evidence. The introduction of new treatments and the withdrawal of certain treatment options require updating of the existing systematic reviews.

The MEDLINE search for the GERD report yielded 6,163 citations and 75 meta-analyses of potential relevance. A search of the Cochrane Database of Systematic Reviews produced 140 additional titles. Given the availability of many prior systematic reviews, it would be more efficient for researchers conducting a new comparative effectiveness review to update previous work rather than starting from scratch unless there are reasons to do so (e.g., poor-quality reviews, unanswered questions, missing data, and new analytic methods). Thus, 37 of the GERD systematic reviews and meta-analyses were retrieved for consideration and seven that met eligibility criteria were used in the report. Among the MEDLINE citations, 327 were identified as potentially relevant new original research and retrieved for further evaluation. The final report included 98 primary studies.

Despite what seems to be a large number of new primary studies and prior systematic reviews, few eligible studies answered the comparative effectiveness question of the three treatment modalities. There were only three RCTs with a total of fewer than 800 patients that compared medical treatment (proton pump inhibitors [PPIs]) with surgery (fundoplication), and only two studies had more than 1 year of follow-up. Only three nonrandomized studies compared surgery (fundoplication) with an endoscopic procedure but these studies were of low methodological quality and could not be relied upon to draw valid conclusions. No studies compared endoscopic procedures with medical therapy.

Most of the available studies were drug trials that compared one drug class (PPIs) with another class (H_2 receptor antagonists), within the same class (between PPIs), between different dosages and dosing regimens within the same class (PPIs), between once daily dosing versus on-demand dosing regiments of PPIs, and between PPIs and over-the-counter PPIs (essentially dosing comparisons). The availability of studies that compared multiple drugs suggests that there was an opportunity for conducting a network meta-analysis of these trials. However, the methodologies for synthesizing these studies and interpreting their results were insufficiently developed at that time. The quality of the evidence addressing the other two key questions was considered weak and derived mostly from observational studies. None of the studies used an acceptable standard or scale for defining the severity of adverse events.

EXAMPLE 10.2: TREATMENT MODALITIES FOR CHRONIC VENOUS ULCERS

Chronic venous leg ulcers affect up to 2-million people annually in the United States and have been estimated to account for up to 3% of total healthcare budgets in developed countries (Zenilman et al., 2013). Management of chronic venous ulcers is complex and often involves multiple-treatment modalities. Compression dressing and debridement are the primary modalities that result in the healing of about one-half of the ulcers. Additional interventions in the form of advanced wound dressings, local or systemic antimicrobials, and venous surgery are needed when the primary treatments fail. Many types of advanced wound dressings and antimicrobial therapies have been developed and their comparative effectiveness has not been established. In the 2013 report, the Johns Hopkins EPC conducted a comparative effectiveness review of treatments for chronic venous ulcers (Zenilman et al., 2013). The report addressed the following questions: (1) What are the additional benefits and harms of advanced wound dressings in conjunction with compression systems? (2) For patients who do not have clinical signs of cellulitis that are being treated with, what are the incremental benefits and harms of using systemic antibiotics? (3) What are the additional benefits and harms of surgical procedures aimed at the underlying venous abnormalities?

The literature search on this topic yielded over 10,000 citations. Anticipating that few comparative studies would be available, the authors decided *a priori* to include studies without a concurrent comparison group if certain criteria (i.e., sample size, timeframe, and reporting of essential information) were met. Even then, only 60 studies met the eligibility criteria and all were included in the report. The majority of included studies were RCTs. However, the researchers found few well-designed RCTs that addressed the comparative effectiveness question. They reported that most RCTs were small and of poor methodological quality that precluded drawing valid conclusions. Many studies did not report statistical analyses beyond simple healing rates; they also did not perform stratification or adjustment to account for potential confounding variables. The reviewers reported that the noncomparative studies were largely limited to convenience populations that made drawing unbiased conclusions difficult. The Hopkins report identified numerous issues in the primary literature that are likely faced by many other teams working on other comparative effectiveness review topics.

The Hopkins report points to a serious inadequacy of the primary literature, the lack of high quality, and coherent research in this area. They found that studies took place in many diverse practice and cultural settings involving a variety of disciplines, including nursing, dermatology, vascular surgery, and internal medicine. While this diversity might suggest greater generalizability of the research findings, the heterogeneity of the methods employed in the studies they found instead suggests little interaction and consensus among clinical disciplines in formulating a common framework to assess the effectiveness and safety of treatments for chronic venous leg ulcers. These limitations include the lack of standard definitions of chronic venous leg ulcers, inconsistent outcome measures, suboptimal comparison groups, and inconsistent duration of interventions. Furthermore, chronic wounds have substantial impact on the patient and his/her family, but quality-of-life assessments were absent in most studies.

EXAMPLE 10.3: PARTICLE BEAM RADIATION THERAPIES FOR CANCER

Radiation therapy has an important role in many cancer treatments and it is often used in conjunction with surgery or chemotherapy. It works by depositing a radiation dose—an amount of energy—in the tumor area in the patient's body, resulting in cellular damage, and hopefully, tumor control. In clinical practice, lethal tumor doses are rarely attainable, because some radiation dose is inevitably delivered to nontumor tissues, causing collateral morbidity.

Many radiation delivery modalities exist: the radiation source may be internal, implanted in the patient's body, or external, directing a beam on the tumor volume. Conventional external radiation therapy with x- or gamma-rays allows only control of the overall dose delivered in various areas in the patient's body. Advances in radiation delivery technology such as intensity-modulated radiation therapy, conformal radiation therapy, and particle beam radiation therapy can maximize dose delivery to the tumor, while minimizing the dose delivered to nontumor tissues (Terasawa et al., 2009). Particle beam radiation therapy requires specialized facilities and is much more costly and far less available than any other alternatives. Only seven such centers were in operation in the United States in 2008.

The comparative effectiveness question, therefore, is which radiation delivery modality is more effective and safe for treating tumors, especially those near critical organs (e.g., base of the skull). Specifically, the technical brief produced by the Tufts EPC in 2009 focused on the comparative effectiveness of particle beam radiation therapy versus other radiation modalities. A technical brief can help insurers such as the Centers for Medicare and Medicaid Services appreciate the maturity of the evidence base, and thus inform their decision making on whether and how to cover the intervention.

Figure 10.1 depicts the results of an assessment of the literature conducted in 2008 on particle beam radiation therapy (Terasawa et al., 2009). In 243 eligible articles, particle beam radiation therapy was used alone or in combination with other interventions for common (e.g., lung, prostate, or breast) or uncommon (e.g., skull-base tumors or uveal melanomas) types of cancer. Of 243 articles, 185 were single-group retrospective studies. Eight RCTs and nine nonrandomized clinical trials compared treatments with or without charged particles. No comparative study reported statistically significant or important differences in overall or cancer-specific survival or in total serious adverse events.

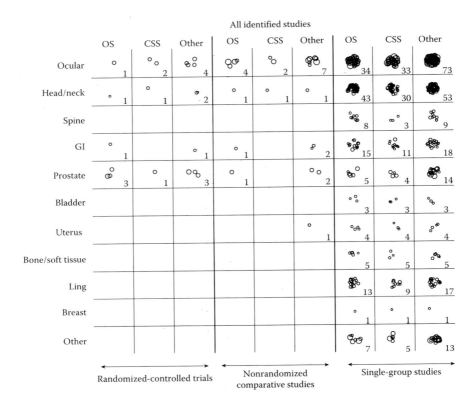

FIGURE 10.1
Each circle represents a study; the size of the circle is proportional to the logarithm of the total number of participants in the study. The number in each cell indicates the total number of studies. Each row shows studies addressing a type of cancer, and the columns show study designs with reported clinical outcomes. The "Other" row includes studies reporting on multiple types of cancer. The "Other" columns include studies that reported clinical outcomes other than OS or CSS (e.g., disease-free survival, progression-free survival, tumor response rate, or quality of life). CSS, cancer-specific survival; GI, gastrointestinal; OS, overall survival. (Reproduced from Trikalinos, T. A. et al. 2009. AHRQ comparative effectiveness technical briefs. *Particle Beam Radiation Therapies for Cancer.* Rockville, MD: Agency for Healthcare Research and Quality (US) (The chapter authors hold the copyright.); (Terasawa, T. et al. 2009. Systematic review: Charged-particle radiation therapy for cancer. *Annals of Internal Medicine*, 151, 556–565.)

The take-home message from the technical brief is that there are very few comparative trials, in common or rare cancers, for any outcome. The interpretation is nuanced: for some tumors and some comparisons, the comparative effectiveness question is answerable without comparative trials. For example, no clinical equipoise exists between conventional photon radiation therapy and particle beam radiation therapy for tumors of the base of the skull: conventional photon-based radiation therapy cannot safely achieve therapeutic doses in the tumor without giving unacceptably high doses to adjacent critical structures, but particle beam radiation therapy can.

In contrast, for other tumor and treatment-comparison combinations, clinical equipoise exists, and these questions should be addressed with comparative trials. In the previous example, both particle beam radiation therapy and intensity-modulated radiation therapy can deliver therapeutic doses to the tumor without destroying nearby critical structures. Other examples where comparative trials are needed pertain to the treatment of common cancers, such as prostate, lung, or breast cancer, where all radiation delivery modalities (including conventional radiation therapy) can achieve therapeutic tumor doses. It has been hypothesized that particle beam radiation therapy may have lower frequency of radiation-induced colitis compared to conventional radiation therapy, because of its superior dose-delivery control. However, at least three RCTs did not demonstrate this, raising questions about whether particle beam radiation therapy for these conditions is worth the substantial extra cost.

Informed by the results of the technical brief, the Centers for Medicare and Medicaid Services decided to cover particle beam radiation therapy on the condition that treated patients are included in approved clinical studies or consent to the collection of additional clinical data, following the so-called Coverage with Evidence Development paradigm.

10.2 Methods of Comparative Effectiveness Review

Much progress has been made in the past three decades in the development of systematic review and meta-analysis methods and numerous articles and textbooks have been published on these topics. Advances have been made in formulating research questions, searching the literature for relevant studies, selecting and critically appraising included studies, and developing statistical methods to combine data and interpret results in meta-analyses. However, researchers have also found large variations in the quality of published systematic reviews and meta-analyses (Jadad et al., 1998). The increasing reliance on using publicly funded comparative effectiveness reviews to inform healthcare decisions mandates that not only the methods be rigorous but that processes be developed to engage patients and stakeholders in a meaningful way to improve the usefulness of these reviews. Users of these products also want to have this information available in a consistent format across topics so that they can be more readily interpreted and applied.

10.2.1 Guidance for Conducting and Reporting Comparative Effectiveness Reviews

To improve the reliability, transparency, and usability of systematic reviews and meta-analyses, several major organizations have published guidance on how to conduct and report this research. The AHRQ EPC program has published a detailed methodological guidance for conducting comparative effectiveness reviews (AHRQ, 2014). The Cochrane Collaboration has continuously updated the *Cochrane Handbook on Systematic Review* and it has also published the *Methodological Expectations of Cochrane Intervention Reviews* (MECIR) (Chandler et al., 2013). The 2011 IOM report on *Standards for Conducting of Systematic Reviews of Comparative Effectiveness Research* made 82 specific recommendations for federally funded systematic reviews (Morton et al., 2011). The recommendations in these guidance documents are based on expert consensus informed by empirical research, current best practices, and guidelines on reporting of clinical studies produced by international workgroups. Examples of the guidelines for reporting systematic reviews and meta-analyses include PRISMA (Preferred Reporting Items for Systematic Reviews and Meta-Analyses) and MOOSE (Meta-analysis Of Observational Studies in Epidemiology). These reporting guidelines can be found on the EQUATOR (Enhancing the QUAlity and Transparency of Health Research) network website (www.equator-network.org).

Most of the recommended practices made by these organizations are similar. The alignment of their recommendations reflects the common goal of these guidance documents to produce systematic reviews that minimize bias, and are relevant and useful to inform important healthcare decisions. Some discrepancies exist and a detailed analysis of the differences between the IOM standards and the AHRQ methods guide has been reported (Lau et al., 2013). For example, the IOM report recommends full, duplicate independent reviews at each step of the process and assessing the strength of evidence of all outcomes. These measures were not recommended in the AHRQ methods guide but are recommended by Cochrane. The difference between the IOM standards and the AHRQ methods guide could be attributed to the desire of the IOM Committee to set a high bar for federally funded systematic reviews, whereas AHRQ as a funding agency also needs to be concerned about delivering a timely product at reasonable costs. Additional research will need to be done before complying with the more rigorous standards either because compliance would require more effort and resources, or because the benefits are uncertain without good evidence (Chang et al., 2013).

Recommendations on conducting comparative effectiveness reviews in general can be grouped into those that focus on processes and infrastructure and those that focus on specific methods of systematic review and meta-analysis. There are already numerous publications on systematic review methodologies. Other chapters of this book also cover network meta-analysis (covered in Chapters 11 and 12), and meta-analysis of studies evaluating the accuracy of diagnostic tests (covered in Chapter 17). We will minimize repeating the same information that could readily be obtained in detail elsewhere. In particular, we will not discuss topics on formulating answerable research questions, searching the literature, selecting studies, and assessing the risk of bias (including publication bias). We will instead focus the discussion on infrastructure and processes necessary to carry out comparative effectiveness reviews and use processes and methods developed for the AHRQ EPC program to illustrate the operationalization of the recommendations. The last part of this section provides an overview of the basic approaches to meta-analysis of summary literature data. This overview will serve as a bridge to the last section of this chapter, which covers IPDMA. IPDMA, in contrast with meta-analysis of summary data, can more readily be used to inform patient-centered outcomes decisions. It is anticipated that individual patient data will increasingly be available in the near future.

The AHRQ EPC program follows three principles in producing comparative effectiveness reviews: (1) reviews must be relevant and timely in order to meet the needs of decision makers; (2) reviews must be objective and scientifically rigorous; and (3) public participation and transparency increase public confidence in the scientific integrity and credibility of reviews and provide further accountability to the EPCs (AHRQ, 2014). In operationalizing these principles, the EPC program has created a continuously updated process to prioritize and refine topics before the review is undertaken, along with an infrastructure to enable these processes. Table 10.1 highlights the key steps and participants in carrying out specific tasks in a comparative effectiveness review under the AHRQ EPC program.

10.2.2 Resources and Infrastructure Needed to Conduct Comparative Effectiveness Reviews

Federally funded comparative effectiveness reviews such as those produced by AHRQ EPCs are major research activities that require a wide range of expertise, significant amounts of resources and time, and a capable infrastructure to support the processes. Adherence to rigorous methodological standards (e.g., independent double-data abstraction, steps to mitigate bias and conflicts of interest, stakeholder engagement, public commenting, and extensive peer reviews) requires even more resources and time. The scope of the EPC comparative effectiveness reviews tends to be large and often needs to assess and synthesize a hundred or more studies.

The 2011 IOM report on standards for systematic review emphasized the importance of establishing a team with appropriate expertise, ensuring user and stakeholder input, and managing bias and conflict of interests. A research team should include individuals with expertise in the following areas: systematic review methodologies, clinical or subject matter, medical literature search/information science, meta-analysis, and statistical methods. The IOM report on standards for systematic reviews also calls for stakeholders and patients participation. An individual with skills to solicit stakeholder and patient input should be part of the team. One person with expertise in several areas may fill multiple roles. Additional team members may include

TABLE 10.1

Key Steps of Conducting a Comparative Effectiveness Review in the AHRQ EPC Program

Steps	Key Participants	Specific Tasks
Determine the need for a new review or update	Funder, stakeholders	Review the existing systematic reviews Search PROSPERO, Cochrane Library Contact potential users of the review
Identify the review team	Funder	Ensure that necessary expertise is available and team members are free of COI
Engage stakeholders	Funder Review team Stakeholders	Identify and recruit stakeholders Seek balanced input Manage COI
Refine research questions	Review team stakeholders	Iterative process to • Create an analytic framework • Develop PICOTS for questions • Define the scope • Establish the eligibility criteria • Formulate the protocol
Register review protocol	Review team	Register the finalized protocol; for example, PROSPERO
Search literature	Review team Technical experts	Search for multiple sources (electronic databases, journals, conference proceedings, reference lists, study registries, and personal contacts)
Select studies and abstract data	Review team	Screen abstracts Retrieve and evaluate full-text articles Apply PICOTS to select studies Dual independent extractions, compare, and resolve all discrepancies

(Continued)

TABLE 10.1 (Continued)

Key Steps of Conducting a Comparative Effectiveness Review in the AHRQ EPC Program

Steps	Key Participants	Specific Tasks
Assess the quality of studies	Review team	Apply the risk of bias tool to assess selection bias, performance bias, detection bias, attrition bias, reporting bias, etc.
Synthesize results	Review team	Organize data to answer research questions
		Perform meta-analysis as appropriate
		Explore reasons (clinical or methodological) for between-study heterogeneity (sensitivity analysis, subgroup analysis, and meta-regression)
Interpret results and grade strength of evidence	Review team	Interpret results based on the treatment effect estimate and on the evaluation of the quality of evidence for the entire body of included studies for each outcome, that is, GRADE system
		Assess the risk of bias: Publication bias, language bias, citation bias, multiple publication bias, selective reporting of outcomes and analyses, and inclusion bias
Draft the report as per standards	Review team	Report findings according to reporting guidelines, that is, PRISMA checklist
Conduct peer review	Review team	Solicit and incorporate peer-review comments
	Stakeholders	
	External reviewers	
Disseminate results	Review team	Publish articles in journals
	Funder	Create summaries for patients, clinicians, and policy makers
	Stakeholders	Use results to make informed decisions

project manager, medical editor, and research assistants. For the systematic review to be credible, members of the research team must be free of real or apparent conflicts of interests. A median of 8 (range 3–18) coauthors were involved in the sample of 50 AHRQ comparative effectiveness reviews described earlier.

The IOM report's recommendation to engage stakeholders and patients in systematic reviews builds upon the increasingly common practice of engaging consumers in clinical research. The Cochrane Collaboration has a long tradition and well-established mechanism of involving patients in systematic reviews (http://consumers.cochrane.org/healthcare-users-cochrane). Consumers are involved in a range of activities that include helping to formulate the systematic review protocol (e.g., identifying outcomes of interest), performing lay person review of the draft systematic review, serving as coauthors, and creating lay summary and helping to disseminate the review. The AHRQ EPC program also has involved stakeholders in various aspects of the evidence review process including topic development, topic refinement, and peer review of its products for over 15 years. However, there is a lack of standardization in the approach and evaluation of their effectiveness and optimal approach (Kreis et al., 2013). A taxonomy of stakeholder engagement for patient-centered outcomes research called the "7Ps" has been proposed as a framework for this activity (Concannon et al., 2012). This taxonomy includes the following categories of participants: patients or public, providers, purchasers, payers, policy makers, product makers, and principal investigators. Applying the 7Ps framework consistently may ensure that an appropriate mix of individuals will be recruited to serve as stakeholders. As yet, there is limited experience operationalizing this framework and an evaluation of the effectiveness of this approach has not yet been reported.

10.2.3 Processes to Identify, Prioritize, and Select Comparative Effectiveness Reviews

Thousands of systematic reviews are published each year. It is increasingly common to see multiple reviews on the same topic conducted by different teams published in the same year. Some of these seeming replications may be justifiable because the questions asked while similar may be sufficiently different to merit additional analyses and new publications. Others may be important updates of previous reviews by including newly published and landmark trials. Unnecessary replications should be minimized because systematic reviews consume significant resources and duplicate publications have minimum added value. There are also many published systematic reviews that concluded that there is no or insufficient evidence to inform the key questions. While finding no evidence has value in pointing to the research needs, this finding is not immediately useful to clinicians and patients. Furthermore, valuable resources and time are expended in such exercises. Therefore, processes to identify, prioritize, and select topics that will likely have sufficient evidence to yield useful answers would be highly desirable before undertaking a review.

In the AHRQ EPC program, topics selected for comparative effectiveness reviews are solicited from the public, prioritized, and vetted to ensure that a comparative effectiveness review is feasible and the results will likely be useful. Processes have been developed and are continuously being refined prior to the commissioning of the review. The major steps include topic nomination, topic development, topic prioritization and selection, and refinement of the systematic review key questions.

Professional societies, health systems, employers, insurers, providers, and consumer groups are invited to submit comparative effectiveness review topics to an AHRQ website. A structured form asks nominators to define the problem and to suggest several key questions, provide information on why the topic is important and how the results of the evidence review will be used to inform decisions, and name other stakeholders who may have an interest in the same topic. If a topic meets the minimum criteria, additional vetting of the topic, often by an EPC, is conducted to assess whether a new review or an update is necessary and that there is likely sufficient evidence to conduct a meaningful review. In addition to PUBMED searches, the PROSPERO registry of systematic review protocols (http://www.crd.york.ac.uk/PROSPERO/) and the clinicaltrials.gov websites are searched for research that has been started but not yet completed.

Nomination information along with data collected in the topic development phase is used by AHRQ to prioritize topics at meetings held at regular intervals. The approved review topic is assigned to an EPC, which is then tasked with refining the topic with input from key informants and patients. The EPC then works with a panel of technical experts comprising clinical experts to refine the key questions and to establish study eligibility criteria. EPCs post key questions online for public comments before they are finalized.

10.2.4 Searching the Literature and Extracting the Data

The largest time component of a systematic review is the search of the literature for relevant papers and subsequent extraction of the data from them. We do not discuss these steps in detail here as there is a voluminous literature detailing the databases and library search strategies to employ, the steps to take to ensure accuracy and reproducibility of the process, and the need for well-trained staff. As noted earlier, the number of citations to screen can be immense and the bookkeeping can be tedious. Typically, it is best to work with a librarian who knows databases and how to search them, to search multiple databases, to search both English and non-English language literature (especially for topics such as Chinese medicine), to have two individuals screen through abstracts found, and to use a sensitive search and screen strategy so as not to miss relevant articles that may appear in nonstandard formats (e.g., data that appear in letters to the editor). Many articles cannot be screened out until the full text is retrieved. Extraction of relevant data on study design, methods, and results requires a well-designed extraction form that may need several passes before it is in final form. Duplicate extraction is ideal, although sometimes beyond the resources of the research team. However, careful checking of at least some of the papers and calibration between reviewers will minimize many errors. Later sections of the chapter describe some of the advantages that having the raw data give and recently developed tools that can reduce the manual burden of data collection.

10.2.5 Assessing Quality: Risk of Bias

As shown in Table 10.1, assessing risk of bias of the individual studies and grading the overall strength of evidence are two key steps in a systematic review. While choices exist for how to tackle both steps, an overall objective should be transparency about what was done and the implications for the results and interpretation of the systematic review. We discuss risk of bias in this section and grading strength of evidence after discussing analytic issues.

For studies of interventions, assessing risk of bias refers to determining how potential bias in the conduct and analysis of a study may have influenced the estimation of the treatment effect. For randomized trials, the Cochrane risk of bias tool helps reviewers think through selection, performance, detection, attrition, reporting, and other biases (Higgins and Green, 2008). Assessing risk of bias for observational studies is particularly challenging given that such studies do not randomize subjects and may not have other internal validity safeguards. CER necessarily encompasses both randomized and observational data. The latter are essential for the assessment of harms, for example, one of the six characteristics of CER as defined by the IOM (Ratner et al., 2009). Furthermore, observational data collected for other purposes are a critical component of CER as described with respect to electronic health records in Chapter 14. Indeed, providing answers to CER questions will often require cross-design synthesis as detailed in Chapter 7.

10.2.6 Meta-Analysis of Comparative Effectiveness Research Summary Data

Once data have been collected and assessed, they need to be analyzed. Sometimes, if the studies are of different types or of insufficient number or have not been quantitatively summarized, the only analysis possible is a qualitative summary of the available information. Such summaries will typically list the types of designs, study patient characteristics, outcomes examined, and so forth but will not attempt to synthesize such information into a summary statistic. When several studies (sometimes as few as two, but usually three or more) report statistical summaries on the same outcome and they are considered alike enough to pool, one can perform a quantitative synthesis or meta-analysis using sufficient statistics from the individual studies. Several advanced meta-analysis methods are discussed elsewhere in the book—including meta-analysis of networks of studies that compare a subset of several interventions (covered in Chapters 11 and 12), and of diagnostic test accuracy (covered in Chapter 17). Cross-design synthesis is discussed in Chapter 7.

For the most part, meta-analysis is a retrospective exercise, in that the analyst has no control over the collection of data, their analysis, and reporting. Thus, refinements in meta-analysis techniques are largely driven by the need to address increasingly complex questions with incompletely reported data, while handling technical and statistical challenges better.

We start with a brief overview of typical pairwise meta-analysis for one outcome (where advances are in estimation and computation), and then discuss its extension to meta-analysis of multiple outcomes, and to analysis of individual participant data.

A typical meta-analysis averages K-independent treatment effects, obtained from as many studies, to compare the effectiveness or safety of two interventions.

To fix some notation, let θ_k be the unobserved population effect and d_k its estimate in study $k = 1, \ldots, K$. In each study, the observed estimate d_k is modeled to follow a normal distribution with mean θ_k and variance σ_k^2:

$$d_k \sim N(\theta_k, \sigma_k^2). \tag{10.1}$$

To *learn* across studies, meta-analysts must make assumptions about how the study population effects θ_k relate between them. The two most common ways of thinking about these assumptions can be described using two generative models, the *equal effect* and the *random effects* model (Hartung et al., 2011).

Under the equal effect model (also called "fixed effect" model), one assumes that all studies estimate a common population effect Θ:

$$\theta_k = \Theta \quad \text{for all} \quad k = 1, \ldots, K. \tag{10.2}$$

This assumption is rather strong, in that it essentially states that the distribution of effect modifiers is the same across all studies. In other words, any diversity in the populations, interventions, or comparisons across the K studies does not affect the treatment effect. See Chapter 8 for a discussion of issues on the heterogeneity of the treatment effects across population characteristics.

The random effects model relaxes the assumption in Equation 10.2, and allows the study-specific effects to differ from each other. However, to learn across studies, we still have to assume that their population effects follow some structure—typically a normal distribution

$$\theta_k \sim N(\Theta, \tau^2) \quad \text{for all} \quad k = 1, \ldots, K, \tag{10.3}$$

where τ^2 is the between-study variance or heterogeneity parameter. The model in Equation 10.3 allows for heterogeneity in the study population effects, albeit in a very specific sense.

The models in Equations 10.1, 10.2 and 10.1, 10.3 are generic, and different specifications can be had for, for example, dichotomous, or count data (Hartung et al., 2011). More importantly, an infinite number of variations exist for the simple random effects model. For example, in Equation 10.3, one can specify a distribution other than a normal, or a mixture of normal distributions (Karabatsos et al., 2015).

With the wide availability of graphical interface-based, user friendly, and open-source software, it is straightforward to fit meta-analysis models in the maximum likelihood or Bayesian framework using state of the science numerical algorithms (Viechtbauer, 2010; Wallace et al., 2012). For practically all evidence synthesis approaches discussed in this chapter, computation is not a major issue.

Arguably, a principled way to choose between the two models mentioned above is to judge their plausibility. It is often easier to argue that the random effects model is more plausible than the equal effect one, in that it allows for between-study variability in the population effects (Borenstein et al., 2010). However, choosing between models becomes more difficult when one considers a larger range of variants (e.g., alternative random effects models, or models in which the effect depends on covariates).

More generally, one can inform model choice by examining model fit. For example, when choosing between the equal and random effects models mentioned above, one can compare the likelihood of the data under each model. This amounts to testing whether the heterogeneity parameter τ^2 is positive. From this viewpoint, the various tests for heterogeneity can be viewed as tests of the fit of the equal effect model. As in regression analysis, tests of model fit can *inform* but, ideally, should not *automatically determine* model choice. This is because model fit tests are generally underpowered for the number of studies typically included in medical meta-analysis. Furthermore, once the model has been chosen on the basis of a statistical test, the distribution of its parameters changes.

Numerous statistics and graphical expositions have been proposed for testing for the presence of statistical heterogeneity, or for quantifying its extent, each conveying different information (Cochran, 1954; Galbraith, 1994; Higgins and Thompson, 2002; Olkin et al., 2012).

10.2.7 Exploration of Between-Study Diversity

More often than not, it is plausible that effect modifiers are distributed differently across studies, or that study results may differ by design or other study-level characteristics. One can use *stratification* (subgroup analyses) or *regression modeling* (meta-regression) to examine the association between the study population effects θ_k and study covariates. Caution is required in the interpretation of findings from stratified or meta-regression analyses. Such findings pertain to the study level, but it can be tempting to misinterpret them as if they pertained to the patient level. For example, consider the treatment effect of using versus not using thrombolytics in patients with acute myocardial infarction. In stratified or meta-regression analyses, one finds that studies with shorter average time between symptom onset and treatment initiation estimate more protective effect sizes for thrombolytics (GISSI, 1987). Strictly speaking, the association holds *at the study level*, but can be confounded by study, that is, studies may differ in unmeasured effect modifiers, and this may explain the association. Thus, the aforementioned association should not be interpreted at the individual patient level: one cannot conclude that *patients* who are treated earlier after symptom onset will benefit more from thrombolysis compared to those who are treated later. It so happens that in this example, the association holds at the individual patient level—but we know that from patient-level analyses or meta-analyses of individual patient data.

10.2.8 Extensions to More Than One Outcome: Multivariate Meta-Analysis

Meta-analysts are often interested in two or more outcomes for the same comparison. For example, one can assess the effectiveness of adding axillary radiation therapy to chemotherapy in women with breast cancer by examining mortality from breast cancer, and mortality from other causes. The relationship between these two outcomes involves correlation: The more women die of breast cancer, the fewer are at risk of dying from other causes. Knowing something about one outcome conveys some information about the other (Trikalinos and Olkin, 2008). More generally, when two outcomes are evaluated in the same patients they can be stochastically dependent (Gleser and Olkin, 2009). It has been argued that it may be advantageous to analyze such outcomes jointly in a single multivariate model, instead of with separate univariate meta-analyses (Gleser and Olkin, 2009; Jackson et al., 2011; Mavridis and Salanti, 2013), in that one can borrow strength between the two outcomes through the correlations, especially if one of the outcomes is missing at random in a substantial number of studies. However, if it is suspected that outcomes are missing not at random, one would have to perform substantive sensitivity analyses to explore the impact of plausible missingness mechanisms.

In simulations and empirically, one does not often find very large differences in the marginal estimates of the summary effect of each outcome with univariate and multivariate meta-analysis (Trikalinos et al., 2014a). However, one does find differences in the confidence or credible intervals of functions of the outcome-specific treatment effects estimates, for example, in calculating quality-adjusted life years in decision analyses (Trikalinos et al., 2014a). Another chapter in this book (Chapter 12) addresses Bayesian network meta-analysis with multiple endpoints.

10.2.9 Extensions to Complex Questions and Data

Meta-analysis methods can address more complex questions. For example, for most, comparative effectiveness questions of more than two alternatives are practical to consider. Network meta-analysis (covered in Chapters 11 and 12) can be used to compare three or more treatments with respect to one (Salanti, 2012) or more (Schmid et al., 2014) outcomes. Meta-analysis can also be used to assess the performance of testing modalities (Rutter and Gatsonis, 2001) and to compare performance in networks of studies of diagnostic tests (Trikalinos et al., 2014b).

10.2.10 Grading the Evidence

In terms of assessing the overall strength of evidence, several approaches exist. Berkman et al. (2013) describe the AHRQ EPC method, which is conceptually similar to that of Grading of Recommendations Assessment, Development, and Evaluation (GRADE) (Guyatt et al., 2011). The IOM standard 4.1 states "Use a prespecified method to evaluate the body of evidence" (Morton et al., 2011). Major healthcare policy decisions often rest on strength of evidence conclusions, for example, those resulting from the United States Preventive Services Task Force (USPSTF, 2016). Work remains regarding evaluating the reliability and validity of different approaches, and in addition, most approaches are time consuming and resource dependent.

The first characteristic of CER as defined by the IOM is that CER "has the objective of directly informing a specific clinical decision from the patient perspective or a health policy decision from the population perspective" (Ratner et al., 2009). These decisions are about the relative effectiveness of different interventions and heterogeneity often exists with respect to effectiveness as discussed in Chapter 8. As stated earlier in this chapter, comparative effectiveness reviews do not by themselves yield recommendations but the decision perspective must be kept in mind when such reviews are conducted. IPDMA discussed later in this chapter endeavors to use patient-level data to address an individual's decision. Indeed, these decisions can be thought of as prediction problems, while systematic reviews are generally descriptive in nature. Chapter 13 addresses prediction in a mathematical modeling context.

10.3 Individual Participant Data Meta-Analysis

When data from individual participants in the studies comprising a meta-analysis are available to the researcher, it is possible to extract much more information from the synthesis than with summary data only. Such IPDMA has become more common as regulators, private companies, and academic consortia mine data from studies conducted in the course of development of drugs or devices or investigation into innovative treatments or safety concerns. This trend continues to increase with government funders and regulators (EMA, NIH, PCORI, FDA, and NICE) requiring those getting public research funds or regulatory approvals to make information available to the public so as to limit the dangers of publication and reporting bias and increase research transparency. Availability of IPD offers several advantages when conducting meta-analyses, including the ability to ask more complex research questions, reconcile different study protocols and harmonize study databases, investigate potential study bias more thoroughly and correct inadequate reporting, carry out more complex analysis, and provide more nuanced interpretations of data. Each of these will now be discussed briefly.

10.3.1 Developing More Complex Research Questions

Medical research is becoming increasingly patient centered, focusing on the needs of individual patient care. The classical RCT seeks to determine the effect of a treatment on a group of individuals compared to another group that receives a different or no treatment. But the treatment will generally not act in the same way on all group members. For example, the effect on men may differ from that on women or a higher dose might act differently from a lower dose. Traditionally, such subgroup differences were studied, if at all, by meta-regression which was necessarily restricted to consideration of study-level factors that varied between, but not within studies (Schmid et al., 2004). For a patient-level characteristic such as age that varies by individual, within-study variation can be accounted for only if data are available at the individual patient level. IPD considerably expands the range of questions that may be asked (Schmid, 1999; Stewart and Tierney, 2002).

For example, after a meta-analysis found that angiotensin-converting enzyme (ACE) inhibitors improved the prognosis of patients with kidney disease but without diabetes (Giatras et al., 1997), investigators wanted to know more about the mechanism of the effect and optimal treatment strategies. ACE inhibitors were known to lower blood pressure and urine protein excretion, both risk factors for kidney disease, but it was not known whether the drugs conferred additional benefits. Did they have the same effect on all patients or was the effect modified by factors that led to differential effects? What doses worked best and which concomitant medications might improve efficacy? Such questions could only be answered with IPD and multivariate statistical analyses that simultaneously accounted for these variables (Jafar et al., 2001).

10.3.2 Study Reconciliation

Application of the population, intervention, comparator, outcomes, timing, and setting (PICOTS) criteria implies that a meta-analysis consists of a set of studies with common inclusion and exclusion criteria. However, such consistency is rare unless studies are carried out under the same research protocol. These differences are most marked if one compares experimental studies under carefully monitored protocols to observational studies in which data are collected under less-controlled conditions. But even within the sets of experimental and observational studies, differences usually prevail. One study might restrict participants to individuals with blood pressures over 140 mmHg, another might use a criterion of 130, and so forth. In meta-analysis using information from study reports only, checking such characteristics relies on the accuracy and completeness of the reported information, which may be inadequate for a thorough appraisal. IPDMAs are better able to reconcile these differences, standardizing criteria and variable definitions, and filling in missing and incomplete data (Stewart, 1995; Stewart and Tierney, 2002).

In the Thrombolytic Predictive Instrument study (Selker et al., 1997), investigators combined data from 12 RCTs and registries of patients presenting to emergency departments with chest pain. Because some studies that restricted the ages of patients were allowed to be included, it was necessary to apply the same restrictions to all studies in order that inferences would not be confounded by the study. Another key set of variables derived from electrocardiograms, but the protocols and timing at which these were taken differed and needed to be reconciled. Missing forms and other data found to be missing were recovered from other sources or from research in original medical records.

Schmid et al. (2003) describe the details of putting together the Angiotensin-Converting Enzyme Inhibition in Progressive Renal Disease (AIPRD) database from 11 RCTs. This consisted of several linked tables including study-level data with protocol information; cross-sectional patient information (demographic, disease history, comorbidity, and previous medication) from 1,860 patients; outcomes with dates; longitudinal lab data (e.g., blood pressure) from 31,345 records; and 28,073 medication profiles from 10 of the 11 studies. The investigators originally constructed a standardized data form for participants to complete, but discovered that many study teams preferred to send their unedited finalized databases. While this provided complete data of larger scope than initially anticipated, it added substantially to the data management burden of the meta-analysis team which then had to standardize variable definitions; reconcile date formats both across different files for the same study and across studies (some studies used exact dates, other visit numbers); determine baseline dates and calibrate these with randomization dates; translate medication text into English and then parse the strings to extract the drug, dose, and dates; standardize dose amount and schedule across drugs; and calibrate different measurement techniques (e.g., use of exact assay vs. a dipstick test) and units. But availability of detailed data did facilitate checking the accuracy of numbers provided in study reports, screening of implausible values, querying trial investigators about potential errors, checking for additional follow-up that may not have been reported in the published literature, imputing missing values, and correcting data errors and omissions. Nevertheless, reconciliation of data from older studies can suffer if the original study teams are no longer together and the principal investigator no longer has access to the data managers and statisticians with the detailed knowledge of the database.

Establishment of a team that includes all of the participating trial principal investigators is a key to a successful collaboration. This structure formalizes the meta-analysis as a separate study and properly credits the individual study investigators for the work that they contribute to the collaborative effort, while ensuring that each study's data will not be shared with other members of the study group or with investigators outside the study group without their consent. In addition, involving the investigators allows them to contribute their expertise to improve the design and conduct of the meta-analysis and encourages them to contribute toward standardizing and reconciling the database. Each article produced by the collaboration originates from its own writing committee generated from volunteers solicited after the proposed article is approved by the team's steering committee. Analyses are often conducted by the Data Coordinating Center (DCC) of the IPDMA that oversees the combined database, but may be done locally with a portion of the database sent out from the DCC (Stewart, 1995).

10.3.3 Investigate Study and Reporting Bias

As discussed earlier in this chapter, checking component studies for characteristics that may indicate study bias is an important function of meta-analysis because it helps to measure the strength of the evidence available for interpreting findings. Identification of such bias can be problematic when information can be taken only from study reports, though, because it relies completely on the quality of the study report. With IPD, however, the availability of the original data allows for verification of the reported summary statistics and study characteristics. It also allows for checking of the validity of the study-analytic methods (Stewart and Tierney, 2002). For instance, while many studies report using the intent to treat (ITT) principle, a recent study examining the disposition of patient withdrawals and number analyzed indicated that use of ITT was unlikely in many of them (Deo et al., 2011). Inspection of the IPD can reconcile such ambiguities.

Publication and outcome-reporting bias can also complicate meta-analytic inferences. Publication bias refers to the unavailability of studies that are not published, usually because of negative results. The discoverable studies are then biased toward a positive result. A special type of publication bias occurs when parts of studies are undiscoverable, even if the study is known. The most common form occurs when investigators report only some of the measured outcomes, often because these gave positive results. Another example occurs when treatment effect modifiers are identified for those factors interacting with treatment, but not for factors for which interaction is not present. With IPD, such reporting bias can be identified and corrected (Ahmed et al., 2012). IPD analysts, however, must be careful of a bias specific to IPDMA caused by the unavailability of IPD for some studies either because data cannot be accessed or investigators are unwilling to contribute their data. In this case, it may be necessary to use analytic techniques that incorporate both types of data, recognizing that between-patient inferences are limited by the lack of IPD data in some of the studies (Riley et al., 2008a). Meta-analysis in which some of the studies are proprietary (e.g., owned by companies that produce a drug or device) is particularly prone to this problem.

10.3.4 Carry Out More Informative Analyses to Obtain More Nuanced Interpretations of Data

Analytically, the primary advantage of IPD lies in the ability to model patient-level as well as study-level factors. While the number of studies with data defines the sample size relevant for analyzing study-level factors, the number of patients is the key value for analysis of patient-level factors. This enables investigation of effect modification through treatment–factor interactions, as well as adjustment for differences among factors among studies (e.g., differences in age distributions by study) and development of models that apply to individual patients. Survival analysis models using time to follow-up can also be developed with IPD. When some studies have IPD and others do not, it is also possible to construct models that use the patient-level data where possible. Although a detailed explanation of the statistical models involved is beyond the scope of this chapter, we briefly outline some of the basic approaches to demonstrate how they can address these issues.

Many of the early IPD analyses focused on using patient follow-up times to estimate within-study hazard ratios that accounted for patient censoring (Peto, 1989). The study hazard ratios were then combined across studies by standard meta-analytic methods to obtain a pooled hazard ratio. This is an example of a two-stage analysis. The first stage combines the data within study and the second stage combines across studies. Such models, however, fail to use the patient-level data from predictors. An improved two-stage model estimates within-study hazard ratios adjusted for potential confounders and then combines these adjusted hazard ratios across studies. This adjustment is especially important for observational studies where the lack of randomization often introduces correlation between treatment and covariate distributions. The two-stage approach can also estimate treatment interactions by first computing the interaction effect within each study and then pooling these effects across studies. However, many important questions require multivariate analysis to estimate several quantities simultaneously. Such analyses require knowledge of correlations that cannot be readily fit into the two-step framework (Riley et al., 2008b).

The need to differentiate between within-study and among-study treatment effects motivates the use of a multilevel, or one-step approach. The simplest multilevel model has two levels. At the patient level (within study),

$$Y_{ij} = \alpha_j + \beta_j X_{ij} + \varepsilon_{ij},$$

where Y_{ij} is the outcome for patient i in study j, X_{ij} is a patient-level covariate, α_j and β_j are study-specific regression coefficients (i.e., each study has its own slope and intercept), and ε_{ij} are independent random within patient deviations from the regression line with mean zero and variance σ^2. The study-level model is written

$$\alpha_j = \alpha_0 + \alpha_1 Z_j + u_\alpha,$$
$$\beta_j = \beta_0 + \beta_1 Z_j + u_\beta,$$

and describes the dependence of the study-specific α_j and β_j on a study-level covariate Z_j with regression coefficients α_0, α_1, β_0 and β_1, as well as error terms u_α and u_β with zero means and variances $\sigma^2_{u_\alpha}$ and $\sigma^2_{u_\beta}$, respectively. Usually, it is also assumed that u_α and u_β are normally distributed. Sometimes, one assumes that α_j and β_j are correlated within study, although they are always assumed to be independent across studies. These models can be easily extended to add additional patient and study-level covariates as well as interactions between them.

Note that the multilevel model can be written as a mixed model by substituting the between-study equations for α_j and β_j into the within-patient equation to obtain

$$Y_{ij} = \alpha_0 + \beta_0 X_{ij} + \alpha_1 Z_j + \beta_1 Z_j * X_{ij} + u_\alpha + u_\beta X_{ij} + \varepsilon_{ij}.$$

From this formulation, it may be seen that α_1 and β_0 are coefficients for the main effects and β_1 is the coefficient for the interaction between a patient-level and study-level effect. To make the intercepts more interpretable, it may be useful to center X_{ij} and Z_j about their means or some other meaningful constant.

A small example will serve as an illustration. Schmid et al. (2004) used results from 11 RCTs to study whether the effect of ACE inhibitor treatment on change in glomerular filtration rate (GFR), a measure of how well the kidneys clear waste from the body, varied with the baseline level of protein in the urine at the start of the study. Treatment received (ACE or control) is a patient-level covariate (X_{ij}) and the average study urine protein level is a study-level covariate (Z_j). Patient GFR level is the outcome (Y_{ij}). This model is mathematically equivalent to a meta-regression. Because IPD is available, however, baseline urine protein (Z_{ij}) is also known for each patient. One can therefore include this factor in the patient-level model, writing $Y_{ij} = \alpha_j + \beta_j X_{ij} + \gamma_j Z_{ij} + \varepsilon_{ij}$. Retaining Z_j in the study-level model would then permit differentiation of the study-level and patient-level effects of baseline urine protein. Alternatively, one could drop the study-level factor and fit a random-effects regression model.

The results of the analysis are conceptually interesting and illustrate the importance of distinguishing between patient-level and study-level effects. Meta-regression found no significant relationship between the average difference in GFR change comparing treated and control patients against the average baseline urine protein level by study. Random effects regression using the patient-level protein level determined that treatment was more beneficial in patients who started the trials with higher levels of protein in the urine. This differential treatment effect was also found in a two-step approach pooling within-study treatment interactions.

Such a difference between study-level and patient-level analyses is called ecological bias. Examination of Figure 10.2, which displays this effect within each study, is instructive in understanding this bias. The average baseline levels are seen to vary little and generally correspond to a fairly low protein level at which the treatment difference is small. Big effects are found only at high levels of protein within the study. Berlin et al. (2002) present another example from five studies examining how patient-level variables modify the effect of antilymphocyte antibody induction therapy in reducing graft failure among renal transplant patients (Berlin et al., 2002). With IPD, induction therapy was found to be substantially more effective when panel-reactive antibodies were elevated; this interaction was not found with meta-regression.

Ecological bias generally occurs when the group-level average does not reflect the patient-level variation that correlates with outcome variation (Figures 10.2 and 10.3). In some cases, as with the GFR–urine protein relationship, this occurs because the averages vary little across studies; in some cases, the within-study distributions may be quite different. For instance, assume treatment efficacy is concentrated in a high-risk subgroup such as the elderly. Studies with higher proportions of high-risk individuals and lower proportions of low-risk individuals will show an effect whereas those with the reversed distribution will not, even though both sets may have the same average of the factor. In such cases, the more interpretable study-level factor may be the proportion of elderly in the study, rather than the mean age.

Simultaneous modeling of the patient-level and study-level forms of a variable may be useful when they reflect different conceptual effects. For instance, low socioeconomic status (SES) is often correlated with poor health outcomes, reflecting the lack of access to health care among the poor and uneducated. Nevertheless, programs targeted at low SES populations may

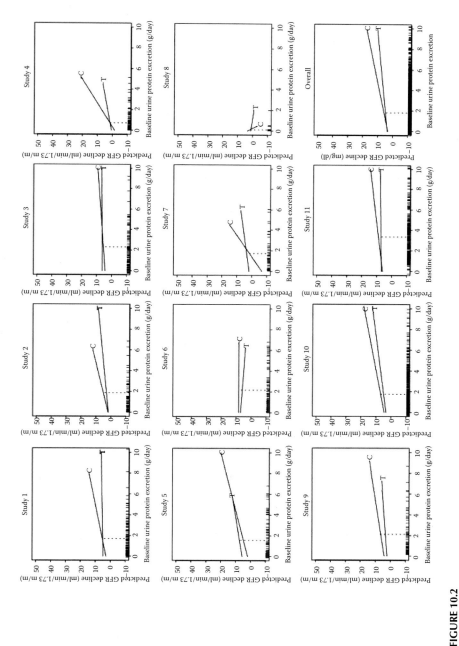

FIGURE 10.2

In each graph, C represents the regression line in the control group, T the regression line in the treatment group. The dotted line indicates the mean level of baseline urine protein in that study and the rug plot shows its distribution in the study.

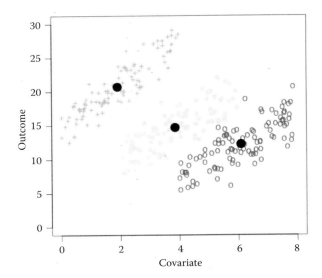

FIGURE 10.3
The different symbols represent data in three separate studies. The solid large black circles represent the average outcome and the average covariate in each study. Outcome and covariate are positively correlated within each study but their averages are negatively correlated across studies.

succeed in improving health. A meta-regression that includes studies both with and without such targeted effects might then find that SES was uncorrelated with health outcomes, whereas the true effect is that within-study lower SES is correlated with poorer outcomes, but across studies, targeted programs are effective. Another example occurs with factors that represent categories of individuals such as sex. Effects for males may differ from those for females, but at the study level where only the proportion of males and females is available these effects may not show up. Furthermore, it is difficult to even interpret the effect of a change in the ratio of males to females. The effect may differ in mixed populations compared to unmixed ones. Changes in male/female mixture proportions may have different effects than comparisons of individual males and females.

Note that under the assumption that the studies with IPD are not systematically different from those without (an assumption that may be unrealistic particularly if the IPD comes from a single source such as a company's proprietary data), the one-step approach can be modified to distinguish between patient and study-level effects even when IPD is only available from some studies (Riley et al., 2008a).

In addition, one can reformulate all the models when the outcomes are discrete categories, counts, or survival times by using different distributional forms for the outcome (e.g., a binomial distribution for a binary outcome) and different link functions for the expectation of the outcome (e.g., a logit function in a logistic regression).

Just as regression models can be used for estimating the effect of variables on responses and for predicting outcomes, meta-analysis using IPD can be used for estimating treatment effects and effect modifiers and also for developing predictive models using data from different databases. For example, Inker et al. (2012) used IPD from 5,352 participants in 13 studies to derive a model for predicting GFR from age, sex, race, serum cystatin, and serum creatinine levels (Inker et al., 2012). This model was validated with data from five additional studies totaling 1,119 participants. Selker et al. (1997) developed five logistic regression models to predict the probability of 30-day and 1-year mortality, stroke, cardiac arrest, and blood transfusion among patients admitted to the emergency department with suspected myocardial infarction (Selker et al., 1997). Such modeling cannot only bring more power to investigate treatment effects in subpopulations, but can also extend the generalizability and robustness of treatment recommendations by incorporating a broad spectrum of patients.

Many of the advantages of IPDMA can be realized through prospectively planning the meta-analysis by designing a series of studies with the same or very similar protocols to be analyzed together upon their completion. Such an approach avoids many of the difficulties of putting together and harmonizing different databases, while increasing the generalizability of the results by applying them in different settings (Berlin and Ghersi, 2005).

Nevertheless, meta-analysis is usually employed to summarize information that has already accumulated from diverse sources. This leads to many challenges and considerable resource needs (Stewart, 1995; Schmid et al., 2003) making IPDMA feasible only for selected important clinical problems, even assuming that the necessary information is available. For example, the controversy about the efficacy of intravenous magnesium in the treatment of acute myocardial infarction arising from the discrepancy between ISIS-4 and a meta-analysis of smaller trials could not be resolved with existing individual patient data because ISIS-4 did not collect data on the timing of administration of magnesium (MAGIC Steering Committee, 2000). Instead, a new trial was needed (MAGIC).

Table 10.2 summarizes the advantages and disadvantages of using IPD rather than summary data to do meta-analysis.

10.4 Summary

Systematic review and meta-analysis have been applied to healthcare topics for over three decades and their value to inform healthcare decisions is no longer debated. The methodologies and processes have advanced to

TABLE 10.2

Comparison of Summary Data versus Individual Patient Data
Meta-Analysis

	Summary Data	Individual Patient
Cost	Cheap	Expensive
Factors	Study level	Patient and study level
Outcomes	Reported	Updated, complete
Data cleaning	Impossible	Possible
Bias	Reporting, ecological	Reporting, retrieval
Interpretation	Study specific	Patient specific

address many early concerns. While these methods are increasingly used to address comparative effectiveness questions, many challenges remain. As the demand for comparative effectiveness information increases, and as data become more readily available, there will also be many opportunities to apply advanced methods such as individual participant meta-analysis to better provide patient-centered information. Here, we summarize major areas where improvements are needed.

10.4.1 Need for Better Primary Studies and Reporting of Information

A frequent conclusion of comparative effectiveness reviews is that there is limited or no direct evidence to answer the research questions. The three comparative effectiveness review examples discussed in this chapter exemplify this problem. All three examples point to the lack of direct comparative effectiveness studies across treatment modalities of interests. These examples also brought out many common issues across topics, not just from the perspective of conducting systematic reviews but for CER and PCOR issues as well. For many problems, there is a lack of relevant studies or the available studies are often of low quality thus limiting the ability to form strong conclusions. Research questions in comparative effectiveness reviews often ask for analyses on population subgroups to assess the possibility of heterogeneity of treatment effects in different patient populations. However, many studies either do not include population subgroups or do not report them to allow these analyses. The lack of head-to-head comparison studies requires the use of indirect evidence that weakens the inferences that could be made.

The chronic venous ulcers comparative effectiveness review points to the lack of consensus in the primary literature on disease definitions and the types of outcomes to be synthesized. This problem speaks to the need for the community including clinical researchers, government regulators, payers, and healthcare products industry, to establish a consensus about how to conduct meaningful studies in this area. The objective would be to develop better standards for disease definition, interventions, comparison groups, and outcome measures. These experts could create templates for study designs that better demonstrate efficacy. A report published by the Center for Medical Technology and Policy, "Methodological Recommendations for Comparative Effectiveness Research on the Treatment of Chronic Wounds," exemplifies this type of activity (Sonnad et al., 2013).

10.4.2 Need to Develop Methods to Optimally Engage Stakeholders and Patients

The increasing emphasis on evidence-based practice and patient-centered decision making mandates that not only the review of evidence be rigorous but that the process be inclusive to involve relevant stakeholders and patients. Interactions with users of the reviews in refining the research questions will ensure the relevance of the systematic reviews and that the results will be useful to decision makers. Optimal methods to achieve desirable end results have yet to be determined. Proposed approaches such as the 7-P approach to identify a stakeholder should be evaluated.

10.4.3 Need to Incorporate Information from Different Designs and to Combine Individual and Aggregate Data

Ideally, a comparative effectiveness review should include all relevant information and in its most granular form. Information about the effectiveness and safety of interventions should be obtained not only from RCTs, but from nonrandomized experimental studies, and from observational studies and even registry analyses. Traditionally, comparative effectiveness reviews have used only evidence from randomized trials to estimate intervention effects. The rationale is that, compared to randomized designs, nonrandomized studies are more susceptible to confounding bias (Higgins and Green, 2008). However, useful information can be obtained from nonrandomized studies that have been carefully analyzed to adjust for residual confounding. Chapters 1 and 2 expand on causally explicit analyses that aim to estimate causal effects from observational data. Schemes that allow learning across designs include approaches that model potential bias (Eddy et al., 1990; Kaizar, 2006, 2015) or that correct study estimates for bias (quantitative bias modeling) (Greenland, 2005; Lash et al., 2014). Cross-design synthesis is also discussed in Chapter 7 of this book.

Furthermore, addressing questions about the heterogeneity of the treatment effect (covered in Chapter 8), for example, how the treatment effect changes across participants with different characteristics, requires modeling interactions between treatment and participant-level factors. For logistical and other reasons, it may be practical to obtain individual patient data for a subset of relevant studies, and have access only to aggregate-level data from other studies. In such cases, one can combine information across studies with individual patient data and aggregate data, as long as attention is given to the fact that aggregate data studies typically report estimates for marginal treatment effects, while analysis of individual participant studies typically focuses on estimates of conditional effects. Schemes for combining information across individual-level and aggregate-level data have been reviewed in the literature (Jackson et al., 2006; Riley et al., 2007, 2008a; Sutton et al., 2008).

10.4.4 Need to Modernize Review Methods

Comparative effectiveness reviews are large, costly, and require a significant amount of time to produce. In the 2015 report to Congressional Committees on CER, the General Accounting Office analyzed 74 AHRQ comparative effectiveness reviews and found the time when a systematic review began to when the findings were disseminated ranged from 1 year to more than 4 years (USGAO, 2015). The time required to produce evidence reviews has probably increased since AHRQ began the EPC program in 1997, this increase can be attributed to additional steps and processes implemented in recent years to ensure rigor, completeness, and inclusiveness. Incorporating all of the 2011 IOM report and future standards without concomitant improvements in the efficiency of the processes will undoubtedly add time and costs.

To produce timely comparative effectiveness reviews without simply adding more people (and hence costs) to the task, systematic review methods and processes must be made more efficient by taking advantage of modern technologies. While researchers have used computer technologies to produce the reviews, such as conducting computerized literature searches, using electronic spreadsheets and database programs to organize studies and abstract data, and using word processors to draft reports, many systematic review processes have remained largely a manual process. Two critical and rate-limiting steps in the systematic review process that currently are mostly performed by humans are screening of citations and abstracting data from eligible full-text articles. Modern tools are beginning to appear to address these areas. For example, Abstractkr, a computer program funded by an AHRQ research grant, uses machine-learning technology to assist researchers to screen abstracts and reduces this mundane task to a fraction of the time previously needed (Wallace et al., 2012). Computer-assisted data abstraction tools are beginning to be developed and evaluated (Ip et al., 2012). Applying these advanced computational methods could significantly increase the efficiency, reduce costs, and at the same time improve the quality of these products.

Finally, comparative effectiveness review has become a global activity that is undertaken by numerous government agencies and independent organizations. Independent efforts by different groups that have similar needs often lead to unnecessary replications. Thus, global collaboration in evidence synthesis would be highly desirable to optimize the utilization of valuable resources. The service provided by the PROSPERO website to prospectively register systematic reviews is an important step toward that direction. Abstracting data from primary articles is probably the most time consuming and costly aspect of a systematic review. Archiving these tediously and expensively collected data and making them freely available to the global research community could allow other groups to reuse these data to answer additional questions and conduct future updates. The Systematic Review Data Repository (SRDR) funded by AHRQ that went into operation in 2012 is one such tool (Ip et al., 2012).

References

Advanced Ovarian Cancer Trialists Group. 1991. Chemotherapy in advanced ovarian cancer: An overview of randomised clinical trials. *British Medical Journal*, 303, 884–893.

Ahmed, I., Sutton, A. J. and Riley, R. D. 2012. Assessment of publication bias, selection bias, and unavailable data in meta-analyses using individual participant data: A database survey. *British Medical Journal*, 344, d7762.

AHRQ. 2014. *Methods Guide for Effectiveness and Comparative Effectiveness Reviews*. AHRQ Publication No. 10(14)-EHC063-EF. Rockville, MD: Agency for Healthcare Research and Quality.

Barza, M., Ioannidis, J. P., Cappelleri, J. C. and Lau, J. 1996. Single or multiple daily doses of aminoglycosides: A meta-analysis. *British Medical Journal*, 312, 338–345.

Bastian, H., Glasziou, P. and Chalmers, I. 2010. Seventy-five trials and eleven systematic reviews a day: How will we ever keep up? *PLoS Medicine*, 7, e1000326.

Berkman, N. D., Lohr, K. N., Ansari, M., Mcdonagh, M., Balk, E., Whitlock, E., Reston, J., Bass, E., Butler, M. and Gartlehner, G. 2013. Grading the strength of a body of evidence when assessing health care interventions for the effective health care program of the Agency for Healthcare Research and Quality: An update methods guide for effectiveness and comparative effectiveness reviews. https://www.ncbi.nlm.nih.gov/books/NBK174881/?report=reader (accessed October 29, 2016).

Berlin, J. A. and Ghersi, D. 2005. Chapter 3. Preventing publication bias: Registries and prospective meta-analysis. In: *Publication Bias in Meta-Analysis: Prevention, Assessment and Adjustments* (Edited by H.R. Rothstein, A.J. Sutton, and M. Borenstein), pp. 35–48. West Sussex, England: John Wiley & Sons, Ltd.

Berlin, J. A., Santanna, J., Schmid, C. H., Szczech, L. A. and Feldman, H. I. 2002. Individual patient-versus group-level data meta-regressions for the investigation of treatment effect modifiers: Ecological bias rears its ugly head. *Statistics in Medicine*, 21, 371–387.

Borenstein, M., Hedges, L. V., Higgins, J. and Rothstein, H. R. 2010. A basic introduction to fixed-effect and random-effects models for meta-analysis. *Research Synthesis Methods*, 1, 97–111.

Brook, R. A., Wahlqvist, P., Kleinman, N. L., Wallander, M. A., Campbell, S. M. and Smeeding, J. E. 2007. Cost of gastro-oesophageal reflux disease to the employer:

A perspective from the United States. *Aliment Pharmacological Therapy*, 26, 889–898.

Chandler, J., Churchill, R., Higgins, J., Lasserson, T. and Tovey, D. 2013. Methodological Expectations of Cochrane Intervention Reviews (MECIR). *Methodological Standards for the Conduct of New Cochrane Intervention Reviews*. Version, 2.

Chang, S. M., Bass, E. B., Berkman, N., Carey, T. S., Kane, R. L., Lau, J. and Ratichek, S. 2013. Challenges in implementing The Institute of Medicine systematic review standards. *Systematic Review*, 2, 69.

Clarke, M., Hopewell, S. and Chalmers, I. 2007. Reports of clinical trials should begin and end with up-to-date systematic reviews of other relevant evidence: A status report. *Journal of Royal Society Medicine*, 100, 187–190.

Cochran, W. G. 1954. The combination of estimates from different experiments. *Biometrics*, 10, 101–129.

Concannon, T. W., Meissner, P., Grunbaum, J. A., Mcelwee, N., Guise, J. M., Santa, J., Conway, P. H., Daudelin, D., Morrato, E. H. and Leslie, L. K. 2012. A new taxonomy for stakeholder engagement in patient-centered outcomes research. *Journal of General Internal Medicine*, 27, 985–991.

Deo, A., Schmid, C. H., Earley, A., Lau, J. and Uhlig, K. 2011. Loss to analysis in randomized controlled trials in CKD. *American Journal of Kidney Diseases*, 58, 349–355.

Eddy, D. M., Hasselblad, V. and Shachter, R. 1990. An introduction to a Bayesian method for meta-analysis the confidence profile method. *Medical Decision Making*, 10, 15–23.

Evidence-Based Medicine Working Group. 1992. Evidence-based medicine. A new approach to teaching the practice of medicine. *Journal of American Medical Association*, 268, 2420–2425.

Galbraith, R. F. 1994. Some applications of radial plots. *Journal of the American Statistical Association*, 89, 1232–1242.

Giatras, I., Lau, J. and Levey, A. S. 1997. Effect of angiotensin-converting enzyme inhibitors on the progression of nondiabetic renal disease: A meta-analysis of randomized trials. *Annals of Internal Medicine*, 127, 337–345.

GISSI. 1987. Long-term effects of intravenous thrombolysis in acute myocardial infarction: Final report of the GISSI study. Gruppo Italiano per lo Studio della Streptochi-nasi nell'Infarto Miocardico (GISSI). [No authors listed] *Lancet*, 2(8564), 871–874.

Gleser, L. J. and Olkin, I. 2009. Stochastically dependent effect sizes. In: *The Handbook of Research Synthesis and Meta-analysis* (edited by H. Cooper, L. V. Hedges, and J. C. Valentine), 2nd ed., pp. 357-Ű376. New York: Russell Sage Foundation.

Greenland, S. 2005. Multiple-bias modelling for analysis of observational data. *Journal of the Royal Statistical Society: Series A (Statistics in Society)*, 168, 267–306.

Guyatt, G. H., Oxman, A. D., Schünemann, H. J., Tugwell, P. and Knottnerus, A. 2011. GRADE guidelines: A new series of articles in the Journal of Clinical Epidemiology. *Journal of Clinical Epidemiology*, 64, 380–382.

Hartung, J., Knapp, G. and Sinha, B. K. 2011. *Statistical Meta-Analysis with Applications*, Hoboken, NJ: John Wiley & Sons.

Higgins, J. and Thompson, S. G. 2002. Quantifying heterogeneity in a meta-analysis. *Statistics in Medicine*, 21, 1539–1558.

Higgins, J. P. and Green, S. 2008. *Cochrane Handbook for Systematic Reviews of Interventions*, Wiley Online Library.

Inker, L. A., Schmid, C. H., Tighiouart, H., Eckfeldt, J. H., Feldman, H. I., Greene, T., Kusek, J. W., Manzi, J., Van Lente, F. and Zhang, Y. L. 2012. Estimating glomerular filtration rate from serum creatinine and cystatin C. *New England Journal of Medicine*, 367, 20–29.

Ip, S., Bonis, P., Tatsioni, A., Raman, G., Chew, P., Kupelnick, B., Fu, L., Devine, D. and Lau, J. 2005. AHRQ comparative effectiveness reviews. *Comparative Effectiveness of Management Strategies for Gastroesophageal Reflux Disease*, Rockville, MD: Agency for Healthcare Research and Quality (US).

Ip, S., Hadar, N., Keefe, S., Parkin, C., Iovin, R., Balk, E. M. and Lau, J. 2012. A web-based archive of systematic review data. *Systematic Review*, 1, 15.

Jackson, C., Best, N. and Richardson, S. 2006. Improving ecological inference using individual-level data. *Statistics in Medicine*, 25, 2136–2159.

Jackson, D., Riley, R. and White, I. R. 2011. Multivariate meta-analysis: Potential and promise. *Statistics in Medicine*, 30, 2481–2498.

Jadad, A., Cook, D., Jones, A., Klassen, T. P., Tugwell, P., Moher, M. and Moher, D. 1998. Methodology and reports of systematic reviews and meta-analyses: A comparison of Cochrane reviews with articles published in paper-based journals. *Journal of American Medical Association*, 280(3), 278–280.

Jafar, T. H., Schmid, C. H., Landa, M., Giatras, I., Toto, R., Remuzzi, G., Maschio, G., Brenner, B. M., Kamper, A. and Zucchelli, P. 2001. Angiotensin-converting enzyme inhibitors and progression of nondiabetic renal disease: A meta-analysis of patient-level data. *Annals of Internal Medicine*, 135, 73–87.

Kaizar, E. E. 2006. *Combining Information from Diverse Sources*, PhD dissertation, Carnegie Mellon University, Pittsburgh, PA.

Kaizar, E. E. 2015. Incorporating both randomized and observational data into a single analysis. *Annual Review of Statistics and Its Application*, 2, 49–72.

Karabatsos, G., Talbott, E. and Walker, S. G. 2015. A Bayesian nonparametric meta-analysis model. *Research Synthesis Methods*, 6, 28–44.

Kreis, J., Puhan, M. A., Schunemann, H. J. and Dickersin, K. 2013. Consumer involvement in systematic reviews of comparative effectiveness research. *Health Expectations*, 16, 323–337.

Lash, T. L., Fox, M. P., Maclehose, R. F., Maldonado, G., Mccandless, L. C. and Greenland, S. 2014. Good practices for quantitative bias analysis. *International Journal of Epidemiology*, 43, 1969–1985.

Lau, J., Chang, S., Berkman, N., Ratichek, S. J., Balshem, H., Brasure, M., and Moher, D. 2013. *EPC Response to IOM Standards for Systematic Reviews, Research White Paper* (Prepared by the Tufts Evidence-based Practice Center, Tufts Medical Center, Boston, MA, under Contract No. HHSA290-2007-10055-I). AHRQ Publication No. 13-EHC006-EF. Rockville, MD: Agency for Healthcare Research and Quality, Available at: http://effectivehealthcare. ahrq.gov/index.cfm/search-for-guides-reviews-and-reports/?productid=1459 &pageaction=displayproduct.

Lau, J., Ioannidis, J. P. A. and Schmid, C. H. 1997. Quantitative synthesis in systematic reviews. *Annual International Medicine*, 127, 820–826.

Lau, J., Ioannidis, J. P. and Schmid, C. H. 1998. Summing up evidence: One answer is not always enough. *Lancet*, 351, 123–127.

MAGIC Steering Committee. 2000. Rationale and design of the magnesium in coronaries (MAGIC) study: A clinical trial to reevaluate the efficacy of early administration of magnesium in acute myocardial infarction. *American Heart Journal*, 139, 10–14.

Mavridis, D. and Salanti, G. 2013. A practical introduction to multivariate meta-analysis. *Statistical Methods in Medical Research*, 22, 133–158.

Morton, S., Levit, L., Berg, A. and Eden, J. 2011. *Finding What Works in Health Care: Standards for Systematic Reviews*, Washington, DC: National Academies Press.

Olkin, I., Dahabreh, I. J. and Trikalinos, T. A. 2012. GOSH—A graphical display of study heterogeneity. *Research Synthesis Methods*, 3, 214–223.

Peto, R. 1989. Effects of adjuvant tamoxifen and of cytotoxic therapy on mortality in early breast cancer. An overview of 61 randomised trials among 28,896 women. *Hormone Research in Paediatrics*, 32, 165–165.

Ratner, R., Eden, J., Wolman, D., Greenfield, S. and Sox, H. 2009. *Initial National Priorities for Comparative Effectiveness Research*. Institute of Medicine. Washington, DC: National Academies Press.

Riley, R. D., Lambert, P. C., Staessen, J. A., Wang, J., Gueyffier, F., Thijs, L. and Boutitie, F. 2008a. Meta-analysis of continuous outcomes combining individual patient data and aggregate data. *Statistics in Medicine*, 27, 1870–1893.

Riley, R. D., Simmonds, M. C. and Look, M. P. 2007. Evidence synthesis combining individual patient data and aggregate data: A systematic review identified current practice and possible methods. *Journal of Clinical Epidemiology*, 60, 431–439.

Riley, R. D., Thompson, J. R. and Abrams, K. R. 2008b. An alternative model for bivariate random-effects meta-analysis when the within-study correlations are unknown. *Biostatistics*, 9, 172–186.

Rutter, C. M. and Gatsonis, C. A. 2001. A hierarchical regression approach to meta-analysis of diagnostic test accuracy evaluations. *Statistics in Medicine*, 20, 2865–2884.

Salanti, G. 2012. Indirect and mixed-treatment comparison, network, or multiple-treatments meta-analysis: Many names, many benefits, many concerns for the next generation evidence synthesis tool. *Research Synthesis Methods*, 3, 80–97.

Schmid, C. H. 1999. Exploring heterogeneity in randomized trials via meta-analysis. *Drug Information Journal*, 33, 211–224.

Schmid, C. H., Landa, M., Jafar, T. H., Giatras, I., Karim, T., Reddy, M., Stark, P. C., Levey, A. S. and Group, A.-C. E. I. I. P. R. D. S. 2003. Constructing a database of individual clinical trials for longitudinal analysis. *Controlled Clinical Trials*, 24, 324–340.

Schmid, C. H., Lau, J., Mcintosh, M. W. and Cappelleri, J. C. 1998. An empirical study of the effect of the control rate as a predictor of treatment efficacy in meta-analysis of clinical trials. *Statistics in Medicine*, 17, 1923–1942.

Schmid, C. H., Stark, P. C., Berlin, J. A., Landais, P. and Lau, J. 2004. Meta-regression detected associations between heterogeneous treatment effects and study-level, but not patient-level, factors. *Journal of Clinical Epidemiology*, 57, 683–697.

Schmid, C. H., Trikalinos, T. A. and Olkin, I. 2014. Bayesian network meta-analysis for unordered categorical outcomes with incomplete data. *Research Synthesis Methods*, 5, 162–185.

Selker, H. P., Griffith, J. L., Beshansky, J. R., Schmid, C. H., Califf, R. M., D'Agostino, R. B., Laks, M. M., Lee, K. L., Maynard, C. and Selvester, R. H. 1997. Patient-specific predictions of outcomes in myocardial infarction for real-time emergency use: A thrombolytic predictive instrument. *Annals of Internal Medicine*, 127, 538–556.

Sonnad, S. S., Goldsack, J. C., Mohr, P. and Tunis, S. 2013. Methodological recommendations for comparative research on the treatment of chronic wounds. *Journal of Wound Care*, 22, 470–480.

Sox, H., Mcneil, B., Eden, J. and Wheatley, B. 2008. *Knowing What Works in Health Care: A Roadmap for the Nation*, Washington, DC: National Academies Press.

Stewart, L. A. 1995. Practical methodology of meta-analyses (overviews) using updated individual patient data. *Statistics in Medicine*, 14, 2057–2079.

Stewart, L. A. and Tierney, J. F. 2002. To IPD or not to IPD? Advantages and disadvantages of systematic reviews using individual patient data. *Evaluation and the Health Professions*, 25, 76–97.

Sutton, A. J., Kendrick, D. and Coupland, C. A. 2008. Meta-analysis of individual- and aggregate-level data. *Statistics in Medicine*, 27, 651–669.

Terasawa, T., Dvorak, T., Ip, S., Raman, G., Lau, J. and Trikalinos, T. A. 2009. Systematic review: Charged-particle radiation therapy for cancer. *Annals of Internal Medicine*, 151, 556–565.

Trikalinos, T. A., Hoaglin, D. C. and Schmid, C. H. 2014a. An empirical comparison of univariate and multivariate meta-analyses for categorical outcomes. *Statistics in Medicine*, 33, 1441–1459.

Trikalinos, T. A., Hoaglin, D. C., Small, K. M., Terrin, N. and Schmid, C. H. 2014b. Methods for the joint meta-analysis of multiple tests. *Research Synthesis Methods*, 5, 294–312.

Trikalinos, T. A. and Olkin, I. 2008. A method for the meta-analysis of mutually exclusive binary outcomes. *Statistics in Medicine*, 27, 4279–4300.

Trikalinos, T. A., Terasawa, T., Ip, S., Raman, G. and Lau, J. 2009. AHRQ comparative effectiveness technical briefs. *Particle Beam Radiation Therapies for Cancer*, Rockville, MD: Agency for Healthcare Research and Quality (US).

United States General Accountability Office. Comparative Effectiveness Research: HHS Needs to Strengthen Dissemination and Data-Capacity Building Efforts. 2015. GAO-15-280.

USPSTF. 2016. *Grade Definitions* [Online]. U.S. Preventive Services Task Force. Available: http://www.uspreventiveservicestaskforce.org/Page/Name/grade-definitions [accessed October 29, 2016].

Viechtbauer, W. 2010. Conducting meta-analyses in R with the metafor package. *Journal of Statistical Software*, 36, 1–48.

Wallace, B. C., Dahabreh, I. J., Trikalinos, T. A., Lau, J., Trow, P. and Schmid, C. H. 2012. Closing the gap between methodologists and end-users: R as a computational back-end. *Journal of Statistical Software*, 49, 1–15.

Zenilman, J., Valle, M. F., Malas, M. B., Maruthur, N., Qazi, U., Suh, Y., Wilson, L. M., Haberl, E. B., Bass, E. B. and Lazarus, G. 2013. AHRQ comparative effectiveness reviews. *Chronic Venous Ulcers: A Comparative Effectiveness Review of Treatment Modalities*, Rockville, MD: Agency for Healthcare Research and Quality (US).

11

Network Meta-Analysis

Orestis Efthimiou, Anna Chaimani, Dimitris Mavridis,
and Georgia Salanti

CONTENTS

ABSTRACT   Meta-analysis is now established in comparative effectiveness research as a valid statistical tool, useful for synthesizing evidence from studies that compare two treatments for the same condition. For the majority of diseases, however, more than two treatments are available and trials might compare different subsets of them. When this is the case, a simple, pairwise meta-analysis cannot provide a definite answer to decision makers as to which intervention is associated with the largest benefit for patients with the target condition. In order to address this very common scenario, a statistical tool has been developed called network meta-analysis (NMA). NMA can be used to jointly analyze the totality of evidence in order to provide estimates for all relative treatment effects, to compare treatments that have never been compared head-to-head, and to obtain a ranking of all competing interventions in order to further facilitate the decision-making process. In this chapter, we introduce the basic concepts and discuss the underlying assumptions of NMA. We present alternative methods for fitting models and for assessing the validity of the underlying assumptions. We especially focus on the various statistical methods that can be applied for checking the consistency of the evidence, a key aspect of NMA. We provide worked examples in order to illustrate all methods presented in the chapter. Finally, we discuss various graphical and tabular options for presenting the results.

11.1 Introduction

Evidence-based practices are crucial in developing and maintaining high-quality medical care. The Institute of Medicine in the United States set a goal that, by the year 2020, 90% of clinical decisions will be evidence-based (Institute of Medicine (US) Roundtable on Evidence-Based Medicine, 2009). The necessity for evidence-based practices calls for comparative effectiveness research (CER) to inform healthcare decisions by providing evidence on the effectiveness, benefits, and harms of available treatment options. An integral part of CER is the quantitative synthesis of the available evidence via meta-analysis. International and national health-care institutions (e.g., World Health Organization [WHO], and National Institute for Health and Clinical Excellence [NICE] in the United Kingdom) often utilize meta-analyses to inform clinical practice. As there is a plethora of interventions available for any clinical condition, traditional meta-analysis that compares two interventions at a time cannot adequately answer important clinical questions: which of the multiple available treatments work best, for which patients, under what circumstances, and which treatments are associated with the optimal balance between benefits and harms.

For many health conditions, there is a large number of competing interventions compared in randomized control trials (RCT) that form a connected network of evidence where information flows directly, indirectly, or both across the available treatment comparisons. Such a body of evidence can be synthesized via network meta-analysis (NMA) (Higgins and Whitehead, 1996; Lu and Ades, 2004; Caldwell et al., 2005; Salanti et al., 2008). The benefits of NMA include estimating the comparative effectiveness of two interventions that have not been compared directly in any of the trials, obtaining more precise and powerful estimates and providing a ranking of treatments. NMA is now an established method in the evidence-based medicine literature and is increasingly used to assess comparative effectiveness of healthcare interventions (Bafeta et al., 2013; Lee, 2014; Nikolakopoulou et al., 2014). This growth has led international organizations to provide guidelines for the appropriate conduct of NMA (e.g., the Decision Support Unit of NICE provides extensive guidance on performing an NMA [2013], the International Society for Pharmacoeconomics and Outcomes Research [ISPOR] has established the Indirect Treatment Comparison Good Research Practices Task force [Hoaglin et al., 2011; Jansen et al., 2011] and the Cochrane Collaboration the "Comparing Multiple Interventions Group" to promote relevant methodology, http://cmimg.cochrane.org/).

The aim of this chapter is to present the current state of the art of NMA. In Section 11.2, we present the datasets used to illustrate the various aspects of the model. Section 11.3 epitomizes the basic concepts and main assumptions underlying NMA and sets the notation that is followed in the rest of the chapter. Section 11.4 presents a synopsis of the modeling techniques that have been developed to fit NMA and Section 11.5 reviews the methods used to evaluate statistically the basic assumption of an NMA model. We review several approaches used to communicate results in Section 11.6. We conclude with a discussion in Section 11.7.

Section III of this volume addresses a number of systematic review and meta-analysis topics in CER. The interested reader is also directed to the first chapter in the section (Chapter 10) for a general background on systematic reviews and basic meta-analysis. As an alternative to this chapter on NMA, Chapter 12 presents a Bayesian approach to NMA with multiple outcomes. Chapter 7 discusses cross-design synthesis in which multiple data sources are combined to address CER decisions.

11.2 Datasets

We use two published datasets to exemplify the presented methods and elucidate the various aspects of NMA. The first example is a network that includes 20 trials evaluating four treatments for heavy menstrual bleeding (Middleton et al., 2010): hysterectomy (which we code as HY), first-generation hysteroscopic and second-generation nonhysteroscopic techniques for endometrial destruction (treatments FGED and SGED, respectively), and the levonorgestrel-releasing intrauterine system Mirena (treatment MI). Each study in this network compares two treatments (two-arm studies). The primary outcome is patient dissatisfaction at 12 months measured as the number of dissatisfied patients out of completers in each study arm. The relative effectiveness is measured by the logarithm of the odds ratio ($\log OR$) along with its 95% confidence interval (CI). Data for this network are shown in Table 11A.1 in Appendix 11A.1. There are 5 studies comparing FGED to HY, 11 studies comparing FGED to SG, 1 study comparing FGED to MI, and 3 studies comparing SGED to MI. There are no studies directly performing the MI vs. HY or the SGED vs. HY comparisons.

The second example is a network that consists of 24 studies comparing four antiplatelet regimens and placebo (coded as PL) for the prevention of serious vascular events after transient ischemic attack or stroke (Thijs et al., 2008). The competing antiplatelet regimens are aspirin (coded as A), the combination of aspirin and dipyridamole (treatment A+DP), thienopyridines (treatment TH), and thienopyridines plus aspirin (coded as TH+A). Eight studies compare PL to A, two studies TH+A to TH, three studies A to A+DP, and four studies A to TH. Each of the comparisons PL vs. A+DP, PL vs. TH, TH+A vs. A, and A+DP vs. TH is evaluated in only one study. There are three additional three-arm studies comparing PL, A+DP, and TH. The data for this network are presented in Table 11A.2 in Appendix 11A.1. Note that there is one study (ID 24) in the dataset with zero events in both arms; this study has been excluded from all analyses and consequently the comparison TH vs. A+DP is not informed directly.

The network graphs for these two datasets are depicted in Figure 11.1. The nodes represent the competing treatments and the edges represent the available direct comparisons. The absence of an edge between two treatments (e.g., between HY and SGED) means that the corresponding comparison was not performed in any of the studies. The thickness of each edge is proportional to the number of the studies in the corresponding comparison. The size of each node corresponds to the total number of patients randomized to the treatment.

11.3 Basic Concepts and Assumptions Underlying NMA

Key concepts in NMA are the indirect estimation of effects and the synthesis of direct and indirect evidence. We may obtain an indirect estimate for the

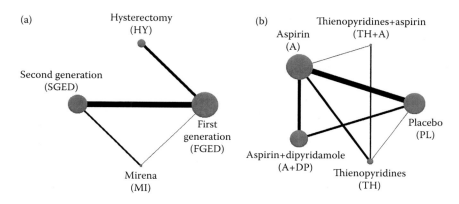

FIGURE 11.1
Heavy menstrual bleeding (a) and serious vascular events network (b). Nodes correspond to treatments; edges correspond to the comparisons reported in studies.

relative effects between two interventions by pooling studies that compare each intervention to a common comparator. Suppose that we have three interventions A, B, and C and that there are studies directly comparing A vs. B and A vs. C. We can get an indirect estimate for the relative effects of B vs. C because both treatments are compared to A (Bucher et al., 1997). This is particularly useful if B and C are not compared directly in any of the studies since it allows us to infer indirectly for their relative effect. In the heavy menstrual bleeding example, we may get an indirect estimate for the relative effectiveness of hysterectomy versus second-generation nonhysteroscopic techniques although there are no studies directly comparing this pair of interventions (see Figure 11.1a). Even when there is direct evidence, synthesizing direct and indirect information via NMA, we get a "mixed" estimate that increases power and precision because more data are being used. In complex networks consisting of many treatments, indirect evidence can be obtained through many different paths and not necessarily via a single common comparator. All these paths are synthesized along with the direct evidence to produce the mixed estimate.

There is controversy around the validity of indirect evidence and its importance when direct evidence is available. Within an RCT, patients are randomized to each of the treatment arms. However, as treatments are not randomized across studies, indirect comparison provides observational evidence and might therefore be subject to bias and confounding (Caldwell et al., 2005). The NICE Decision Support Unit (2013) and the Cochrane Handbook (Higgins and Green, 2013) express a preference for direct evidence, highlighting the observational nature of indirect evidence, and encourage the use of indirect evidence as a supplemental analysis. However, the gain in precision by using indirect evidence may be substantial (Cooper et al., 2011), while indirect evidence can be occasionally less biased than direct evidence (Song et al., 2012). This will be the case, for example, when placebo-controlled trials of a new treatment are biased to the same extent as placebo-controlled trials of an older treatment (e.g., due to sponsorship bias). In this case, when computing the indirect comparison of new versus older treatment, the two biases will cancel out and the corresponding estimate will be unbiased, while there might still be bias in studies directly comparing these two treatments (Song et al., 2008).

Suppose that A is the reference treatment (e.g., placebo) and there are two new active interventions B and C. New treatments are commonly compared to placebo for regulatory purposes. However, placebo-controlled studies are not directly relevant to decision making, as policy makers are often interested in the direct comparison of active agents (Sutton and Higgins, 2008). In the menstrual bleeding example, there is only one study comparing first-generation hysteroscopic techniques to Mirena and the uncertainty is large using only direct evidence ($OR = 0.35$ with a 95% CI ranging from 0.06 to 1.95).

NMA, as any statistical model, is built on assumptions. The key assumption in NMA is that of similarity (Song et al., 2003) or transitivity (Salanti, 2012), implying that there are no differences in the distribution of the effect modifiers across treatment comparisons. This assumption *can be tested statistically* but also *conceptually and epidemiologically* (Salanti, 2012). In practice, the transitivity assumption can be evaluated by comparing the distribution of the potential effect modifiers across the different sets of studies grouped by comparison (Jansen and Naci, 2013). Suppose that the A vs. B studies involve younger patients than the A vs. C studies. If age is an effect modifier, the two types of studies will provide an invalid indirect comparison for B vs. C due to confounding by age. Another example where the transitivity assumption is doubtful is when the common comparator, say A, differs systematically between A vs. B and A vs. C trials. Treatment A may be given in different doses or in different modalities. When comparing different fluoride treatments for the prevention of dental caries, an indirect estimate between fluoride toothpaste and fluoride rinse via placebo may not hold because placebo modality differs between the two comparisons (Salanti et al., 2009). A thorough review of the transitivity assumption and examples where it might be violated are given elsewhere (Salanti, 2012; Donegan et al., 2013). The statistical manifestation of transitivity is called consistency. Consistency states that direct and indirect evidence are in agreement and can be evaluated statistically by comparing the two sources of evidence (direct and indirect). A network can be checked for consistency only when it includes *closed loops*, that is, only in the presence of polygons in the network graph. In Section 11.5, we discuss in depth various alternative methods for assessing the consistency of a network.

11.4 Models for NMA and Fitting Options

Several modeling strategies have been suggested to fit NMA models. All approaches described in this section are equivalent and their choice usually depends on the availability of suitable software routines and the technical expertise of the researchers. Different approaches may lead to slightly different estimates: for example, fitting an NMA model in a frequentist setting may give somewhat different results than fitting the model following a Bayesian approach (see Chapter 12). These small differences, however, should not be seen as a limitation of the model nor should they deter decision makers from using the results of an NMA.

We discuss the available software options for fitting each method in Appendix 11B.1.

11.4.1 Notation and Setup of the Model

Let us consider a network comprising N studies that involve T different treatments and let us assume that t_i treatments are compared in study i. NMA synthesizes all available data to estimate simultaneously any relative treatment effect (e.g., odds ratios and mean differences) for each pair of the T treatments.

11.4.1.1 Parameters Denoting Relative Treatment Effects

Let us denote with μ_{CB} the parameter underlying the true relative treatment effect of C vs. B; that is, the effect of treatment C minus the effect of treatment B. The assumption of consistency in the network implies that

$$\mu_{CB} = \mu_{CA} - \mu_{BA} \tag{11.1}$$

Equation 11.1 suggests that not all relative effects need to be estimated from the data. Consider a vector of dimension $T - 1$ that includes the true effects of all treatments relative to a (randomly selected) reference treatment A, $\mu = (\mu_{BA}, \mu_{CA}, \dots, \mu_{TA})'$. This vector includes only a subset of pairwise relative effects, usually called "basic parameters" or "basic contrasts." For brevity, we denote the vector of basic parameters as $\mu = (\mu_B, \mu_C, \dots, \mu_T)'$. Equation 11.1 suggests that all possible treatment comparisons can be written as linear functions of elements in μ. Note that the choice of basic parameters is arbitrary; different sets of $T - 1$ parameters can be used as long as the elements of μ are independent and every treatment in the network is included in at least one basic contrast.

11.4.1.2 Data Reported in Studies

The parameters $\mu = (\mu_B, \mu_C, \ldots, \mu_T)'$ can be estimated from the study data. A study with t_i arms estimates a total of $\binom{t_i}{2}$ relative treatment effects. However, $t_i - 1$ (observed) treatment effects suffice to express all $\binom{t_i}{2}$ estimates because the consistency Equation 11.1 holds by definition within a trial. Therefore, from a study with t_i arms, we need to estimate $t_i - 1$ study-specific treatment effects that we include in a vector denoted by y_i and a $(t_i - 1) \times (t_i - 1)$ variance–covariance matrix S_i between the elements of y_i. These observed treatment effects estimate some of the parameters in μ or their linear combinations. We assume that within-study variances and covariances are adequately estimated by their sample counterparts. If $t_i = 2\,\forall i$, then each study provides information about a single effect size y_i and its variance s_i^2.

The stacked vector $y = (y_1, y_2, \ldots, y_N)'$ comprises the y_i vectors ($i = 1, \ldots, N$) of the effect sizes reported in the N trials and has length $\sum_{i=1}^{N}(t_i - 1)$. The random error terms associated with within-study variation in treatment effects are denoted by $\varepsilon = (\varepsilon_1, \varepsilon_2, \ldots, \varepsilon_N)'$ and are assumed to follow a multivariate normal distribution with zero means and a block-diagonal covariance matrix with S_i in the diagonal, $\varepsilon_i \sim N(0, diag(S_i))$. For a two-arm study i, only one y_i and the corresponding ε_i are relevant. For a three-arm study i comparing treatments A, B, and C, the corresponding vector of effect sizes is $y_i = (y_{iBA}, y_{iCA})'$ and the vector of error terms is $y_i = (\varepsilon_{iBA}, \varepsilon_{iCA})'$. The within-study variance–covariance matrix is

$$S_i = \begin{pmatrix} s_{iBA}^2 & cov(y_{iBA}, y_{iCA}) \\ cov(y_{iBA}, y_{iCA}) & s_{iCA}^2 \end{pmatrix}$$

There are formulae available for estimating the sample covariance between various effect size measures (e.g., log odds ratio and mean difference) (Higgins and Whitehead, 1996; Franchini et al., 2012).

11.4.1.3 Random Effects Meta-Analysis and Heterogeneity

The vector of data y is used to estimate the parameters in μ. In the estimation, the random errors ε need to be taken into account. In addition, variation in treatment effects due to differences in study-level characteristics can be accounted for. More specifically, in a meta-analysis model, we assume that either there is only random variation within studies (fixed effects) or that there is random variation in the treatment effects both within and across studies (random effects). For the random effects model, the vector of parameters associated with variation in treatment effects across studies is $\delta = (\delta_1, \delta_2, \ldots, \delta_N)'$. It is assumed to be normally distributed with zero means and a block-diagonal variance–covariance matrix with the study-specific matrices $\boldsymbol{\Delta}_i$ in its diagonal, $\boldsymbol{\Delta} = diag(\boldsymbol{\Delta}_i)$. Between-study variance (hetero-geneity) refers to deviations of the study-specific underlying treatment effects from their mean value due to unobserved patient or trial characteristics and is known as heterogeneity. The extent of heterogeneity is crucial for a meta-analysis, pairwise or NMA; large values will lead to difficulties in interpreting results and may even prohibit data synthesis.

Accurate estimation of the heterogeneity variance requires a moderate to large number of studies. In cases of few studies available, accounting for heterogeneity might prove challenging and further assumptions might be needed. For further discussion of heterogeneity in pairwise meta-analysis, see Chapter 10. Chapter 8 discusses heterogeneity of treatment effects and its relevance to CER.

In this chapter, the heterogeneity corresponding to a comparison B vs. A is denoted by τ_{AB}^2. A commonly employed and convenient assumption is that of equal heterogeneities across treatment comparisons, $\tau_{XY}^2 = \tau^2$ for any treatments X and Y (Higgins and Whitehead, 1996). This assumption is made because there are usually few available studies per treatment comparison. In the simple case where there are only two-arm studies and we assume the same heterogeneity across treatment comparisons, we may write $\boldsymbol{\Delta} = diag(\tau^2)$.

For a three-arm study i comparing A vs. B vs. C, $\delta_i = (\delta_{iBA}, \delta_{iCA})'$ and if we assume the same heterogeneity across different comparisons, the study-specific heterogeneity variance–covariance matrix takes the following form:

$$\boldsymbol{\Delta}_i = \begin{pmatrix} \tau^2 & \tau^2/2 \\ \tau^2/2 & \tau^2 \end{pmatrix} \tag{11.2}$$

The off-diagonal elements in this matrix are shown to be equal to $\tau^2/2$ after using the consistency Equation 11.1 at the random effects level (Higgins and Whitehead, 1996).

Note that the equal heterogeneities assumption might be considered a strong assumption that may not always be realistic. Lu and Ades suggested that the consistency equations impose restrictions on heterogeneities, so that they cannot be completely independent (Lu and Ades, 2009). More specifically, heterogeneity for a comparison C vs. B is bounded by the heterogeneities of the basic parameters: $\left|\tau_{CA}^2 - \tau_{BA}^2\right| \leq \tau_{CB}^2 \leq \left|\tau_{CA}^2 + \tau_{BA}^2\right|$. Accounting for these constraints requires further re-parameterization of the between-studies variance–covariance matrix, which makes the approach rather cumbersome.

11.4.2 Network Meta-Analysis as a Meta-Regression Model

This approach, first presented by Lumley (2002), treats the different treatment comparisons as covariates in a meta-regression model. Lumley considered this approach for networks including only two-arm trials but an extension to incorporate multiarm trials is straightforward. The model is described by the following equation:

$$y = X\mu + \varepsilon + \delta \tag{11.3}$$

where X is a design matrix of $\sum_{t=1}^{N}(t_i - 1)$ rows and $T - 1$ columns. Each study contributes $t_i - 1$ rows in the design matrix X and each column corresponds to one of the $T - 1$ basic parameters. If the treatment comparison in study i is one of the basic contrasts (e.g., BA), the element in the corresponding row assumes value 1 (in the column that corresponds to BA) and all other elements assume a zero value. If a study comparison is not one of the basic contrasts (e.g., CB), all entries in the corresponding row are zero with the exception of the columns that compare each of the two treatments with the reference treatment (CA and BA). In this case, we embed the consistency Equation 11.1 in the design matrix by assigning values -1 and 1 to the columns BA and CA, respectively.

The basic parameters are then estimated as $\hat{\mu} = (X^T W X)^{-1} X^T W y$. The variance–covariance matrix of the estimates is given by $var(\hat{\mu}) = (X^T W X)^{-1}$, where W is the weight matrix, with $W = (S + \Delta)^{-1}$. There are various alternative ways to estimate Δ, including likelihood methods (maximum likelihood or restricted maximum likelihood) or the method of moments (Berkey et al., 1998; van Houwelingen et al., 2002; Jackson et al., 2010).

Lu et al. (2011) suggested that NMA can be performed as a linear model using a two-stage approach. In the first step, we perform a traditional meta-analysis of each pair of interventions that has been compared in at least one study. Let us denote with $\hat{\mu}^{dir}$ the vector that contains all estimates of direct treatment effects. These pairwise direct estimates are used as the dependent variable in a meta-regression model at the second stage of the analysis:

$$\hat{\mu}^{dir} = Z\mu + \varepsilon^* + \delta^* \tag{11.4}$$

where Z is a design matrix that describes the set of treatments compared in each observed pairwise direct summary estimate in $\hat{\mu}^{dir}$ and ε^*, δ^* are the random effects and random errors, respectively, with the star super index used to differentiate them from the corresponding quantities in Equation 11.3.

Rucker showed how to apply graph-theoretical methods, commonly used in analyzing electrical networks, to perform a fixed-effects NMA (Rucker, 2012). A common problem with multiarm trials in random effects models is the modeling of the between-studies variance–covariance matrix. Recently, a package in R (R Core Team, 2014) (netmeta) became available that extends the framework of graph-theoretical methods to random effects NMA (Rucker et al., 2016). The idea is to extract from the multiarm studies in the network all possible pairwise comparisons and then adjust their variances in such a way that allows treating the elements of y_i as if they were independent.

EXAMPLE 11.1: WORKED EXAMPLE—ANALYSIS OF THE HEAVY MENSTRUAL BLEEDING NETWORK USING META-REGRESSION

We use the heavy menstrual bleeding network to illustrate how NMA can be expressed as a meta-regression model.

We start by constructing the rows of the design matrix X (each row corresponds to a study). All 20 studies have two arms so the design matrix has 20 rows and 3 columns. We take hysterectomy (HY) to be the reference treatment and the basic contrasts are FGED vs. HY, SGED vs. HY, and MI vs. HY. In Table 11.1, we present 4 of the 20 studies of the network and we conventionally name them Study 1 through 4 in order to exemplify the way of identifying the entries in the design matrix.

The model in Equation 11.3 for these four studies would be written as follows:

$$
\begin{pmatrix} y_1 \\ y_2 \\ y_3 \\ y_4 \\ \vdots \end{pmatrix} = \begin{pmatrix} 1 & 0 & 0 \\ 1 & -1 & 0 \\ 1 & 0 & -1 \\ 0 & -1 & 1 \\ \vdots & \vdots & \vdots \end{pmatrix} \begin{pmatrix} \mu_{FGEDvsHY} \\ \mu_{SGEDvsHY} \\ \mu_{MIvsHY} \end{pmatrix} + \begin{pmatrix} \varepsilon_1 \\ \varepsilon_2 \\ \varepsilon_3 \\ \varepsilon_4 \\ \vdots \end{pmatrix} + \begin{pmatrix} \delta_1 \\ \delta_2 \\ \delta_3 \\ \delta_4 \\ \vdots \end{pmatrix}
$$

We model the rest of the studies in the same way and we obtain the summary estimates for the basic contrasts $\hat{\mu} = (\hat{\mu}_{FGEDvsHY}, \hat{\mu}_{SGEDvsHY}, \hat{\mu}_{MIvsHY})$ and the common between-study variance $\hat{\tau}^2$.

The NMA estimates for all treatment comparisons are presented in Table 11.2. The model was fit using the `metareg` command in Stata (StataCorp, 2013) and Δ was estimated using restricted maximum likelihood (Raudenbush and Bryk, 1985). The standard `metareg` output gives the estimates for the basic parameters and their standard errors. The estimates for all other relative treatment effects are derived from the consistency equations (can be obtained in Stata using the `lincom` command). The NMA model suggests there is no statistical heterogeneity in the network ($\tau^2 = 0$).

TABLE 11.1

Example from Four Studies in the Heavy Menstrual Bleeding Network

Study	Comparison	Design Matrix Columns (Basic Parameters)		
		FGED vs. HY	SGED vs. HY	MI vs. HY
1	FGED vs. HY	1	0	0
2	FGED vs. SGED	1	−1	0
3	FGED vs. MI	1	0	−1
4	MI vs. SGED	0	−1	1
$\vdots$	$\vdots$	$\vdots$	$\vdots$	$\vdots$

TABLE 11.2

League Table for the Heavy Menstrual Bleeding Network

HY	2.61 (1.55, 4.42)	–	–
2.61 (1.49, 4.60)	FGED	0.82 (0.60, 1.12)	2.85 (0.51, 15.79)
2.23 (1.16, 4.26)	0.85 (0.61, 1.18)	SGED	0.74 (0.25, 2.25)
2.31 (0.88, 6.09)	0.89 (0.40, 1.94)	1.04	MI (0.50, 2.18)

Note: Diagonal cells contain the names of the four competing treatments. Off-diagonal cells in the lower triangle report the network summary odds of the treatment in the row versus the treatment in the column. Values in the upper triangle report the respective direct summary odds ratios (column vs. row), corresponding to a random effects pairwise meta-analysis. For example, the direct odds ratio estimate for SGED vs. FGED is 0.82 while the network summary is 0.85.

NMA allows us to compare treatments that were not directly compared in any of the studies (e.g., SGED vs. HY and MI vs. HY). All NMA estimates are comparable with the ones obtained from the simple pairwise meta-analysis of direct studies with the exception of the MI vs. FGED comparison. This was reported in just one (relatively small) study, leading to a wide confidence interval for the odds ratio. Using NMA, we achieve a significant increase in precision for this comparison by exploiting the indirect evidence in the network.

11.4.3 Network Meta-Analysis as a Hierarchical Model

Hierarchical models offer increased flexibility in NMA modeling. For two-arm studies, we assume

$$y_i \sim N(\theta_i, s_i^2) \tag{11.5}$$

Note that the normality assumption is plausible even for skewed distributed outcomes due to the central limit theorem, when the study sizes are not too small (Dias et al., 2013).

The underlying study-specific treatment effects for each comparison can be assumed to be either fixed and equal to the common summary effect, $\theta_i = \mu_{BA}$ for a study comparing A to B (fixed-effect model), or coming from a common distribution (conventionally a normal distribution, though other distributions have been suggested [Lee and Thompson, 2008])

$$\theta_i \sim N(\mu_{BA}, \tau_{BA}^2) \tag{11.6}$$

Equation 11.5 can be alternatively written as $y_i = \mu_{BA} + \varepsilon_i + \delta_i$, with $\varepsilon_i \sim N(0, s_{iBA}^2)$ and $\delta_i \sim N(0, \tau_{BA}^2)$. For a three-arm trial comparing A vs. B vs. C, we model $y_i \sim N(\theta_i, S_i)$, where $y_i = (y_{iBA}, y_{iCA})'$ and $\theta_i = (\theta_{iBA}, \theta_{iCA})'$. Then we assume $\theta_i \sim N((\mu_{BA}, \mu_{CA})', \Delta_i)$. Studies with more treatment arms are treated similarly.

For studies not including the reference treatment, the consistency equations must be used. For a C vs. B study, for example, Equation 11.6 would be written as $\theta_i \sim N(\mu_{CA} - \mu_{BA}, \tau_{CB}^2)$.

It is possible to use the exact likelihood of the data, if arm-level data are available. Dias et al. (2013) describe a generalized linear model framework that can be used for various kinds of data and different choices of the likelihood. The likelihood is defined in terms of (unknown) parameters γ and a link function g that maps these parameters to the $(-\infty, +\infty)$ range. For a two-arm B vs. A study, for example, the model is written as

$$g(\gamma_{iA}) = u_i$$

$$g(\gamma_{iB}) = u_i + \theta_{iBA}$$

The link function g can be the logit (for dichotomous data following a binomial likelihood), the identity function (for continuous data following a normal likelihood), and so on. The rest of the model is similar to the previous model for study-level data omitting Equation 11.6 onwards.

For example, if the outcome is dichotomous and we assume a binomial likelihood for the number of events in each arm, we have

$$r_{it} \sim Binomial(p_{it}, n_{it}) \tag{11.7}$$

In this formula, n_{it} is the total number of patients in the t arm of study i and p_{it} is the probability of an event in this arm (to be identified with the γ parameter). Then, to derive the study-specific underlying treatment effects θ_{iBA} (log odds ratio of treatment B over A), we use the logit link function

$$logit(p_{iA}) = u_i$$

$$logit(p_{iB}) = u_i + \theta_{iBA} \tag{11.8}$$

For a comprehensive review of likelihood distributions for different types of data (continuous, rates, etc.) and alternative link functions, we refer the reader to Dias et al. (2013).

EXAMPLE 11.2: WORKED EXAMPLE—ANALYSIS OF THE SERIOUS VASCULAR EVENTS NETWORK USING A HIERARCHICAL MODEL

The data for this network are presented in Table 11A.2 in Appendix 11A.1. Since the outcome is dichotomous and arm-level data are available, we can use Equations 11.7 and 11.8. We fit the model in a Bayesian software (WinBUGS [Lunn et al., 2000, 2009]) using the code provided online at http://mtm.uoi.gr/index.php/how-to-do-an-mtm

We employ a normal prior distribution truncated on $(0, +\infty)$ for τ, the heterogeneity standard deviation, and noninformative normal prior distributions with zero mean and large variance for the basic parameters, $N(0, 10^3)$.

TABLE 11.3

League Table for the Network of Serious Vascular Events

Placebo	0.86 (0.78, 0.96)	0.77 (0.58, 1.03)	0.65 (0.57, 0.76)	–
0.85 (0.77, 0.93)	Aspirin	0.94 (0.85, 1.04)	0.79 (0.70, 0.90)	0.83 (0.67, 1.03)
0.79 (0.69, 0.91)	0.93 (0.83, 1.04)	Thienopyridines	–	0.97 (0.84, 1.10)
0.67 (0.58, 0.75)	0.78 (0.70, 0.88)	0.83 (0.72, 0.99)	Aspirin and dipyridamole	–
0.73 (0.61, 0.87)	0.85 (0.73, 1.00)	0.92 (0.80, 1.06)	1.09 (0.91, 1.33)	Thienopyridines and aspirin

Note: Diagonal cells contain the names of the four competing treatments. Off-diagonal cells in the lower triangle report the network summary odds of the treatment in the row versus the treatment in the column along with their 95% credible intervals. Values in the upper triangle report the respective direct summary odds ratios (column vs. row)

The network estimates for the relative treatment effects in terms of odds ratios are presented in Table 11.3 along with the respective direct estimates. The heterogeneity standard deviation was estimated to be 0.04 (credible interval 0.00–0.13).

Although the point estimates are similar between the results of network and pairwise meta-analysis, the network estimates are more precise for most of the comparisons. This can be seen by comparing the upper and lower triangles of Table 11.3.

11.4.4 Network Meta-Analysis as a Multivariate Meta-Analysis Model

White et al. (2012) suggested treating the different comparisons as different outcomes and employing standard multiple outcomes (multivariate meta-analysis) techniques to fit the model (Jackson et al., 2011; Mavridis and Salanti, 2013). The $T - 1$ vector of basic parameters μ represents all the available "outcomes." If there are studies that do not include the reference treatment, a data augmentation technique is used to "impute" minimal information to the reference arm. This reflects the consistency assumption, which implies that the missing arm is "missing at random" and all comparisons in the network can be expressed via the basic contrasts. In this way, we ensure that each study reports at least one basic parameter. The model can be written as a multivariate meta-analysis model:

$$y = X^*\mu + \varepsilon + \delta \tag{11.9}$$

where the design matrix X^* refers now to the treatments being compared in each study. Note that the y vector in this equation has a different dimension than the y in Equation 11.3. This also holds for the random errors and random effects vectors.

EXAMPLE 11.3: WORKED EXAMPLE—NMA OF THE SERIOUS VASCULAR EVENTS NETWORK USING MULTIVARIATE META-ANALYSIS

The network includes five treatments and hence four basic parameters are necessary for the analysis. Choosing placebo (PL) as the reference, the basic parameters are $\mu_{TH+AvsPL}$, $\mu_{A+DPvsPL}$, μ_{AvsPL}, and μ_{THvsPL}. For studies including the reference treatment, the log odds ratios corresponding to the basic parameters can be readily estimated. For the studies that do not include placebo, we impute a placebo arm giving it minimal information as described below.

Consider the first two trials presented in Table 11.4. Trial 1 compares treatments PL, A, and A+DP. Thus, the observed log odds ratios y_{1AvsPL} and $y_{1A+DPvsPL}$ with their standard errors and their covariance are the required information from this study.

Trial 2 compares treatments A and TH+A and we need to impute a reference placebo arm PL. It has been recommended to impute 0.001 for the number of events and 0.01 for the total number of randomized patients (White et al., 2012); however, smaller values can be imputed as well. Consequently, two pairwise log odds ratios y_{2AvsPL} and $y_{2TH+AvsPL}$ with their standard errors and their covariance can be estimated as shown in Table 11.4. In the model for the subset of these two studies, we identify

$$\mathbf{y} = (y_{1AvsPL}, y_{1A+DPvsPL}, y_{2AvsPL}, y_{2TH+AvsPL}, \ldots)'$$

$$\boldsymbol{\mu} = (\mu_{TH+AvsPL}, \mu_{AvsPL}, \mu_{A+DPvsPL}, \mu_{THvsPL})'$$

$$\boldsymbol{\varepsilon} = (\varepsilon_{1AvsPL}, \varepsilon_{1A+DPvsPL}, \varepsilon_{2AvsPL}, \varepsilon_{2TH+AvsPL}, \ldots)'$$

$$\boldsymbol{\delta} = (\delta_{1AvsPL}, \delta_{1A+DPvsPL}, \delta_{2AvsPL}, \delta_{2TH+AvsPL}, \ldots)'$$

$$X^* = \begin{pmatrix} 0 & 1 & 0 & 0 \\ 0 & 0 & 1 & 0 \\ 0 & 1 & 0 & 0 \\ 1 & 0 & 0 & 0 \\ \vdots & \vdots & \vdots & \vdots \end{pmatrix}$$

TABLE 11.4

Two Trials from the Serious Vascular Events Network

Study Number	Number of Arms	Treatments	Data in Each Trial
1	3	Reported: PL, A, A+DP No imputation needed	y_{1AvsPL}, s^2_{1AvsPL} $y_{1A+DPvsPL}, s^2_{1A+DPvsPL}$ $cov(y_{1AvsPL}, y_{1A+DPvsPL})$
2	2	Reported: A, TH+A A placebo arm needs to be imputed	y_{2AvsPL}, s^2_{2AvsPL} $y_{2TH+AvsPL}, s^2_{2TH+AvsPL}$ $cov(y_{2AvsPL}, y_{2TH+AvsPL})$

The random errors are assumed to follow a (multivariate) normal distribution:

$$\varepsilon \sim N\left(0, \begin{pmatrix} S_1 & 0 & \cdots \\ 0 & S_2 & \cdots \\ \vdots & \vdots & \ddots \end{pmatrix}\right)$$

with

$$S_1 = \begin{pmatrix} s^2_{1AvsPL} & cov(y_{1AvsPL}, y_{1A+DPvsPL}) \\ cov(y_{1AvsPL}, y_{1A+DPvsPL}) & s^2_{1A+DPvsPL} \end{pmatrix}$$

and similarly for S_2, and so on.

If equal heterogeneities are assumed, the random effects are distributed as

$$\delta \sim N\left(0, \begin{pmatrix} \Delta_1 & 0 & \cdots \\ 0 & \Delta_2 & \cdots \\ \vdots & \vdots & \ddots \end{pmatrix}\right)$$

where Δ_1 and Δ_2 are defined by Equation 11.2.

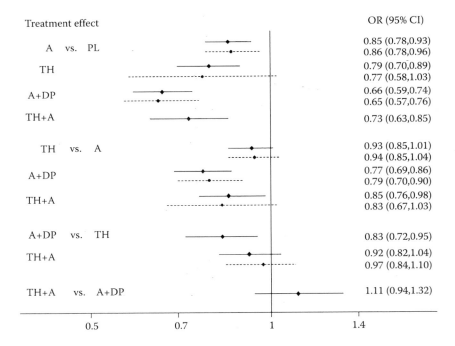

FIGURE 11.2

Forest plot of the summary odds ratios for the serious vascular events network. Thick lines correspond to the network estimates (derived from the multivariate meta-analysis approach) while dashed lines to the direct summary estimates. The horizontal lines are the respective 95% CI.

After fitting the model in Stata using the `mvmeta` command (White, 2011), we obtain the estimates for the odds ratios presented in Figure 11.2. The heterogeneity variance was estimated using restricted maximum likelihood to be almost zero (10^{-8}), whereas the hierarchical model gave a slightly larger estimate. Comparing the NMA results in Figure 11.2 to the corresponding (network) estimates of Table 11.3, we see that the two approaches gave similar point estimates of relative effects. The credible intervals of the hierarchical model, though, are somewhat wider than the respective confidence intervals from the multivariate approach. This occurs because the latter approach ignores uncertainty in the estimation of heterogeneity.

11.5 Methods to Evaluate Statistically the Inconsistency in a Network

The assumption of consistency in the network (e.g., that all pieces of evidence are in agreement) underlies the NMA methodology. When the distribution of effect modifiers is not comparable across comparisons, then this might create statistical disagreement between direct and indirect sources of evidence, usually called inconsistency (or incoherence) (Lu and Ades, 2006). In this section, we discuss methods to evaluate the presence and extent of inconsistency in a network of interventions. Inconsistency can be explored both *locally* (in a specific loop of evidence) and *globally* with an omnibus test evaluating the presence of inconsistency in the entire network.

11.5.1 Local Approaches for Inconsistency

11.5.1.1 Loop-Specific Approach

The loop-specific method is a straightforward approach to estimate inconsistency in a closed loop of evidence. Consider a triangular network consisting of treatments A, B, and C, for which there are data available on all pairwise comparisons (A vs. B, A vs. C, and B vs. C). Comparisons may be informed by two-arm and/or multiarm studies. An indirect relative effect μ_{CB}^{ind} can be estimated via Equation 11.1 as $\hat{\mu}_{CB}^{ind} = \hat{\mu}_{CA}^{dir} - \hat{\mu}_{BA}^{ind}$ with estimated variance $\hat{v}_{CB}^{ind} = \hat{v}_{CA}^{dir} + \hat{v}_{BA}^{ind}$.

Differences between direct and indirect estimates for a specific comparison are called inconsistency factors (Lu and Ades, 2006) and there is only one inconsistency factor per loop. As the direction of inconsistency is of no importance, we estimate the absolute inconsistency factor as

$$\hat{W}_{ABC} = |\hat{\mu}_{CB}^{dir} - \hat{\mu}_{CA}^{ind}| \tag{11.10}$$

It can be shown that the inconsistency factor within a loop is invariant to the comparison used in Equation 11.10 (Lu and Ades, 2006). Thus, *w* pertains to the entire loop and not to a specific comparison, hence the ABC subscript. The variance of $\hat{w}_{ABC}$ is

$$var(\hat{w}_{ABC}) = \hat{v}_{BC}^{dir} + \hat{v}_{BC}^{ind}$$

A 95% CI can be obtained as $\hat{W}_{ABC} \pm 1.96\sqrt{var(\hat{w}_{ABC})}$ and a z-test assessing the null hypothesis $w_{ABC} = 0$ (Bucher et al., 1997) is

$$z = \frac{\hat{w}_{ABC}}{\sqrt{var(\hat{w}_{ABC})}} \sim N(0,1)$$

This method can be extended to a full network that includes many closed loops (triangular, quadrilateral, etc.), where the consistency assumption is evaluated separately for each independent loop (e.g., loops that include nested loops of lower order do not need to be evaluated).

Despite ease of implementation, this approach has important limitations. Direct evidence on each treatment comparison is not compared to all available indirect information but only to the indirect evidence from a specific loop. Also, some treatment comparisons can be included in more than one loop leading to inconsistency factors being dependent across loops while there are multiple testing issues. The method also fails to account for the correlations induced by multiarm studies. Song et al. (2012) conducted a simulation study and found that this approach has low power to detect inconsistency. This implies that there might be loops with statistically nonsignificant but clinically important inconsistency. Thus, loops with inconsistency factors that are statistically nonsignificant but large in magnitude (depending on the studied clinical condition) should also be considered as potential sources of important inconsistency. Another issue that limits the usefulness of this method—and this also holds for all methods to detect inconsistency—is the trade-off with heterogeneity. Note that different assumptions for heterogeneity may be employed and are likely to affect results; researchers can assume a common heterogeneity parameter for the entire network, a common heterogeneity within each loop but different across loops, or a different heterogeneity for each comparison (Veroniki et al., 2013). The choice between the various approaches might impact substantially on the inference about inconsistency. Veroniki et al. (2013) found empirically that there are between 2% and 9% chances for a loop to be inconsistent in a network, the variability depending primarily on the assumption about heterogeneity.

EXAMPLE 11.4: WORKED EXAMPLE—INCONSISTENCY OF THE HEAVY MENSTRUAL BLEEDING NETWORK USING THE LOOP-SPECIFIC APPROACH

The heavy menstrual bleeding network includes only one triangular loop SGED vs. MI vs. FGED (see Figure 11.1). The independent pairwise meta-analyses for the three comparisons in this loop give the direct summary estimates and standard errors presented in Table 11.5.

TABLE 11.5

Pairwise, Random Effect Meta-Analyses for All Available
Direct Comparisons in the Menstrual Bleeding Network

Comparison	Studies	*lnOR*	*SE(lnOR)*	$\hat{\tau}^2$
FGED vs. HY	5	0.96	0.27	0.00
SGED vs. FGED	11	−0.20	0.16	0.00
MI vs. FGED	1	1.05	0.87	−
MI vs. SGED	3	−0.30	0.57	0.50

The indirect estimates for the comparison MI vs. SG are estimated as
$\hat{\mu}_{MIvsSGED}^{ind} = \hat{\mu}_{MIvsFGED}^{dir} - \hat{\mu}_{SGEDvsFGED}^{dir} = 1.25$ with $\hat{v}_{MIvsSGED}^{ind} = 0.78$.
The inconsistency factor of this loop is the difference between $\hat{\mu}_{MIvsSGED}^{dir}$
and $\hat{\mu}_{MIvsSGED}^{ind}$, $\hat{W}_{SGEDvsMIvsFGED}$, with variance $var(\hat{W}_{SGEDvsMIvsFGED}) =$
1.10. The 95% CI of $\hat{W}_{SGEDvsMIvsFGED}$ is $(−0.51, 3.61)$ and the *p*-value
of the z-test (for the null hypothesis $\hat{\mu}_{MIvsSGED}^{dir} = \hat{\mu}_{MIvsSGED}^{ind}$) is 0.14.
Based on the confidence interval (which includes the zero value) or the
p-value (larger than 0.05), we would conclude that there might not be
important inconsistency in this loop. However, caution is needed when
interpreting inconsistency factors due to the limitations of the approach
described earlier in this section. Investigators should not solely focus on
p-values and statistical significance, but should consider whether a ratio
of odds ratios, $\exp(\hat{W}_{SGEDvsMIvsFGED}) = 4.71$, is large enough to suggest
important discrepancies between direct and indirect estimates for heavy
menstrual bleeding (in the target population). In this example, we used a
comparison-specific heterogeneity, as can be seen in Table 11.5. Caution is
needed, since using another assumption (e.g., loop-specific τ) might lead
to a different inference for the inconsistency factors as it will impact on
the precision of their estimation.

11.5.1.2 Composite Test for Inconsistency

Caldwell et al. (2010) suggested a χ^2 composite test for inconsistency. The difference with the loop-specific approach is that it accounts for many indirect estimates of the same comparison. Suppose that the comparison A vs. B is included in L loops that only have the A vs. B comparison in common; these loops provide L indirect estimates for the relative effect A vs. B. For example, in the serious vascular events network (Figure 11.1b) the loops A vs. PL vs. TH and A vs. PL vs. A+DP would give two independent indirect estimates for the comparison A vs. PL.

Generally, the estimated direct summary effect $\hat{\mu}_{BA}^{dir}$ and the L independent summary indirect estimates $\hat{\mu}_{BA}^{ind_1}, \ldots, \hat{\mu}_{BA}^{ind_L}$ can be synthesized in the "mixed" estimate:

$$\hat{\mu}_{BA} = \frac{\frac{1}{\hat{v}_{BA}^{dir}} \hat{\mu}_{BA}^{dir} + \sum_{i=1}^{L} \frac{1}{\hat{v}_{BA}^{ind_i}} \hat{\mu}_{BA}^{ind_i}}{\frac{1}{\hat{v}_{BA}^{dir}} + \sum_{i=1}^{L} \frac{1}{\hat{v}_{BA}^{ind_i}}}$$

Then the statistic

$$T_{BA} = \frac{1}{\hat{v}_{BA}^{dir}} \left(\hat{\mu}_{BA}^{dir} - \hat{\mu}_{BA} \right)^2 + \sum_{i=1}^{L} \frac{1}{\hat{v}_{BA}^{ind_i}} \left(\hat{\mu}_{BA}^{ind_i} - \hat{\mu}_{BA} \right)$$

follows a χ_L^2 distribution under the hypothesis that all available estimates for this comparison (BA), direct and indirect coming from different loops, are in agreement. This composite test, however, fails to account for the correlations between different estimates in the presence of multiarm trials and can be applied as an omnibus test for inconsistency only for a collection of loops sharing a common comparison.

> **EXAMPLE 11.5: WORKED EXAMPLE—COMPOSITE TEST FOR INCONSISTENCY IN THE SERIOUS VASCULAR EVENTS NETWORK**
>
> We estimate the logOR and its variance for the comparison A vs. PL to be $\hat{\mu}_{AvsPL}^{dir} = -0.15$ and $\hat{v}_{AvsPL}^{dir} = 0.0026$, respectively. There are also two independent indirect estimates for this comparison coming from the loops A vs. PL vs. A+DP and A vs. PL vs. TH with mean and variance $\hat{\mu}_{AvsPL}^{ind_1} = -0.22$, $\hat{v}_{AvsPL}^{ind_1} = 0.0084$ from the first loop and $\hat{\mu}_{AvsPL}^{ind_2} = 0.21$, $\hat{v}_{AvsPL}^{ind_2} = 0.0284$ from the second loop. The weighted average of these three estimates is $\hat{\mu}_{AvsPL} = -0.17$ and consequently $T_{AvsPL} = 0.51$ with a p-value 0.77. This finding suggests that the three different sources of evidence for the comparison A vs. PL might not disagree. However, we again need to be aware of the lack of sufficient power of this test and the absence of statistically significant inconsistency should not be misinterpreted as evidence of consistency. Note that in this example we have disregarded the fact that some of the studies in the network are three-arm trials.

11.5.1.3 Node-Splitting Approach

Dias et al. (2010) suggested a method that separates evidence on a particular comparison (node) into "direct" and "indirect." They called their method "node splitting." The method excludes one direct comparison at a time and estimates the indirect treatment effect for the excluded comparison from the rest of the network. Thus, two estimates are obtained for the relative treatment effect of each comparison B vs. A; a direct one coming from all studies comparing treatments B and A, and an indirect one coming from an NMA of all studies after excluding those that compare B to A. The null hypothesis $H_0 : \mu_{BA}^{dir} = \mu_{BA}^{ind}$ can be evaluated using a z-test.

The main drawback of this method is that it is computationally intensive for large complex networks and, similarly to the previous approaches, it cannot correctly handle multiarm studies. This is because the same study may inform both direct and indirect evidence, when the split node is included in a multiarm trial.

An equivalent approach, also suggested by Dias et al. (2010), is the "back-calculation" method. In this approach, the complete dataset is used to produce a network estimate for each pairwise comparison. Then, it is assumed that each network estimate is a weighted average of the direct estimate and the indirect estimate from the rest of the network. This allows us to back-calculate an indirect estimate as

$$\hat{\mu}_{BA}^{ind} = \left(\frac{\hat{\mu}_{BA}}{\hat{v}_{BA}} - \frac{\hat{\mu}_{BA}^{dir}}{\hat{v}_{BA}^{dir}} \right) \hat{v}_{BA}^{ind}$$

The variance of the indirect estimate is given by

$$\frac{1}{\hat{v}_{BA}^{ind}} = \frac{1}{\hat{v}_{BA}} - \frac{1}{\hat{v}_{BA}^{dir}}$$

Then the difference between the direct and indirect estimates is calculated and using a z-test we can infer about the magnitude and the statistical significance of inconsistency for that particular comparison. If the method is performed in a Bayesian framework, a comparison of the posterior distributions of direct and indirect treatment effects can be used to assess visually the magnitude of inconsistency.

EXAMPLE 11.6: WORKED EXAMPLE—NODE SPLITTING ON THE SERIOUS VASCULAR EVENTS NETWORK

We focus on the comparison A vs. PL for which we have estimated $\hat{\mu}_{AvsPL}^{dir} = -0.15$, $\hat{v}_{AvsPL}^{dir} = 0.0026$ (see Section 11.5.1.2). Then, to estimate the indirect relative effect, we exclude the studies that compare directly the two interventions (A and PL). Using the remaining data, we perform NMA and we estimate the indirect relative effect $\hat{\mu}_{AvsPL}^{ind} = 0.21$, $\hat{v}_{AvsPL}^{ind} = 0.0063$. Then, the inconsistency factor is the difference between these two estimates $\hat{w}_{AvsPL} = 0.06$ with $var(\hat{w}_{AvsPL}) = 0.0089$. The estimated z-statistic $z = \frac{0.06}{\sqrt{0.0089}} = 0.64$ gives a p-value 0.52, suggesting no statistically significant difference between direct and indirect estimates for the A vs. PL comparison. To infer about all 10 comparisons in the network, we need to repeat this procedure for each comparison. Note that, as in the two previous approaches, the lack of statistically significant inconsistency is not evidence for the absence of inconsistency and large inconsistency factors need exploration.

11.5.2 Global Approaches for Inconsistency

11.5.2.1 Lu and Ades Model

The Lu and Ades model (Lu and Ades, 2006) is an NMA model where the consistency assumption is "relaxed" by adding an extra term in the consistency equations to reflect the possible disagreement between different sources of evidence. For example, the consistency equation for the ABC loop under the Lu and Ades model becomes $\mu_{BA} = \mu_{CA} - \mu_{BA} + w_{ABC}$. For each closed loop in the network, there is a different w parameter added in the model; these parameters are the inconsistency factors. We can treat the various inconsistency factors as being independent and estimate each one separately; a large w value suggests important inconsistency in the respective loop. Inference for inconsistency in the entire network is based on a χ^2 test for evaluating the hypothesis that all inconsistency factors are zero. Alternatively, we can assume that the different inconsistency factors are exchangeable, with an aim to increase power in their estimation, that is, we assume that they follow a normal distribution with zero mean and inconsistency variance σ^2, $w_{XYZ} \sim N(0, \sigma^2)$. Comparing σ^2 with τ^2 can help draw inference about the "extra" variability due to inconsistency in the entire network.

In the absence of multiarm studies, the maximum number of potential inconsistencies in the network ("inconsistency degrees of freedom," *ICDF*) is computed as $ICDF = C - T + 1$, where C is the number of pairwise comparisons with data and T the total number of competing treatments. Multiarm studies are always internally consistent, so for a network including multiarm studies, the number of possible inconsistency factors would be $ICDF = C - T + 1 + S$, where S is "the number of independent inconsistency relations in which the corresponding parameters are supported by no more than two independent sources of evidence" (Lu and Ades, 2006). Calculating S can be difficult for networks with many multiarm studies, which renders this approach cumbersome for large complex networks. Also note that the parameterization of multiarm studies (i.e., which comparisons to be included in the model, see Section 11.4.1.2) often impacts on the results of this model and inference about the presence of inconsistency in the network.

The Lu and Ades inconsistency model (as well as the design-by-treatment model described in the next paragraph) can in principle be fit using any of the approaches described in Section 11.4.

EXAMPLE 11.7: WORKED EXAMPLE—ASSESSING INCONSISTENCY IN THE SERIOUS VASCULAR EVENTS NETWORK USING THE LU AND ADES MODEL AND THE MULTIVARIATE META-ANALYSIS APPROACH

First, we need to calculate the required number of inconsistency factors. It is easy to see from Figure 11.1 that the number C of pairwise comparisons present in the network equals 7 (note that the A+DP vs. TH comparison is excluded, as described in Section 11.2). There are five treatments and S equals zero, since all loops in the network are informed by more than two independent sources. Hence, the required number of inconsistency factors is $ICDF = C - T + 1 + S = 7 - 5 + 1 - 0 = 3$. The $ICDF$ also corresponds to the number of loops in the network. Then, the consistency equations in the three loops expressed as functions of the basic parameters (assuming placebo is the common reference) are relaxed to include the three inconsistency factors:

$$\mu_{AvsA+DP} = \mu_{AvsPL} - \mu_{A+DPvsPL} + w_{A+DPvsAvsPL}$$

$$\mu_{THvsA} = \mu_{THvsPL} - \mu_{AvsPL} + w_{THvsPLvsA}$$

$$\mu_{THvsTH+A} = \mu_{THvsA} - \mu_{TH+AvsA} + w_{AvsTH+AvsTH}$$

$$= \mu_{THvsPL} - \mu_{TH+AvsPL} + w_{AvsTH+AvsTH}$$

We will now see how to fit this model in the multivariate meta-analysis framework presented in Section 11.4.4 after including the inconsistency factors as covariates. We start by extending our dataset to include three dummy covariates, one for each inconsistency factor, $w_{A+DPvsAvsPL}$, $w_{THvsPLvsA}$, and $w_{AvsTH+AvsTH}$. We initially set the values of these covariates to be equal to zero. We then start "building" the network by adding studies, starting from the studies reporting the basic parameters. Whenever there is a loop forming, we set the value of the corresponding dummy covariate equal to one, for example, studies comparing A+DP vs. A close the A+DP vs. A vs. PL loop and, thus, all A+DP vs. A studies inform the $w_{A+DPvsAvsPL}$ inconsistency factor; studies comparing TH vs. A inform $w_{THvsPLvsA}$, and so on.

To illustrate the method, let us choose three studies from the network, shown in Table 11.6.

TABLE 11.6

Three Studies from the Serious Vascular Events Network

Study ID	Comparisons
2	TH vs. A (PL arm imputed)
8	TH+A vs. A (PL arm imputed)
15	A vs. PL

TABLE 11.7

Inconsistency Factors for the Serious Vascular
Events Network, Using the Lu and Ades Model

Inconsistency Factors	Estimate (95% CI)
$w_{A+DPvsAvsPL}$	0.08 (−0.15, 0.32)
$w_{THvsPLvsA}$	−0.05 (−0.36, 0.27)
$w_{AvsTH+AvsTH}$	−0.01 (−0.40, 0.38)

The first two studies do not include the reference treatment; a reference
arm is imputed. Equation 11.9 is modified as follows for this subset of
studies when the inconsistency factors are included:

$$
\begin{pmatrix} y_{2THvsPL} \\ y_{2AvsPL} \\ y_{8TH+AvsPL} \\ y_{8AvsPL} \\ y_{15AvsPL} \end{pmatrix} = \begin{pmatrix} 0 & 0 & 0 & 1 \\ 0 & 1 & 0 & 0 \\ 1 & 0 & 0 & 0 \\ 0 & 1 & 0 & 0 \\ 0 & 1 & 0 & 0 \end{pmatrix} \begin{pmatrix} \mu_{TH+AvsPL} \\ \mu_{AvsPL} \\ \mu_{A+DPvsPL} \\ \mu_{THvsPL} \end{pmatrix}
$$

$$
+ \begin{pmatrix} 0 & 1 & 0 \\ 0 & 0 & 0 \\ 0 & 0 & 1 \\ 0 & 0 & 0 \\ 0 & 0 & 0 \end{pmatrix} \begin{pmatrix} w_{A+DPvsAvsPL} \\ w_{THvsPLvsA} \\ w_{AvsTH+AvsTH} \end{pmatrix} + \varepsilon + \delta
$$

After fitting the model in Stata using the `mvmeta` command, we get
the estimates for the covariates (inconsistency factors) presented in
Table 11.7.

Note that none of the inconsistency factors was found to be statistically
important, as one can see in their respective confidence intervals, while
an omnibus χ^2-test for all inconsistency terms being simultaneously zero
gives a *p*-value of 0.88. Thus, we conclude that there is no evidence of
inconsistency in the network as a whole.

However, the results should be interpreted with caution, as there are
multiarm studies present in the example and as we discussed, different
parameterizations may alter the inference for inconsistency. The design-
by-treatment model described in the following section is a better option
in this case.

11.5.2.2 Design-by-Treatment Interaction Model

Higgins et al. (2012) and White et al. (2012) extended the Lu and Ades
model presented in Section 11.5.2.1 by introducing the concept of design
inconsistency. More specifically, their model considers disagreement between
direct and indirect evidence and also disagreement that may arise between
estimates for a specific pairwise comparison computed from studies with

different designs. The term "design" refers to the set of treatments being compared in each study, for example, a study comparing A to B is an AB design, while a three-arm A vs. B vs. C study is considered to be an ABC design. This means that the summary estimate for the A vs. B comparison obtained from two-arm studies (A vs. B studies) may differ from the estimate obtained from the synthesis of three-arm studies A vs. B vs. C. This source of disagreement is called design inconsistency.

The Lu and Ades model presented in the previous section is a special case of the design-by-treatment model. When there are no multiarm trials in the network, there can be no design inconsistency but only loop inconsistency and the two models are equivalent. The w factors are again assumed to be either fixed and independent or random, $w_i \sim N(0, \sigma^2)$ (Jackson et al., 2014). The number of identifiable inconsistency factors equals $\sum_d (T_d - 1) - (T - 1)$, where T_d is the number of treatments compared in design d and the sum goes through all available designs.

Also, Jackson et al. (2014) present an I^2 statistics to quantify inconsistency of a random effects NMA model.

EXAMPLE 11.8: WORKED EXAMPLE—ASSESSING INCONSISTENCY IN THE SERIOUS VASCULAR EVENTS NETWORK USING THE DESIGN-BY-TREATMENT MODEL AND THE MULTIVARIATE META-ANALYSIS APPROACH

In the example of the previous section, we assessed only the presence of loop inconsistency; now, we consider both loop and design inconsistency. This implies that inconsistency factors are placed wherever there is potential for disagreement between comparisons forming a loop, or between two designs including the same comparison. The easiest way to determine these factors is to go through the list of available designs and add an inconsistency factor for each loop of evidence that is formed (loop inconsistency) or when the same comparison is estimated in different designs (design inconsistency). Note that the number of studies under each design (which can be read from Table 11A.2 in Appendix 11A.1) is irrelevant to the parameterization of the network in terms of inconsistency factors.

We can now fit NMA as a hierarchical model (Section 11.4.3) or as a multivariate meta-analysis model (Section 11.4.4) including five inconsistency factors (for designs 3, 6, 7, 8). Care is needed when assigning the inconsistency factors to the study designs. Parameterization can be difficult, particularly for complex and large networks with many multiarm trials, as discrimination between loop and design inconsistency is not always straightforward. For example, we may choose to include the inconsistency factor introduced by design 3 (TH+A vs. A) in Table 11.8, in either the TH+A vs. PL basic parameter, or the A vs. PL, but not both. Similarly, design 8 (A vs. PL vs. A+DP) introduces two inconsistency factors that we must include in both the A vs. PL and A+DP vs. PL basic parameters of the model. Nevertheless, inference about the presence of

TABLE 11.8

Inconsistency Factors for the Serious Vascular Events Network (Design-by-Treatment Model)

Design	Design Code	Potential Inconsistencies (w)	Explanation
TH vs. A	1	–	
TH vs. TH+A	2	–	
			Loop inconsistency
TH+A vs. A	3	1	Closed loop with designs 1, 2
A+DP vs. PL	4	–	
A+DP vs. A	5	–	
			Loop inconsistency
A vs. PL	6	1	Closed loop with designs 4, 5
			Loop inconsistency
TH vs. PL	7	1	Closed loop with designs 1, 6
			Design inconsistency
A vs. PL vs. A+DP	8	1	A vs. PL also estimated in design 6
		1	A+DP vs. PL also estimated design 4

inconsistency in the entire network (based on a χ^2-test) is invariant to the choice of parameterization.

We fit the model in Stata using the `mvmeta` command as described in the previous example with the two additional inconsistency factors. None of the inconsistency factors was found to be statistically significant and the χ^2 omnibus test does not suggest that there is important inconsistency in the network as a whole (p-value 0.89). Heterogeneity was estimated to be very small (10^{-8}).

The reader should keep in mind, however, that inference on the presence or absence of inconsistency should also consider the findings of local approaches.

11.5.2.3 Q-Statistic in NMA

The Q-statistic for inconsistency is a by-product of the two-stage method to fit NMA models and it is an analogous to the Q-statistic for heterogeneity in pairwise meta-analysis.

For simplicity, we assume that there are only two-arm studies in the network. In the first stage of the analysis, we estimate the direct mean effect $\hat{\mu}_{BA}^{dir}$ for each comparison B vs. A. Then, a comparison-specific Q-statistic for heterogeneity would be

$$Q_{BA}^{het} = \sum_{i=1}^{N_{BA}} \frac{1}{s_i^2} \left(y_i - \hat{\mu}_{BA}^{dir} \right)^2$$

where N_{BA} denotes the number of studies comparing A to B. Q^{het}_{BA} represents the distances between the observed effects in studies (y_i) and the pooled direct effect $\hat{\mu}^{dir}_{BA}$ for the comparison B vs. A. Under the null hypothesis of homogeneity in the AB comparisons, this statistic follows a χ^2 distribution with $N_{BA} - 1$ degrees of freedom. According to Krahn et al. (2013), the sum of all the within-comparisons $\sum_{k=1}^{C} Q^{het}_k$ is the Q-statistic for heterogeneity in the network of trials (Q^{het}) and follows a χ^2 distribution with $N - C$ degrees of freedom.

A similar Q-statistic can be estimated at the second stage of the analysis as described in Section 11.4.2. After estimating the NMA summary effect $\hat{\mu}^{dir}_k$ and the variance $\hat{v}^{dir}_k$ for each one of the $k = 1, \ldots, C$ available pairwise direct comparisons, we can estimate the following Q-statistic for inconsistency:

$$
Q^{inc} = \left[\left(\hat{\mu}^{dir}_1 \cdots \hat{\mu}^{dir}_C \right) - \left(\hat{\mu}_1 \cdots \hat{\mu}_C \right) \right]
\begin{pmatrix}
1/\hat{v}^{dir}_1 & \cdots & 0 \\
\vdots & \ddots & \vdots \\
0 & \cdots & 1/\hat{v}^{dir}_C
\end{pmatrix}
$$

$$
\times \left[\begin{pmatrix} \hat{\mu}^{dir}_1 \\ \vdots \\ \hat{\mu}^{dir}_C \end{pmatrix} - \begin{pmatrix} \hat{\mu}_1 \\ \vdots \\ \hat{\mu}_C \end{pmatrix} \right]
$$

This represents the (weighted) distances between the direct summary estimates $\hat{\mu}^{dir}_k$ and the network summary estimates $\hat{\mu}_k$ for each comparison AB. Under the null hypothesis of consistency, Q^{inc} follows a χ^2 distribution with $C - T + 1$ degrees of freedom.

Krahn et al. (2013) further suggested that the total Q-statistic for both stages of the analysis is the sum of the Q-statistic for heterogeneity and inconsistency:

$$
Q^{tot} = Q^{het} + Q^{inc}
$$

Under the null hypothesis of consistency and homogeneity in the network, Q^{tot} follows a χ^2 distribution with $N - T + 1$ degrees of freedom.

Note that all the above Q-statistics have been extended to account for the inclusion of multiarm trials. For details on these extensions, see Krahn et al. (2013) and Lu et al. (2011).

EXAMPLE 11.9: WORKED EXAMPLE—Q-STATISTIC FOR THE NMA OF THE MENSTRUAL BLEEDING NETWORK

Using Equations 11.30 through 11.32, we derive that Q^{tot} is equal to 27.28. This is decomposed into Q^{het}, which measures the heterogeneity within each comparison, estimated equal to 24.96 (with 16 degrees of freedom, corresponding to a p-value 0.07) and the inconsistency Q^{inc} estimated to 2.32 (with 1 degree of freedom, p-value 0.13). These results suggest that neither heterogeneity nor inconsistency is statistically significant in this network.

11.5.3 Overview of Methods

In Table 11.9, we provide a summary of the presented methods for evaluating inconsistency in a network, along with their main characteristics.

Song et al. (2012) performed a simulation study to explore the statistical properties of the loop-specific, node-splitting, and Lu and Ades models to infer about inconsistency. They found that even though all methods are generally unbiased, they have low power. Hence, the absence of statistically significant inconsistency should not be interpreted as evidence of absence of inconsistency.

Also, inconsistency is closely related to heterogeneity. The assumptions for heterogeneity and the method used to evaluate it might affect inference on inconsistency. Large values of heterogeneity in the network may hinder the search for inconsistency. Therefore, the consistency assumption should always be assessed, both epidemiologically (e.g., by comparing the distribution of potential effect modifiers across comparisons (Salanti, 2012; Cipriani et al., 2013) and statistically.

Empirical evidence evaluating the prevalence of statistical inconsistency in published networks showed that often the consistency assumption is violated. More specifically, Song et al. (2011) performed a meta-epidemiological study, including 112 independent, triangular, published networks. They used the loop-specific approach and found statistically significant inconsistency in 16 cases (14%, 95% CI 9%–22%). Veroniki et al. (2013) assessed the inconsistency in published networks including four or more competing treatments and at least one closed loop. Inconsistency was evaluated using the loop-specific approach and the design-by-treatment model. In a total of 303 loops

TABLE 11.9

Summary of Methods for Evaluating the Inconsistency in a Network of Interventions

Method	Identifies Spots of Inconsistency	Can Infer about the Entire Network	Sensitive to Parameterization of Multiarm Studies
Loop-specific approach	Yes	No	Yes
Composite test	Yes	No	Yes
Node splitting and back-calculation	Yes	No	Yes
Lu and Ades model	Yes	Yes	Yes
Design-by-treatment	Yes	Yes	No
Q-statistic	No	Yes	No

(from 40 networks), statistically significant inconsistency was detected in 2%–9% of the loops depending on the effect measure and the method used for estimating heterogeneity. Using the design-by-treatment interaction model, about one-eighth of the networks were found to be inconsistent.

Both local and global tests should be ideally employed for the evaluation of consistency. In the presence of inconsistency, after checking for data extraction errors, researchers should try to explore it and find its possible sources. If sufficient studies are available, network meta-regression can be used with the potential effect modifiers as covariates. For example, small-study effects are a quite common source of both heterogeneity and inconsistency in NMA (Chaimani and Salanti, 2012; Chaimani et al., 2013b). When significant inconsistency is found, results should be interpreted with great caution considering that pooling these studies is invalid.

11.6 Presentation of Data and Results in Network Meta-Analysis

Reporting and presenting all aspects of NMA can be challenging, particularly for large complex networks. In this section, we describe graphical and tabular options that may facilitate a concise presentation of the evidence base, evaluation, and presentation of the assumptions and the results.

11.6.1 Presentation of the Evidence Base

11.6.1.1 Network Graph

Network graphs are one of the most commonly used tool to present the competing interventions (represented by nodes) and the pairwise comparisons evaluated in at least one study (represented by edges) in a network of trials. In Section 11.2, we presented the network graphs for the two examples of this chapter (Figure 11.1). The use of different weighting and coloring schemes for the edges has been suggested to reveal differences between the different pairwise comparisons, such as the number of included studies, baseline characteristics of the patients, or limitations in the design of the studies (Chaimani et al., 2013a).

11.6.1.2 Contribution Plot

Each direct comparison contributes to a different degree to the estimation of the NMA summary treatment effects. It has been shown that the contribution of each direct comparison to the network estimate depends on its variance and the structure of the network (Lu et al., 2011; Krahn et al., 2013). The contribution of each direct estimate to the network estimates can be expressed

| | | Direct comparisons in the network | | | |
		FGEDvsHY	FGEDvsMI	FGEDvsSGED	MIvsSGED
Mixed estimates					
	FGEDvsHY	100.0			
	FGEDvsMI		18.4	40.8	40.8
	FGEDvsSGED		2.2	95.6	2.2
	MIvsSGED		22.4	22.4	55.2
Indirect estimates					
	HYvsMI	37.2	11.5	25.6	25.6
	HYvsSGED	49.4	1.1	48.3	1.1
Entire network		30.9	9.8	37.3	22.0
Included studies		5	1	11	3

Network meta-analysis estimates (vertical axis label)

FIGURE 11.3
Contribution plot for the serious vascular events network. The size of each square is proportional to the weight attached to each direct summary effect (horizontal axis) for the estimation of each network summary effects (vertical axis). The numbers re-express the weights as percentages.

as a percentage and presented in a matrix form (Chaimani et al., 2013a; Krahn et al., 2013). The columns of this "contribution matrix" correspond to the available direct comparisons and the rows to all possible pairwise comparisons (direct and indirect) between pairs of interventions. Cells in this $\binom{T}{2} \times C$ matrix refer to the contribution of each comparison to the entire network. These are estimated using the "two-stage approach" for NMA (see Section 11.4.2). More specifically, a least square solution for Equation 11.4 gives that

$$\hat{\mu} = (Z^T W^{dir} Z)^{-1} Z^T W^{dir} \hat{\mu}^{dir}$$

with W^{dir} the inverse of the variance–covariance matrix of the direct estimates $\hat{\mu}^{dir}$. Hence, the matrix $H = (Z^T W^{dir} Z)^{-1} Z^T W^{dir}$ that maps the direct estimates into the network estimates contains the weight of each direct comparison in the estimation. These weights can be expressed as percentages by taking the ratio of their absolute value over the total of the respective row. The sum of each column of the matrix gives the weight of each direct comparison in all comparisons and this divided by the sum of all column totals is the percentage contribution of each direct comparison in the entire network.

EXAMPLE 11.10

Figure 11.3 presents the contribution plot for the heavy menstrual bleeding network. According to the graph, the network summary effect of FGED vs. HY is not informed indirectly by any other comparison; hence, we expect that network estimate would equal the direct estimate (100% contribution from the direct estimate). On the other hand, to estimate the NMA effect for the comparison FGED vs. MI, 18.4% of the information comes from the respective direct estimate, 40.8% comes from FGED vs. SGED, and 40.8% comes from MI vs. SGED. The most influential direct comparison for the entire network is FGED vs. SGED; this is because of the "central" position of this comparison (see Figure 11.1) and the relatively larger number of included studies compared with the other three comparisons.

11.6.2 Presenting the Assumptions of the Analysis

As pointed out earlier in this chapter, all models for NMA presented in Section 11.4 rely on the assumption of consistency. In Section 11.5, we described different approaches that can be used to assess whether important inconsistency is present in the data. This section focuses on tools that can offer a visual representation for some of these approaches and may supplement the ease of their interpretation.

11.6.2.1 Inconsistency Plot

The estimated inconsistency factors for all closed loops of a network derived from the loop-specific approach (Section 11.5.1.1) can be presented jointly in a forest plot (Song et al., 2003). Horizontal lines represent the inconsistency factor confidence intervals and these can be used to detect any loops with important inconsistency.

EXAMPLE 11.11

To illustrate the interpretation of this graph, we present in Figure 11.4 the inconsistency plot for the serious vascular events network. The network includes three triangular loops. To facilitate interpretation, we present the inconsistency factors on the exponential scale, which is the ratio of odds ratios (ROR) between direct and indirect estimates in each loop. The confidence intervals (horizontal lines) are truncated to the null value (here the value 1) as we are not interested in the direction of inconsistency but only in its magnitude. The graph suggests that there might be no inconsistency in the network as none of the inconsistency factor appears to be statistically significant. Despite the negative findings, there may be low power to detect inconsistency and we need to consider whether an ROR around 1.5 (the upper limit of the confidence intervals) is large enough to suggest disagreement between direct and indirect estimates for the clinical setting and outcome of this network. Note that in this example we

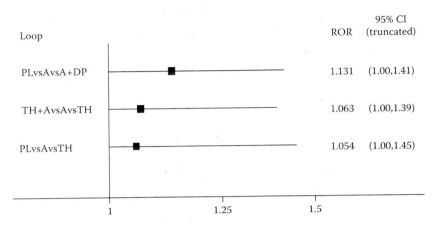

FIGURE 11.4
Inconsistency plot for the serious vascular events network assuming a common heterogeneity for the entire network.

assumed a common heterogeneity variance for the entire network. More specifically, we used the heterogeneity estimated from the hierarchical model $\tau^2 = 0.002$ (see Section 11.4.3).

11.6.3 Presenting the Results

The most important output of NMA is the summary relative treatment effects between pairs of interventions, which can be presented using several graphical or tabular ways. We have already seen in Figure 11.2 a forest plot that presents all NMA effect estimates and also the results from pairwise meta-analyses. In the presence of many competing interventions, however, presenting all estimated effects in a concise and comprehensible way is a challenging issue.

The relative ranking of treatments can be used as a supplementary output to facilitate the presentation and interpretation of results. Also note that deriving a treatment hierarchy based on the studied outcome is often one of the objectives of systematic reviews. An advantage of relative ranking measures is that they offer a compact way of summarizing the findings of NMA. However, focusing on ranking measures can be misleading as they are associated with much uncertainty. Ranking measures should be interpreted with caution and always in conjunction with the relative treatment effects.

Treatment hierarchy can be derived using several approaches, such as ordering the means of the estimated treatment effects, using ranking probabilities (Salanti et al., 2011), or employing multidimensional scaling techniques (Chaimani et al., 2013a). In this section, we present measures related with ranking probabilities, which is probably the most common approach. A ranking probability p_{tj} is the probability that treatment t is ranked at the jth place ($j = 1, \ldots, T$) according to the studied outcome. Inferences on the relative ranking of the treatments should not be limited on just comparing the probabilities of each treatment being the best (p_{t1}), as this method can give misleading results. A better approach is to incorporate information about all p_{tj}, that is, about the probabilities of each treatment being at each possible rank: first best, second best, third best, $\ldots T$th best.

Two different but equivalent approaches are the mean ranks or the surface under the cumulative ranking curves. The mean rank of a treatment t is the weighted average of the probabilities for all possible ranks estimated as

$$m\,(rank_t) = \sum_{j=1}^{T} p_{tj} \times j$$

The surface under the cumulative ranking curve (SUCRA) for a treatment can also be expressed as a percentage; it is interpreted as the percentage of the effectiveness or safety that this treatment has obtained compared to a treatment that would be ranked first without uncertainty and is estimated by the formula

$$\text{SUCRA}_t = \frac{\sum_{j=1}^{T-1} cum_{tj}}{T-1}$$

where cum_{tj} is the cumulative probability that treatment t would be within the first j places (Salanti et al., 2011).

The ranking probabilities for each treatment can be presented graphically in a system of coordinate axes plotted against the possible ranks ("rankograms"). Mean ranks and SUCRA values can be given in a separate table or can be presented in the league table along with the relative effects.

EXAMPLE 11.12

In Figure 11.5, we present the rankograms for the treatments in the serious vascular events network. The graphs suggest that the combination of aspirin and dipyridamole has the highest probability of being the best and placebo has the highest probability of being the last. Looking at the mean ranks or the SUCRA values in Table 11.10, we can infer about the treatment hierarchy for the studied outcome.

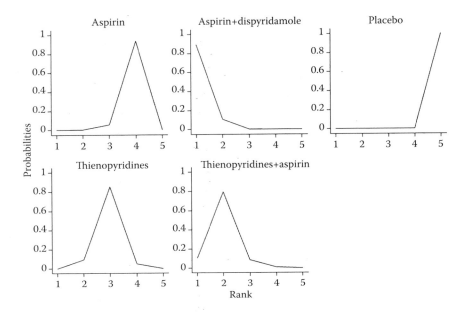

FIGURE 11.5
Plots of the ranking probabilities (rankograms) for the serious vascular events network. The horizontal axis contains the possible ranks and the vertical axis the ranking probabilities. Each curve connects the points that show the estimated probabilities of being at each specific rank for every treatment.

TABLE 11.10

SUCRA Values and Mean Ranks for the Five
Treatments of the Serious Vascular Events Example

Treatment	Mean Rank	SUCRA
Placebo	5.0	0.0
Thienopyridines+aspirin	2.0	75.1
Aspirin	3.9	26.6
Aspirin+dipyridamole	1.1	97.2
Thienopyridines	3.0	51.1

Note: Larger SUCRA values and smaller mean ranks denote better treatments.

11.7 Discussion

The plethora of available treatment options and the sparse direct evidence between treatments have necessitated the use of NMA. The assumption of transitivity required to fit NMA demands that the distributions of effect modifiers are similar across treatment comparisons. If this assumption is plausible, and when the various pieces of direct and indirect evidence are in statistical agreement (consistency), NMA is a valid statistical tool and constitutes a powerful addition to the arsenal of CER. The results provided by NMA are usually more precise than those obtained by conventional, pairwise meta-analyses and NMA can also provide a ranking of the treatments according to studied outcome. Thus, the use of NMA enhances CER by allowing more informed decisions to be drawn on how competing treatments compare with each other in terms of effectiveness and on which of the available options is associated with the greater benefit or harm for the patients.

Despite the benefits of NMA with respect to the purposes of CER, this methodology is far from an established practice. Its complexity, lack of user-friendly software, and low trust in indirect evidence discourage systematic reviewers from widely adopting this technique. In this chapter, we reviewed the literature on NMA putting emphasis on statistical models, methods to evaluate statistically the assumption of consistency, and ways to present the results derived from NMA. We epitomized the available software options to fit and visualize NMA.

NMA is an active research field and, despite the rapid development of the relevant methodology, further research is still needed to cover gaps in the current knowledge. For instance, methods to correct NMA estimates for publication bias or for analyzing simultaneously multiple outcomes are still under investigation (Mavridis et al., 2013; Efthimiou et al., 2014, 2015). In addition, methods for evaluating the quality of evidence (e.g., GRADE guidelines [Guyatt et al., 2011]) need to be extended into the context of NMA.

Appendix 11A.1: Data for the Worked Examples in This Chapter

The data from the menstrual bleeding network is given in Table 11A.1.

TABLE 11A.1

Data from the Menstrual Bleeding Network

Study ID	Treatment	Events	Patients Randomized
1	FGED	13	107
1	HY	7	103
2	FGED	5	38
2	HY	2	39
3	FGED	7	106
3	HY	2	50

(Continued)

TABLE 11A.1 (*Continued*)

Data from the Menstrual Bleeding Network

Study ID	Treatment	Events	Patients Randomized
4	FGED	13	104
4	HY	4	93
5	FGED	19	99
5	HY	6	97
6	FGED	3	16
6	SGED	2	27
7	FGED	1	101
7	SGED	3	201
8	FGED	5	55
8	SGED	3	56
9	FGED	10	72
9	SGED	16	156
10	FGED	3	33
10	SGED	4	37
11	FGED	13	58
11	SGED	15	75
12	FGED	5	82
12	SGED	11	154
13	FGED	14	38
13	SGED	7	37
14	FGED	19	48
14	SGED	15	45
15	FGED	33	128
15	SGED	29	121
16	FGED	1	120
16	SGED	5	125
17	MI	5	34
17	FGED	2	35
18	MI	5	25
18	SGED	5	28
19	MI	2	37
19	SGED	9	39
20	MI	10	32
20	SGED	9	35

The data from the serious vascular events network is given in Table 11A.2.

TABLE 11A.2

Data from the Serious Vascular Events Network

Study ID	Treatment	Events	Patients Randomized
1	PL	46	204
1	A	31	198
1	A+DP	30	202
2	A	112	907
2	TH	133	902
3	A	488	3,195
3	TH	453	3,233
4	A	395	1,540
4	TH	370	1,529
5	A	22	164
5	TH	12	165
6	TH+A	445	3,797
6	TH	473	3,802
7	TH+A	10	132
7	TH	10	138
8	TH+A	175	2,160
8	A	207	2,160
9	A+DP	183	1,250
9	PL	263	1,250
10	A+DP	246	1,650
10	PL	361	1,649
10	A	314	1,649
11	A+DP	12	137
11	A	11	147
11	PL	16	155
12	A+DP	6	88
12	A	3	95
13	A+DP	149	1,363
13	A	192	1,376
14	A+DP	79	448
14	A	85	442
15	A	26	162
15	PL	35	157
16	A	59	253
16	PL	55	252
17	A	32	144

(Continued)

TABLE 11A.2 (*Continued*)

Data from the Serious Vascular Events Network

Study ID	Treatment	Events	Patients Randomized
17	PL	30	139
18	A	23	101
18	PL	27	102
19	A	21	150
19	PL	21	151
20	A	2	30
20	PL	5	30
21	A	342	1,622
21	PL	193	814
22	A	183	676
22	PL	193	684
23	PL	139	541
23	TH	112	531
24	A+DP	0	11
24	TH	0	11

Appendix 11B.1: Software Options for NMA

In this appendix, we discuss the available software options for fitting the various models and methods presented in this chapter. Recently developed commands in Stata may help popularize the method among nonstatisticians (Harbord and Higgins, 2004; White, 2011; White et al., 2012). Chaimani et al. present and explain a series of graphical tools aiming to make NMA accessible and understandable to researchers without a strong statistical background (Chaimani et al., 2013a; Chaimani and Salanti, 2015). BUGS software (WinBUGS and OpenBUGS) (Lunn et al., 2000, 2009) are widely used for analyses in Bayesian framework and programming codes for most models can be found in the literature or online (see, e.g., www.bris.ac.uk/social-community-medicine/projects/mpes or http://www.mtm.uoi.gr).

R is a popular choice as a free software environment for statistical computing and there are various packages available for fitting models in a non-Bayesian setting. GeMTC software (van Valkenhoef et al., 2012), available as an R package as well as a stand-alone graphical user interface, can be used to implement various NMA. SAS is also an option although not very widely used for NMA (Jones et al., 2011; Carlin et al., 2013; Hong et al., 2013). In Table 11B.1, we give a brief summary of the more popular methods for fitting each model.

TABLE 11B.1

Available Software and Routines for Implementing the Methods Presented in This Chapter

Subject	Section	Software Available
NMA as meta-regression	11.4.2	BUGS (e.g., WinBUGS, OpenBUGS) Stata (`metareg` command: without multiarm studies; `mvmeta` command, either as a stand-alone command or via the package `network`: with multiarm studies; `lincom` command can be used in both cases to obtain estimates for the functional parameters) R (`rma` command from `metafor` package: without multiarm studies; `netmeta` package: with multiarm studies)
Hierarchical NMA model	11.4.3	BUGS code available at http://www.mtm.uoi.gr, http://www.bris.ac.uk/social-community-medicine/projects/mpes/ GeMTC software
NMA as a multivariate meta-analysis	11.4.4	Stata (`mvmeta` command, `lincom`) BUGS R (`mvmeta` package: cannot incorporate the assumption of a common heterogeneity across comparisons)
Loop-specific approach for inconsistency	11.5.1.1	BUGS Stata (`network graphs` package) R (routines available at http://mtm.uoi.gr/index.php/how-to-do-an-mtm)
Composite test for inconsistency	11.5.1.1	No routine available
Node-splitting approach	11.5.1.3	BUGS codes available at http://www.bristol.ac.uk/cobm/research/mpes GeMTC software Stata (`network` package)
Lu and Ades model	11.5.2.1	BUGS (can incorporate either the assumption of fixed-independent inconsistency factors or of random inconsistency factors; the parameterization needs to be done manually) Stata (`mvmeta` command: can incorporate only the assumption of fixed-independent inconsistency factors; the parameterization needs to be done manually) GeMTC software

(Continued)

TABLE 11B.1 (*Continued*)

Available Software and Routines for Implementing the Methods Presented in This Chapter

Subject	Section	Software Available
Design-by-treatment model	11.5.2.2	Stata (`mvmeta` command: can incorporate only the assumption of fixed-independent inconsistency factors, the parameterization can be done automatically using the package `network`) BUGS (can incorporate either the assumption of fixed-independent inconsistency factors or of random inconsistency factors, the parameterization needs to be done manually)
Q-statistic in NMA	11.5.2.3	R (`netmeta`)
Presentation options (graphs)	11.6	Stata (`network graphs` package)

References

Bafeta, A. et al. 2013. Analysis of the systematic reviews process in reports of network meta-analyses: Methodological systematic review. *BMJ*, 347, f3675.

Berkey, C.S. et al. 1998. Meta-analysis of multiple outcomes by regression with random effects. *Stat. Med.*, 17, 2537–2550.

Bucher, H.C. et al. 1997. The results of direct and indirect treatment comparisons in meta-analysis of randomized controlled trials. *J. Clin. Epidemiol.*, 50, 683–691.

Caldwell, D.M., Ades, A.E. and Higgins, J.P. 2005. Simultaneous comparison of multiple treatments: Combining direct and indirect evidence. *BMJ*, 331, 897–900.

Caldwell, D.M., Welton, N.J. and Ades, A.E. 2010. Mixed treatment comparison analysis provides internally coherent treatment effect estimates based on overviews of reviews and can reveal inconsistency. *J. Clin. Epidemiol.*, 63, 875–882.

Carlin, B.P. et al. 2013. Case study comparing Bayesian and frequentist approaches for multiple treatment comparisons. (Prepared by the Minnesota Evidence-Based Practice Center under Contract No. 290-2007-10064-I2). AHRQ, Publication No. 12(13)-EHC103-EF. Rockville, MD: Agency for Healthcare Research and Quality.

Chaimani, A. and Salanti, G. 2012. Using network meta-analysis to evaluate the existence of small-study effects in a network of interventions. *Res. Synth. Method*, 3, 161–176.

Chaimani, A. and Salanti, G. 2015. Visualizing assumptions and results in network meta-analysis: The network graphs package. *Stata J.* 15, 905–950.

Chaimani, A. et al. 2013a. Graphical tools for network meta-analysis in STATA. *PLoS One*, 8, e76654.

Chaimani, A. et al. 2013b. Effects of study precision and risk of bias in networks of interventions: A network meta-epidemiological study. *Int. J. Epidemiol.*, 42, 1120–1131.

Cipriani, A. et al. 2013. Conceptual and technical challenges in network meta-analysis. *Ann. Intern. Med.*, 159, 130–137.

Cooper, N.J. et al. 2011. How valuable are multiple treatment comparison methods in evidence-based health-care evaluation? *Value Health*, 14, 371–380.

Dias, S. et al. 2010. Checking consistency in mixed treatment comparison meta-analysis. *Stat. Med.*, 29, 932–944.

Dias, S. et al. 2013. Evidence synthesis for decision making 2: A generalized linear modeling framework for pairwise and network meta-analysis of randomized controlled trials. *Med. Dec. Making*, 33, 607–617.

Donegan, S., Williamson, P., D'Alessandro, U., and Tudur Smith, C. 2013. Assessing key assumptions of network meta-analysis: A review of methods. *Res Syn Method*, 4, 291–323.

Efthimiou, O. et al. 2014. An approach for modelling multiple correlated outcomes in a network of interventions using odds ratios. *Stat. Med.*, 33, 2275–2287.

Efthimiou, O., Mavridis, D., Riley, R.D., Cipriani, A., and Salanti, G. 2015. Joint synthesis of multiple correlated outcomes in networks of interventions. *Biostatistics*, 16, 84–97.

Franchini, A.J. et al. 2012. Accounting for correlation in network meta-analysis with multi-arm trials. *Res. Synth. Method*, 3, 142–160.

Guyatt, G.H., Oxman, A.D., Schünemann, H.J., Tugwell, P., and Knottnerus, A. 2011. GRADE guidelines: A new series of articles in the Journal of Clinical Epidemiology. *J. Clin. Epidemiol.*, 64:380–382.

Harbord, R. and Higgins, J.P.T. 2004. METAREG: Stata module to perform meta-analysis regression. Boston College Department of Economics.

Higgins, J.P.T. and Green, S.e. 2013. *Cochrane Handbook for Systematic Reviews of Interventions*, Version 5.1.0 [updated March 2011]. The Cochrane Collaboration, 2011. Available from www.cochrane-handbook.org

Higgins, J.P.T. and Whitehead, A. 1996. Borrowing strength from external trials in a meta-analysis. *Stat. Med.*, 15, 2733–2749.

Higgins, J.P.T. et al. 2012. Consistency and inconsistency in network meta-analysis: Concepts and models for multi-arm studies. *Res. Synth. Method*, 3, 98–110.

Hoaglin, D.C. et al. 2011. Conducting indirect-treatment-comparison and network-meta-analysis studies: Report of the ISPOR task force on indirect treatment comparisons good research practices: Part 2. *Value Health*, 14, 429–437.

Hong, H., Carlin, B.P., Shamliyan, T.A., Wyman, J.F., Ramakrishnan, R., Sainfort, F., and Kane, R.L. 2013. Comparing Bayesian and frequentist approaches for multiple outcome mixed treatment comparisons. *Med Decis Making*, 33, 702–714.

Institute of Medicine (US) Roundtable on Evidence-Based Medicine. 2009. *Leadership Commitments to Improve Value in Healthcare: Finding Common Ground: Workshop Summary*. Washington, DC: National Academies Press (US).

Jackson, D., Riley, R. and White, I.R. 2011. Multivariate meta-analysis: Potential and promise. *Stat. Med.*, 30, 2481–2498.

Jackson, D., White, I.R. and Thompson, S.G. 2010. Extending DerSimonian and Laird's methodology to perform multivariate random effects meta-analyses. *Stat. Med.*, 29, 1282–1297.

Jackson, D. et al. 2014. A design-by-treatment interaction model for network meta-analysis with random inconsistency effects. *Stat. Med.*, 33, 3639–3654.

Jansen, J. and Naci, H. 2013. Is network meta-analysis as valid as standard pairwise meta-analysis? It all depends on the distribution of effect modifiers. *BMC Med.*, 11, 159.

Jansen, J.P. et al. 2011. Interpreting indirect treatment comparisons and network meta-analysis for health-care decision making: Report of the ISPOR task force on indirect treatment comparisons good research practices: Part 1. *Value Health*, 14, 417–428.

Jones, B. et al. 2011. Statistical approaches for conducting network meta-analysis in drug development. *Pharm. Stat.*, 10, 523–531.

Krahn, U., Binder, H. and Konig, J. 2013. A graphical tool for locating inconsistency in network meta-analyses. *BMC Med. Res. Methodol.*, 13, 35.

Lee, A.W. 2014. Review of mixed treatment comparisons in published systematic reviews shows marked increase since 2009. *J Clin. Epidemiol.* 67, 138–143.

Lee, K.J. and Thompson, S.G. 2008. Flexible parametric models for random-effects distributions. *Stat. Med.*, 27, 418–434.

Lu, G. and Ades, A.E. 2004. Combination of direct and indirect evidence in mixed treatment comparisons. *Stat. Med.*, 23, 3105–3124.

Lu, G. and Ades, A.E. 2006. Assessing evidence inconsistency in mixed treatment comparisons. *J. Am. Stat. Assoc.*, 101, 447–459.

Lu, G. and Ades, A. 2009. Modeling between-trial variance structure in mixed treatment comparisons. *Biostatistics*, 10, 792–805.

Lu, G. et al. 2011. Linear inference for mixed treatment comparison meta-analysis: A two-stage approach. *Res. Synth. Method*, 2, 43–60.

Lumley, T. 2002. Network meta-analysis for indirect treatment comparisons. *Stat. Med.*, 21, 2313–2324.

Lunn, D.J., Thomas, A. and Spiegelhalter, D. 2000. WinBUGS—A Bayesian modelling framework: Concepts, structure, and extensibility. *Stat. Comput.*, 10, 325–337.

Lunn, D.J. et al. 2009. The BUGS project: Evolution, critique and future directions. *Stat. Med.*, 28, 3049–3067.

Mavridis, D. and Salanti, G. 2013. A practical introduction to multivariate meta-analysis. *Stat. Methods Med. Res.*, 22, 133–158.

Mavridis, D. et al. 2013. A fully Bayesian application of the Copas selection model for publication bias extended to network meta-analysis. *Stat. Med.*, 32, 51–66.

Middleton, L.J. et al. 2010. Hysterectomy, endometrial destruction, and levonorgestrel releasing intrauterine system (Mirena) for heavy menstrual bleeding: Systematic review and meta-analysis of data from individual patients. *BMJ*, 341, c3929.

NICE. 2013. Evidence Synthesis, http://www.nicedsu.org.uk/Evidence-Synthesis-TSD-series%282391675%29.htm. National Institute of Health and Clinical Excellence.

Nikolakopoulou, A., Chaimani, A., Veroniki, A.A., Vasiliadis, H.S., Schmid, C.H., and Salanti, G. 2014. Characteristics of networks of interventions: A description of a database of 186 published networks. *PLoS ONE* 9, e86754.

Raudenbush, S.W. and Bryk, A.S. 1985. Empirical Bayes meta-analysis. *J. Educ. Behav. Stat.*, 10, 75–98.

R Core Team. 2014. *R: A Language and Environment for Statistical Computing*. R Foundation for Statistical Computing, Vienna, Austria. http://www.R-project.org

Rucker, G. 2012. Network meta-analysis, electrical networks and graph theory. *Res. Synth. Method*, 3, 312–324.

Rücker, G., Schwarzer, G., Krahn, U., and Künig, J. 2016. netmeta: Network Meta-Analysis using Frequentist Methods. R package version 0.9-1. https://CRAN.R-project.org/package=netmeta

Salanti, G. 2012. Indirect and mixed-treatment comparison, network, or multiple-treatments meta-analysis: Many names, many benefits, many concerns for the next generation evidence synthesis tool. *Res. Synth. Method*, 3, 80–97.

Salanti, G., Ades, A.E. and Ioannidis, J.P. 2011. Graphical methods and numerical summaries for presenting results from multiple-treatment meta-analysis: An overview and tutorial. *J. Clin. Epidemiol.*, 64, 163–171.

Salanti, G., Marinho, V. and Higgins, J.P.T. 2009. A case study of multiple-treatments meta-analysis demonstrates that covariates should be considered. *J. Clin. Epidemiol.* 62, 857–864.

Salanti, G. et al. 2008. Evaluation of networks of randomized trials. *Stat. Methods Med. Res.*, 17, 279–301.

Song, F., Harvey, I. and Lilford, R. 2008. Adjusted indirect comparison may be less biased than direct comparison for evaluating new pharmaceutical interventions. *J. Clin. Epidemiol.*, 61, 455–463.

Song, F., Altman, D.G., Glenny, A.M., and Deeks, J.J. 2003. Validity of indirect comparison for estimating efficacy of competing interventions: Empirical evidence from published meta-analyses. *BMJ*, 326, 472.

Song, F. et al. 2011. Inconsistency between direct and indirect comparisons of competing interventions: Meta-epidemiological study. *BMJ*, 343, d4909.

Song, F. et al. 2012. Simulation evaluation of statistical properties of methods for indirect and mixed treatment comparisons. *BMC Med. Res. Methodol.*, 12, 138.

StataCorp. 2013. Stata Statistical Software: Release 13.

Sutton, A.J. and Higgins, J.P.T. 2008. Recent developments in meta-analysis. *Stat. Med.*, 27, 625–650.

Thijs, V., Lemmens, R. and Fieuws, S. 2008. Network meta-analysis: Simultaneous meta-analysis of common antiplatelet regimens after transient ischaemic attack or stroke. *Eur. Heart J.*, 29, 1086–1092.

van Houwelingen, H.C., Arends, L.R. and Stijnen, T. 2002. Advanced methods in meta-analysis: Multivariate approach and meta-regression. *Stat. Med.*, 21, 589–624.

van Valkenhoef, G. et al. 2012. Automating network meta-analysis. *Res. Synth. Method*, 3, 285–299.

Veroniki, A.A. et al. 2013. Evaluation of inconsistency in networks of interventions. *Int. J. Epidemiol.*, 42, 332–345.

White, I.R. 2011. Multivariate random-effects meta-regression: Updates to mvmeta. *Stata J.*, 11, 255–270.

White, I.R. et al. 2012. Consistency and inconsistency in network meta-analysis: Model estimation using multivariate meta-regression. *Res. Synth. Method*, 3, 111–125.

12

Bayesian Network Meta-Analysis for Multiple Endpoints

Hwanhee Hong, Karen L. Price, Haoda Fu, and Bradley P. Carlin

CONTENTS

ABSTRACT Network meta-analysis (NMA) is a statistical technique to assess various treatment effects and compare their benefits or harms simultaneously in a systematic review. In comparative effectiveness research, NMA offers useful information to help patients and their caregivers make better decisions on their health care. Recently, many systematic reviews collecting various endpoints and methods for integrating such multivariate evidence jointly in NMA have been developed. In this chapter, we introduce Bayesian NMA methods under a missing data framework incorporating multiple outcomes by accounting for their inherent correlations. We utilize two different parameterizations which can be applied separately based on the scientific question of interest. In addition, we provide two decision-making tools, best and acceptability probabilities. We illustrate our methods using a real diabetes data example including two outcomes, and a simulation study validates the performance of our methods in terms of model selection and coverage probability. We close this chapter with a brief summary and discussion of potential future work.

12.1 Introduction

In many biomedical settings, researchers want to synthesize all previous study findings about key aspects of efficacy or safety of certain treatments. *Meta-analysis* is a statistical technique to assess treatment effects inferentially in comparative effective research (CER) using a systematic review, by combining the results from several independent studies (DerSimonian and Laird 1986; Whitehead 2003). Meta-analysis is conducted in a systematic review to compare two treatments, but only when the individual study results are comparable. *Network meta-analysis* (NMA) extends this methodology to compare multiple treatments. Recently, incorporating *individual patient data* has garnered attention because this approach enables us to make personalized decisions based on a patient's clinical characteristics (Hong et al. 2015).

One limitation of traditional meta-analysis is that only two treatments can be compared at a time to obtain a relative effect (e.g., between placebo and an experimental drug). However, to understand the performance of all possible interventions comprehensively, we have to compare them to one another. NMA, also called *mixed treatment comparisons* (MTC), extends traditional meta-analysis to incorporate multiple treatments simultaneously when none of the studies investigates all the treatments at the same time (Hoaglin et al. 2011; Jansen et al. 2011). Since few studies are typically available to provide evidence of *direct* head-to-head comparisons, we have to depend on *indirect* comparisons. The biggest assumption in meta-analysis and NMA is exchangeability among studies; that is, any ranking of the true treatment effects across studies is equally likely *a priori*. In addition, populations in selected studies should be similar to the target population to obtain a valid clinical interpretation (Ades et al. 2012). Visit Section 11.3 in Chapter 11 for a detailed discussion of assumptions underlying NMA.

Bayesian hierarchical statistical meta-analysis for NMA with a single outcome has been investigated actively. The methods and BUGS code of Lu and Ades (LA) (2004, 2006) allowed Bayesian NMA models for a single binary outcome to gain popularity, and subsequent papers by the National Institute for Health and Care Excellence (NICE) group in the United Kingdom (e.g., Dias et al. 2013) show the extension of these models to other types of outcomes (continuous, count, etc.). Recently, developing Bayesian NMA methods for *multiple* outcomes is getting attention (Bujkiewicz et al. 2013; Efthimiou et al. 2014, 2015; Hong et al. 2012, 2016; Schmid et al. 2014; Wei and Higgins 2013). For example, our motivating diabetes data, which will be discussed in depth in Section 12.2, include two efficacy outcomes, fasting blood glucose (BG) and hemoglobin A1c (HbA1c); the dataset in Hong et al. (2016) also includes two efficacy outcomes related to knee osteoarthritis, pain, and disability scores. In fact, many randomized-controlled trials (RCTs) measure several secondary, often patient-centered outcomes, rather than a single primary outcome such as death. NMA can analyze multiple outcomes and deliver more sophisticated results by incorporating all measurements and their correlations.

Another issue which has not had as much attention is the sparsity of NMA data. Since most RCTs include only two or three treatment arms, often including a control group (typically, "usual care" in CER), many potential arms are missing. For example, Table 12.1 presents our motivating dataset wherein the empty cells correspond to missing arms. We can calculate the missingness rate of this dataset by taking the ratio of the number of empty cells and the number of all cells which is 54/90 or 60%. Obviously this problem worsens as the total number of treatments increases. When missingness is not completely at random and depends on some observed or unobserved information, ignoring the problem can yield biased results (Little and Rubin 2002). Current widely used NMA models often ignore such missing components. However, we can borrow strength across missing and observed data by imputing the missing values in a Bayesian hierarchical model with correlations across arms and outcomes using Markov chain Monte Carlo (MCMC) algorithms.

In this chapter, we review existing LA-style NMA models, and also discuss more recent Bayesian missing data approaches for bivariate continuous outcomes, using an application to type 2 diabetes data as motivation. We interpret and compare our data-analytic findings across models having various assumptions using a sensible treatment-ranking system. We also provide a simulation study to investigate the performance of the different models in terms of correct model selection and confidence interval coverage probability when the model is correctly specified or misspecified.

12.2 Motivating Example

Diabetes mellitus, or simply diabetes, is a disease characterized by elevated BG. It is a major cause of kidney failure, nonacute lower-limb amputations, blindness, heart disease, and stroke. As a result, diabetes is one of the leading causes of death worldwide. On the basis of data from the Centers for Disease Control and Prevention (http://www.cdc.gov/diabetes/pubs), in 2011, diabetes affected 25.8-million American people, a roughly 8.3% of the U.S. population. New cases are diagnosed at a rate of roughly 1-million people per year. There are two common types of diabetes: Type-1 diabetes mellitus (T1DM) and Type-2 diabetes mellitus (T2DM). T1DM results from body's failure to produce insulin. T2DM is caused by inadequate insulin secretion, failing to properly use insulin, or increased insulin resistance. An important goal of treating diabetes patients is to lower their BG, but we also want to avoid further hypoglycemic episodes as well as long-term complications. For T2DM patients, treatments often start with improved diet and exercise.

TABLE 12.1

Type 2 Diabetes Data with Respect to Fasting BG Change and HbA1c Changes

Study	Placebo			Gliclazide			Metformin			Pioglitazone			Rosiglitazone		
	$Y_{ik\ell}$	$s_{ik\ell}$	$n_{ik\ell}$	$Y_{ik\ell}$	$s_{ik\ell}$	$n_{ik\ell}$	$Y_{ik\ell}$	$s_{ik\ell}$	$n_{ik\ell}$	$Y_{ik\ell}$	$s_{ik\ell}$	$n_{ik\ell}$	$Y_{ik\ell}$	$s_{ik\ell}$	$n_{ik\ell}$
Fasting BG change (mmol/L)															
1							−2.79	2.62	525	−2.96	2.42	522			
2				−2.93	2.83	564				−2.79	2.48	563			
3							−3.15	3.13	295	−2.92	2.42	293			
4				−2.26	2.87	291				−2.43	2.66	284			
5							−3.03	3.20	90	−2.61	2.85	100	−2.24	2.03	50
6										−2.14	2.28	51			
7				−2.90	3.13	272				−2.53	2.44	240			
8	0.26	4.70	134							−1.90	5.00	125			
9	1.56	5.90	8							−3.81	3.78	20			
HbA1c change (%)															
1							−1.81	1.12	525	−1.56	1.12	522			
2				−1.82	1.10	564				−1.60	1.04	563			
3							−1.75	1.02	295	−1.50	0.99	293			
4				−1.40	0.99	291				−1.24	0.96	284			
5							−1.51	1.11	90	−1.25	1.10	100	−0.75	0.76	50
6										−0.96	1.01	51			
7				−1.70	1.18	272				−1.45	1.04	240			
8	−0.24	0.90	134							−0.80	1.01	125			
9	1.19	0.90	8							−1.11	1.56	20			

Note: $Y_{ik\ell}$ is the sample mean, $s_{ik\ell}$ is the sample standard deviation, and $n_{ik\ell}$ is the sample size for the kth treatment with respect to the ℓth outcome in the ith study.

When glycemic control can no longer be achieved with these tools alone, oral antihyperglycemic agents are added (Nathan et al. 2009).

The diabetes NMA dataset contains nine trials. All of these trials were multicenter, double-blind, randomized clinical trials for T2DM patients who had failed on diet and exercise alone. All studies are phase II or III trials of pioglitazone for patients using mono-therapy. The treatments are all oral antihyperglycemic agents: metformin, gliclazide, pioglitazone, and rosiglitazone. Two important efficacy measurements for the treatment of diabetes are considered: fasting BG, and HbA1c. Fasting BG values are measured before patients have breakfast, and is often the first test done to check for diabetes; it is also used to adjust the dose for many diabetes medications. HbA1c values instead measure the average level of BG over the previous 3 months, and indicate how well patients are controlling their diabetes. Each study measured fasting BG change and HbA1c change between pre-treatment (baseline) and after a 6-month treatment period. Thus, the two outcomes indicate how much a drug lowers fasting BG and HbA1c in 6 months. Table 12.1 displays the data with respect to these two outcomes. Each study reports the sample mean ($Y_{ik\ell}$), sample standard deviation ($s_{ik\ell}$), and sample size ($n_{ik\ell}$) of its arms for fasting BG change and HbA1c change. Figure 12.1 exhibits the network between drugs, which is the same for the two outcomes. In Figure 12.1, the size of each node corresponds to the number of trials considering the drug, while the thickness of each edge represents the total number of patients for the relation. The number of studies for the relation is provided on each edge.

We make two comments regarding our example. First, we consider clinical outcomes in our illustrative example, though CER usually focuses on patient-centered outcomes, such as quality of life. The same statistical NMA models can be applied with patient-centered outcomes if all studies report comparable measurements. Second, in CER, the standard of care is often considered to be a reference treatment while placebo is the most common control arm in RCTs for pharmaceutical drugs. However, every trial of our diabetes data

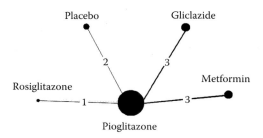

FIGURE 12.1
Network graph of Diabetes II data. The size of each node corresponds to the number of trials considering the drug, while the thickness of each edge represents the total number of patients for the relation. The number of studies for the relation is provided on each edge.

includes the pioglitazone arm, leading to the star network in Figure 12.1. This is because these NMA data were provided by Eli Lilly Company and resulted from their interest in investigating pioglitazone, one of their products. We recommend selecting the most frequently observed treatment as the reference treatment in NMA analysis, to reduce statistical modeling and computational complexities. Therefore, we select pioglitazone as the reference treatment, rather than placebo in our data analysis.

12.3 Bayesian Models for Multiple Endpoints NMA Analysis

We consider L continuous outcomes compared over K treatments from I studies. Specifically, our diabetes data have $L = 2$, $K = 5$, and $I = 9$. For each continuous outcome, we assume we can potentially observe the sample mean ($Y_{ik\ell}$), standard deviation ($s_{ik\ell}$), and sample size ($n_{ik\ell}$) in the kth treatment arm from the ith study with respect to the ℓth outcome. We assign $\ell = 1$ for the fasting BG outcome and 2 for the HbA1c outcome.

We can write the likelihood of $Y_{ik\ell}$ in two ways, depending on whether we assume the study-specific standard deviation is known or unknown. First, the likelihood assuming standard deviations σ_ℓ^2 is known and simply set equal to $s_{ik\ell}^2$ can be written as

$$Y_{ik\ell} \mid \Delta_{ik\ell} \sim N\left(\Delta_{ik\ell}, \frac{s_{ik\ell}^2}{n_{ik\ell}}\right), \quad i = 1,\ldots,I,\ k = 1,\ldots,K,\ l = 1,\ldots,L, \quad (12.1)$$

where $\Delta_{ik\ell}$ is the true population mean and we consider $k = 1$ to be the reference treatment (pioglitazone in our example). Clearly Equation 12.1 is an approximation and relies on the $s_{ik\ell}^2$ being good estimates. Alternatively, we can consider the $s_{ik\ell}$ as separate data from $Y_{ik\ell}$, and assume they estimate a common true outcome-specific standard deviation σ_ℓ

$$Y_{ik\ell} \mid \Delta_{ik\ell}, \sigma_\ell \overset{ind}{\sim} N\left(\Delta_{ik\ell}, \frac{\sigma_\ell^2}{n_{ik\ell}}\right) \quad (12.2)$$

$$\text{and } (n_{ik\ell} - 1)s_{ik\ell}^2 \mid \sigma_\ell \sim Gamma\left(\frac{n_{ik\ell} - 1}{2}, \frac{1}{2\sigma_\ell^2}\right), \quad (12.3)$$

with Equations 12.2 and 12.3 statistically independent. Section 8.3 of Spiegelhalter et al. (2004) shows how this model is justified: Basu's theorem guarantees the independence, and the Gamma distribution comes from the multiple of the chi-square distributions for the sample variances. Since LA develop NMA models under the first likelihood, we denote it as *LA style*, whereas we refer to the second likelihood as *SAM style*, following the preceding reference. We remark that all models in this section can be easily extended to binary or count events by replacing the normal likelihood with an appropriate alternate distribution and link function.

In the remainder of this section, we will present 10 different NMA models under various assumptions. Table 12.2 offers a brief summary of the assumptions made across the 10 models.

12.3.1 Contrast-Based Models

12.3.1.1 Nonimputation Approach

For NMA, we can readily fit a fixed effects model which assumes that treatment effects are the same across all studies. The model can be written as

$$\Delta_{ik\ell} = \alpha_{iB\ell} + d_{Bk\ell}, \tag{12.4}$$

where B represents a baseline treatment (usually placebo), $\alpha_{iB\ell}$ is the baseline treatment effect in the ith study, and $d_{Bk\ell}$ is the fixed mean contrast between treatment k and the baseline treatment with $d_{Bk\ell} \equiv 0$ when $k = B$ for outcome ℓ. We refer to Equation 12.4 as a *contrast-based* (CB) model. Setting $B = 1$, we can infer treatment effects with $d_{1k\ell}$, which compares the kth treatment to the reference treatment. Under the consistency assumption, we can define $d_{Bk\ell} = d_{1k\ell} - d_{1B\ell}$ and compare treatment effects through $d_{1k\ell}$, not $d_{Bk\ell}$. Alternatively, the fixed mean *absolute* effect can be calculated as $E(\alpha_{i1\ell}) + d_{1k\ell}$, where $E(\alpha_{i1\ell})$ is interpreted as the average effect of the reference treatment for outcome ℓ. We denote the fixed effects model under the SAM likelihood as SAMFE, and under the LA likelihood as LAFE.

Next, to allow for variability of treatment effects between studies, we can add *random* effects respecifying model (12.4) to

$$\Delta_{ik\ell} = \alpha_{iB\ell} + \delta_{iBk\ell}, \tag{12.5}$$

where $\delta_{iBk\ell}$ is the random contrast between treatment k and B in the ith study for outcome ℓ, and where we take $\delta_{i1k\ell} = 0$. One constraint in this CB random effects model is that $\alpha_{iB\ell}$ and $\delta_{iBk\ell}$ are considered to be independent, that is, this model does not incorporate any correlation between the baseline effect and the effect contrast. Specifically, we assume that the random contrasts independently follow a normal distribution, such as

$$\delta_{iBk\ell} \overset{ind}{\sim} N\left(d_{1k\ell} - d_{1B\ell}, \tau_\ell^2\right), \tag{12.6}$$

where τ_ℓ is an outcome-specific variance. In this random effects model, we assume homogeneous variance τ_ℓ^2 across all K treatments; for the specification of heterogeneous variance random effects model,

TABLE 12.2

Summary of Model Assumptions

	Likelihood	Parameterization	Treatment Effect	Missing Arm Imputation	Treatment-Wise Correlation	Outcome-Wise Correlation
SAMFE	SAM style	CB	Fixed effect	No	No	No
LAFE	LA style	CB	Fixed effect	No	No	No
SAMRE	SAM style	CB	Random effect	No	Yes	No
LARE	LA style	CB	Random effect	No	Yes	No
CBRE1	LA style	CB	Random effect	Yes	Yes	No
CBRE2	LA style	CB	Random effect	Yes	No	Yes
CBRE3	LA style	CB	Random effect	Yes	Yes	Yes
ABRE1	LA style	AB	Random effect	Yes	Yes	No
ABRE2	LA style	AB	Random effect	Yes	No	Yes
ABRE3	LA style	AB	Random effect	Yes	Yes	Yes

see Lu and Ades (2006). As before, the random effects model under the SAM likelihood will be called the SAMRE model, and that under the LA likelihood will be called the LARE model.

12.3.1.2 Missing Data Framework

A common issue with NMA data is that they feature many missing arms, because most trials are designed for just two or three study arms among all possible treatments (which often exceed five in number). The resulting sparsity of NMA data can lead to biased estimates when the missingness does not occur randomly (Little and Rubin 2002). Another common issue, especially problematic for CB models, is the frequent lack of a common baseline treatment across studies. This makes it hard to interpret the $\alpha_{iB\ell}$ or use them in decision making. To try to avoid misleading results, we can instead impute unobserved arms by considering them as unknown parameters in the Bayesian model. Under this *missing data framework*, all studies are assumed to have a common (though possibly missing) baseline treatment, that is, B in Equation 12.5 is always 1. Another advantage of an imputation approach is that we can easily consider correlations between all treatments and/or outcomes under various assumptions. In our preliminary analysis, we found the SAM likelihood to provide rather implausible sample standard deviation estimates for our random effects models and exhibit poorer deviance information criterion (DIC) performance than models under the LA likelihood. The additional parameter σ_ℓ in the SAM likelihood might lead to large $\overline{D}$ (see Table 12.3), because it is a parameter to be estimated in Equation 12.2 and simultaneously a hyperparameter in Equation 12.3. As such, we will consider only the LA likelihood in our missing data framework. In addition, fixed effects model cannot be applied in the missing data framework because we impute random effects. Thus, we develop our approach using only random effects models.

TABLE 12.3

Model Comparisons with DIC for the Diabetes II Data Analysis

	SAMFE	LAFE	SAMRE	LARE	CBRE1
p_D	25.6	26.0	33.0	32.1	30.9
$\overline{D}$	53.6	47.0	45.1	42.7	37.2
DIC	79.2	73.0	78.1	74.8	68.1

	CBRE2	CBRE3	ABRE1	ABRE2	ABRE3
p_D	30.5	29.0	32.3	31.2	28.9
$\overline{D}$	37.4	35.0	34.9	34.9	34.6
DIC	67.9	64.0	67.2	66.1	63.5

Note: DIC is the sum of $\overline{D}$, a measure of goodness of fit, and p_D, an effective number of model parameters. Smaller DIC values indicate better models.

In this approach, the random effects model has the same form as in Equation 12.5 with $B = 1$, and the independent specification of the $\delta_{i1k\ell}$ in Equation 12.6 is replaced with a matrix form. If we first assume independence between outcomes but not treatments, Equation 12.6 would be rewritten as

$$\delta_{i\ell}^{Trt} \sim MVN\left(\mathbf{d}_{\ell}^{Trt}, \Sigma_{\ell}^{Trt}\right), \tag{12.7}$$

where $\delta_{i\ell}^{Trt} = (\delta_{i12\ell}, \dots, \delta_{i1K\ell})^T$, $\mathbf{d}_{\ell}^{Trt} = (d_{12\ell}, \dots, d_{1K\ell})^T$, and Σ_{ℓ}^{Trt} is a $(K-1) \times (K-1)$ unstructured covariance matrix for $\ell = 1, \dots, L$. Note that since $\delta_{i11\ell}^{Trt}$ and $d_{11\ell}^{Trt}$ are always 0 by definitions, they are not included in $\delta_{i\ell}$ and $\mathbf{d}_{\ell}$. Here, Σ_{ℓ}^{Trt} captures the correlation of random contrasts between treatments independently and uniquely for each outcome ℓ. We refer to this model as a *contrast-based random effects* model assuming independence between outcomes (CBRE1).

Next, suppose we instead allow correlation between outcomes but insist an independence between treatments. Then, the matrix specification of the $\delta_{i1k\ell}$ in Equation 12.7 will change to

$$\delta_{ik}^{Out} \sim MVN(\mathbf{d}_{k}^{Out}, \Sigma_{k}^{Out}), \tag{12.8}$$

where $\delta_{ik}^{Out} = (\delta_{i1k1}, \dots, \delta_{i1kL})^T$, $\mathbf{d}_{k}^{Out} = (d_{1k1}, \dots, d_{1kL})^T$, and Σ_{k}^{Out} is an $L \times L$ unstructured covariance matrix for $k = 2, \dots, K$. In this model, the covariance matrix Σ_{k}^{Out} accounts for all the relationships among the random contrasts between outcomes. We call this model CBRE2. Note that we can also use the same Σ_{k}^{Out} for all k, if such an assumption is reasonable.

Finally, we can incorporate *both* between-treatment and between-outcome correlations by allowing two independent sets of random effects. Under this assumption, model (12.5) is rewritten as

$$\Delta_{ik\ell} = \alpha_{i1\ell} + d_{1k\ell} + \nu_{ik} + \omega_{i\ell}, \tag{12.9}$$

where $\nu_i = (\nu_{i2}, \dots, \nu_{iK})^T \sim MVN(\mathbf{0}, \mathbf{R}^{Trt})$, $\omega_i = (\omega_{i1}, \dots, \omega_{iL})^T \sim MVN(\mathbf{0}, \mathbf{R}^{Out})$, and the ν_{ik} and $\omega_{i\ell}$ are assumed to be independent. Here, $\mathbf{R}^{Trt}$ and $\mathbf{R}^{Out}$ are $(K-1) \times (K-1)$ and $L \times L$ unstructured covariance matrices capturing correlations between treatments and outcomes, respectively. We denote this model by CBRE3.

12.3.2 Arm-Based Models

The primary parameter of interest in a CB model is a *relative* effect, such as a mean difference and log odds ratio between two treatments for continuous and binary outcomes, respectively. An alternative parametrization is the so-called *arm-based* (AB) method, which attempts to deal with *absolute* rather than relative effects. The AB approach delivers a pure treatment effect with a more straightforward interpretation. The choice of AB or CB parameterization depends on the questions of interest. In our diabetes data example, the objective of treatment is to lower HbA1c to a certain level; as such, a patient might want to know the expected posttreatment decrease in HbA1c, not the net decrease compared to the reference treatment. In this case, AB models could deliver more appropriate information for decision makers. Compared to CB models, AB models are less constrained because CB models assume independence between baseline and relative treatment effects while AB models do not. However, AB models do require somewhat stronger assumptions regarding the similarity and exchangeability of all populations (and not merely effects relative to baseline), in order to permit meaningful clinical inference. That is, the target populations of studies in NMA data should be similar. This assumption cannot be tested statistically, but can be investigated empirically by comparing baseline sample characteristics of all studies.

In this approach, we respecify Equation 12.5 as

$$\Delta_{ik\ell} = \mu_{k\ell} + \eta_{ik\ell},\qquad(12.10)$$

where $\mu_{k\ell}$ is the fixed mean effect of treatment k with respect to outcome ℓ, and $\eta_{ik\ell}$ is the study-specific random effect. Again, we will introduce AB models only under the LA likelihood within the missing data framework.

Similar to CB models, we begin by assuming independent random effects between outcomes, where the random effects $\eta_{ik\ell}$ in Equation 12.10 can be modeled as $(\eta_{i1\ell}, \ldots, \eta_{iK\ell})^T \sim MVN(\mathbf{0}, \Lambda_\ell^{Trt})$, with Λ_ℓ^{Trt} a $K \times K$ unstructured covariance matrix capturing relations among random effects between treatments, for $\ell = 1, \ldots, L$. We denote this model as ABRE1. Next, we can instead allow dependence of random effects between outcomes but independence between treatments by defining $(\eta_{ik1}, \ldots, \eta_{ikL})^T \sim MVN(\mathbf{0}, \Lambda_k^{Out})$, where Λ_k^{Out} is an $L \times L$ unstructured covariance matrix capturing correlations between outcomes, for $k = 1, \ldots, K$. We refer to this model as ABRE2, where again we can use the same Λ^{Out} for all k assuming homogeneous variance for random effects across treatments within each outcome. Finally, we can allow both correlation sources by rewriting the mean structure (12.10) as $\Delta_{ik\ell} = \mu_{k\ell} + \nu_{ik} + \omega_{i\ell}$, where $(\nu_{i1}, \ldots, \nu_{iK})^T \sim MVN(\mathbf{0}, \mathbf{D}^{Trt})$, $(\omega_{i1}, \ldots, \omega_{iL})^T \sim MVN(\mathbf{0}, \mathbf{D}^{Out})$, and ν_{ik} and $\omega_{i\ell}$ are independent. Here, $\mathbf{D}^{Trt}$ and $\mathbf{D}^{Out}$ are $K \times K$ and $L \times L$ unstructured covariance matrices.

12.3.3 Prior Distribution Selection and Computational Notes

In applied Bayesian analysis, we often utilize *noninformative* prior distributions that allow the data to drive the posterior information. For models under the nonimputation method, we use a vague normal prior distribution, namely $N(0, 100^2)$, for the $\alpha_{iB\ell}$ and $d_{Bk\ell}$, and a vague Uniform distribution, $Uniform(0.01, 10)$, for the τ_ℓ. We can certainly adopt other priors for τ_ℓ, such as an inverse gamma or half-normal distribution, but Gelman (2006) shows that a Uniform prior works fairly well unless the number of studies is small (say, <5). In the SAM likelihood, the common sample standard deviation, σ, is often assigned a log-Uniform priors, that is, $log(\sigma) \sim Uniform(-10, 10)$ (Gelman 2006).

Models under the missing data framework, CBREs and ABREs, also use a vague normal prior distribution for the $\alpha_{iB\ell}$, $d_{Bk\ell}$, and $\mu_{k\ell}$, while all inverse covariance matrices follow a $Wishart(\Omega, \gamma)$ with a mean of $\gamma\Omega^{-1}$ and γ taken to be the matrix dimension, the smallest value yielding for a proper Wishart prior. For our data analysis, we select Ω to be the identity matrix, a noninformative specification that still ensures MCMC convergence. In this chapter, we use only noninformative priors since we lack expert opinions or historical data needed to inform a prior. However, informative priors could be incorporated when there is auxiliary information providing strong evidence for an effect size or its distribution, though this appears fairly rare in CER.

OpenBUGS or WinBUGS (Lunn et al. 2000) is readily used for NMA Bayesian data analysis. We typically obtain 50,000 MCMC samples after a 50,000-iteration burn-in with two parallel sampling chains. To check MCMC convergence, we used standard diagnostics, including trace plots and lag 1 sample autocorrelations (Carlin and Louis 2009, Section 3.4). For simulation studies, we used the rjags package in R, where we call JAGS (Plummer et al. 2003) 500 times from R, once for each simulated dataset. JAGS is a C++-based version of the BUGS language popular with developers.

12.3.4 Decision Making with Multiple Endpoints

To identify the best treatment, we can certainly compare the posteriors of the $d_{1k\ell}$ or $\mu_{k\ell}$, but those quantities only give outcome-specific information. In this section, we will introduce a Bayesian probability-based decision-making tool that enables us to combine across multiple outcomes. Suppose $\theta_k^{(\ell)}$ is the marginal posterior absolute effect under treatment k for outcome ℓ. Denoting the data on outcome ℓ by $y^{(\ell)}$, we can calculate the posterior probability of being the best treatment under each outcome when the outcome has a positive interpretation (e.g., positive responses in a quality-of-life questionnaire) as

$$Pr\{k \text{ is the best treatment}|y^{(\ell)}\} = Pr\{\text{rank}(\theta_k^{(\ell)}) = 1|y^{(\ell)}\}. \tag{12.11}$$

We denote this probability by "Best1." For a negative outcome (e.g., the number of adverse events such as dry mouth), we simply change 1 to K on the right-hand side of Equation 12.11. Similarly, one can calculate the probability of being the first or second-best treatment, denoted by "Best12," by replacing the right-hand side of Equation 12.11 with $Pr\{\text{rank}(\theta_k^{(\ell)}) = 1 \text{ or } 2|y^{(\ell)}\}$, where again small ranks indicate best treatments.

Next, to combine these univariate probabilities over all the endpoints and obtain one omnibus measure of "best," we might utilize an overall, weighted score. Suppose that $T_k^{(\ell)} = \theta_k^{(\ell)}$ for positive outcomes and $T_k^{(\ell)} = -\theta_k^{(\ell)}$ for negative outcomes, so that high values of $T_k^{(\ell)}$ indicate the best condition. Define the overall score as

$$S_k = \sum_\ell w^{(\ell)} T_k^{(\ell)}, \qquad (12.12)$$

where $w^{(\ell)}$ is the weight for outcome ℓ, and $\sum_\ell w^{(\ell)} = 1$. This score can be used to obtain overall Best1 and Best12 probabilities by replacing $\theta_k^{(\ell)}$ by S_k in Equation 12.11. Sensible weights can be chosen by physicians or public health professionals based on their relative preferences among outcomes; they are not estimated from the data. For example, if a patient were more concerned about possible adverse events from a treatment than its benefits, she might prefer a large weight on a safety outcome. In addition, we can compare Best probabilities estimated under various weights to investigate how robust those probabilities are to this choice, and illustrate such results in Section 12.4.

Another tool for decision making is to identify an *acceptable* drug, using a metric that captures whether a treatment performs better or worse than a certain level. This might be useful in CER for physicians or patients to rule out an acceptable treatment, specifically when nonpharmaceutical or educational treatments are compared. Most pharmaceutical drugs investigated using RCTs are approved by Food and Drug Administration (FDA), so that they should have significantly more efficacy than placebo. Recall that the mean absolute effect for treatment k with respect to an outcome ℓ is $\mu_{k\ell}$, and this can be obtained by the sum of the mean reference treatment effect and $d_{1k\ell}$ under the CB parameterization. Thus, we may define drug k as *acceptable* for a specific outcome ℓ if

$$Pr\{\mu_{k\ell} > \mu_{k\ell}^*\} > p_\ell^A, \qquad (12.13)$$

where larger values of $\mu_{1k\ell}$ mean better performance, $\mu_{k\ell}^*$ is a prespecified constant chosen to reflect clinical significance, and p_ℓ^A is also a fixed probability, typically fairly large (say, 0.9) (Chuang-Stein et al. 2011). The inequality sign would be flipped when smaller values of $\mu_{k\ell}$ indicate better drugs. The left-hand side probability in Equation 12.13 can be easily calculated under our MCMC-based Bayesian framework.

12.4 Analysis of Diabetes Data

We fit the 10 different models listed in Table 12.2: four nonimputation models (two fixed effects and two random effects models under the SAM and LA likelihood specifications), and six random effects models under the missing data framework (three CB and three AB models under various correlation assumptions). We consider three correlation assumptions for each of the CB and AB models: independence between outcomes but dependence between treatments, dependence between outcomes but independence between treatments, and dependence both between treatments and between outcomes (but not between treatments and outcomes). Table 12.3 shows results for Bayesian model selection using the DIC. DIC is the sum of $\overline{D}$, a measure of goodness of fit, and p_D, an effective number of model parameters (Spiegelhalter et al. 2002). Smaller DIC values indicate better models, with a DIC difference of five or more considered to be practically meaningful. For all CB and AB models, we calculate $\overline{D}$ using only the observed data (not the imputed data). For the nonimputation approach, models under SAM likelihood give the largest DIC values, with p_D differences of roughly 1 between SAM and LA fixed and random effects models, resulting from additional population variance parameters. Moving to the CBRE and ABRE models, we observe large drops in $\overline{D}$, with CBRE3 and ABRE3 giving the smallest DIC values (about 10 units smaller than those of the nonimputation models). Generally, model-based imputation of unobserved arms yielded better DIC performance than ignoring such arms for these diabetes data.

Figure 12.2 displays point and interval estimate of absolute treatment effects (i.e., mean changes) for each outcome. For both outcomes, the four nonimputation models produce significantly narrower 95% credible intervals than all CB and AB models, due to their failure to capture all sources of data uncertainty. Note that SAMRE gives slightly wider credible intervals than LARE, since SAMRE contains more parameters to be estimated. As we expected, the estimates for pioglitazone are the most precise, with narrow 95% credible intervals (since all nine studies investigate pioglitazone), while those for placebo and rosiglitazone have relatively wide intervals and are less consistent across models. In addition, placebo and rosiglitazone are not significantly effective in decreasing HbA1c (only two and one studies investigate placebo and rosiglitazone), and rosiglitazone is also not significantly effective for fasting BG change under CBRE1. Gliclazide, metformin, and pioglitazone help to decrease BG with respect to both outcomes, but do not differ significantly from each other (note the overlapping 95% credible intervals).

The estimated sample standard deviations under SAMFE and SAMRE are the same in each outcome ($\hat{\sigma}_1 = 2.876$ and $\hat{\sigma}_2 = 1.063$), and the posterior distributions appear perfectly Gaussian with 95% credible intervals equal to $\pm 1.96 * \text{sd}(\hat{\sigma}_\ell)$, where "sd" stands for standard deviation, revealing that the posterior standard deviations σ_ℓ are unaffected by the presence of random effects. The posterior median of random effect variability τ_ℓ in Equation 12.6 is estimated as follows: $(\hat{\tau}_1, \hat{\tau}_2) = (0.29, 0.30)$ under SAMRE, and $(\hat{\tau}_1, \hat{\tau}_2) = (0.25, 0.11)$ under LARE. Overall, CB and AB models give a bit larger variability estimates, likely because they incorporate additional uncertainty from

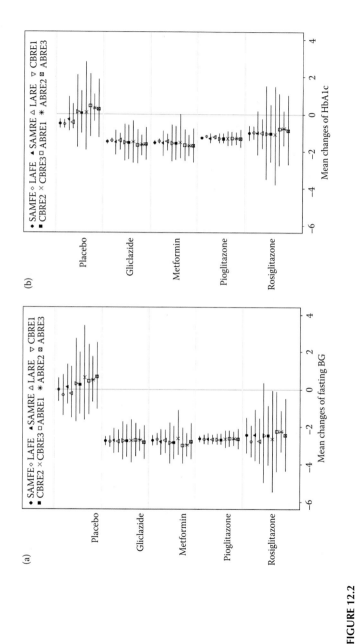

FIGURE 12.2
Interval plots for the Diabetes II data analysis: (a) Fasting BG change; (b) HbA1c change. The estimated absolute treatment effects with associated 95% BCIs are plotted under 10 different models.

the missing data. CBRE1 can be compared to LARE equivalently because both models assume independence between outcomes, although only CBRE1 allows unstructured correlation between treatments. Note that CBRE1 estimates the variability for each treatment, and the square roots of the diagonal elements of $\hat{\Sigma}_\ell^{Trt}$ in Equation 12.7 are between 0.5 and 0.8 for both outcomes, where 0.8 is the variability of the contrast between rosiglitazone and pioglitazone, estimated from only one study. The between-treatment correlation is estimated as 0.27 (-0.41, 0.75) and 0.36 (-0.29, 0.77) under the CBRE2 and ABRE2 models, respectively, indicating a weak positive linear relationship.

Table 12.4 shows Best12 probabilities (as defined in Section 12.3.4) and associated standard errors (in parentheses) to help find the best drug under simultaneous consideration of both the fasting BG and HbA1c outcomes using models such as LAFE, LARE, and ABRE3. We specify S_k in Equation 12.12 as $S_k = wT_k^{(FBG)} + (1 - w)T_k^{(HbA1c)}$, where FBG stands for fasting BG, and consider three different weights: $w = 0.5$ for an equal weight on both outcomes, $w = 0.8$ for heavier weighting on the short-term fasting BG measure, and $w = 0.2$ for heavier weighting on HbA1c, the longer-term measure. Again, the weight is chosen by a patient or physician based on personal

TABLE 12.4

Best12 Probabilities under the LAFE, LARE, and ABRE3 Models

	$w = 0.5$	$w = 0.8$	$w = 0.2$
Lu and Ades fixed effects model (LAFE)			
Placebo	0.000 (0.00)	0.000 (0.00)	0.000 (0.00)
Gliclazide	**0.916** (0.28)	**0.842** (0.36)	0.981 (0.14)
Metformin	0.803 (0.40)	0.478 (0.50)	**0.985** (0.12)
Pioglitazone	0.023 (0.15)	0.187 (0.39)	0.000 (0.00)
Rosiglitazone	0.258 (0.44)	0.493 (0.50)	0.034 (0.18)
Lu and Ades random effects model (LARE)			
Placebo	0.000 (0.01)	0.000 (0.02)	0.001 (0.03)
Gliclazide	**0.779** (0.41)	**0.692** (0.46)	0.880 (0.33)
Metformin	0.767 (0.42)	0.590 (0.49)	**0.903** (0.30)
Pioglitazone	0.138 (0.34)	0.241 (0.43)	0.080 (0.27)
Rosiglitazone	0.316 (0.46)	0.478 (0.50)	0.137 (0.34)
Arm-based random effects model 3 (ABRE3)			
Placebo	0.001 (0.03)	0.000 (0.02)	0.005 (0.07)
Gliclazide	0.686 (0.46)	**0.662** (0.47)	0.708 (0.45)
Metformin	**0.711** (0.45)	0.647 (0.48)	**0.762** (0.43)
Pioglitazone	0.317 (0.47)	0.353 (0.48)	0.284 (0.45)
Rosiglitazone	0.285 (0.45)	0.338 (0.47)	0.241 (0.43)

Note: Associated standard errors are in parentheses. Three different weights are incorporated ($w = 0.2, 0.5$, and 0.8). The highest Best12 probabilities in each model are in bold.

TABLE 12.5

Acceptability Probabilities under the LAFE, LARE, and ABRE3 Models When $\mu_{k1}^* = -2$ and $\mu_{k2}^* = -1$

	Fasting BG Change			HbA1c Change		
	LAFE	**LARE**	**ABRE3**	**LAFE**	**LARE**	**ABRE3**
Placebo	0.001	0.004	0.002	0.000	0.007	0.043
Gliclazide	**1.000**	**0.987**	**0.967**	**1.000**	**0.978**	**0.920**
Metformin	**1.000**	**0.988**	**0.950**	**1.000**	**0.981**	**0.937**
Pioglitazone	**1.000**	**1.000**	**0.989**	**1.000**	**1.000**	**0.900**
Rosiglitazone	**0.965**	**0.915**	0.704	0.434	0.477	0.437

Note: If a calculated acceptability probability for a certain drug is greater than 0.9, the performance of the drug exceeds our threshold, indicating that the drug is acceptable under the criteria. Acceptability probabilities larger than 0.9 are in bold.

preference. Under LA-style models, gliclazide is the winner when $w = 0.5$ or 0.8 and metformin is the winner when $w = 0.2$, while under ABRE3, metformin is the winner when $w = 0.2$ or 0.5 followed by gliclazide. The fixed effects model produces somewhat more extreme Best12 probabilities than the other two random effects model. In addition, the difference of Best12 probabilities for gliclazide and metformin is 0.364 under LAFE, while the difference is just 0.102 and 0.015 for LARE and ABRE3, respectively. Still, it is clear from the table and Figure 12.2 that these two drugs are essentially tied for "best." Note that the weights are chosen by the investigator to reflect his/her preferences. Thus, when this choice has a big effect, that just means the "winning" drug is not the same for all outcomes.

Table 12.5 exhibits acceptability probabilities ($Pr\{\mu_{k\ell} > \mu_{k\ell}^*\}$) for each outcome under the LAFE, LARE, and ABRE3 models. Note that we set $\mu_{k\ell}^*$ and p_ℓ^A in Equation 12.13 somewhat arbitrarily to illustrate the approach, although in practice, these values should be carefully specified to have clinical meaning. Since smaller $\mu_{k\ell}$ values mean better performance in our diabetes data, the left-hand side in Equation 12.13 should be rewritten as $Pr\{\mu_{k\ell} < \mu_{k\ell}^*\}$, and we set μ_{k1}^* and μ_{k2}^* to -2 and -1, respectively. We consider the cutpoint p_ℓ^A to be 0.9. That is, if a calculated acceptability probability for a certain drug is greater than 0.9, the performance of the drug exceeds our threshold, indicating that it is acceptable under the criteria. For example, if the probability is 1, the drug would be acceptable no matter what cutpoint p_ℓ^A is used under our choice of $\mu_{k\ell}^*$. For all models agree that gliclazide, metformin, and pioglitazone are acceptable for both outcomes under our criteria, though for HBA1c change, the probability for pioglitazone in ABRE3 is marginally less than 0.9 before rounding. Placebo is not acceptable for either outcome across all models. Rosiglitazone is not acceptable for the HbA1c outcome whereas for fasting BG change, acceptability varies somewhat across models.

12.5 Simulation Study

Although we fit 10 different NMA models to the diabetes data and choose the best-fitting model in terms of DIC, we cannot guarantee that the selected model is "the" correctly specified model for our data. Thus, we might want a more robust model that consistently performs well even when the model is misspecified. To investigate the robustness of our four main models (LARE, SAMRE, CBRE3, and ABRE3), we create four different datasets under each framework, then fit all four models to each; that is, 16 scenarios are considered. We adopt the same star network as in Figure 12.1 (comparing five treatments with respect to two outcomes), and the same sample sizes and standard deviations. Estimated parameter values from our diabetes data analysis, such as posterior medians of fixed mean and covariance matrices from the four fitted models, are regarded as the true parameter values for our simulated datasets. A total of 500 simulated datasets were generated, and we consider a small number of studies (nine, the same as in the diabetes data) and a large number of studies (45, augmenting the small number of studies scenario by a factor of 5). Note that our parameter of interest is the mean treatment effect. To avoid excessive uncertainty in the treatment effects, we use informative priors for the random variance parameters. That is, prior distributions for τ_ℓ or covariance matrices have mean values set equal to the truth (i.e., estimated values from our data analysis) with relatively small variabilities.

Table 12.6 displays three quantities from the simulation: the probability each model is selected as best using DIC and the coverage probability of the 95% Bayesian credible interval (BCI) for a mean effect of the baseline treatment for the fasting BG outcome. Note that all diagonals of all four blocks in the table correspond to scenarios where the model is correctly specified. For the first quantity, we estimate the probability of having the smallest DIC among the four models from 500 simulated datasets, so that the rows sum to 1 and diagonal values should be close to 1. When $I = 9$, LARE gives about a 50% correct model selection probability, whereas we obtain 0.734 and 0.666 for CBRE3 and ABRE3, respectively. This trend gets clearer with the larger number of studies; ABRE3 now delivers the highest probability of being the best model when the true model is ABRE3, while LARE and CBRE3 have only about a 50% chance of being the best-fitting model under their true data. SAMRE performs worst, with the lowest diagonal quantities for both small and large numbers of studies.

For the coverage probabilities, although there are 10 absolute mean effect parameters (five treatments and two outcomes), we only report the coverage probability of baseline treatment for the first outcome; the others display similar patterns. Here, the diagonal values should be close to 0.95, the nominal coverage probability. LARE shows a bit lower coverage probability than 0.95; it also tends to yield lower coverage for other nonbaseline treatment

TABLE 12.6

Results of Simulation Study

Data	Fitted Model							
	Small Number of Studies ($I = 9$)				Large Number of Studies ($I = 45$)			
Pr(model selected as best using DIC)								
	LARE	SAMRE	CBRE3	ABRE3	LARE	SAMRE	CBRE3	ABRE3
LARE	0.484	0.062	0.318	0.136	0.544	0.002	0.276	0.178
SAMRE	0.568	0.056	0.274	0.102	0.992	0.008	0.062	0.008
CBRE3	0.046	0.034	0.734	0.186	0.000	0.000	0.530	0.470
ABRE3	0.010	0.030	0.294	0.666	0.000	0.000	0.082	0.918
Coverage probability of 95% BCI for mean effect of baseline treatment for Outcome 1								
	LARE	SAMRE	CBRE3	ABRE3	LARE	SAMRE	CBRE3	ABRE3
LARE	0.764	0.956	0.980	0.982	0.778	0.958	0.978	0.990
SAMRE	0.918	0.958	1.000	1.000	0.910	0.968	1.000	1.000
CBRE3	0.710	0.950	0.984	0.990	0.700	0.946	0.946	0.984
ABRE3	0.662	0.932	0.954	0.946	0.622	0.938	0.938	0.956

Note: Three quantities from the simulation are reported: the probability each model is selected as best using DIC and the coverage probability of the 95% BCI for a mean effect of the baseline treatment for the fasting BG outcome.

estimates. However, the baseline treatment effect parameters have the poorest coverage, and this is not resolved when the number of studies is large. This might be because the fixed baseline effect parameter $\alpha_{iB\ell}$ does not estimate the baseline effect well in LARE, resulting in higher type 1 error than it should be. CBRE3 gives higher than 0.95 coverage probability under CBRE3 data when $I = 9$, but improves to 0.946 when $I = 45$. SAMRE and ABRE3 show coverage probabilities close to 0.95 under their true data assumption for both small and large numbers of studies, partially rehabilitating SAMRE after its poor DIC performance. In practice, the LA-style likelihood (assuming sample standard deviations are known) is commonly utilized in NMA. Our simulation results for SAMRE are hard to interpret, and further investigation is needed.

12.6 Discussion and Future Work

In this chapter, we introduced various Bayesian hierarchical modeling for NMA and compared with the existing method. Our proposed contrast- and AB random effects models incorporate information from observed and missing data, and enable us to fit multiple outcomes, possibly inducing some correlation. A simulation study shows that the models under the missing data framework perform better even when a model is misspecified, and deliver more robust results for decision making. Although we have only shown Bayesian NMA models with bivariate continuous outcomes, one can easily apply our methods to other types of outcomes (e.g., binary or count) by using a proper likelihood and link function (e.g., logit or log) (Dias et al. 2013). Additionally, more than two outcomes can be easily incorporated, though this increases the dimension of the covariance matrix containing outcome-wise correlation information. It can be difficult to satisfy the positive definiteness condition for the covariance matrix in MCMC, but the use of an inverse Wishart prior makes it possible.

In the diabetes data analysis, we found a trend that AB and CB random effects models produced a lot wider credible intervals than those from LA models. This can be expected because AB and CB models incorporate more uncertainty, though it depends on which assumptions are made for AB and CB models. Hong et al. (2016) fit another real, much larger, NMA data set having two continuous outcomes, and show that LA models can produce wider credible intervals than the CBRE2 and ABRE2 models for several treatment effects. This might be because CBRE2 and ABRE2 have relatively fewer parameters for the covariance matrix of random effects (i.e., the dimension of the covariance matrix is lower than the CB and AB models under the other two assumptions). SAMRE performs unexpectedly poorly in the data analysis and simulation studies including random effects that do not significantly affect the estimates of sample standard deviations in the data analysis, and the Gibbs sampling algorithm for SAMRE is extremely slow. Our analysis has some limitations. First, all the analyses were conducted under consistency assumption, and *inconsistency*, traditionally defined as discrepancy between direct and indirect comparisons, was not presented in this chapter. Recently, other researchers (Dias et al. 2011; Higgins et al. 2012; Lu and Ades 2006; Piepho et al. 2012; Presanis et al. 2013) have stated that inconsistency is observed when the characteristics of samples from independent studies are different (such as when different baseline severity of disease or various levels of drug dosage are not accounted for in the models), and propose various methods for modeling such inconsistency. These modeling techniques include node splitting, estimating w-factors, and allowing design-by-treatment interactions. These methods are discussed in depth in Section 11.5 of Chapter 11. Second, we only utilize noninformative priors in our data analysis. However, (weakly) informative priors can be used when we have some information from historical or observational studies. For example, if correlation between outcomes is well known and observed from external sources, we can construct an informative inverse Wishart prior by specifying its parameters appropriately. Hong et al. (2016) conducted such sensitivity analyses by applying various informative inverse Wishart priors, but found that they did not decrease DIC values nor change the ranking of treatments in their example.

NMA is an important statistical modeling approach to synthesize evidence in CER. A flexible Bayesian framework helps stakeholders make better decisions by providing various decision-making tools, and more importantly allows us to incorporate multiple outcomes and their inherent relationships. Future work looks to extend existing methods to mixed types of outcomes (say, a binary safety outcome paired with a continuous efficacy outcome). Another needed future model enhancement is to the case of differential borrowing of strength across nonexchangeable subgroups, say determined by similarities across trials or treatments. In addition, the future direction in CER might be combining evidence from experimental (RCTs) and nonexperimental (observational) studies. Finally, one might extend the models to incorporate both aggregated and individual patient-level data, potentially permitting the borrowing of strength from patient-level covariates to investigate how those personal clinical characteristics impact estimated treatment effects. Such methods could be implemented in user-friendly web-based software to help patients and their caregivers make personalized decisions incorporating modern approaches to CER.

Acknowledgment

This chapter was supported by Eli Lilly and Company through the Lilly Research Award Program (LRAP).

References

Ades, A. E., Caldwell, D. M., Reken, S., Welton, N. J., Sutton, A. J., and Dias, S. 2012. NICE DSU Technical Support Document 7: Evidence synthesis of treatment efficacy in decision making: A reviewers checklist. Available from http://www.nicedsu.org.uk

Bujkiewicz S., Thompson J. R., Sutton A. J., Cooper N. J., Harrison M. J., Symmons D. P. M., and Abrams K. R. 2013. Multivariate meta-analysis of mixed outcomes: A Bayesian approach. *Statistics in Medicine*, 32:3926–3943.

Carlin, B. P. and Louis, T. A. 2009. *Bayesian Methods for Data Analysis*, 3rd Edition, Boca Raton, FL: Chapman & Hall/CRC.

Chuang-Stein, C., Kirby, S., French, J., Kowalski, K., Marshall, S., Smith, M. K., Bycott, P., and Beltangady, M. 2011. A quantitative approach for making go/no-go decisions in drug development. *Drug Information Journal*, 45:187–202.

DerSimonian, R. and Laird, N. 1986. Meta-analysis in clinical trials. *Controlled Clinical Trials*, 7:177–188.

Dias, S., Sutton, A. B., Ades, A. E., and Welton, N. J. 2013. A generalized linear modeling framework for pairwise and network meta-analysis of randomized controlled trials. *Medical Decision Making*, 33:607–617.

Dias, S., Welton, N. J., Sutton, A. J., Caldwell, D. M., Lu, G., and Ades, A. E. 2011. NICE DSU Technical Support Document 4: Inconsistency in networks of evidence based on randomised controlled trials. Last updated April 2012; available from http://www.nicedsu.org.uk

Efthimiou, O., Mavridis, D., Cipriani, A., Leucht, S., Bagos, P., and Salanti, G. 2014. An approach for modelling multiple correlated outcomes in a network of interventions using odds ratios. *Statistics in Medicine*, 33:2275–2287.

Efthimiou, O., Mavridis, D., Riley, R. D., Cipriani, A., and Salanti, G. 2015. Joint synthesis of multiple correlated outcomes in networks of interventions. *Biostatistics*, 16(1):84–97.

Gelman, A. 2006. Prior distributions for variance parameters in hierarchical models. *Bayesian Analysis*, 1:515–533.

Higgins, J. P. T., Jackson, D., Barrett, J. K., Lu, G., Ades, A. E., and White, I. R. 2012. Consistency and inconsistency in network meta-analysis: Concepts and models for multi-arm studies. *Research Synthesis Methods*, 3:98–110.

Hoaglin, D. C., Hawkins, N., Jansen, J. P., Scott, D. A., Itzler, R., Cappelleri, J. C., Boersma, C. et al. 2011. Conducting indirect-treatment-comparison and network-meta-analysis studies: Report of the ISPOR task force on indirect treatment comparisons good research practices: Part 2. *Value Health*, 14:429–437.

Hong, H., Carlin, B. P., Shamliyan, T., Wyman, J. F., Ramakrishnan, R., Sainfort, F., and Kane, R. L. 2012. Comparing Bayesian and frequentist approaches for multiple outcome mixed treatment comparisons. *Medical Decision Making*, 33:702–714.

Hong, H., Fu, H., Price, K. L., and Carlin, B. P. 2015. Incorporation of individual patient data in network meta-analysis for multiple continuous endpoints, with application to diabetes treatment. *Statistics in Medicine*, 34(20):2794–2819.

Hong, H., Chu, H., Zhang, J., and Carlin, B. P. 2016. A Bayesian missing data framework for generalized multiple outcome mixed treatment comparisons (with discussion and rejoinder). *Research Synthesis Methods*, 7:6–33.

Jansen, J. P., Fleurence, R., Devine, B., Itzler, R., Barrett, A., Hawkins, N., Lee, K., Boersma, C., Annemans, L., and Cappelleri, J. C. 2011. Interpreting indirect treatment comparisons and network meta-analysis for health-care decision making: Report of the ISPOR task force on indirect treatment comparisons good research practices: Part 1. *Value Health*, 14:417–428.

Little, R. J. and Rubin, D. B. 2002. *Statistical Analysis with Missing Data*, 2nd Edition, New York: Wiley.

Lu, G. and Ades, A.E. 2004. Combination of direct and indirect evidence in mixed treatment comparisons. *Statistics in Medicine*, 23(20):3105–3124.

Lu, G. and Ades, A. E. 2006. Assessing evidence inconsistency in mixed treatment comparisons. *Journal of the American Statistical Association*, 101:447–459.

Lunn, D., Thomas, A., Best, N., and Spiegelhalter, D. J. 2000. WinBUGS—A Bayesian modelling framework: Concepts, structure, and extensibility. *Statistics and Computing*, 10:325–337.

Nathan, D., Buse, J., Davidson, M., Ferrannini, E., Holman, R., Sherwin, R., and Zinman, B. 2009. Medical management of hyperglycemia in type 2 diabetes: A consensus algorithm for the initiation and adjustment of therapy a consensus statement of the American Diabetes Association and the European Association for the Study of Diabetes. *Diabetes Care*, 32:193–203.

Piepho, H. P., Williams, E. R., and Madden, L. V. 2012. The use of two-way linear mixed models in multitreatment meta-analysis. *Biometrics*, 68:1269–1277.

Plummer, M. 2003. JAGS: A program for analysis of Bayesian graphical models using Gibbs sampling. In *Proceedings of the 3rd International Workshop on Distributed Statistical Computing*, pp. 202. Citeseer.

Presanis, A. M., Ohlssen, D., Spiegelhalter, D. J., and De Angelis, D. 2013. Conflict diagnostics in directed acyclic graphs, with applications in Bayesian evidence synthesis. *Statistical Science*, 28:376–397.

Schmid, C. H., Trikalinos, T. A., and Olkin, I. 2014. Bayesian network meta-analysis for unordered categorical outcomes with incomplete data. *Research Synthesis Methods*, 5:162–185.

Spiegelhalter, D. J., Abrams, K. R., and Myles, J. P. 2004. *Bayesian Approaches to Clinical Trials and Health-Care Evaluation*, England: Wiley.

Spiegelhalter, D. J., Best, N. G., Carlin, B. P., and Linde, A. v. d. 2002. Bayesian measures of model complexity and fit. *Journal of the Royal Statistical Society, Series B*, 64:583–639.

Wei, Y. and Higgins, J. P. T. 2013. Estimating within-study covariances in multivariate meta-analysis with multiple outcomes. *Statistics in Medicine*, 32:1191–1205.

Whitehead, A. 2003. *Meta-Analysis of Controlled Clinical Trials*, New York: John Wiley.

13

Mathematical Modeling

Mark S. Roberts, Kenneth J. Smith, and Jagpreet Chhatwal

CONTENTS

ABSTRACT　Mathematical models are being increasingly used to evaluate the future impacts of various therapies for particular problems, and to inform many types of clinical and policy decisions facing clinicians, patients, and policy makers in healthcare today. One advantage of mathematical models is that they can incorporate evidence from many different sources and provide a framework to integrate this knowledge and estimate an optimal decision under various different conditions. The purpose of this chapter is to provide an overview of the use of mathematical modeling in comparative effectiveness research, with a concentration on the commonly used methods, including simple decision trees, time-varying state transition (often called Markov) models, and microsimulation. Several examples are described, and references to more complete expositions on the methodology are provided.

13.1 Introduction

> Comparative effectiveness research is designed to inform health-care decisions by providing evidence on the effectiveness, benefits, and harms of different treatment options.—AHRQ Effective Healthcare Program.

Comparative effectiveness research strives to provide evidence for making the optimal decision across a range of plausible or available alternatives in real clinical situations. The overall goal is to provide useful information to patients and clinicians that facilitates making optimal clinical decisions about the appropriate choice in each particular patient's situation. Unfortunately, applying the current evidence base is often fraught with difficulty as the specific choices being evaluated may not have been tested in a specific study. The tenets of evidence-based medicine strongly recommend the use of randomized-controlled trials (RCTs) [1], but such trials often do not compare all of the possible alternatives, and are typically designed for the purpose of FDA approval and not for the development of evidence to inform the specific, complex decisions that are made within specific clinical situations. Meta-analyses of these RCTs have many of the same limitations. If the underlying RCTs do not compare all of the appropriate alternatives, meta-analyses cannot as well; see Chapters 11 and 12. Observational trials can be used in evidence-based recommendation, but their strength is considered less compelling than RCTs [2]. Chapter 7 discusses combining information across design.

Decision analysis is another method that can be used to structure and summarize the current knowledge about a particular set of decisions that must be made. Decision analysis is a methodology through which the best available evidence is combined into a structured representation of the decision problem, and the decision that maximizes the value of the specified outcome is chosen as the best strategy. For the purpose of this chapter, we define a "decision model" as a specific application of decision analysis that quantifies the specific choices and outcomes that can occur over a set of choices. The PCORI (Patient-Centered Outcomes Research Institute) methods committee has embraced mathematical modeling as an analytic methodology for the conduct of comparative effectiveness [3,4].

13.1.1 Decision-Making Paradigm: Predicting the Downstream Consequences of Decisions

The basic goal of any methodology used to conduct comparative effectiveness research is to provide the best information and evidence available to help the decision maker estimate the downstream events and outcomes implied by making various decisions. This is illustrated in Figure 13.1, in which a set of clinical strategies are illustrated. Each choice produces a set of downstream consequences that must be predicted in order to make the optimal decision. The choices represented in the figure are arbitrary: they could be choices of different medications in a particular clinical situation (e.g., which of many lipid-lowering drugs should be used in a particular

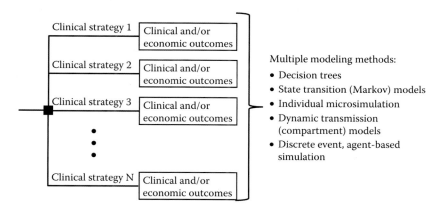

FIGURE 13.1
Basic structure of a clinical decision problem.

patient with a particular set of clinical characteristics), different surgical interventions for a particular clinical condition (such as a choice between cardiac catheterization or coronary artery bypass surgery for coronary artery disease), or any set of decisions that must be made. A wide array of consequences may be important in understanding how to make the optimal decision, including life expectancy, quality-adjusted life expectancy, the likelihood of certain complications, as well as the expected cost of each strategy. There are many methodologies that can be used to provide evidence for estimating the likelihood of downstream events given the various choices made. The most obvious would be the RCT, provided all of the relevant clinical strategies were represented as an arm in a trial. The use of RCTs to make these predictions is described in Chapters 4 through 6. However, other methods, including observational statistical methods, which are the subject of Chapters 1 through 3, can often be used when RCTs are not available. However, RCTs and other observational methods are not always possible or practical to answer many treatment decisions facing patients and clinicians today.

Using a decision modeling to predict the outcomes that can occur after making specific clinical choices implies the use of a mathematical model to represent all of the downstream events and outcomes that can occur given each of the choices. In this use, it may be useful to consider a decision model as a framework on which to place all of the current knowledge we have about a particular problem, whether this knowledge comes from physiologic studies, observational studies, or RCTs. There are a series of modeling methodologies that can be used to represent the outcomes that occur as the result of choosing a specific strategy, including decision trees, state transition models, microsimulation techniques, discrete-event simulation, agent-based simulation, and compartment models. The following section will describe these methods in more detail.

13.2 Basic Steps in Developing a Decision Model

The development of any decision model involves a series of steps that when complete assure an easily describable, transparent representation of a particular problem and its solution. In late 2012, the Society for Medical Decision Making (SMDM) and the International Society for Pharmacoeconomics and Outcomes Research (ISPOR) published a series of papers describing best practices in mathematical modeling for the purpose of healthcare policy decision making. The reader is referred to these papers for more detailed descriptions of methodological best practices [5–11].

Figure 13.2 illustrates the general steps required to develop a decision model to address a particular problem. The relative importance of different steps may vary depending upon the purpose of the model, the number of stakeholders or interested parties who wish to use the model results, and the

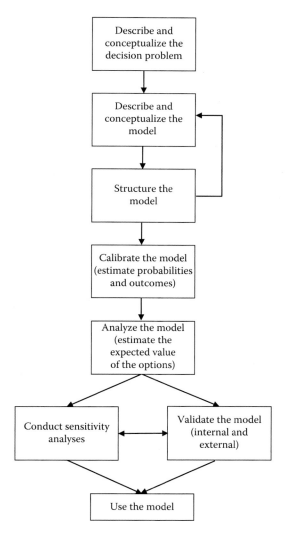

FIGURE 13.2
Steps in developing a decision model.

complexity of the particular problem being modeled. However, each of these steps is important in the development of a complete, transparent, and useful model to answer a particular comparative effectiveness question.

13.2.1 Conceptualize the Problem

The first step in any study utilizing any methodology is to conceptualize and understand the problem being addressed [10]. For most comparative effectiveness studies, the problem is to decide the optimal therapy among multiple possible choices for a specific condition. However, the scope and scale of the problem being addressed, the specifics of the population to be represented, the exact characteristics of the strategies being compared, the perspective of the stakeholder(s), and the relevant outcomes to be included in the analysis are all important characteristics to be included in the conceptualization of the problem. It is strongly advised that this phase of the development of decision analysis should always include content experts in the disease or situation that is being modeled and represented.

13.2.2 Conceptualizing the Model

Once the characteristics of the problem have been agreed upon and described, the appropriate modeling method to be used to represent the problem can be decided [10]. Each modeling method has strengths and weaknesses with respect to particular characteristics of a disease or intervention or population being evaluated. In general, the choice of modeling type relies on whether or not the analysis is expected to represent individuals or groups, and whether interactions between patients are an important component of the analysis. For example, if one were considering choices between alternative therapies for patients with HIV disease where the goal was to maximize the life expectancy of an individual patient, representing the impact on the epidemic is not crucial answering that decision [12,13]. However, if the comparative effectiveness decision involves strategies to reduce the incidence of HIV disease through various treatments or prevention programs, then modeling the interaction between patients and the impact of the various interventions on transmission is crucial to obtaining a realistic answer [7].

Similarly, deciding the appropriate level of detail to include in the model is difficult. Very simple models are easy to develop, have rapid turnaround times for changes and enhancements, but often do not include characteristics of the disease that experts feel is important to have face validity. Complex models, although they may have more external face validity, are often sometimes so complicated to build, debug, and validate that they become onerous as an analytic and investigative tool. An excellent review of the importance of validity notes that transparency is an important foundation to validation [5].

13.2.3 Specifying Type of Model to Be Used

As noted in Figure 13.1, there are many modeling methods that can be used to create a representation of a clinical or policy decision. A review of all of the modeling types is beyond the scope of this chapter, and the reader is referred to the series of modeling recommendations made by ISPOR and SMDM [5–11]. However, the following is a very brief summary of the characteristics of modeling types and the situations in which they are useful.

13.2.3.1 Decision Trees

These are useful for relatively simple problems where the difference in outcomes is easily summarized by a single parameter such as a life expectancy, where the specific time course of events in the future is not important, and when the outcome for the entire population is important.

13.2.3.2 State Transition (Markov) Models

These are useful when the clinical condition can be described as a series of health states and very useful when interventions affect the likelihood of certain states occurring. They provide outcomes that are aggregated for the entire population.

13.2.3.3 Individual Microsimulation

Typically developed as an expansion of a state transition model, microsimulation allows for individual characteristics of patients in the model to be followed and affects the transitions that the individual makes in the model. It is useful when data on individuals are important.

13.2.3.4 Dynamic Transmission (Compartment) Models

Used primarily for the representation of infectious diseases, these models represent the probability of transmitting a disease as a function of the particular disease, the number of people in a cohort who are infectious, and the proportion of the cohort that is susceptible.

13.2.3.5 Discrete-Event, Agent-Based Simulation

These modeling methods can be modified to represent virtually any other form of decision model; however, they are particularly useful when individuals within the model interact, or when there are specific capacity constraints in the delivery of a particular therapy.

13.2.4 Structure the Model

Once a specific model type has been decided upon, the actual structure of the problem must be built into the model. The process of moving from a conceptual model of the problem to a mathematical model in a software tool or a set of equations is an engineering problem, in that the conceptualization of the model that represents the problem will imply a certain structure for that modeling type. The mechanisms by which this is done vary by the modeling type. For simple decision trees, this amounts to drawing the decision tree that represents the particular problem. For state transition or Markov processes, this process involves delineating and describing all of the various states that are relevant to the description of the problem. For individual microsimulation and more complex modeling methods, this process includes describing the variables that will be followed along with each individual in the model, how those variables will be affected by time, and the model and any interactions that might occur between patients. This process will be described in more detail in the examples below.

13.2.5 Analyze the Model

Analyzing the model simply means calculating the expected value of each of the specified strategies. Typically, this process is done by a computer using either specific decision analytic software or a more generic tool such as Excel. The difficulty in this step is directly proportional to the complexity of the model, simple models in standard software packages are typically computationally evaluated in seconds, complex microsimulations may take days to run on even powerful desktop computers, and even more complex agent-based models that require interactions between individuals (such as many models of pandemics and epidemics and entire countries) may require hours and hours of computation on a supercomputer.

13.2.6 Conduct Sensitivity Analysis

For most decision models, the specific "answer" is less relevant than how that answer changes when parameters or assumptions in the model are varied. Each estimate used in parameterizing a model, such as a probability or an outcome, is a point estimate typically from a study or distribution that has variability in it. Sometimes this variability is well understood and even measured, for example, if the parameter comes from a study report with a mean and 95% confidence limits. Sometimes the variability is less well described, for example, when the estimate comes from an expert panel. However, just as an RCT would not reproduce exactly the same answer between arms of the study if run a second time, a decision model is entirely dependent upon the value of the parameters that have been used to calibrate the model. Therefore, understanding how sensitive the answer (or value of each strategy) is to changes in the inputs and assumptions of the model is crucial to understanding the stability of the models results under different conditions or assumptions, as well as in providing confidence that the model accurately reflects the underlying true state of the world [6].

The process of sensitivity analysis is simply the reanalysis of the decision model under different assumptions or values for input parameters. In its simplest form, a single parameter would be varied across a reasonable or relevant range, and the expected value of each strategy would be calculated under each possible value for that variable. This is called a one-way sensitivity analysis. A one-way sensitivity analysis is described in the example at the end of this chapter. More complicated sensitivity analyses can involve varying more than one input variable simultaneously, which can create two-, three-, or multiway sensitivity analysis.

Although one-way and multiway sensitivity analyses are useful in understanding the impact of changes in a variable on the outcome of interest for the various strategies, they are in "deterministic" in that the answer to the decision model is conditional upon the specific values of each parameter in the model. The analysis of a decision model makes a statement: "*if* the parameters of interest are related as described by the structure of the model, and the parameters have the values included in the model, *then* the expected value of each outcome strategy is. . .." This type of statement gives no estimate of how variable that answer is to the multiple levels of uncertainty in the development of the model. To accommodate this problem, many modelers will use probabilistic sensitivity analysis to gain an understanding of how likely various outcomes are given estimated uncertainty in the input parameters.

A more detailed description of probabilistic sensitivity analysis can be found in many references [14–16]. Briefly, the basic methodology of probabilistic sensitivity analysis is to analyze the model literally tens of thousands of times, and for each iteration, specific values for each variable are drawn from a distribution representing that variable's uncertainty. For example, a mortality rate for a procedure might be derived from a study that provided a mean and 95% confidence limits around estimated mortality. A probabilistic sensitivity analysis would define a distribution with that mean and that 95% confidence limits, and would use a distribution that met all of the other criteria for a probability distribution. The model is run multiple times and at each iteration a different value from each probability distribution is sampled and the expected value of each strategy is determined. Correlations between variables can be built into this kind of analysis, and variables in the model that are found to be dependent upon each other can have those correlational dependencies represented in a probabilistic sensitivity analysis.

Finally, there is uncertainty about the structure of the model itself. Does the model include the appropriate choices, does it estimate the consequences of each choice for a sufficient period of time, and does it represent all of the relevant outcomes that can occur after each choice? There are no specific recommendations on how extensive an evaluation should be conducted on model uncertainty [6] but the inclusion of content-based experts during the development of the model can help identify those components of the problem in which model uncertainly is important [10].

In addition to describing the impact of various input parameters on the outcomes, and in providing confidence in the models results, another use of sensitivity analysis is in the development and "debugging" of a model. It is often the case that the model developer will know the expected answer of which strategy is optimal under various simplifying and perhaps extreme assumptions. If the modeler conducts a sensitivity analysis using those specific values, and the model returns an unexpected result, it is often an indication that the model has a conceptual or technical error in its construction.

13.2.7 Validate the Model

Validating the model is one of the most important attributes in providing confidence that the model represents the real-world clinical situation for which it was designed. Detailed essays on model validation are found elsewhere [5,17]; here, we briefly describe the purpose of different types of validation.

One of the first steps in making sure that a model is working as designed is whether or not it can reproduce the expected outcomes from the data on which it was calibrated. This process is often called verification and is simply an assurance that the model is behaving as it was designed. A much stronger test of the model's validity is when a model is shown to be able to predict the outcomes from studies that were not used in model creation. Examples of this type of external validation can be found in HIV disease [18,19], liver disease, cardiovascular disease [20], and many others.

13.3 Types of Modeling Methods

As demonstrated in Figure 13.1, the goal of the decision model is to create a representation of the events that occur after making a decision. There are multiple modeling methodologies that can be used to create estimates of the downstream events conditional upon various choices made. These modeling methods will be briefly reviewed here; the reader is referred to the reference list at the end of the chapter for more information regarding each of the specific methods [10,11,21].

For all types of modeling methods, the goal of the representation is similar: provide an unbiased, robust estimate of the likely downstream consequences of the various policy decisions, which when combined with the values for those downstream consequences can produce an expected value of the outcomes of interest such that the choice with the highest expected value can be made. Similar to many other analytic methodologies, some modeling methods are more appropriate for particular kinds of problems than others. A detailed discussion of the specific attributes of a modeling problem that imply the use of a particular method is beyond the scope of this chapter. The reader is referred to several references for a more detailed description of how to match the specific problem to an appropriate modeling method. In this chapter, we will briefly describe the methods of branch and node decision trees, state transition or Markov processes, microsimulation, discrete-event and agent-based simulation, and differential equations or compartment models. We will then review several comparative effectiveness studies that used decision analysis, and end the chapter with a simple worked example.

13.3.1 Basic Branch and Node Decision Trees

The simplest version of a decision analytic problem, branch and node decision trees, starts with a specific choice (called a decision node) followed by a series of stochastically determined chance nodes that describes the probabilistic events that occur after making a decision. At the end of a path of probabilistic events, an outcome occurs that is represented by a value, such as a probability of survival or a life expectancy. Each branch of the decision node will have an expected value of the outcome and the highest expected value is the optimal strategy.

Figure 13.3 represents a simple decision tree that describes the decision whether to screen a population for HIV disease. This tree is modified from a cost-effectiveness study of HIV screening by Sanders [22]. The decision is whether to screen a particular population, characterized by its prevalence of HIV. In the screening branch, some portion of the people will be HIV positive, the probability given by the prevalence of HIV, and some will not be positive indicated as one minus the prevalence. In those patients who are HIV positive, the probability that the test is positive will be the sensitivity of the test, and the probability that the test will be negative is one minus the sensitivity or the false-negative rate. For patients who are HIV negative, the probability that the test will be negative is provided by the specificity, and the probability that the test will be positive is given by one minus the specificity or the false-positive rate. On the nose screening arm, a portion of the population given by the prevalence will be HIV positive; one minus that prevalence will be HIV negative. It is assumed that if a patient is screened

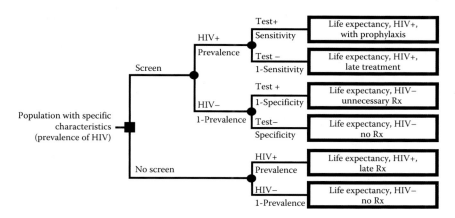

FIGURE 13.3
Simple branch and node decision tree evaluating whether to screen for HIV disease.

and found to be HIV positive, they are started on appropriate antiretroviral therapy and prophylaxis. In the nose screening arm, those who are HIV positive will eventually be detected through the development of symptoms, but they will not experience the benefit of early and prophylactic therapy.

In this case, the individual path is represented by a life expectancy. In the case of the true-positive test result (Screen → HIV+ → Test+), the patient will have the life expectancy of a patient of that age with HIV disease that is treated early. In the case of the false-negative test (Screen → HIV+ → Test−), the patient will not receive the benefit of early therapy, and have the life expectancy of an HIV-positive individual who is treated late after the development of symptoms. For the true-negative result (Screen → HIV− → Test−), the patient will have the life expectancy of a similar aged patient without HIV disease. For the false-positive test (Screen → HIV− → Test+), this analysis had assumed that there was some life expectancy decrement to being falsely labeled as HIV positive. It is very likely that this life expectancy decrement is no longer true in the case of HIV disease, as treatments are no longer made based on an HIV test alone. Clinicians would obtain a CD4 count, a viral load, and other tests, and it would be quickly determined that the patient was actually not HIV positive. However, for the purpose of this example and in the Saunders paper [22], there was considered to be a small negative consequence to the false-positive HIV test.

On the no screen arm, the paths are relatively straightforward as well. For those who are HIV positive (No Screen → HIV+), they will have the same life expectancy as the false-negative test in the screen arm, as they will not be detected until they develop symptoms. For those without HIV disease (No Screen → HIV−), they will have the life expectancy of a similarly aged patient.

It is important to note that the simplistic view of the screening problem can be made more complicated. The screening could be done in various populations, it could be done in various intervals, negative tests could be rescreened at a different interval, and there could be follow-on tests once the HIV test was positive. The level of detail that should be included in a decision model is one of the most complicated and difficult decisions in building a model.

13.3.2 State Transition (Markov) Models

Note that in this simple example, a tremendous amount of complexity is represented by a single number, the life expectancy of a patient at the terminal node of a particular path. For example, after a patient is found to have a positive test and is treated for HIV disease (Screen → HIV+ → Test+), a complex set of future decisions and events will occur. At diagnosis, the patient will have a particular viral load and CD4 count. Depending upon the recommendations being followed, the patient may not have a CD4 count that would suggest the need for treatment. As time goes on, the patient's

CD4 count might decline, various infections or complications of HIV disease might occur, resistance to the antiretroviral therapy might develop, and treatment regimens might change. These future events would be extremely difficult (if not impossible) to describe in a series of sequential branches and nodes.

Therefore, for decision problems that represent recurrent events, or for which the decision changes the probability of one or more future events that can occur over time, representation as a branch and node decision tree becomes quite complicated, and models representing complex future events may become nearly impossible to create because of the large number of branches required to represent multiple events over time. In these situations, where policy or treatment choices may change the probability of a future event, or where the outcome of interest may recur multiple times, it is often quite useful to represent the problem as a series of clinical states that a person may occupy, and represent the transitions between those states as probabilities.

Such models are called state transition or Markov models. In these models, the model world is divided into a series of mutually exclusive and collectively exhaustive states in which the patient may be found. That they are mutually exclusive means the patient may be in only one state; that they are collectively exhaustive means the patient must be in at least one state. Multiple references describe the methodologies for building state transition models in detail [9,23,24]; here, we will present a brief review of the methodology.

Continuing the HIV example, early models of HIV disease made an important distinction between people who were simply HIV positive and those who had an AIDS-defining illness. Although this definition is no longer of significant clinical importance, we will use it as a simplifying representation of HIV disease for the purpose of describing a Markov process. In this simplistic view, patients may be HIV positive, have developed AIDS, or have died. This is represented in Figure 13.4, which represents a three-state Markov process that has the characteristics of being mutually exclusive and collectively exhaustive. Patients may be HIV positive (HIV+), have developed an AIDS-defining illness (AIDS), or have died (DEAD). For an

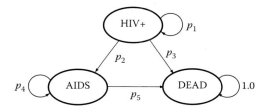

FIGURE 13.4
State transition model of a simple representation of the progression of HIV disease.

HIV-positive patient, there will be some probability that they will simply remain HIV positive (p_1), some probability (p_2) that the patient will develop an AIDS-defining illness in each time period, and some probability that the patient will die (p_3). Once the patient has developed an AIDS-defining illness, there is some probability that they will remain alive (p_4) and some probability that they will die (p_5). In this case, the likelihood of dying once an AIDS-defining illness has developed is likely to be higher than the probability of dying prior to the development of AIDS. Once the patient has died, they may not leave the dead state and the probability of remaining in that state is 1.0.

Although there are mathematical solutions to a state transition model under several simplifying assumptions, such as the transition probabilities remain constant over time, most state transition models in the current literature today are solved by a method called "cohort simulation" where a cohort of an arbitrary size is entered into the model, and transitions between states occur at specific discrete time cycles (typically measured in months or years) and the membership in each state is calculated for each time period. This is graphically represented in Figure 13.5, which depicts the three states of HIV positive, AIDS, and DEAD, and illustrates a population starting in the HIV-positive state at the beginning of the model. After one time period, some people will have progressed from HIV to AIDS, some may have died with HIV disease but without an AIDS-defining illness, but most patients will simply have remained alive in the HIV-positive state.

As time continues, members of the cohort travel through the various states in the model, and eventually, after sufficient time has passed, all members

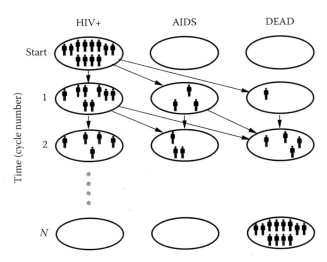

FIGURE 13.5
Basic mechanics of cohort simulation top evaluate a state transition model.

of the cohort have died and are in the "DEAD" state. The life expectancy of the entire cohort is simply the sum over all time periods in the model of the proportion of the cohort residing in each state times the value of being found in that state. A more detailed description of preference weights for outcome states is beyond the scope of this chapter, and the reader is referred to other references for more details [9,23]. For the purpose of this example, assume that we have a utility measure that represents the quality of life of being in a state that ranges between a low of zero for the state of death, and a high of one for a state of perfect health. Then, the expected value or cumulative utility of the cohort of patients represented by the state transition model in Figure 13.5 is

$$\text{Cumulative utility} = \sum_{t=1}^{T}\sum_{i=1}^{n} f_{i,t}q_{i,t},$$

where $f_{i,t}$ is the proportion of the cohort in state i at time t, and $q_{i,t}$ is the utility weight of being found in state i at time t.

The membership of the cohort in each individual state can be represented graphically, as illustrated in Figure 13.6. This illustrates that in standard state transition or Markov processes, the analysis evaluates a single cohort that is initially distributed across the states in the model (typically the entire cohort will be in one state at the beginning of the simulation, but that is not necessary) and progresses through transitions from one state to another over time. If there is an absorbing state, a state from which a member of the cohort may not leave, such as death, eventually, all of the cohort will induct into that state. It is important to note that the state membership in the HIV-positive state represented in this figure exhibits an exponential decline because in this simple model, the transition probabilities were assumed to be constant

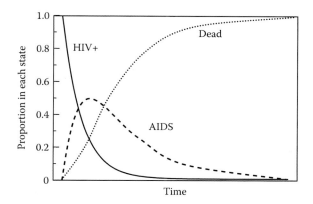

FIGURE 13.6
Cohort membership over time in a state transition or Markov model from Figure 13.3.

over time. Because the analysis is carried out in a discrete time cycles and analytic solutions are not required, the standard Markovian assumption of constant probabilities is not typically necessary, and when clinical states and their transitions are simulated, the probabilities may easily be changed based on the amount of time that has passed in the model.

To incorporate such a state transition model into the decision model described in Figure 13.3, each terminal node of the branch and node decision tree would be replaced by a state transition model that would represent the life expectancy implied by finding oneself at that terminal path in the tree.

13.3.2.1 Adding Clinical Detail

The representation of the life expectancy of a patient with HIV disease is in reality substantially more complicated than illustrated in Figure 13.4. In fact, currently, the distinction between being HIV positive and having an AIDS-defining illness has become substantially less important as the importance of knowing biologic parameters such as the CD4 count and viral load have become aggressively more important in determining the appropriate treatment. Therefore, most models that would be built to represent HIV disease would have a significantly more complicated representation of the progression of HIV disease.

The first obvious expansion is to describe states with respect to the CD4 count of the particular individual. Because the initiation of treatment is dependent on the level of the CD4 count, and the development of complications to HIV disease is also related to the CD4 count, one can imagine the desire to divide the representation of somebody with HIV disease into states representing the level of that patient's CD4 count. Again, for simplicity, we describe dividing the states into three levels, a CD4 count greater than 500, a CD4 count between 350 and 500, and a CD4 count below 350. One can imagine significantly more complicated and detailed representations of categories of CD4 count that might be appropriate (Figure 13.7).

In this situation, the same representation of disease progression would be attached to the true-positive path (HIV+ → Test+) as well as the false-negative path (HIV+ → Test−) as patients will still progress through their disease through these states. What will be different between the two versions of the state transition process will be the probabilities that a patient will transition between those states. Under the true-positive path, the model assumes that the patient will be treated appropriately with antiretrovirals, and the probabilities representing progression between states of CD4 count will be different (lower probabilities of progression to a lower CD4 count state) than in the false-negative path, where a patient has HIV disease but it is unknown and therefore the patient is not on treatment.

Of course, there are a very large number of other characteristics that one could consider important to include in a model of the progression of HIV disease. Figure 13.8 describes an additional expansion of the complexity of

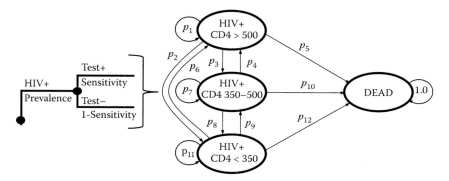

FIGURE 13.7
Representation of outcomes as a state transition (Markov) process. The HIV+ state is divided into different states based on the patient's CD4 count.

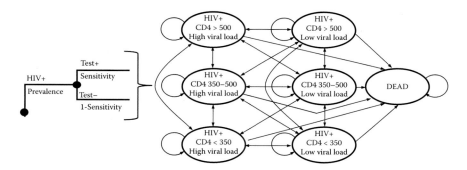

FIGURE 13.8
Representation of outcomes as a state transition (Markov) process. The HIV+ state is divided into different states based on the patient's CD4 count, and also subdivided by viral load.

this HIV model, by adding levels of viral load (high or low) to each CD4 count level. Again the reason for doing this would be to be able to represent the transitions between CD4 count states as a function of whether the viral load was higher or lower. In addition, appropriate treatment with antiretroviral agents might shift the proportion of people who have high viral loads as viral replication is suppressed.

As is obvious from the illustrations between Figures 13.7 and 13.8, substantial clinical realism can be included in a state transition model by increasing the number of states representing the clinical or biological processes in the model. In fact, the HIV progression model by Sanders [22] on which this example is based contains substantially more detail than we have described here. Because these state transition models require all of the individuals within a state to be treated the same way, heterogeneity in history, or in patient characteristics such as clinical comorbidity, age, and so on all have to be incorporated into the state space that describes the disease. This can cause an explosion in the number of states required to represent a problem with a relatively modest amount of clinical detail. For example, consider a situation in which one wanted to represent five levels of CD4 count, five levels of viral load (e.g., log 10 units), the presence or absence of coinfection with hepatitis C, and keeping track of whether the person was on their first, second, or third cycle of antiretroviral therapy. This modest amount of clinical detail would require a model with 150 states ($5 * 5 * 2 * 3$). Models representing more realistic clinical detail have required many thousands of states. It is the standard "Markovian" property that transition probabilities must be path independent and that the probability of transition to another state can only depend upon membership in that state that requires state transition models to grow so large. This is the impetus for the use of microsimulation techniques (described below) that release these assumptions by representing specific individuals in the model rather than cohorts, which mitigates the effect of having to treat the entire portion of the cohort in any given state the same.

13.3.3 Microsimulation Models

Microsimulation models follow individual patients, one at a time, as they traverse the model, rather than following an entire cohort, as typically performed in standard decision analysis trees or Markov models. Following a single individual through the model allows them to be tagged with specific historical details, which can then modify the likelihood of future events based on that individual's past history and present clinical picture. This model structure avoids the Markov "state explosion" problem outlined in the prior section and allows a much less complex model to be built. The cost of this modeling flexibility is that microsimulation models typically need to be run hundreds of thousands of times or more to capture the variability seen in a patient group, rather than the single run afforded by a cohort simulation.

Returning to the example in the previous section, where the number of Markov states exploded as clinical detail was added, we can use microsimulation to model this scenario in a much more compact structure (Figure 13.9). Here, a patient with HIV disease has variables, commonly referred to as "tracker variables," attached to him/her that track CD4 count, viral load, hepatitis C status, and the antiretroviral therapy cycle currently prescribed.

In the figure, the patient begins the model in the HIV-positive (HIV+) state, with CD4 counts and viral load categorized based on that patient's clinical status, with the antiretroviral therapy status also noted. Based on transition probabilities over time, the patient can become hepatitis C positive, following the arrow to HIV+, Hep C+ state in the figure. If this occurs, then the variable tracking hepatitis C status changes to denote this, with the subsequent risk of returning to the newly diagnosed hepatitis C state becoming 0, since the patient is now tagged as already having hepatitis C. Other variables could

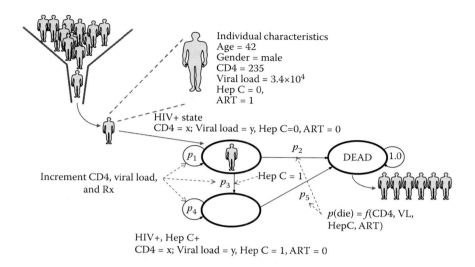

FIGURE 13.9
Microsimulation. Individuals proceed through the model 1 person at a time, each person being characterized by a set of clinical variables. These variables can be altered based on where the patient is in the model and the duration of time that has transpired, and specific transitions can be functionally dependent upon these clinical characteristics.

be created to track the status of hepatitis C progression as a function of other clinical parameters over time.

HIV disease progression risk in this model becomes a function of time since diagnosis, CD4 count, viral load, current retroviral therapy, time on that therapy, prior therapies, and hepatitis C status. As the individual's time in the model continues, CD4 counts and viral loads are updated, based on those same clinical factors, along with the patient's adherence with therapy and the risk of antiviral resistance. Disease progression can be modeled as a function of those variables or as a state, as it is in State 3 in the figure. In either case, the risk of worsening disease status or of death can be derived from tracker variable values for clinical characteristics, with risk of further progression and of death increasing as clinical features worsen. The patient is followed over time in this fashion, typically until death. At this point, a new patient enters the model, and the process is repeated.

In microsimulation models, patients progress through the model based on random draws from probability distributions representing the occurrence of events or progression. In this way, patients with the same clinical features at the start of the model can follow different paths due to those random draws, representing the range of outcomes that can occur based on likelihood of those outcomes.

In addition, individual patient characteristics at the start of the model can vary, capturing differences in clinical characteristics within patient groups.

For example, a different patient could start the HIV model already hepatitis C positive, on her second cycle of antiretroviral therapy, and with different CD4 and viral load levels. This ability to model individual patient characteristics is a strength, compared to cohort simulation (where average patient characteristics are modeled), particularly when cohort or subgroup averages do not adequately capture variability or heterogeneity within patient groups.

Any number of individual patient characteristics can be tagged for each patient modeled. Demographic data such as age, gender, and race could be added to the characteristics tagged in our example, as could clinical features, such as liver function test results, and risk factors for disease progression, like continued intravenous drug use, unsafe sexual practices, or unstable support systems. However, added characteristics, in order to be meaningful in the modeling process, must have fairly specific data available to support their inclusion. It is not helpful to tag patients with characteristics whose numeric contribution to risk is not well known, more speculative, or not specific enough. It is possible to have patient characteristics that are so specific that the effect of that set of characteristics on the modeled disease cannot be ascertained.

To summarize, microsimulation, which follows individuals through a modeling structure, is useful when multiple clinical and/or demographic characteristics are important to follow in the model. The ability to tag individuals with tracker variables allows a more compact modeling structure to be used. However, these models are computationally intensive, typically requiring 100,000 individuals or more to run through the model to adequately capture the characteristics of the population being modeled.

13.3.4 Discrete-Event and Agent-Based Models

Developed originally in computer sciences and industrial engineering, discrete-event simulation and agent-based modeling expand the capability of mathematical models applied to health care through representation of interactions between individuals in the model with each other, with other components of the model such as clinical resources such as emergency rooms, hospitals, physicians, or other components of the healthcare delivery systems. Excellent reviews of these modeling types are found in the recent ISPOR–SMDM reviews [7,8] and the general literature [25].

In discrete-event simulation, entities (e.g., patients) are generally passive and do not adapt their behavior to, or learn from, the environment. Agent-based models are more flexible than discrete-event models, where agents (e.g., patients, care providers) interact with environment and can learn from other agents [26]. Agent-based models also allow simulation of complex social networks, which could be critical in controlling the spread of an infectious disease. Another unique property of agent-based models is that they can capture emergent phenomena that result from the interactions of individual entities. By definition, an emergent phenomenon evolves in an unpredictable way as the process evolves. For example, how individual-level decision to vaccinate or to stay at home when sick during the influenza season affects the peak of influenza epidemic [27].

13.3.5 Infectious Disease (Compartment) Models

Infectious disease models, also referred to as compartmental, dynamic transmission, or equation-based models, can account for persons with an infection being a risk factor for that disease and for disease incidence being directly related to infection prevalence, thus capturing the dynamic nature of infectious disease [7]. The previously described modeling structures typically model disease incidence more statically, based on constant or time-based risk and cannot easily vary disease incidence based on the number of persons with disease, and thus are not well suited to capturing the dynamics of infectious disease epidemiology.

A common infectious disease model is the SIR model, which has three compartments: "S," which represents the portion of the population that is Susceptible to the disease; "I," who are infected and Infectious; and "R," those who were infected, have Recovered, and are now immune. The likelihood (or force) of infection, that is, transitioning between S and I compartments, is a function of the number of infected individuals, the relative infectiousness of the disease, and likelihood of contact sufficient to transmit the disease between infected and susceptible individuals. These models are typically defined by differential equations describing the dynamics of flow between compartments based on the force of infection in the population and the duration of the infectious period. These models can be evaluated deterministically or stochastically, depending on the disease modeled and the needs of the modeling exercise.

13.3.6 Hybrids

Many complex models are constructed of more than one modeling type, where each component of the model uses the most appropriate method to represent that particular component of the problem. Modern computing methods of object-oriented programming allow for this technique. Most decision models start with a basic decision tree and may use one or more modeling types to estimate downstream events that occur after the decision (Figure 13.1). Detailed exposition is beyond the scope of this chapter, but an excellent example of such a hybrid model is the Archimedes model [20,28,29].

13.4 Examples of Decision Models Used in Comparative Effectiveness

Because decision models can easily evaluate multiple outcomes simultaneously, it is often used to conduct cost-effectiveness analyses of a particular series of interventions. For this volume, we are concerned with the use of decision models for the purpose of comparative effectiveness exclusive of the decision's impact on cost. We review a few examples of decision models that have examined complex treatment decisions for the purpose of understanding the optimal choice of therapy.

13.4.1 Use of Virtual Colonoscopy

There have been several decision analytic models to examine various decisions regarding the use of virtual colonoscopy. Hur et al. built a detailed state transition model of the growth and progression of small polyps found on virtual colonoscopy to evaluate the optimal management of these polyps [30]. They examined to strategies and immediate real colonoscopy compared to a repeat virtual colonoscopy 3 years later to assess polyp progression. Their results supported a strategy of immediate colonoscopy and biopsy over repeat virtual colonoscopy. These results were robust to multiple sensitivity analyses, and estimated that as many as 734 cancers per hundred thousand patients with diminutive polyps could be prevented using the optimal strategy.

13.4.2 First-Line Therapy for Follicular Lymphoma

Olin et al. evaluated three different strategies for the initial treatment of follicular lymphoma, a particularly aggressive cancer [31]. Three different chemotherapeutic regimens were compared in patients with this disease (rituximab, cyclophosphamide, vincristine, and prednisone [RCVP], rituximab, cyclophosphamide, doxorubicin, vincristine, and prednisone [RCHOP], rituximab- and fludarabine [RFlu]). Because of the absence of a three-arm randomized control comparing these directly, the authors used phase 1 and phase 2 trial data to predict the results of what was essentially a virtual RCT between all three chemotherapies. These data were used to calibrate a detailed multistate model of the progression of disease under different treatment conditions. The authors concluded that RCHOP was the most appropriate first-line therapy for most patients, although they were able to make predictions regarding what characteristics would determine which of the therapies was optimal in different patients. This particular decision analysis is interesting because the results of the decision analysis were virtually identical to the results of a three-arm RCT published 3 years later [32].

13.5 Decision Analysis Worked Example

Although decision models can be made for situations with an arbitrary number of choices, for simplicity of description, we will describe decision and analytic methodologies comparing only two choices. For the purpose of description and illustration, we will use a relatively simple example of a woman with multiple medical comorbidities, who is found to have a large aneurism of the ascending aorta. The question is whether or not it makes sense to operate upon the woman or pursue watchful waiting. The case is real, and was a woman admitted by the author while in medical school, but illustrates many of the advantages of decision modeling in the context of clinical decision making. We use this case for several reasons. First, it is highly unlikely that there would ever be an RCT answering this particular therapeutic question. The woman has multiple comorbidities and would be excluded from virtually all surgical intervention trials. Second, the case illustrates how decisions can be made quite patient specific in decision analytic methods through the inclusion of patient preferences for the outcome states. Finally, it is a simple case that can illustrate all of the components of building a decision model.

Case description: The patient is a 50-year-old female with a past medical history of poorly treated hypertension, CREST syndrome, and primary biliary cirrhosis who was admitted to the hospital for evaluation of a large mediastinal mass observed on chest x-ray. An x-ray taken 18 months earlier revealed no mass. The woman was asymptomatic and had an unremarkable physical exam, except for uncontrolled hypertension. CT scan revealed that the mass was a saccular aneurism of the ascending aorta involving the innominate (brachiocephalic) and left common carotid arteries. A cardiac catheterization revealed that she had two vessel coronary artery diseases. The primary medicine team felt that the aneurism was growing (it had not been there 18 months previously) and would likely rupture; therefore, surgical repair was indicated. However, the cardiothoracic surgery consult suggested that she had too many chronic diseases, and that the risk of the operation was too high.

13.5.1 Basic Structure and Definitions of a Decision Analysis (Branches/Nodes/Outcomes)

The following sections will describe the decision tree constructed to answer this specific clinical question, describe where to find data sources to calibrate a decision model, illustrate the basic mechanics of finding the optimal solution in the decision problem, and demonstrate the value of sensitivity analysis.

13.5.2 Branches and Nodes

Decision trees are constructed from primitive elements that can be combined to form complex models of clinical and biological processes. Figure 13.10 illustrates a simple decision tree constructed to represent this particular clinical problem. In general, decision trees will start with a particular clinical situation, and the decisions that must be made. Decision nodes are represented by a square and in this simple example, there are two options being considered: operating on the aneurism (Surgery) or watchful waiting (No Surgery). Under the surgical strategy, we assume quite simple postsurgical sequelae; either the patient dies from the operation (Operative death) or the patient survives (Operative Success) and is left with the risk of death from her primary biliary cirrhosis and her coronary disease. These outcomes are not under the control of the decision maker, and happen stochastically: they are represented by a chance node or a circle. The end of each path is called a terminal node, typically represented by a box. In this case, the termination of operative death is that the patient is dead, the termination of the operative success is that the patient remains alive with the risk of death of primary biliary cirrhosis, and coronary artery disease, the termination of the watchful waiting or no surgery arm is that the patient has the risk of death of primary biliary cirrhosis, coronary artery disease, and ascending aortic aneurysm. The appropriate level of detail to include in a decision analysis is not trivial, and depends upon who is the decision maker for this particular decision, the availability of data to understand and calibrate a more detailed model, and the purpose of making the decision. In this case, one can imagine adding significant amounts of detail to the postsurgical component of this tree, which might include representing a series of complications that can occur. Some of

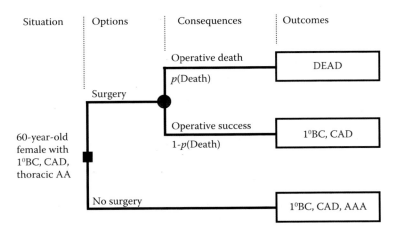

FIGURE 13.10
Decision tree for patient with ascending aortic aneurism. 1^0BC = primary biliary cirrhosis, CAD = coronary artery disease, AAA = ascending aortic aneurism.

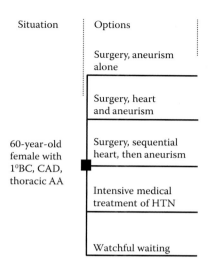

FIGURE 13.11
Adding multiple different possible treatment strategies.

those complications, such as a perioperative stroke or a perioperative heart attack, might very well affect her long-term survival.

Similarly, one can imagine adding a significant amount of detail to the possible treatment strategies. One could consider fixing the heart either independently or sequentially rather than just operating on the aneurysm. One could also imagine a strategy of intensive medical therapy for her hypertension, which might significantly decrease the rate of progression or probability of rupture of the aneurysm. Figure 13.11 illustrates one possible series of expanded strategies to be represented in this model.

13.5.3 Probabilities and Outcomes

One of the most important components of a decision analysis is calibrating the decision model to real data. Data can come from multiple sources, the purpose is to define as unbiased as possible estimates of the particular parameters included in the model. Typically, there are two types of data that are required: probabilities and values for outcomes.

In this simple example, we need only one probability, the risk of operative death for a 60-year-old female with primary biliary cirrhosis, hypertension, coronary artery disease, and CREST syndrome who undergoes a repair of an ascending aortic aneurysm. A literature search in MEDLINE will not find the specific mortality needed. When this problem was initially evaluated by the author in the 1980s, most of the data in the literature on mortality from operations on aneurysms of the ascending aorta came from Dr. Michael E. DeBakey's group in Texas. At that time, the average reported mortality was between 8% and 10%. However, the description in these sources of the level of illness of the patients indicated that the patients who experienced this mortality were substantially healthier than the patient considered in this decision problem. Therefore, after consultation with a cardiologist, to whom the case was described, the addition of the coronary disease, liver disease, and hypertension was felt by the cardiologist to raise the operative mortality to approximately 15%.

The values for the outcome states are equally important. There are two values required for this particular problem—the life expectancy of a 67-year-old woman with coronary disease, hypertension, and primary biliary cirrhosis, and the life expectancy of the same woman if she also has an ascending aortic aneurysm. Once again, it is very difficult to find specific literature that accurately represents the life expectancy of a person with this combination of illnesses.

It is possible to find the excess mortality inferred by coronary disease, by hypertension, and by primary biliary cirrhosis. Making several simplifying assumptions that the risk of death from these diseases is independent, one can combine the forces of mortality to create an estimate of the overall mortality from all three diseases. This method is called the declining exponential approximation of life expectancy (the DEALE) [33,34] which produces an estimate of the overall life expectancy assuming simultaneous effect of independent multiple sources of mortality. Using this method and literature that estimated the risk of death from these three diseases, the life expectancy of a 67-year-old woman with coronary disease, hypertension, and primary biliary cirrhosis was estimated to be 6.7 years.

To find the risk of death under the watchful waiting or no surgery strategy, there was a set of references in the literature that described a cohort of patients who had ascending aortic aneurysms but who refused surgery. Although it is possible that the people in this observational cohort who did not choose surgery may not be similar to those who chose surgery, and might have characteristics that make them sicker or more likely to die than those who chose surgery, this cohort was the closest the author could find to providing an estimate for this population. These aneurysms tend to burst at rates approaching 50% per year, and if they burst outside of the hospital to have a mortality rate that typically exceeds 95%. Using these data, the life expectancy of the watchful waiting arm was estimated to be 2.3 years.

Many criticisms of decision analysis arise from the process described above to calibrate the model. Data explicitly describing the probabilities and outcomes represented in the decision tree are often not directly available from the literature or from national databases. Sometimes, ad hoc procedures are necessary to create the best estimate for the particular situation represented in a decision tree. By "best," a modeler typically needs an unbiased estimate of the particular probability or outcome and a measure of the variability of that estimate for the purpose of sensitivity analysis. If this is not available in the literature, expert panels or Delphi methods can be used to make estimates of the necessary parameters.

13.5.4 Mechanics: Expected Value of the Outcomes

Once the probabilities and outcomes have been appropriately estimated and entered into the tree, the value of each choice in the decision tree is calculated. The goal of analyzing a decision tree is to estimate the expected value of the outcome across the different choices that can be made in a particular decision. In this case, the goal would be to calculate the life expectancy of the surgical strategy compared to the life expectancy of the watchful waiting strategy. The process is called "averaging out and rolling back" and is illustrated in Figure 13.12. Each chance node is replaced with the expected value of the outcome at that chance node. In this case, if the patient is operated upon, she has a 15% chance of dying (in which case her life expectancy is zero) and an 85% chance of surviving the operation and living on average 6.7 years. The expected value of that chance node is then

$$LE = 5.7 \text{ years} = (0.15 * 0 \text{ years}) + (0.85 * 6.7 \text{ years}).$$

Because that is the only chance node in this strategy, 5.7 years is the value of the surgical arm. There are no chance nodes on the watchful waiting arm; the value of watchful waiting was estimated to be 2.3 years. Because 5.7 years is larger than 2.3 years, the choice that maximizes life expectancy is to operate upon the aneurysm.

Essentially, no matter how large or complex a decision model becomes, the process for calculating the expected value of each strategy is the same. Every

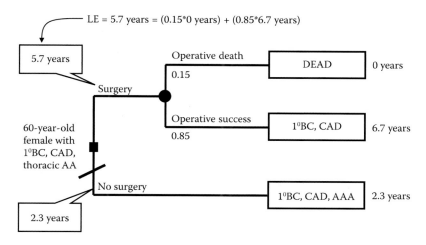

FIGURE 13.12
"Averaging out and folding back": calculating the expected value of each branch.

chance node is evaluated and replaced with its expectation; those expectations are folded back at each branch until the expected value of each initial strategy on the decision node is determined. The branch with the highest expected value is considered the optimal strategy.

13.5.5 Sensitivity Analysis

One of the most valuable attributes of a decision model is the ability to test the impact of the assumptions that you made in creating the model on the outcomes or answers that the model produces. The data that are used to calibrate a decision model, which means to estimate specific values for the probabilities and outcomes, may come from many different sources and have different levels of precision depending upon the type of study or dataset that was used to create that estimate. For all decision models, virtually all of the data that are used to calibrate the probabilities and outcomes is only an estimate of the true parameter, and is estimated with some degree of uncertainty. For example, in this case, we estimated that the probability of operative death for this woman was 15%. That may be too high or too low an estimate for this particular individual. Higher levels of mortality would decrease the value of the surgical arm, whereas lower values of mortality would increase the value of the surgical strategy. When the data to calibrate a model are derived from the published literature, the specific value of a probability or outcome estimate will vary depending upon the type of study used and the sample size that produced the specific estimate.

The value of representing this as a model is that all possible ranges of mortality can be included in the model and the value of each strategy can be calculated under multiple different assumptions about the value of any specific variable. When only one variable is changed, this is termed a one-way sensitivity analysis, and indicates the value of each strategy across tested values for that particular variable. This is illustrated in Figure 13.13 for our problem with the aneurysm. The probability of operative death was varied across its entire possible range, from 0% to 100%. For each value of operative mortality, the tree is reevaluated (the averaging out and folding back process is repeated), which produces an expected value of the outcome for each strategy. If the operative mortality were zero, the value of the surgical arm would be 6.7 years (the life expectancy of a woman with her comorbidities and no aneurysm), whereas if the operative mortality were 100%, the value of the surgical arm would be zero (as all patients would die during the operation). In this simple decision tree, the value of the surgical option is a straight line between 6.7 and zero across operative mortality. In more complicated models, a sensitivity analysis will not necessarily be a straight line: it is only true in this case because of the simplicity of the model itself. The life expectancy of the watchful waiting arm does not vary across values of operative mortality because the patient does not undergo an operation on

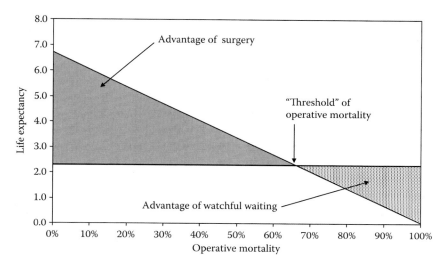

FIGURE 13.13
One-way sensitivity analysis illustrating the expected value of each strategy across all possible values for operative mortality.

the watchful waiting arm. Therefore, across all ranges of operative mortality, the value of the watchful waiting arm is 2.3 years.

These two lines, which represent the life expectancy for this woman under two different strategies across various assumptions about the operative mortality, define several parameters of interest. First, the operative mortality at which the lines cross is called the threshold mortality and indicates that mortality at which the optimal strategy switches from surgery to watchful waiting. Operative mortality is below the threshold that favors surgery, and the shaded area between the value of the surgical arm and the value of the watchful waiting arm indicates the benefits to a surgical strategy. For operative mortalities above the threshold, the shaded area to the right indicates the amount of benefit derived from watchful waiting under those operative mortalities.

13.6 Value of Information Analysis

As discussed in earlier sections, uncertainty is almost always present in parameters used to build mathematical models. Therefore, model outputs are typically based on some uncertainty in model inputs. Under such situation, it is natural for stakeholders to ask these questions: how much does the uncertainty matter in making a decision based on model's recommendations? In other words, should one make a decision based on uncertain information or should more information be collected to reduce uncertainty in model parameters and then make a decision? If more information is needed, then what kind of new evidence is most valuable, and is evidence needed for some subgroups or the entire population being considered?

Consider a case of quadrivalent human papillomavirus (qHPV) vaccine, which has been approved in the United States for the prevention of HPV infection in boys and young men between 11 and 26 years of age. However, the vaccine has not been approved among men aged 27 years or older (hereinafter, older men). Emerging evidence based on observational studies (which could have high uncertainty) suggests that the vaccine is also effective as an adjuvant anal cancer prevention strategy in older men who have sex with men (MSM) if given along with the treatment for high-grade squamous intraepithelial lesions (HSIL) [35]. It is believed that the vaccine can decrease the risk of invasive anal cancer either by slowing disease progression or by decreasing subsequent HPV infection [35–37]. Mathematical models, based on observational studies, have shown that such a strategy would be cost-effective [38,39].

Though observational data have shown benefits of adjuvant qHPV vaccination, no RCT, the gold standard for the evaluation of any intervention, has evaluated the benefits of such a strategy. Health policy stakeholders must, therefore, choose either to maintain the current policy recommendations, that is, not to vaccinate older MSM who have been diagnosed and treated for HSIL, or to vaccinate them based on the limited existing information on vaccine effectiveness in this population. If RCTs show that qHPV vaccination is efficacious in reducing the incidence of anal cancer in these men, waiting several years before implementation of the vaccination policy would result in an opportunity lost to reduce anal cancer burden because some patients would develop anal cancer, who otherwise would have not with vaccination in place. However, if trials show that adjuvant vaccination of older MSM does not effectively reduce HSIL recurrence and prevent anal cancer, then premature implementation of a vaccination policy would result in unnecessary use of healthcare resources without yielding any substantial benefits.

Such trade-offs can be evaluated by conducting a value of information (VOI) analysis, which provides a unique perspective on the need of conducting future research before making a policy decision, and an indication of the amount that society should be willing to spend on research about unknown factors, for example, vaccine efficacy and disease progression.

VOI analysis provides an analytical framework to systematically evaluate the need for further evidence before making a decision to adopt a technology or intervention based on current evidence. VOI analysis has been successfully used in engineering and risk analysis [40–42], and has recently been used to evaluate healthcare technologies [43–45]. VOI analysis has a significant potential to inform prioritization of future research and provide the best value from limited research dollars, for example, by helping to determine whether available resources should be spent on conducting a randomized control trial to resolve uncertainty about the efficacy of a new vaccine or on conducting an epidemiological study to estimate the prevalence and natural history of a disease. VOI, based on Bayesian decision theory, provides a methodological framework to establish the value of acquiring additional information (by conducting additional research) compared with making decision with uncertain information [46,47].

By using mathematical models to include long-term outcomes, VOI accounts for uncertainty in the health benefits and risks associated with alternative interventions, the ability of research findings to alter that uncertainty, and the long-term impact of new research on population health [44,48].

13.6.1 Expected Value of Perfect Information

In decision theory, the expected value of perfect information (EVPI) is defined as the maximum price that one would be willing to pay in order to gain access to perfect information. The EVPI is equal to the difference of expected value given perfect information (EV|PI) and expected value (EV) of a strategy. Below we describe a nonparametric approach, which is the most common approach, to conduct VOI analysis. If i denotes alternative interventions (or strategies), R_i denotes the net benefit (NB) of choosing intervention i, and θ denotes the uncertain model parameters, then, EV, EV|PI, and EVPI can be found by

$$EV = \max_i E_\theta[R_i(\theta)], \tag{13.1}$$

$$EV|PI = E_\theta\left[\max_i R_i(\theta)\right], \tag{13.2}$$

and

$$EVPI = EV|PI - EV = E_\theta\left[\max_i R_i(\theta)\right] - \max_i E_\theta[R_i(\theta)]$$

$$= E_\theta\left[\max_i R_i(\theta) - \max_i E_\theta[R_i(\theta)]\right], \tag{13.3}$$

where E_θ denotes the expectation with respect to θ. An alternative interpretation of EVPI is the expected lost opportunity cost, where the lost opportunity cost is defined as the difference between the expected NB of parameter-specific best policy (i.e., $E_\theta[\max_i E[R_i(\theta)]]$) and the expected optimal policy (i.e., $\max_i E_\theta[R_i(\theta)]$).

Table 13.1 illustrates the estimation of EVPI for a hypothetical case with two interventions A and B. The table represents simulated net benefit of 10 iterations from the probabalistic sensitivity analysis (PSA). Note that PSA of a decision analytic model is a necessary step for VOI analysis [45]. With

TABLE 13.1

Calculation of EVPI Using PSA Outcomes

Iteration (*i*)	Net Benefit (NB)		Optimal Choice	Maximum NB	Opportunity Loss
	A	B			
1	12,000	11,000	A	12,000	0
2	11,000	12,000	B	12,000	1,000
3	15,000	13,000	A	15,000	0
4	12,000	11,000	A	12,000	0
5	11,000	12,000	B	12,000	1,000
6	14,000	12,000	A	14,000	0
7	9,000	10,000	B	10,000	1,000
8	12,000	11,000	A	12,000	0
9	13,000	14,000	B	14,000	1,000
10	11,000	9,000	A	11,000	0
Expectation	12,000	11,500		12,400	400

current information, the expected NB of A (12,000) is greater than that of B (11,500). Therefore, the optimal decision using available evidence is to select intervention A. However, with perfect information, that is, with resolution of uncertainty from PSA runs, the optimal decision does not always remain A. For instance, in iteration 2, the NB of B is greater than that of A; therefore, the optimal decision would have been B if the uncertainty in parameters was resolved as in iteration 2. Because A was selected based on current information, opportunity loss in this case would have been 1,000 (i.e., difference between the NB of the selected intervention and the maximum NB obtained with perfect information). Similarly, for iteration 5, the NB of B was higher than that of A. However, we will not know in advance which of these possibilities will turn out to represent the true value of the parameter; therefore, the expected NB with perfect information is the expectation of the maximum NB, that is, 12,400. The EVPI is the difference between the maximum NB and the NB obtained with current information, that is, $12400 - 12000 = 400$. Note that the EVPI is also equivalent to expected opportunity loss. Here, we presented a case of two alternatives; however, the same approach can be used when there are more than two alternatives.

The EVPI is typically estimated over the entire population and for the duration of the technology's lifetime. For example, if a new vaccine being considered is expected to remain in practice for 10 years before being replaced by another vaccine, then the EVPI needs to be estimated for a 10-year time horizon. The following equation shows the estimation of population-level EVPI from individual-level EVPI:

$$\text{Population EVPI} = \text{EVPI} . \sum_{t=1,2,\ldots,T} \frac{I_t}{(1+r)^t},$$

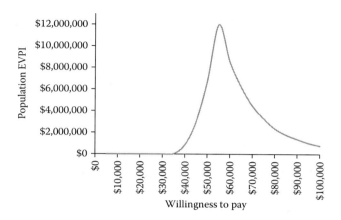

FIGURE 13.14
Population EVPI curve at varying willingness-to-pay thresholds.

where I_t is the incidence over the time period t and r is the discount rate.

Figure 13.14 presents a hypothetical EVPI curve that is obtained by varying willingness-to-pay threshold from $0 to $100,000. The peak of the curve represents the maximum amount one should be willing to pay to get the perfect information. If the EVPI exceeds the total cost of conducting further research, then it is *potentially* cost-effective to conduct additional research. For example, if additional research to gain further evidence will cost $2 million, then it is potentially cost-effective to conduct additional research before making a decision if willingness-to-pay threshold is $50,000. However, if the cost of additional research exceeds the EVPI, then future research should not be conducted because the returns from research will not offset the cost of conducting additional research.

Therefore, the value of further research depends on the population size that could benefit from additional research, time horizon being considered, and uncertainty surrounding the current estimates of net-benefit under existing evidence.

13.6.2 Expected Value of Partial Perfect Information

While the EVPI is useful in answering if further research is needed, one is often interested in knowing what kind of research is needed, if so. To answer such a question, one would need to estimate the EVPI of different subset of parameters. Such an analysis will estimate the benefit of reducing parameter estimation uncertainty for a subset of parameters, the parameters of interest φ. The analysis of the VOI for a subset of model input parameters is called expected value of parameter perfect information (EVPPI, also known as the expected value of partial perfect information), and is conducted in a very similar way to the EVPI. In particular, EVPPI is found by

$$\text{EVPPI} = E_\varphi\left[\max_i E_{\theta|\varphi}[R_i(\theta)]\right] - \max_i E_\theta[R_i(\theta)], \qquad (13.4)$$

where $E_{\theta|\varphi}$ represents the conditional expectation with respect to θ, given the realization for φ. Though the calculation of EVPPI is conceptually very similar to that of EVPI, the computational burden is very high because of two loops (inner and outer) of expectation. For individual-level models, the estimation of EVPPI will require three levels of loops. Therefore, for complex decision analytic models, EVPPI may not be practical. In such a case, approximation algorithms can be used to reduce the computational burden [49,50].

13.6.3 Research Prioritization Using VOI Analysis

VOI analysis can be used as a tool by governments, funding agencies, and research institutions to systematically prioritize future research that maximizes the returns [51]. VOI analysis provides an objective approach to assess future research needs within a disease area or across multiple disease areas. For example, should a funding agency prioritize research in understanding the effects of delaying hepatitis C treatment, or resolving uncertainty around the efficacy of new therapies in selected patient groups [52]. Such a decision can be made based on the value of EVPPI for different parameters or group of parameters. Depending on the cost of future research, one can determine what kind of future research will provide the maximum value. United Kingdom's National Institute for Health and Care Excellence (NICE) in the past commissioned a pilot study of VOI analysis to provide recommendations on institute's research. In the United States, VOI analysis was recommended to prioritize future research by multiple funding agencies, including the Agency for Healthcare Research and Quality (AHRQ) and the PCORI [53–55].

13.7 Summary

The purpose of comparative effectiveness research is to provide patients and clinicians with actionable information regarding the potential outcomes of choices that must be made in clinical situations. It is often the case that the choices facing patients and clinicians are far more numerous than the strategies that are directly compared in the medical literature. For example, a new antihypertensive medication may be compared in an RCT to a placebo, and be demonstrated to be beneficial. However, the decision facing a patient and his/her doctor is not whether to choose that medication or nothing, which is the choice represented in the RCT. Rather, the decision is which antihypertensive medication out of a large number of possibilities would be the best choice for a particular patient with a specific set of characteristics.

Decision models provide a useful mechanism for representing multiple diagnostic or treatment strategies in a particular clinical situation. One advantage of decision models is that multiple different sources of data can be integrated into a single representation of the outcomes and events that occur after different strategies are chosen. Therefore, unlike the RCT, which is often quite limited in scope or number of strategies compared, a decision model can represent multiple strategies simultaneously, and can integrate data from multiple sources to provide estimates of what outcomes are likely to occur after different choices are made.

There are multiple types of decision models that can be used to represent specific clinical situations, and they vary in the level of complexity, the time horizon, and multiple other characteristics of the specific set of therapies that is being compared.

References

1. Guyatt GH, Haynes RB, Jaeschke RZ et al. Users' Guides to the Medical Literature: XXV. Evidence-based medicine: Principles for applying the users' guides to patient care. Evidence-Based Medicine Working Group. *JAMA* 2000;284:1290–6.
2. Evidence-Based Medicine Working Group. Evidence-based medicine. A new approach to teaching the practice of medicine. *JAMA* 1992;268:2420–5.
3. Sox HC, Goodman SN. The methods of comparative effectiveness research. *Annual Review of Public Health* 2012;33:425–45.
4. Patient-Centered Outcomes Research Institute. The PCORI Methodology Report, 2012. Retrieved from: http://www.pcori.org/content/pcori-methodology-report. (Accessed January 18, 2015).
5. Eddy DM, Hollingworth W, Caro JJ et al. Model transparency and validation: A report of the ISPOR-SMDM Modeling Good Research Practices Task Force-7. *Medical Decision Making: An International Journal of the Society for Medical Decision Making* 2012;32:733–43.
6. Briggs AH, Weinstein MC, Fenwick EA et al. Model parameter estimation and uncertainty analysis: A report of the ISPOR-SMDM Modeling Good Research Practices Task Force Working Group-6. *Medical Decision Making: An International Journal of the Society for Medical Decision Making* 2012;32:722–32.
7. Pitman R, Fisman D, Zaric GS et al. Dynamic transmission modeling: A report of the ISPOR-SMDM Modeling Good Research Practices Task Force Working Group-5. *Medical Decision Making: An International Journal of the Society for Medical Decision Making* 2012;32:712–21.
8. Karnon J, Stahl J, Brennan A, Caro JJ, Mar J, Moller J. Modeling using discrete event simulation: A report of the ISPOR-SMDM Modeling Good Research Practices Task Force-4. *Medical Decision Making: An International Journal of the Society for Medical Decision Making* 2012;32:701–11.

9. Siebert U, Alagoz O, Bayoumi AM et al. State-transition modeling: A report of the ISPOR-SMDM Modeling Good Research Practices Task Force-3. *Medical Decision Making: An International Journal of the Society for Medical Decision Making* 2012;32:690–700.

10. Roberts M, Russell LB, Paltiel AD et al. Conceptualizing a model: A report of the ISPOR-SMDM Modeling Good Research Practices Task Force-2. *Medical Decision Making: An International Journal of the Society for Medical Decision Making* 2012;32:678–89.

11. Caro JJ, Briggs AH, Siebert U, Kuntz KM, Force I-SMGRPT. Modeling good research practices—Overview: A report of the ISPOR-SMDM Modeling Good Research Practices Task Force-1. *Medical Decision Making: An International Journal of the Society for Medical Decision Making* 2012;32:667–77.

12. Freedberg KA, Tosteson AN, Cohen CJ, Cotton DJ. Primary prophylaxis for *Pneumocystis carinii* pneumonia in HIV-infected people with CD4 counts below $200/mm^3$: A cost-effectiveness analysis. *Journal of Acquired Immune Deficiency Syndromes* 1991;4:521–31.

13. Freedberg KA, Tosteson AN, Cotton DJ, Goldman L. Optimal management strategies for HIV-infected patients who present with cough or dyspnea: A cost-effective analysis. *Journal of General Internal Medicine* 1992;7:261–72.

14. Doubilet P, Begg CB, Weinstein MC, Braun P, McNeil BJ. Probabilistic sensitivity analysis using Monte Carlo simulation. A practical approach. *Medical Decision Making: An International Journal of the Society for Medical Decision Making* 1985;5:157–77.

15. Briggs AH, Ades AE, Price MJ. Probabilistic sensitivity analysis for decision trees with multiple branches: Use of the Dirichlet distribution in a Bayesian framework. *Medical Decision Making: An International Journal of the Society for Medical Decision Making* 2003;23:341–50.

16. Ades AE, Claxton K, Sculpher M. Evidence synthesis, parameter correlation and probabilistic sensitivity analysis. *Health Economics* 2006;15:373–81.

17. Kim LG, Thompson SG. Uncertainty and validation of health economic decision models. *Health Economics* 2010;19:43–55.

18. Braithwaite RS, Shechter S, Chang CC, Schaefer A, Roberts MS. Estimating the rate of accumulating drug resistance mutations in the HIV genome. *Value in Health: The Journal of the International Society for Pharmacoeconomics and Outcomes Research* 2007;10:204–13.

19. Braithwaite RS, Shechter S, Roberts MS et al. Explaining variability in the relationship between antiretroviral adherence and HIV mutation accumulation. *The Journal of Antimicrobial Chemotherapy* 2006;58:1036–43.

20. Schlessinger L, Eddy DM. Archimedes: A new model for simulating health care systems—The mathematical formulation. *Journal of Biomedical Informatics* 2002;35:37–50.

21. Stahl JE. Modelling methods for pharmacoeconomics and health technology assessment: An overview and guide. *PharmacoEconomics* 2008;26:131–48.

22. Sanders GD, Bayoumi AM, Sundaram V et al. Cost-effectiveness of screening for HIV in the era of highly active antiretroviral therapy. *The New England Journal of Medicine* 2005;352:570–85.

23. Sonnenberg FA, Beck JR. Markov models in medical decision making: A practical guide. *Medical Decision Making: An International Journal of the Society for Medical Decision Making* 1993;13:322–38.

24. Roberts M, Sonnenberg F. Decision modeling techniques. In: Chapman G, Sonnenberg F, eds. *Decision Making in Health Care: Theory, Psychology, Applications.* New York: Cambridge University Press. 2000.
25. Bonabeau E. Agent-based modeling: Methods and techniques for simulating human systems. *PNAS* 2015;112:7280–7.
26. Chhatwal J, He T. Economic evaluations with agent-based modelling: An introduction. *PharmacoEconomics* 2015;33:423–33.
27. Grefenstette JJ, Brown ST, Rosenfeld R et al. FRED (a Framework for Reconstructing Epidemic Dynamics): An open-source software system for modeling infectious diseases and control strategies using census-based populations. *BMC Public Health* 2013;13:940.
28. Eddy DM, Schlessinger L. Validation of the Archimedes diabetes model. *Diabetes Care* 2003;26:3102–10.
29. Eddy DM, Schlessinger L. Archimedes: A trial-validated model of diabetes. *Diabetes Care* 2003;26:3093–101.
30. Hur C, Chung DC, Schoen RE, Gazelle GS. The management of small polyps found by virtual colonoscopy: Results of a decision analysis. *Clinical Gastroenterology and Hepatology: The Official Clinical Practice Journal of the American Gastroenterological Association* 2007;5:237–44.
31. Olin RL, Kanetsky PA, Ten Have TR, Nasta SD, Schuster SJ, Andreadis C. Determinants of the optimal first-line therapy for follicular lymphoma: A decision analysis. *American Journal of Hematology* 2010;85:255–60.
32. Olin RL, Andreadis C. David versus Goliath: Decision analysis predicts results of a large clinical trial in follicular lymphoma. *Journal of Clinical Oncology: Official Journal of the American Society of Clinical Oncology* 2013;31:3608–9.
33. Beck JR, Kassirer JP, Pauker SG. A convenient approximation of life expectancy (the "DEALE"). I. Validation of the method. *American Journal of Medicine* 1982;73(6):883–8.
34. Beck JR, Pauker SG, Gottlieb JE, Klein K, Kassirer JP. A convenient approximation of life expectancy (the "DEALE"). II. Use in medical decision-making. *American Journal of Medicine* 1982 Dec;73(6):889–97.
35. Swedish KA, Factor SH, Goldstone SE. Prevention of recurrent high-grade anal neoplasia with quadrivalent human papillomavirus vaccination of men who have sex with men: A nonconcurrent cohort study. *Clinical Infectious Diseases* 2012;54:891–8.
36. Swedish KA, Goldstone SE. Prevention of anal condyloma with quadrivalent human papillomavirus vaccination of older men who have sex with men. *PLoS One* 2014;9:e93393.
37. Joura EA, Garland SM, Paavonen J et al. Effect of the human papillomavirus (HPV) quadrivalent vaccine in a subgroup of women with cervical and vulvar disease: Retrospective pooled analysis of trial data. *BMJ* 2012;344: e1401.
38. Deshmukh AA, Chhatwal J, Chiao EY, Nyitray AG, Das P, Cantor SB. Long-term outcomes of adding HPV vaccine to the anal intraepithelial neoplasia treatment regimen in hiv-positive men who have sex with men. *Clinical Infectious Diseases* 2015; 61(10):1527–35.
39. Deshmukh AA, Chiao EY, Das P, Cantor SB. Clinical effectiveness and cost-effectiveness of quadrivalent human papillomavirus vaccination in

HIV-negative men who have sex with men to prevent recurrent high-grade anal intraepithelial neoplasia. *Vaccine* 2014;32:6941–7.

40. Yokota F, Thompson KM. Value of information analysis in environmental health risk management decisions: Past, present, and future. *Risk Analysis* 2004;24: 635–50.

41. Howard RA. Information value theory. *IEEE Transactions on Systems Science and Cybernetics* 1966;2:22–6.

42. Howard RA. Value of information lotteries. *IEEE Transactions on Systems Science and Cybernetics* 1967;3:54–60.

43. Claxton K, Cohen JT, Neumann PJ. When is evidence sufficient? *Health Affairs (Millwood)* 2005;24:93–101.

44. Claxton K, Neumann PJ, Araki S, Weinstein MC. Bayesian value-of-information analysis. *International Journal of Technology Assessment in Health Care* 2001;17: 38–55.

45. Briggs A, Sculpher M, Claxton K. *Decision Modelling for Health Economic Evaluation.* New York, NY: Oxford University Press. 2006.

46. Chhatwal J, Elbasha EH. *Transformation of Transition Rates and Probabilities in Discrete-Time Markov Chains: What about Competing Risks?* Chicago, IL: Society for Medical Decision Making. 2011.

47. Marino S, Hogue IB, Ray CJ, Kirschner DE. A methodology for performing global uncertainty and sensitivity analysis in systems biology. *Journal of Theoretical Biology* 2008;254:178–96.

48. Raiffa H, Schlaifer R. *Applied Statistical Decision Theory.* Boston, MA: Harvard Business School Publications. 1961.

49. Jalal H, Goldhaber-Fiebert JD, Kuntz KM. Computing expected value of partial sample information from probabilistic sensitivity analysis using linear regression metamodeling. *Medical Decision Making: An International Journal of the Society for Medical Decision Making* 2015;35:584–95.

50. Strong M, Oakley JE, Brennan A. Estimating multiparameter partial expected value of perfect information from a probabilistic sensitivity analysis sample: A nonparametric regression approach. *Medical Decision Making: An International Journal of the Society for Medical Decision Making* 2014;34:311–26.

51. Minelli C, Baio G. Value of information: A tool to improve research prioritization and reduce waste. *PLoS Medicine* 2015;12:e1001882.

52. PCORI Board Approves Providing up to $50 Million for CER on Hepatitis C. Retrieved from: http://www.pcori.org/news-release/pcori-board-approves-providing-50-million-cer-hepatitis-c (Accessed December 22, 2015).

53. Myers E, Sanders GD, Ravi D et al. *Evaluating the Potential Use of Modeling and Value-of-Information Analysis for Future Research Prioritization within the Evidence-Based Practice Center Program.* Rockville, MD. 2011.

54. Myers E, McBroom A, Shen L, Posey R, Gray M. Value of information analysis for patient-centered outcomes research prioritization. Duke Evidence-Based Practice Center for Patient-Centered Outcomes Research Institute. 2012.

55. Rein DB. Value of information and research prioritization. White Paper for the Patient-Centered Outcomes Research Institute: NORC at the University of Chicago. 2012.

Section IV

Special Topics

14

On the Use of Electronic Health Records

Sebastien J-P.A. Haneuse and Susan M. Shortreed

CONTENTS

ABSTRACT Electronic health records (EHRs) provide a huge opportunity for comparative effectiveness research (CER). As electronic renderings of health and health-related information, EHRs give researchers unprecedented access to data that can help address questions that would otherwise be very difficult to answer. Crucially, as data collected from EHRs often reflect large and diverse populations of individuals seeking care, EHR-based CER studies can be used to help guide patient decision-making in real-world settings. Notwithstanding their potential benefits, however, the use of EHR data for research purposes requires care. Specifically, since EHRs are typically implemented to support clinical and/or billing systems, researchers interested in using EHR data for CER face challenges regarding (i) accessing the data, (ii) ensuring the data are research quality, and (iii) the control of confounding bias. Adding to these challenges is that, since there is no single universally accepted format, EHRs vary substantially in their structure and in the information they contain. This chapter reviews the current methods for addressing these challenges, focusing on the context of observational CER. While many of these methods borrow from the existing literature, novel methods that consider issues specific to EHRs, including their complex, high-dimensional nature, have been developed in recent years. Progress has not been uniform, however, and the gaps that remain represent opportunities for the development of new innovative methods.

14.1 Introduction

Medical and public health research is undergoing a "Big Data" revolution with recent technological advances giving biomedical researchers the ability to collect and analyze enormous amounts of diverse and often complex health-related data. One central component of this revolution has been the strong push toward the use of electronic health records (EHRs). While electronic health databases, particularly in the form of administrative claims databases, have been in use for decades, 2009 represented a watershed in the commitment to the use of EHRs. Crucially, the American Recovery and Reinvestment Act set aside $19.2 billion in incentives and grants to stimulate physicians and hospitals to develop and adopt EHR systems [6,139]. In parallel to this financial commitment by the U.S. federal government, the 2009 Institute of Medicine report on initial priorities for comparative effectiveness research (CER) called for "large-scale clinical and administrative data networks that enable observational studies of patient care while protecting patient privacy and data security" [67]. In the same year, the Federal Coordinating Center for Comparative Effectiveness Research released a report highlighting health information technology data infrastructure as a major category of investment for their strategic framework for CER [37] and the National Institutes of Health directly called for widened use of EHR for secondary research purposes [98]. Since 2010, the Electronic Data Methods Forum, set up with support from the Agency for Healthcare Research and Quality, has sought to facilitate collaborations toward the advancement of EHR as a research resource [65]. Most recently, in 2013, the Patient-Centered Outcomes Research Institute (PCORI) has invested more than 100 million dollar in 11 clinical data research networks, referred to as PCORnet, to build infrastructure between EHR systems that touch patients in every U.S. state [41].

TABLE 14.1

Summary of Potential Benefits and Challenges Associated with the Used EHR Data for CER

Benefits	Challenges
• Rich data on large populations over long time frames • Real-world clinical settings • Relatively inexpensive • Potential near real-time access	• Heterogeneity across EHR systems • Processing text-based clinical notes • Linkage in the absence of unique patient identifiers • Incomplete/missing data • Measurement error and misclassification • Confounding bias

That EHR data present an appealing opportunity for CER is well recognized [44,131,155,156]. Relative to data obtained via dedicated research designs, EHR data enjoy numerous benefits that have the potential to improve CER and, eventually, provide a stronger basis for guiding decision-making in clinical contexts (see Table 14.1). First, EHRs often contain rich data on a broad range of factors for relatively large populations over a long period of time. The Centers for Medicare and Medicaid Services (CMS) data systems, for example, maintain administrative claims data on 33.3 million Medicare fee-for-service beneficiaries who received care in 2012 [22]. This wealth of information is particularly useful when interest lies in addressing questions that could not feasibly or ethically be conducted otherwise, including studies of very rare outcomes, of minority populations and when interest lies with establishing noninferiority [77]. Second, since EHRs document "real-world" health care, they provide a ready infrastructure for the study of nonstandard treatment and protocols, as well as for when treatments are used off-label [62]. Third, by building on an existing infrastructure, the "collection" of data from EHR systems is relatively inexpensive. Finally, the near real-time access to data as it accrues has the potential to be very useful as a basis for recruitment in prospective or surveillance studies such as the Mini-Sentinel Initiative [108].

Notwithstanding the potential benefits of EHR data for CER, researchers face a number of practical and methodologic challenges. These challenges include those that are inherent to all studies of comparative effectiveness (the reader is referred to Chapters 1 and 9 for overviews) as well as a number of challenges that are specific to the use of EHR data (see Table 14.1). As we elaborate upon in the remainder of this chapter, the challenges specific to EHR-based CER arise primarily because the data are typically collected for clinical and/or billing purposes, and not with any specific research agenda in mind. Furthermore, since there is no uniformly accepted definition of "electronic health record" [33,70], the type and quality of data that researchers have access to across and within studies can be incredibly heterogeneous [62].

As such, while future EHR systems may be specifically designed with secondary research agendas in the mind [88], the use of EHR data for CER is not straightforward. With this in mind, the challenges are placed under three broad headings:

1. Accessing EHR data
2. Ensuring EHR data is research quality
3. Controlling confounding bias in EHR-based CER

As we discuss these challenges, we focus on observational CER studies. While randomized trials clearly represent the "gold standard" in terms of establishing causality, they suffer from important conceptual and practical drawbacks, and researchers are increasingly recognizing the value of observational study designs as discussed in Chapters 1 through 3 [44,62,103,131]. The remainder of the chapter is as follows. Section 14.2 highlights heterogeneity in EHR data by providing an overview of the various types of data sources that researchers might consider using. Section 14.3 provides a brief description of an ongoing comparative effectiveness study of antidepressant medications that is used to illustrate concepts introduced and discussed in this chapter. Sections 14.4 through 14.6 describe the methodologic challenges that researchers may face when attempting to use EHR data for CER along with solutions currently available. Finally, Section 14.7 provides concluding remarks, including avenues for future methodologic research.

14.2 Electronic Health Records Data

Arguably, the prevailing view of EHRs is that they are electronic renditions of the traditional paper-based medical chart [33]. While reasonable in many settings, this view fails to encompass the heterogeneity researchers find in nature and the complexity of EHRs [62,131]. Recognizing this heterogeneity is critical as researchers decide among methods for dealing with challenges that they may face, or as they develop new methods. Prior to describing these methods, this section provides an overview of the variety of EHR resources available to comparative effectiveness researchers also summarized in Table 14.2.

14.2.1 Administrative Databases

Among the most widely used EHR research resources are healthcare utilization or administrative claims/billing databases [131]. These databases, maintained by both public and private insurance entities, constitute an electronic record of health-related activities that generate a claim or bill, including hospitalizations, visits to a healthcare provider, the receipt of a procedure,

TABLE 14.2

Summary of Types of EHR Data Sources/Systems, along with Primary Positive/Negative Attributes

---

Administrative databases:
  + Large, often diverse populations
  − Lack of detailed clinical information
Registries:
  + Detailed clinical information
  − Tend to focus on specific diseases/conditions
Integrated healthcare systems:
  + Linked billing and clinical information
  − Populations defined by local geography and demographics
Hospitals and tertiary healthcare systems:
  + Detailed clinical information
  − Open cohorts
Linked EHR data systems:
  + Detailed clinical information on huge populations
  − Complexity of logistics and analysis

---

and the filling of a prescription. The largest such database in the United States is the federally funded Medicare program, which provides insurance for 97% of individuals aged 65 years or older, patients with end-stage renal disease, and some disabled persons. For each submitted claim, Current Procedural Terminology (CPT) codes and International Classification of Diseases, Ninth Revision (ICD-9) diagnostic codes are used to describe the nature of the billed service. In addition, each claim typically includes demographic information on the patient, an encrypted provider number, and dates of service. Similarly, the Canadian Institute for Health Information maintains the Discharge Abstract Database, which captures administrative, clinical, and demographic information on all separations (discharges, transfers, and deaths) from all Canadian hospitals [19].

Beyond these public entities, a number of private commercial entities have developed very large administrative databases that facilitate research through the provision of de-identified, individual-level healthcare claims data. Examples include the MarketScan Research Database, maintained by Truven Health Analytics, with information on more than 180 million unique individuals since 1995 [148] and the HealthCore Integrated Research Database covering nearly 43 million individuals across 14 states [54].

14.2.2 Registries

One important drawback of administrative databases is that they only consistently include information on health-related activities that generate a claim or bill. Consequently, the scope and detail of data generated is geared specifically toward billing purposes and, as such, may be limited when employed for CER. A second, widely used form of EHR data arises from disease-specific registries. The Surveillance, Epidemiology, and End Results (SEER) Program of the National Cancer Institute, for example, collects data from 17 tumor registries, covering approximately 28% of the U.S. population and 97% of incidence cases in the registries catchment areas [97]. Information routinely collected by SEER includes data on demographics, tumor characteristics and stage at diagnosis, initial treatment regimens, and follow-up for vital status. A second example of a large, national registry is the United States Renal Data System, funded by the National Institute of Diabetes and Digestive and Kidney Diseases, that collects, analyzes, and distributes information on the end-stage renal disease population in the United States, including treatments and outcomes [99]. Other examples include the CORRONA database, a nationwide prospective registry of patients with rheumatoid arthritis in the United States [72] and the Bariatric Surgery Registry at Kaiser Permanente Southern California [137]. Finally, beyond the United States, many countries provide universal health care and are able to use unique personal identifiers to link systems to build registries that contain complete and comprehensive electronic health data; most prominent among these are Scandinavian countries, including Denmark [32], Norway [101], and Sweden [144].

14.2.3 Integrated Healthcare Systems

While registries provide greater clinical detail than most administrative databases, other than registries associated with national healthcare systems, they focus on specific diseases and/or health conditions. In contrast, integrated health organizations that simultaneously provide insurance coverage and healthcare maintain databases that collect a wide range of health-related information on entire populations. An example of such an organization is Group Health Cooperative, which provides comprehensive health care on a prepaid basis to approximately 600,000 individuals in Washington State and Idaho [125]. As part of their administrative systems, Group Health maintains electronic databases that record information on health plan enrollment, healthcare use including laboratory values, procedures, diagnoses, and pharmacy dispensings. Since 2005, a fully integrated EHR system based on EpicCare (Epic Systems Corporation of Madison, Wisconsin) documents all patient care at Group Health clinics, including vital signs such as height, weight, and body mass index (BMI). Collectively, these electronic systems provide a detailed record of a patient's health both prior to and after diagnosis of any given condition. This, in turn, gives comparative effectiveness researchers opportunities to investigate questions of disease prevention among healthy individuals as well as treatment options among sick patients.

In addition to Group Health, many integrated health organizations maintain comprehensive EHRs. Examples include Kaiser Permanente

Southern California, Kaiser Permanente Northern California, Harvard Pilgrim in Boston, Massachusetts, and the Henry Ford Health System in Detroit, Michigan. These systems, together with 13 others, are members of the HMO Research Network (HMORN) which, collectively, covers 13.7 million lives in the United States [63]. Beyond these entities, another example of a large integrated healthcare system is the Veterans Health Administration (VA). Providing care for nearly 9 million veterans in the United States, the VA runs an information resource center (VIReC) to facilitate research using their extensive EHR systems in collaboration with VA researchers [150].

14.2.4 Hospital and Tertiary Healthcare Systems

A key advantage of integrated organizations, such as the VA and those in the HMORN, is that the linkage between insurance and health care provides incentives for patients to receive all of their care within a single system. While patients can, of course, disenroll from their plans, for the most part, this linkage provides researchers with (essentially) closed cohorts of patients with little risk of relevant information being recorded outside of the organization's EHR. Most patients in the United States, however, receive care outside such systems. In particular, most patients have health insurance through one organization and receive health care from another. Most prominent among such health insurers is the federal government, specifically with the Medicaid and Medicare programs. With the decoupling of insurance and health care, patients are free to choose whichever hospital they would like to receive their care at, on an as-needed basis. Many of these "stand-alone" hospital systems maintain comprehensive EHRs. Examples with established track records for research include Brigham and Women's Hospital, Boston, Massachusetts; Vanderbilt Medical Center, Nashville, Tennessee; and Mayo Clinic, Rochester, Minnesota.

14.2.5 Linked EHR Data

Finally, in addition to the vast number of stand-alone resources available to CER researchers, there are many ongoing systematic efforts to directly bridge gaps across differing EHR systems to enable biomedical research. One established resource in the HMORNs Virtual Data Warehouse (VDW) [66]. Briefly, the VDW consists of a collection of dataset standards and automated procedures that allow data retrieval programs to be developed at one of the HMORN sites and run seamlessly at 15 of them. This provides the comparative effectiveness researcher with an efficient framework for the quick extraction of large, detailed datasets for multisite studies without the need for site-specific customization. Other similar systems maintained by the HMORN include the Center for Education and Research on Therapeutics (CERT) [109] and the Cancer Research Network (CRN) [96]. Beyond the HMORN, the National Cancer Institute maintains the SEER-Medicare Linked

Database, which reflects the linkage of the two large component EHR data resources to provide researchers with comprehensive health-related information on 1.6 million Medicare beneficiaries who developed cancer, both prior to and after diagnosis. Other initiatives, recently funded by the federal government, include the Electronic Medical Records and Genomics (eMERGE) Network, a consortium of nine institutions with linkages between DNA repositories and EHR systems [92] and the Mini-Sentinel Initiative, which collates EHR data from 18 participating organizations to create an active surveillance system to monitor and evaluate safety of FDA-regulated medical products [93].

14.3 Comparative Effectiveness of Antidepressant Medication on Weight Change

To ground the discussion of methodologic challenges that can arise when using EHR-derived data for CER, we describe an ongoing comparative study of antidepressant medication. Jointly, depression and obesity represent major public health concerns with substantial impact on medical morbidity, healthcare spending, and quality of life [40,140]. While the processes underlying their impact on health outcomes are the subject of much recent research [36,84,102,151,160], there is a growing body of clinical evidence suggesting that the choice of antidepressant drug therapy may influence changes in weight over time [136]. With climbing rates of obesity [40,104] and antidepressant agents, the most commonly prescribed drugs in the United States [105], understanding the impact of different antidepressant drugs on weight change over time is crucial to helping patients and physicians make informed decisions regarding treatment. The primary goal of the study, therefore, is to evaluate the comparative effects of different medications on subsequent weight changes over time.

The setting for the study is Group Health (see Section 14.2.3). To study the relationship between antidepressant drug therapy and weight change, we considered all adult Group Health enrollees, aged 18–65 years, with a diagnosis of depressive disorder (ICD-9 = 296.2x, 296.3x, 311, or 300.4) and who initiated a new monotherapy episode of antidepressant drug treatment between January 2006 and November 2009. A new monotherapy episode was defined as a dispensing for a single medication, without any other antidepressant medication dispensing in the prior 9 months. Following data abstraction from the EHR, $n = 16,277$ patients satisfying the inclusion/exclusion criteria were identified. For each patient, we extracted all records in the EHR, censoring follow-up at the first of 720 days posttreatment initiation, disenrollment from their Group Health plan, November 1, 2009, or death.

14.4 Challenge #1: Accessing EHR Data

A key motivation for using EHR data for CER is that, from the perspective of the researcher, the data infrastructure already exists. That is, the data exist in an electronic format in some health systems-specific repository or across multiple such systems [2,5]. Unfortunately, that the data exist does not mean that they are easily extracted. In particular, as in the antidepressants study described in Section 14.3, relevant electronic health-related data may reside in numerous places within any given system; demographic information, laboratory measurements, clinical notes, pharmacy prescription data, and billing claims may all be stored in separate purpose-built databases. Furthermore, if these systems/databases were developed independently or over different time frames, they may not be structured around some common, unique patient identifier. As such, in contrast to databases that are developed and built specifically for research purposes, the first practical challenge of an EHR-based study is the extraction of data into a format that is suitable for the intended analysis and is compatible with the intended analysis software. Specifically, prior to assessments of data quality and analyses, researchers may face two practical challenges:

1. Coding and classification of clinical information from text-based notes
2. The linkage of information from multiple sources when a unique patient identifier is unavailable

14.4.1 Coding and Classification of Text-Based Notes

Ultimately, for information in the EHR to be used in quantitative analyses, it must be translated into discrete data elements. In many instances, however, the information contained in the EHR consists of unstructured text-based clinical notes [5]. Examples include detailed history notes, notes on recommendations given to a patient, preoperative assessments of a patient about to undergo surgery, notes on the interpretation of a radiology report, and discharge summaries. In the antidepressant study, a patient's clinical notes could supplement the EHR by providing information on their history of depression, prior medication use, and current smoking status. It might also provide important information on missingness in the EHR; if standard practice is that weight is measured at a primary care visit and yet one is not recorded in the EHR, the clinical notes could provide insight.

Taking full advantage of data contained in clinical notes requires the accurate translation of free text into discrete data elements suitable for analyses. This represents an incredibly difficult task with specific challenges, including spelling/grammatical error identification, the identification of specific words/phrases and their categorization, disambiguation of homographs (i.e., words with multiple meanings), negation and uncertainty identification, and relationship extraction. Toward addressing these challenges, the theory of natural language processing (NLP) provides a framework for information retrieval and processing [95]. With a rich history in the fields of artificial intelligence and linguistics, early NLP algorithms were based on sets of rules derived from formal theories of grammar. More recently, statistical methods from the machine-learning literature have been used to develop and evaluate NLP algorithms; specific methods include support vector machines, conditional random fields, and hidden Markov models [87]. For any given method, learning can be *supervised* when "truth" is known and results can be validated. If the truth is not known, the learning process is *unsupervised* and relies on the discovery and recognition of patterns.

Regardless of the approach used, an important consideration is that of overfitting where the algorithm performs poorly outside of the data setting used to develop it. One strategy for minimizing this is cross-validation, which repeatedly randomly partitions the data into a training portion and a validation subsample; validation results are then averaged across the rounds and used as a basis for choosing a final algorithm [52].

In the context of EHR-based CER, NLP has most successfully been applied when interest lies in the determination of some specific data element, such as a diagnosis. An initial goal of the eMERGE network, for example, was to investigate the feasibility of genome-wide association studies with phenotype information obtained from each institution's EHR. To supplement billing codes, laboratory measurements, test results, and clinical documentation, NLP was used to increase both sensitivity and specificity in the identification of patients with specific phenotypes [34]. An important caveat, however, is that NLP algorithms are typically not generalizable beyond the settings in which they were trained [138]. That a significant investment of time and resources is required to develop an NLP algorithm, the lack of generalizability has been used as a rationale for not pursing information in text-based fields at all [2]. Nevertheless, there are ongoing efforts to develop NLP platforms that interface with EHR systems and are usable for CER [53].

14.4.2 Linkage in the Absence of Unique Patient Identifiers

In many settings, a patient's electronic health data is not stored in a single database. Consider, for example, a Medicare enrollee who has a cancer diagnosis. While CMS databases track healthcare-related claims and billing information, detailed information on their medical history, diagnosis, treatment, and follow-up is not. If the Medicare enrollee resides in one of the SEER registry catchment areas, this information is captured albeit in a different database. Given a unique patient identifier common to both databases, the linkage of information would be trivial (barring data entry mistakes). Unfortunately, however, since the CMS and SEER programs were developed and are administered by two different federal entities, there is no built-in common identifier for the individual. Fortunately, to resolve this, the National Cancer Institute and CMS began a collaborative effort in 1991 to link the two databases [153].

The field of record linkage provides a framework for merging patient data from multiple sources when no "gold standard" identifier is available [49,79]. For the most part, algorithms in record linkage work by constructing a score (based on some metric) that quantifies the extent to which two records are from the same patient. The numeric score is then evaluated against some predetermined threshold and a final decision of whether or not the two records are from the same patient is made. Typically, methods for linkage fall into one of two broad classes: *deterministic rules* and *probabilistic models.*

Deterministic rules consider two records to be linked if they both satisfy prespecified threshold conditions for a collection of fields. The SEER-Medicare linkage algorithm, for example, starts out by asking whether or not a valid social security number (SSN) is available in both records. If it is, the records are (deterministically) linked if the records are complete matches on any of the following collections:

1. SSN and first name and last name
2. SSN and first name and month of birth and sex
3. SSN and last name and month of birth and sex

If a valid SSN is not available as a basis for matching, additional collections are considered, which include year of birth, day of birth, middle initial, month and year of death, and individual digits of the SSN, if available [110]. In practice, linkage decisions can be based on requiring an exact match for each field or can permit certain fields to only partially match; matching based on first and last names in SEER-Medicare, for example, only considers the first six positions. Although deterministic rules are relatively easy to implement, they tend to be ad hoc and difficult to generalize as a universal methodology, and their accuracy can be very sensitive to data quality [79].

Instead of relying on the specification of a set of rules, probabilistic methods rely on some underlying statistical model for the agreement between two records across a set collection of fields. Given estimates for the parameters that index the model, distance metrics are evaluated for each pair of records and compared to some predetermined threshold. As with statistical methods for NLP, probabilistic linkage models can be *supervised* when the truth is known or *unsupervised* if the truth is not known. One specific unsupervised methodology that has been extensively used for record linkage is latent class models. Briefly, the unknown linkage status of two records (i.e., linked or not linked) is treated as a latent variable. Mixture models are then used to characterize the relationship between the unobserved latent variable and the observed matching status of the various individual fields; matching patterns across the fields are viewed as arising from mixtures of matches and nonmatches. Specification of the mixture models includes the classic Fellegi–Sunter model, which assumes conditional independence among fields given the latent class [38], log-linear models for the expected number of distinct matching patterns [76], and probit latent class models that permit general correlation structures among the individual fields [159]. Beyond these unsupervised methods, approaches have been proposed that make use of "gold standard" clerical review data. Larsen and Rubin [76], for example, developed a strategy that iterates between identifying specific records for clerical review and re-estimation of the mixture model parameters.

14.5 Challenge #2: Ensuring EHR Data Is Research Quality

In addition to information encoded in free-text fields, EHRs typically contain a wealth of information stored in structured fields. Examples include a patient's gender and age, anthropomorphic measurements such as weight and height, results from laboratory tests, diagnosis codes, and prescriptions. Fortunately, in contrast to free text, information stored in these fields is typically relatively easy to extract and export into a format that can then be used for analysis. That these data can be readily extracted, however, does not mean that they are suitable for CER. In particular, since priorities between clinical and billing contexts often differ from those of research contexts, an often-cited criticism of EHR-derived data is that they are not of the same quality as data obtained from dedicated research studies [155]. Crucially, since EHR data accrue outside the context of any particular research study agenda or protocol, researchers have no *a priori* control over data collection, including the timing of measurements, as well as on definitions and standards of measurement to be used.

To understand the limitations of EHR-derived data, researchers often conduct internal quality assessments. Over the last 20 years, numerous literature reviews have sought to synthesis the performance of such quality assessment studies [23,64,145,146,156]. Broadly, one finds that there is substantial variation in quality across EHR systems and that this variation is determined by the complex interplay of patient-, healthcare provider-, and organizational-level factors and decisions. To address this complexity, a number of classification schemes have been developed to provide researchers with a structured approach to defining "quality" in any given EHR setting—Hersh et al. [61], for example, recently developed a set of quality-related caveats on the use of EHR in CER.

While recognizing the multifaceted nature of "quality," in this chapter, we focus on two general themes:

1. Completeness of EHR data, or lack thereof
2. Accuracy of EHR, or lack thereof

Both themes lend themselves to the application of statistical methods that have been published in the literature. In the remainder of this section, we consider them in turn, providing details on the challenges that arise specifically in the context of EHR-based CER and on existing methods that researchers can employ.

14.5.1 Incomplete Data

Returning to the antidepressants study, Figure 14.1 provides a summary of weight-related information for six patients over the course of the first 720

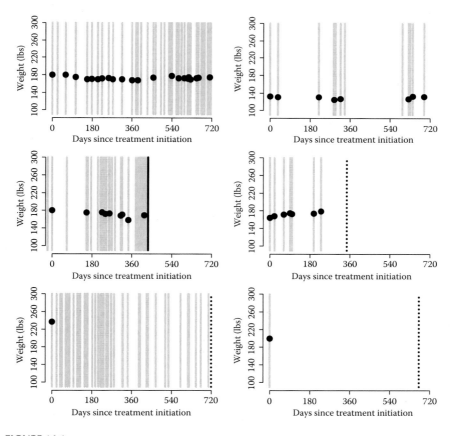

FIGURE 14.1

Observed weight information up to 720 days posttreatment initiation in the Group Health EHR for six patients identified as satisfying the inclusion/exclusion criteria of the antidepressant's comparative effective study. Gray lines indicate an encounter with the healthcare system; a dotted black line indicates follow-up was censored on November 1, 2009; a solid black line indicates follow-up was censored due to disenrollment. Black dots indicate that a weight measurement was obtained and recorded in the EHR.

days posttreatment initiation. In each panel, a vertical gray line indicates that an encounter with the healthcare system took place on that date; a black dot indicates that a weight measurement was obtained and recorded in the EHR. For the first of these patients, represented by the top-left panel, we see that their interactions with the Group Health healthcare system were intense. Over the 2-year follow-up period, they had a total of 87 encounters from which a total of 31 weight measurements were recorded in the EHR. Since these measurements are distributed throughout the 720 days, they provide rich data on the patient's weight trajectory over time.

In contrast, the patients represented by the remaining panels have relatively sparse information. Consider, for example, the top-right panel. This patient only had 24 encounters over the 2-year period, with only 8 weight measurements recorded in the EHR. Furthermore, these measurements are recorded at irregular time points, with two long time periods during which no weight-related activity was observed. The patient in the middle-left panel has a similar quantity of information (specifically, 31 encounters and 9 weight measurements) although the activity took place entirely within just over 1 year; at day 433, the patient disenrolled from Group Health. The remaining panels describe patients whose follow-up time was censored due to the end of the study observation period (i.e., November 1, 2009), although their activity in the EHR in terms of encounters and weight measurements is very different.

Collectively, the six panels in Figure 14.1 highlight the notion that, while a patient's weight trajectory progresses smoothly in time, the information available in the EHR consists of a series of "snap-shots" that vary substantially in both frequency and timing. In principle, one could use a linear mixed effects model for longitudinal data to analyze the observed weight measurements [39,75]. Such an analysis is appealing in that correlation within a subject is accounted for through the use of random effects and that observations are not required to be measured at regular intervals in time. The validity of results, however, requires assumptions regarding the frequency and timing of the observed data. In particular, validity requires the "missing at random" (MAR) assumption, which states that the process by which the observed data are generated depends solely on factors that are completely observed within the EHR [82]. If, for example, the timing of any given measurement is dictated solely by when the previous measurement occurred, then MAR would hold. If the timing depends solely on comorbid conditions and other patient-level characteristics (e.g., gender, age) that are measured in the EHR then, again, MAR would hold. Finally, if the timing depends on decisions made by the physician or the healthcare system or both and that these decisions are documented in the EHR or elsewhere, then, again, MAR would hold. If, however, the timing and frequency are determined (even in part) by factors that are not measured in the EHR, then MAR will not hold. The observed data are then said to be "missing not-at-random" (MNAR). In the context of the antidepressants study, the observed data would be MNAR if patients who had recently gained or lost weight systematically decided not to engage with the healthcare system and/or refused to be weighed. For completeness, we note that a third scenario is where the observed data are "missing completely at random" (MCAR), which corresponds to the irregular frequency and timing of data in the EHR being unrelated to any patient-, physician-, or organizational-level factors.

Determining whether or not the observed data are MCAR, MAR, or MNAR is crucial: if an assumption is made but fails to hold, analyses may be subject to bias with downstream consequences for the validity of conclusions and guidance on clinical decision-making. It is important to note that this bias is distinct from confounding bias. In particular, while confounding bias concerns the establishment of *internal validity*, regarding causation, bias that arises in the missing data context speaks to the *external validity* and the ability to generalize beyond the sample to the intended patient population of interest [50]. To emphasize this distinction, and the fact that both types of bias can arise in any given comparative effectiveness study, we refer to bias due to missing data as "selection bias" [57]. Methods for the control of confounding bias in EHR-based CER are reviewed in Section 14.6.

To identify and control selection bias, a detailed understanding of the process by which the EHR data was generated and recorded is required. Unfortunately, understanding this process, sometimes referred to as the *provenance* [130], can be a difficult task since

- Measurement requires active engagement with the clinical system and is rarely passive (i.e., does not continue once a condition has been treated or a patient disenrolls) so that it is difficult to distinguish between a missing value and a negative value.
- Patients do not necessarily receive care consistent with standards at their institution and those standards may change over time.
- Patients may receive care at multiple organizations/facilities so that the absence of information does not mean that care is not being received.
- The EHR system may be unable to record the measurement of interest by design.
- The design and structure of the EHR system may change over time, as can coding policies/procedures.
- With finite time during routine healthcare encounters, whether or not a measurement is taken and recorded may be tied to clinical priorities such as those determined by the presenting condition.

In practice, any given EHR-based comparative effectiveness study may or may not suffer from any or all of these issues. As issues are identified, however, researchers must consider which patient-, healthcare provider-, organizational-level factors influence them [5,23,61,103,145]. The extent to which each of these factors is available to researchers determines, in large part, whether or not the observed data are MAR or MNAR.

Given a detailed understanding of the data provenance, researchers have at their disposal a vast literature on the analysis of missing/incomplete data with which to perform statistical adjustments for selection bias. In general, the two most common approaches to handling missing data are multiple imputation (MI) [82,123] and inverse-probability weighting (IPW) [78,119]. Interestingly, while these methods are pervasive in the statistical literature, there is a general paucity of papers that are specifically developed to the context of EHR-based CER. One notable exception is a paper by Wells et al. [157], which reviews the use of MI in EHR-based studies, focusing on MI by chained equations [18,158], and gives a number of broad recommendations for accommodating the high-dimensional nature of EHR data. The paper also provides a review of software implementations of MI.

The extent to which either MI or IPW provides valid results, however, hinges on the appropriateness of the MAR assumption. In particular, if an important determinant of provenance is not available, then the observed data are MNAR. In the antidepressants study, for example, Group Health does not uniformly collect information on socioeconomic status in their EHR. If patients across different socioeconomic statuses interact with the healthcare system in systematically different ways, one would not be able to perform the necessary adjustments using either MI or IPW. Consequently, residual selection bias would likely remain, even after adjustment for known determinants of provenance. One long-term solution is to modify the EHR to collect broader and/or more detailed information, beyond that collected for clinical and administrative purposes, specifically with secondary research agenda in mind. Recently proposed distributed health data networks aim to achieve this on a national scale [88]. In the short term, researchers faced with EHR data that are MNAR can perform sensitivity analyses in an effort to understand how robust their results are under various scenarios for the way in which the missing determinant impacts provenance. While frameworks for sensitivity analyses in missing data analyses have been developed [20,31], none have been developed specifically for EHR-based studies and how best to do this remains an open question.

14.5.2 Inaccurate Data

A second theme regarding quality of EHR-derived data is the extent to which the extracted information provides an accurate representation of the patient's true state at the time the measurement was recorded or, perhaps less ambitiously, an accurate representation of what would have been collected had a dedicated study been conducted. In practice, while standards of care are typically established at institutions that maintain EHR systems, measurements obtained during routine clinical care may be subject to a broad range of practical phenomena that affect their accuracy and, ultimately, their suitability for research purposes. In the antidepressants study, for example, weight measurements in the EHR may have been taken with or without extra clothing and shoes or may be self-reported if there was insufficient time during the clinical visit [3].

More generally, as others have pointed out, the notion of "accuracy" is multifaceted, with potential problems arising at the level of the patient, healthcare provider, and organization [5,23,61,103,156]. In particular, comparative effectiveness researchers should consider:

- *The potential impact of the timing of measurements.* Glucose measurements in studies of type 2 diabetes mellitus, for example, are generally preferred to have been obtained when the patient has fasted to ensure that recent meals do not influence the observed value. Similarly, circulating melatonin levels are typically measured from urine specimens, which are generally preferred to have been obtained in the morning prior to the first void after sleep. If the fasting status or timing of the measurement is not known or difficult to ascertain from the EHR, the observed values may not be an accurate representation of what the researcher would actually hope to have access to.

- *How coding policies and procedures vary across institutions and over time.* In many settings, the International Classification of Diseases (ICD) system is used to classify and record diagnoses. Maintained by the World Health Organization, the system was last updated in 1994, expanding the 17,000 codes in the ICD-9 system to over 155,000 codes in the International Classification of Diseases, Tenth Revision (ICD-10) systems; the next planned update is due to be published in 2017. While the United States currently uses ICD-9 codes to classify and record diagnosis, on October 1, 2015, all U.S. healthcare agencies will be required by the Department of Health and Human Safety to use ICD-10 codes to classify and record diagnoses. This change will affect many EMR-based CER studies, as the collection of health outcome data relying ICD codes will have to be modified. Unfortunately, while similarities exist, there is no road map that clearly walks between ICD-9 and ICD-10 codes. As previous countries have made this transition successfully, however, U.S.-based researchers may be able to borrow from earlier international work in this area as well as develop new and improved algorithms for utilizing ICD-9 and ICD-10 codes in the same study without jeopardizing validity.

- *Information obtained directly from patients may be inconsistently collected and subject to recall bias.* While much of the EHR, including anthropomorphic and laboratory measurements, can be obtained with a degree of objective accuracy, some values may rely on the patient's direct input. Examples include family history, diagnosis dates for prevalent conditions, and past and present medication use. While recall bias is a well-known challenge, the extent to which the information is accurate also depends on the effort undertaken by the healthcare provider in obtaining it. As such, variation in recall-related accuracy may arise within an institution across patients and providers as well as over time.

- *Technological advances that may have changed how biomarkers are measured.* For certain biomarkers, such as CD4 count and human immunodeficiency virus (HIV) viral load, measurement technologies may have lower and upper limits of detection as well as inherent measurement error variation. As comparative effectiveness researchers wait for these technologies to evolve and become more uniformly adopted, they must contend with the resulting variation in accuracy over time and across institutions.

- *Some inaccuracies may be purposeful.* Many electronic health systems record diagnoses for both clinical and billing purposes; in some of these, the coding polices at the level of the organization may be geared toward optimal reimbursement. Jackson et al. [69], for example, found that the ICD-9 codes used for billing purposes in claims databases suffered substantial inaccuracies when compared to gold standard information from a medical chart review. Furthermore, in some settings, physicians may employ specific coding policies if there are downstream consequences for the patient [103].

In the event that information obtained from an EHR are thought or found to be inaccurate, comparative effectiveness researchers have at their disposal a number of ways forward. In the long term, researchers are working to establish common standards for EHR coding to ensure that clinical protocols are better aligned with the rigor of typical research protocols. Raebel et al., for example, propose a unifying set of definitions for prescription adherence [112]. In the short term, researchers may perform validation studies on small samples of their populations evaluating standard measures of accuracy, including sensitivity, specificity, positive predictive values, and negative predictive values [107]. Recent examples in the CER literature include a quality assessment of EHR data for classifying newly diagnosed from preexisting type 2 diabetes patients [73] and a validation study of accuracy of EHR-based information on the measurement of lipid management adherence [30].

If such validation studies indicate that the observed data are either sufficiently accurate for direct use or that the inaccuracies are nondifferential with respect to treatment choice and the outcome of interest, then researchers can proceed without adjustment with the only caveat being the possibility that the observed results will be attenuated toward the null. Results from these studies can either be interpreted as stand-alone or used together with established statistical methods for the adjustment of measurement error and misclassification. Two accessible but comprehensive overviews of these methods, including likelihood-based methods, regression calibration, and SIMEX, are given by Buonaccorsi [16] and Gustafson [48]; two additional references, specific to methods for measurement error, are texts by Fuller [42] and Carroll et al. [21].

As with the application of existing solutions for missing data, however, current methods for measurement error and misclassification do not explicitly account for the inherent complexity of EHR-derived data. The extent to which these methods fail to adjust for inaccuracies in EHR-derived data as well as the development of new methods that acknowledge the complex provenance of measurements are currently open areas of research.

14.6 Challenge #3: Confounding Bias in EHR-Based CER

Finally, even if appropriate information can be extracted from the EHR and it is of sufficient quality to be used for research purposes, the most-often cited challenge associated with the use of EHR data for CER is the potential for confounding bias [71]. While randomized trials are the established gold standard for assessing causation as it relates to comparing alternative treatment options, treatment is never randomly assigned in the clinical contexts that EHR systems represent. This, in turn, raises the possibility that observed differences in outcomes across different treatment choices may be spurious in the sense that they are driven by other factors that influence treatment choice. In the antidepressants study, for example, recent work has shown that the choice of antidepressant medication in clinical contexts can be driven, in part, by the patient's weight trajectory immediately prior to the diagnosis of depression [7]. Furthermore, a patient's pretreatment initiation weight trajectory is also likely to be associated with subsequent weight changes. Consequently, if variation in pretreatment weight trajectory is not accounted for in the primary comparative analyses, the results may be spurious and the ability to interpret the results as representing causal compromised.

Outside of the specific context of EHR-based CER, there is a vast literature on methods for unbiased estimation of causal treatment effects from observational data, as discussed in the first three chapters of this book [60,106]. These methods generally have two steps:

1. Identify a set of risk factors such that adjustment for these factors eliminates confounding bias.

2. Use a statistical technique to estimate the desired causal effect.

Undertaking the first of these steps in an EHR-based comparative effectiveness study is nontrivial, however, because it requires evaluating potentially hundreds of patient-, healthcare provider-, and organizational-level factors that may influence the often-complex decision of treatment choice. Fortunately, recent work has sought to directly address this issue. As we describe the methods, we first consider the setting where all potential confounders are available in the EHR. We then consider methods for the setting where one or more important factors are not available, a setting typically referred to as unmeasured confounding.

14.6.1 Confounding Bias When All Potential Confounders Are Measured

Suppose all potential confounders are measured in the EHR and that, likely in collaboration with subject-matter experts, a subset of these risk factors can be identified as being sufficient for the control of confounding [47]. Given this information, by far the most common approach for the statistical control of confounding bias is to include each of these factors into the outcome regression model, along with indicators for treatment choice. This approach is referred to as *regression adjustment*. Intuitively, by conditioning on these factors in the model one "breaks" or "controls" for their association with the outcome so that they no longer confound the association of interest. An alternative is to break or control their association with treatment choice so that, again, they no longer confound the association of interest. The latter approach requires building a model for treatment choice, as a function of potential confounders, generally referred to as a *propensity score* model [120]. As discussed in Chapter 1, given this model, one can then use the fitted propensity score values as balancing scores so that, under certain assumptions, the causal effect of interest can be identified without bias; commonly implemented approaches include stratification [83,121], matching [74,124], and inverse probability weighing [58].

In practice, notwithstanding the current enthusiasm for propensity score adjustment, the two approaches generally work equally well as methods for the control of confounding [141]. In studies of rare outcomes, researchers may prefer propensity score adjustment because it avoids the loss of degrees of freedom associated with including additional covariates into a model for the outcome. In an EHR-based study, however, sample size may be less of an issue. Given their similar performance in most settings, arguably, if one is to choose between the two methods, then the most reasonable approach to doing so is to determine whether or not more is known about determinants of the outcome, including the functional form of the association, or if more is known about determinants of treatment choice. If the former is the case, regression adjustment will likely be more successful; if the latter, propensity score adjustment should be pursued. If one is unable or unwilling to choose between the two approaches, recent doubly robust methods integrate them to provide a framework within which researchers can have the best of both worlds [4,43,149].

While many comparative effectiveness studies consider point treatments (i.e., treatments that are allocated at a single point in time), an important strength of EHR data is the rich longitudinal data that is available on patients. This provides researchers with unique opportunities to evaluate treatments that vary over time, perhaps dynamically in response to how the patient reacts to treatment as well as to changes in other factors. Evaluating causal effects for such time-varying treatment choices, however, is considerably more complex than evaluating causal effects for point treatments [60]. Consider, for example, a modification to the antidepressants study for which interest lies with not just the choice of medication but also the dosing of each drug. Assuming the relevant information is available in the EHR, it is reasonable to suppose that decisions over time regarding the choice and dose of medication in clinical contexts is driven by prior choices/doses as well as how the patient is responding to those choices/doses. The interplay between these decisions can result in *time-dependent confounding bias*. Unfortunately, the direct application of standard methods in the presence of time-dependent confounding does not resolve confounding bias [58]. Two strategies that permit the control of time-dependent confounding include those based on marginal structural models [27,56,115,118] and on structural nested mean models [116,117]. The reader can consult Chapters 1 and 3 for further discussion.

As emphasized at the beginning of this section, regardless of the analytic approach used to account for confounding bias, the distinguishing challenge in EHR-based CER is that the available data is often so rich that it is difficult, if not impossible, to choose a succinct set of patient-, healthcare provider-, and organizational-level variables such that their control will eliminate confounding. Although one could, in principle, guarantee the control of confounding by including any and all possible confounders into an outcome regression or propensity score model, overadjustment is undesirable in that it can lead to significant losses of statistical power [46,122,128]. While methods for variable selection for outcome regression models are well established [52], the recent literature has seen numerous methods proposed for variable selection specific to marginal structural models [14] as well as for propensity score-based analyses including high-dimensional propensity scores [133,147] and Bayesian methods that aim to explicitly account for all sources of uncertainty [152,161].

14.6.2 Unmeasured Confounding

While advances in analysis methods for conducting EHR-based CER have been made, most rely on the assumption that information is readily available on all potential confounders. Also known as the assumption of no unmeasured confounding, the extent to which it holds is particularly tenuous in EHR-based CER since healthcare decisions are often complex and made considering patient, healthcare provider, and organizational preferences. Even with the rich information available in an EHR, it is possible that one or more factors that induce confounding bias are not measured. When an important confounder is missing from the observed data, researchers currently have at their disposal three strategies for moving forward.

Instrumental variable (IV) analysis has enjoyed recent enthusiasm in the comparative effectiveness literature. See Chapter 2 for a detailed discussion of this approach. Briefly, an IV is a variable that is associated with treatment choice but has no direct effect on the outcome of interest [1]. If such a variable can be identified, the potentially confounded association between treatment choice and the outcome can be adjusted by (i) the relationship between the IV and treatment choice and (ii) the lack of a relationship between IV and the outcome, other than through treatment. From this we see that IV analyses permit the estimation of causal effects without the need to identify and control potential confounders of treatment. This is clearly an appealing property, especially in the complex setting of EHR-based CER. However, the fact that the variable under consideration is indeed a true IV is a very strong assumption that cannot be empirically verified [59,90]. Hence, IV analyses avoid the unverifiable assumption of no unmeasured confounding with a different unverifiable assumption. In practice, this has translated to relatively few variables being posited as plausible IVs in CER settings, with the most prominent being provider prescribing preferences in the context of pharmacoepidemiological studies [25,113]. From an inferential perspective, if the variable under consideration is a plausible IV, standard errors and statistical power are related to the strength of the association between the IV and treatment choice. If this association is weak, IV analyses can be subject to bias and inflated standard errors [8,68,90]. Recent work, however, has sought to mitigate this problem [13,17,24,94].

IV analyses are particularly useful when the unmeasured confounders are themselves unknown; that is, the factors driving treatment choice are not completely understood. In the somewhat more straightforward setting where the potential confounders are known but not measured, it is sometimes possible to collect additional, detailed information on a subsample of patients to supplement the information known on the larger analysis sample [35,134]. While the subsample can be chosen at random, statistical efficiency/power gains can often be obtained by stratified and/or outcome-dependent sampling [9,10,28,51,154], including in longitudinal settings [126,127]. Recently, a number of calibration-based methods have also been developed in an effort to make as much use of the broad information typically available on the larger patient population, beyond that specifically used to define the sampling frame for the subsample [11,12,81,142,143]. If it is unknown whether or not an important covariate not available in the EHR is truly a confounder, it may be possible to use detailed survey information on a subset of individuals to assess the likelihood of unmeasured confounding [135]. Finally, when the validity of the unmeasured confounding assumption is questionable and alternative methods cannot be used to make inference, researchers can appeal to recently developed study designs that can lessen the impact of unmeasured confounding. New user designs are common in pharmacoepidemiological studies when individuals in prevalent user cohorts are thought to be different from all potential users of the drugs. For example, if substantial side effects are likely to begin soon after drug initiation, individuals who remain on the drug long term may in fact be healthier than all potential takers or resistant to harms [55,114]. Alternatively, instead of narrowing the treatment group definition, a well-chosen comparator group [100] or a restricted study population [111,131,132] can lessen the effects of unmeasured differences between exposure groups. A design-based approach to accounting for unmeasured differences between those who receive a therapy versus those who do not are self-controlled and cross over designs [86,89]. These study designs are most effective when the risk window of interest is short and time-dependent confound is of minimal concern.

Finally, when design and analytic strategies cannot be used to reduce unmeasured confounding to negligible levels, sensitivity analyses can be used to evaluate the impact of violations of the unmeasured confounding assumption on effect estimates and corresponding confidence intervals [129,131]. In particular, sensitivity analyses can bound effect estimates between "worst" and "best" case scenarios [45,85,120], under a specific hypothesized scenario [15,26,80] or over a range of plausible scenarios [91].

14.7 Concluding Remarks

Recent investments in EHR systems have given researchers unprecedented access to rich health-related information, which have the potential to help address many important CER questions that could otherwise not be addressed. Indeed, since EHR systems typically represent real-world contexts, they, arguably, have the greatest potential to provide the most relevant information to inform current questions of comparative effectiveness. Furthermore, ongoing initiatives, such as distributed data health networks [88], have the potential to embed informatics-based CER within healthcare systems providing the opportunity for "learning healthcare systems" to evolve. As researchers plan and conduct EHR-based CER studies, however, the data available and analyses conducted must be carefully scrutinized if conclusions drawn are to be translated into practical guidance for decision-making. While such scrutiny should be applied to any study, observational or randomized, EHR-based studies may require greater scrutiny because of the complex and high-dimensional nature of the data [145]. These attributes, in turn, lead to a number of challenges that CER researchers must consider, including how to extract data from the EHR system, the extent to which EHR data are complete and/or accurate, and the control of confounding bias. Recent developments in the methodology literature have sought to directly address these challenges but, as discussed in this chapter, there are numerous open methodologic questions that remain.

We conclude by noting that while EHR data seems incredible as a potential CER resource, that the data are often so rich may itself be a hindrance in efficient research. In particular, that an EHR has so much information means that researchers may be able to pursue a broader range of scientific questions than would typically be the case. This, in turn, can often lead to a loss of focus with respect to scientific goals and researchers finding themselves in a position where they are performing analyses over and over again. With this mind, we believe that a useful general strategy for EHR-based CER is for researchers to perform a thought experiment prior to any data extraction/analyses in which they consider what the "ideal study" would have looked like had the researchers had the opportunity to design and implement it, akin to the discussion in Chapter 3 [29,55,130]. This thought experiment could proceed in the same way that one typically proceeds when developing a standard study protocol: set out the scientific specific aims and hypotheses, decide upon the population of primary interest, identify relevant covariates (i.e., outcomes, exposures, and adjustment variables), determine their operational definitions, set a measurement schedule (i.e., baseline/study entry and a series of regular follow-up visits), and outline an analytic plan. Collectively, these details provide a foundation for rigorous and reproducible CER in much the same way that a grant proposal does so that EHR-based studies have the best chance of truly informing clinical decision-making in the real world.

References

1. J. Angrist, G. Imbens, and D. Rubin. Identification of causal effects using instrumental variables. *Journal of the American Statistical Association*, 91(434):444–455, 1996.
2. M. Apte, M. Neidell, E. F. Yoko, D. Caplan, S. Glied, and E. Larson. Using electronically available inpatient hospital data for research. *Clinical and Translational Science*, 4(5):338–345, 2011.
3. D. Arterburn, L. Ichikawa, E. Ludman, B. Operskalski, J. Linde, E. Anderson, P. Rohde, R. Jeffery, and G. Simon. Validity of clinical body weight measures as substitutes for missing data in a randomized trial. *Obesity Research & Clinical Practice*, 2(4):277–281, 2008.
4. H. Bang and J. Robins. Doubly robust estimation in missing data and causal inference models. *Biometrics*, 61(4):962–973, 2005.
5. K. Bayley, T. Belnap, L. Savitz, A. Masica, N. Shah, and N. Fleming. Challenges in using electronic health record data for CER: Experience of 4 learning organizations and solutions applied. *Medical Care*, 51(8 Suppl 3):S80–S86, 2013.
6. D. Blumenthal. Stimulating the adoption of health information technology. *New England Journal of Medicine*, 360(15):1477–1479, 2009.

7. D. Boudreau, D. Arterburn, A. Bogart, S. Haneuse, M. Theis, E. Westbrook, and G. Simon. Influence of body mass index on the choice of therapy for depression and follow-up care. *Obesity*, 21(3):E303–E313, 2013.

8. J. Bound, D. Jaeger, and R. Baker. Problems with instrumental variables estimation when the correlation between the instruments and the endogenous explanatory variable is weak. *Journal of the American Statistical Association*, 90(430):443–450, 1995.

9. N. Breslow and N. Chatterjee. Design and analysis of two-phase studies with binary outcome applied to Wilms tumour prognosis. *Journal of the Royal Statistical Society: Series C*, 48(4):457–468, 1999.

10. N. Breslow and R. Holubkov. Weighted likelihood, pseudo-likelihood and maximum likelihood methods for logistic regression analysis of two-stage data. *Statistics in Medicine*, 16(1):103–116, 1997.

11. N. Breslow, T. Lumley, C. Ballantyne, L. Chambless, and M. Kulich. Improved Horvitz–Thompson estimation of model parameters from two-phase stratified samples: Applications in epidemiology. *Statistics in Biosciences*, 1(1):32–49, 2009.

12. N. Breslow, T. Lumley, C. Ballantyne, L. Chambless, and M. Kulich. Using the whole cohort in the analysis of case-cohort data. *American Journal of Epidemiology*, 169(11):1398–1405, 2009.

13. A. Brookhard, J. Rassen, and S. Schneeweiss. Instrumental variable methods in comparative safety and effectiveness research. *Pharmacoepidemiology and Drug Safety*, 19(6):537–554, 2010.

14. A. Brookhart and M. van der Laan. A semiparametric model selection criterion with applications to the marginal structural model. *Computational Statistics & Data Analysis*, 50(2):475–498, 2006.

15. B. A. Brumback, M. A. Hernán, S. J. P. A. Haneuse, and J. M. Robins. Sensitivity analyses for unmeasured confounding assuming a marginal structural model for repeated measures. *Statistics in Medicine*, 23(5):749–767, 2004.

16. J. Buonaccorsi. *Measurement Error: Models, Methods, and Applications*. CRC Press, Boca Raton, 2010.

17. S. Burgess and S. Thompson. Improving bias and coverage in instrumental variable analysis with weak instruments for continuous and binary outcomes. *Statistics in Medicine*, 31(15):1582–1600, 2012.

18. S. Buuren and K. Groothuis-Oudshoorn. MICE: Multivariate imputation by chained equations in R. *Journal of Statistical Software*, 45(3), 2011.

19. Canadian Institute for Health Information. Discharge Abstract Database. http://www.cihi.ca/ (accessed December 2, 2013).

20. J. Carpenter, M. Kenward, and I. White. Sensitivity analysis after multiple imputation under missing at random: A weighting approach. *Statistical Methods in Medical Research*, 16(3):259–275, 2007.

21. R. Carroll, D. Ruppert, L. Stefanski, and C. Crainiceanu. *Measurement Error in Nonlinear Models: A Modern Perspective*. CRC Press, Boca Raton, 2012.

22. Centers for Medicare and Medicaid Services. CMS Fast Facts. http://www.cms.gov/Research-Statistics-Data-and-Systems (accessed December 2, 2013).

23. K. Chan, J. Fowles, and J. Weiner. Review: Electronic health records and the reliability and validity of quality measures: A review of the literature. *Medical Care Research and Review*, 67(5):503–527, 2010.

24. J. Chao and N. Swanson. Consistent estimation with a large number of weak instruments. *Econometrica*, 73(5):1673–1692, 2005.

25. Y. Chen and B. Briesacher. Use of instrumental variable in prescription drug research with observational data: A systematic review. *Journal of Clinical Epidemiology*, 64(6):687–700, 2011.

26. Y. Chiba, T. Sato, and S. Greenland. Bounds on potential risks and causal risk differences under assumptions about confounding parameters. *Statistics in Medicine*, 26(28):5125–5135, 2007.

27. S. Cole, M. Hernán, J. Margolick, M. Cohen, and J. Robins. Marginal structural models for estimating the effect of highly active antiretroviral therapy initiation on CD4 cell count. *American Journal of Epidemiology*, 162(5):471–478, 2005.

28. J.-P. Collet, D. Schaubel, J. Hanley, C. Sharpe, and J.-F. Boivin. Controlling confounding when studying large pharmacoepidemiologic databases: A case study of the two-stage sampling design. *Epidemiology*, 9(3):309–315, 1998.

29. G. Danaei, L. García Rodríguez, O. Fernández Cantero, R. Logan, and M. Hernán. Observational data for comparative effectiveness research: An emulation of randomised trials of statins and primary prevention of coronary heart disease. *Statistical Methods in Medical Research*, 22(1):70–96, 2013.

30. C. Danford, A. M. Navar-Boggan, J. Stafford, C. McCarver, E. Peterson, and T. Wang. The feasibility and accuracy of evaluating lipid management performance metrics using an electronic health record. *American Heart Journal*, 166(4):701–708, 2013.

31. M. Daniels and J. Hogan. *Missing Data in Longitudinal Studies: Strategies for Bayesian Modeling and Sensitivity Analysis*. CRC Press, Boca Raton, 2008.

32. Danish National Patient Registry. http://www.biobankdenmark.dk/ (accessed December 2, 2013).

33. B. Dean, J. Lam, J. Natoli, Q. Butler, D. Aguilar, and R. Nordyke. Review: Use of electronic medical records for health outcomes research a literature review. *Medical Care Research and Review*, 66(6):611–638, 2009.

34. J. Denny. Mining electronic health records in the genomic era. *PLoS Computational Biology*, 8(12):e1002823, 2012.

35. P. Eng, J. Seeger, J. Loughlin, C. Clifford, B. Mentor, and A. Walker. Supplementary data collection with case-cohort analysis to address potential confounding in a cohort study of thromboembolism in oral contraceptive initiators matched on claims-based propensity scores. *Pharmacoepidemiology and Drug Safety*, 17(3):297–305, 2008.

36. M. Faith, M. Butryn, T. Wadden, A. Fabricatore, A. Nguyen, and S. Heymsfield. Evidence for prospective associations among depression and obesity in population-based studies. *Obesity Reviews*, 12(5):e438–e453, 2011.

37. Federal Coordinating Council for Comparative Effectiveness Research. Report to The President and The Congress, 2009. US Department of Health and Human Services.

38. I. Fellegi and A. Sunter. A theory for record linkage. *Journal of the American Statistical Association*, 64(328):1183–1210, 1969.

39. G. Fitzmaurice, N. Laird, and J. Ware. *Applied Longitudinal Analysis*. John Wiley & Sons, Hoboken, NJ, 2012.

40. K. Flegal, M. Carroll, C. Ogden, and L. Curtin. Prevalence and trends in obesity among US adults, 1999–2008. *Journal of the American Medical Association*, 303(3):235–241, 2010.

41. R. L. Fleurence, L. H. Curtis, R. M. Califf, R. Platt, J. V. Selby, and J. S. Brown. Launching PCORnet, A national patient-centered clinical research network. *Journal of the American Medical Informatics Association*, 21:578–582, 2014.

42. W. Fuller. *Measurement Error Models*. John Wiley & Sons, 2006.

43. M. Funk, D. Westreich, C. Wiesen, T. Stürmer, A. Brookhard, and M. Davidian. Doubly robust estimation of causal effects. *American Journal of Epidemiology*, 173(7):761–767, 2011.

44. B. Gallego, A. Dunn, and E. Coiera. Role of electronic health records in comparative effectiveness research. *Journal of Comparative Effectiveness Research*, 2(6):529–532, 2013.

45. P. Gilbert, R. Bosch, and M. Hudgens. Sensitivity analysis for the assessment of causal vaccine effects on viral load in HIV vaccine trials. *Biometrics*, 59(3):531–541, 2003.

46. S. Greenland. Invited commentary: Variable selection versus shrinkage in the control of multiple confounders. *American Journal of Epidemiology*, 167(5):523–529, 2008.

47. S. Greenland, J. Pearl, and J. Robins. Causal diagrams for epidemiologic research. *Epidemiology*, 10(1):37–48, 1999.

48. P. Gustafson. *Measurement Error and Misclassification in Statistics and Epidemiology: Impacts and Bayesian Adjustments*. CRC Press, Boca Raton, 2003.

49. R. Gutman, C. Afendulis, and A. Zaslavsky. A Bayesian procedure for file linking to analyze end-of-life medical costs. *Journal of the American Statistical Association*, 108(501):34–47, 2013.

50. S. Haneuse. Distinguishing selection bias and confounding bias in comparative effectiveness research. *Medical Care*, 54(4):e23–e29, 2016.

51. J. Hanley and N. Denukuri. Efficient sampling approaches to address confounding in database studies. *Statistical Methods in Medical Research*, 18:81–105, 2009.

52. T. Hastie, R. Tibshirani, and J. Friedman. *The Elements of Statistical Learning*, volume 2. Springer, New York, 2009.

53. B. Hazlehurst. *Clinical Effectiveness Research with Natural Language Processing of EMR*. Kaiser Foundation Research Institute (R01 HS19828-01).

54. HealthCore, Inc. HealthCore Integrated Research Database. http://www.healthcore.com/home/research_enviro.php (accessed December 2, 2013).

55. M. Hernán, A. Alonso, R. Logan, F. Grodstein, K. Michels, M. Stampfer, W. Willett, J. Manson, and J. Robins. Observational studies analyzed like randomized experiments: An application to postmenopausal hormone therapy and coronary heart disease. *Epidemiology*, 19(6):766, 2008.

56. M. Hernán, B. Brumback, and J. Robins. Estimating the causal effect of zidovudine on CD4 count with a marginal structural model for repeated measures. *Statistics in Medicine*, 21(12):1689–1709, 2002.

57. M. Hernán, S. Hernandez-Diaz, and J. Robins. A structural approach to selection bias. *Epidemiology*, 15(5):615–625, 2004.

58. M. Hernán and J. Robins. Estimating causal effects from epidemiological data. *Journal of Epidemiology and Community Health*, 60(7):578–586, 2006.

59. M. Hernán and J. Robins. Instruments for causal inference: An epidemiologist's dream? *Epidemiology*, 17(4):360–372, 2006.

60. M. Hernán and J. Robins. *Causal Inference*. CRC Press, Boca Raton, 2010.

61. W. Hersh, M. Weiner, P. Embi, J. Logan, P. Payne, E. Bernstam, H. Lehmann et al. Caveats for the use of operational electronic health record data in comparative effectiveness research. *Medical Care*, 51(8 Suppl 3):S30–S37, 2013.

62. D. Hershman and J. Wright. Comparative effectiveness research in oncology methodology: Observational data. *Journal of Clinical Oncology*, 30(34):4215–4222, 2012.

63. HMO Research Network. HMORN Health Plan Characteristics. http:// www.hmoresearchnetwork.org/en/Tools & Materials/Proposal Writing/ HMORN_Population+Characteristics.doc (accessed December 2, 2013).

64. W. Hogan and M. Wagner. Accuracy of data in computer-based patient records. *Journal of the American Medical Informatics Association*, 4(5):342–355, 1997.

65. E. Holve and N. Calonge. Lessons from the electronic data methods forum: Collaboration at the frontier of comparative effectiveness research, patient-centered outcomes research, and quality improvement. *Medical Care*, 51(8 Suppl 3):S1–S3, 2013.

66. M. Hornbrook, G. Hart, J. Ellis, D. Bachman, G. Ansell, S. Greene, E. Wagner et al. Building a virtual cancer research organization. *JNCI Monographs*, 2005(35):12–25, 2005.

67. Institute of Medicine (IOM). *Initial National Priorities for Comparative Effectiveness Research*, The National Academies Press, Washington, DC, 2009.

68. R. Ionescu-Ittu, J. Delaney, and M. Abrahamowicz. Bias–variance trade-off in pharmacoepidemiological studies using physician-preference-based instrumental variables: A simulation study. *Pharmacoepidemiology and Drug Safety*, 18(7):562–571, 2009.

69. M. Jackson, J. Nelson, and L. Jackson. Why do covariates defined by international classification of Diseases codes fail to remove confounding in pharmacoepidemiologic studies among seniors? *Pharmacoepidemiology and Drug Safety*, 20:858–865, 2011.

70. A. Jha, T. Ferris, K. Donelan, C. DesRoches, A. Shields, S. Rosenbaum, and D. Blumenthal. How common are electronic health records in the United States? A summary of the evidence. *Health Affairs*, 25(6):w496–w507, 2006.

71. M. Johnson, W. Crown, B. Martin, C. Dormuth, and U. Siebert. Good research practices for comparative effectiveness research: Analytic methods to improve causal inference from nonrandomized studies of treatment effects using secondary data sources: The ISPOR good research practices for retrospective database analysis task force report? Part III. *Value in Health*, 12(8):1062–1073, 2009.

72. J. M. Kremer. The CORRONA database. *Autoimmunity Reviews*, 5(1):46–54, 2006.

73. R. Kudyakov, J. Bowen, E. Ewen, S. West, Y. Daoud, N. Fleming, and A. Masica. Electronic health record use to classify patients with newly diagnosed versus preexisting type 2 diabetes: Infrastructure for comparative effectiveness research and population health management. *Population Health Management*, 15(1):3–11, 2012.

74. L. Kupper, J. Karon, D. Kleinbaum, H. Morgenstern, and D. Lewis. Matching in epidemiologic studies: Validity and efficiency considerations. *Biometrics*, 37(2):271–291, 1981.

75. N. Laird and J. Ware. Random-effects models for longitudinal data. *Biometrics*, 38(4):963–974, 1982.

76. M. Larsen and D. Rubin. Iterative automated record linkage using mixture models. *Journal of the American Statistical Association*, 96(453):32–41, 2001.

77. A. Leon. Challenges in designing comparative-effectiveness trials for antidepressants. *Clinical Pharmacology & Therapeutics*, 91(2):165–167, 2012.

78. L. Li, C. Shen, X. Li, and J. Robins. On weighting approaches for missing data. *Statistical Methods in Medical Research*, 22(1):14–30, 2013.

79. X. Li and C. Shen. Linkage of patient records from disparate sources. *Statistical Methods in Medical Research*, 22(1):31–38, 2013.

80. D. Lin, B. Psaty, and R. Kronmal. Assessing the sensitivity of regression results to unmeasured confounders in observational studies. *Biometrics*, 54(3):948–963, 1998.

81. H. W. Lin and Y. H. Chen. Adjustment for missing confounders in studies based on observational databases: 2-stage calibration combining propensity scores from primary and validation data. *American Journal of Epidemiology*, 180(3):308–317, 2014.

82. R. Little and D. Rubin. *Statistical Analysis with Missing Data*. Wiley, Hoboken, NJ, 2002.

83. J. Lunceford and M. Davidian. Stratification and weighting via the propensity score in estimation of causal treatment effects: A comparative study. *Statistics in Medicine*, 23(19):2937–2960, 2004.

84. F. Luppino, L. de Wit, P. Bouvy, T. Stijnen, P. Cuijpers, B. Penninx, and F. Zitman. Overweight, obesity, and depression: A systematic review and meta-analysis of longitudinal studies. *Archives of General Psychiatry*, 67(3):220, 2010.

85. R. MacLehose, S. Kaufman, J. Kaufman, and C. Poole. Bounding causal effects under uncontrolled confounding using counterfactuals. *Epidemiology*, 16(4):548–555, 2005.

86. M. Maclure. The case-crossover design: A method for studying transient effects on the risk of acute events. *American Journal of Epidemiology*, 133(2):144–153, 1991.

87. C. Manning and H. Scheutze. *Foundations of Statistical Natural Language Process*. The MIT Press, 1999.

88. J. Maro, R. Platt, J. Holmes, B. Strom, S. Hennessy, R. Lazarus, and J. Brown. Design of a national distributed health data network. *Annals of Internal Medicine*, 151(5):341–344, 2009.

89. R. Marshall and R. Jackson. Analysis of case-crossover designs. *Statistics in Medicine*, 12(24):2333–2341, 1993.

90. E. Martens, W. Pestman, A. de Boer, S. Belitser, and O. Klungel. Instrumental variables: Application and limitations. *Epidemiology*, 17(3):260–267, 2006.

91. L. McCandless, P. Gustafson, and A. Levy. Bayesian sensitivity analysis for unmeasured confounding in observational studies. *Statistics in Medicine*, 26(11):2331–2347, 2007.

92. C. McCarty, R. Chisholm, C. Chute, I. Kullo, G. Jarvik, E. Larson, R. Li et al. The eMERGE network: A consortium of biorepositories linked to electronic medical records data for conducting genomic studies. *BMC Medical Genomics*, 4(1):13, 2011.

93. D. McGraw, K. Rosati, and B. Evans. A policy framework for public health uses of electronic health data. *Pharmacoepidemiology and Drug Safety*, 21(S1):18–22, 2012.

94. M. Moreira. Tests with correct size when instruments can be arbitrarily weak. *Journal of Econometrics*, 152(2):131–140, 2009.

95. P. Nadkarni, L. Ohno-Machado, and W. Chapman. Natural language processing: An introduction. *Journal of the American Medical Informatics Association*, 18(5):544–551, 2011.

96. National Cancer Institute. Cancer Research Network. http://crn.cancer.gov/ (accessed December 2, 2013).

97. National Cancer Institute. Surveillance, Epidemiology, and End Results Program. http://seer.cancer.gov/ (accessed December 2, 2013).

98. National Center for Research Resources. Widening the Use of Electronic Health Record Data for Research, 2009. http://videocast.nih.gov/summary.asp? (accessed November 27, 2013).

99. National Institute of Diabetes and Digestive and Kidney Diseases. United States Renal Data System. http://www.usrds.org/ (accessed December 2, 2013).

100. J. Nelson, S. Shortreed, O. Yu, D. Peterson, R. Baxter, B. Fireman, N. Lewis et al. on behalf of the Vaccine Safety Datalink project. Integrating database knowledge and epidemiological design to improve the implementation of data mining methods that evaluate vaccine safety in large healthcare databases. *Statistical Analysis and Data Mining: The ASA Data Science Journal* 7(5):337–351, 2014.

101. Norwegian Institute of Public Health. http://www.fhi.no/eway/ (accessed December 2, 2013).

102. C. Onyike, R. Crum, H. Lee, C. Lyketsos, and W. Eaton. Is obesity associated with major depression? Results from the Third National Health and Nutrition Examination Survey. *American Journal of Epidemiology*, 158(12):1139–1147, 2003.

103. J. Overhage and L. Overhage. Sensible use of observational clinical data. *Statistical Methods in Medical Research*, 22(1):7–13, 2013.

104. S. Patten, J. Williams, D. Lavorato, S. Khaled, and A. Bulloch. Weight gain in relation to major depression and antidepressant medication use. *Journal of Affective Disorders*, 134(1):288–293, 2011.

105. R. Paulose-Ram, M. Safran, B. Jonas, Q. Gu, and D. Orwig. Trends in psychotropic medication use among US adults. *Pharmacoepidemiology and Drug Safety*, 16(5):560–570, 2007.

106. J. Pearl. *Causality: Models, Reasoning and Inference*. Cambridge University Press, New York, 2009.

107. M. Pepe. *The Statistical Evaluation of Medical Tests for Classification and Prediction*. Oxford University Press, New York, 2003.

108. R. Platt and R. Carnahan. The US Food and Drug Administration's mini-sentinel program. *Pharmacoepidemiology and Drug Safety*, 21(S1):1–303, 2012.

109. R. Platt, R. Davis, J. Finkelstein, A. Go, J. Gurwitz, D. Roblin, S. Soumerai et al. Multicenter epidemiologic and health services research on therapeutics in the HMO research network center for education and research on therapeutics. *Pharmacoepidemiology and Drug Safety*, 10(5):373–377, 2001.

110. A. Potosky, G. Riley, J. Lubitz, R. Mentnech, and L. Kessler. Potential for cancer related health services research using a linked Medicare-tumor registry database. *Medical Care*, 31(8):749–756, 1993.

111. B. Psaty and D. Siscovick. Minimizing bias due to confounding by indication in comparative effectiveness research: The importance of restriction. *Journal of the American Medical Association*, 304(8):897–898, 2010.

112. M. Raebel, J. Schmittdiel, A. Karter, J. Konieczny, and J. Steiner. Standardizing terminology and definitions of medication adherence and persistence in

research employing electronic databases. *Medical Care*, 51(8 Suppl 3):S11–S21, 2013.

113. J. Rassen, A. Brookhart, R. Glynn, M. Mittleman, and S. Schneeweiss. Instrumental variables II: Instrumental variable application—In 25 variations, the physician prescribing preference generally was strong and reduced covariate imbalance. *Journal of Clinical Epidemiology*, 62(12):1233–1241, 2009.

114. W. Ray. Evaluating medication effects outside of clinical trials: New-user designs. *American Journal of Epidemiology*, 158(9):915–920, 2003.

115. J. Robins. A new approach to causal inference in mortality studies with a sustained exposure period? Application to control of the healthy worker survivor effect. *Mathematical Modelling*, 7(9):1393–1512, 1986.

116. J. Robins. Correcting for non-compliance in randomized trials using structural nested mean models. *Communications in Statistics—Theory and Methods*, 23(8):2379–2412, 1994.

117. J. Robins. Marginal structural models verses structural nested models as tools for causal inference. In M. E. Halloran and D. Berry, editors, *Statistical Models in Epidemiology, the Environment, and Clinical Trials*. Springer, New York, 95–134, 2000.

118. J. Robins, M. Hernán, and B. Brumback. Marginal structural models and causal inference in epidemiology. *Epidemiology*, 11(5):550–560, 2000.

119. J. Robins, A. Rotnitzky, and L. P. Zhao. Estimation of regression coefficients when some regressors are not always observed. *Journal of the American Statistical Association*, 89(427):846–866, 1994.

120. P. Rosenbaum and D. Rubin. The central role of the propensity score in observational studies for causal effects. *Biometrika*, 70(1):41–55, 1983.

121. P. Rosenbaum and D. Rubin. Reducing bias in observational studies using subclassification on the propensity score. *Journal of the American Statistical Association*, 79(387):516–524, 1984.

122. A. Rotnitzky, L. Li, and X. Li. A note on overadjustment in inverse probability weighted estimation. *Biometrika*, 97(4):1–5, 2010.

123. D. Rubin and N. Schenker. Multiple imputation in healthcare databases: An overview and some applications. *Statistics in Medicine*, 10(4):585–598, 1991.

124. D. Rubin and N. Thomas. Matching using estimated propensity scores: Relating theory to practice. *Biometrics*, 52(1):249–264, 1996.

125. K. Saunders, R. David, and A. Stergachis. Group health cooperative. In B. L. Strom, editor, *Pharmacoepidemiology*. John Wiley & Sons, Chichester, UK, 4th edition, 2007.

126. J. Schildcrout and P. Heagerty. Regression analysis of longitudinal binary data with time-dependent environmental covariates: Bias and efficiency. *Biostatistics*, 6(4):633–652, 2005.

127. J. Schildcrout and P. Heagerty. On outcome-dependent sampling designs for longitudinal binary response data with time-varying covariates. *Biostatistics*, 9(4):735–749, 2008.

128. E. Schisterman, S. Cole, and R. Platt. Overadjustment bias and unnecessary adjustment in epidemiologic studies. *Epidemiology*, 20(4):488, 2009.

129. S. Schneeweiss. Sensitivity analysis and external adjustment for unmeasured confounders in epidemiologic database studies of therapeutics. *Pharmacoepidemiology and Drug Safety*, 15(5):291–303, 2006.

130. S. Schneeweiss. Understanding secondary databases: A commentary on "Sources of bias for health state characteristics in secondary databases." *Journal of Clinical Epidemiology*, 60(7):648, 2007.

131. S. Schneeweiss and J. Avorn. A review of uses of health care utilization databases for epidemiologic research on therapeutics. *Journal of Clinical Epidemiology*, 58(4):323–337, 2005.

132. S. Schneeweiss, A. Patrick, T. Stürmer, M. Brookhart, J. Avorn, M. Maclure, K. Rothman, and R. Glynn. Increasing levels of restriction in pharmacoepidemiologic database studies of elderly and comparison with randomized trial results. *Medical Care*, 45(10 Suppl):S131, 2007.

133. S. Schneeweiss, J. Rassen, R. Glynn, J. Avorn, H. Mogun, and A. Brookhard. High-dimensional propensity score adjustment in studies of treatment effects using health care claims data. *Epidemiology*, 20(4):512, 2009.

134. S. Schneeweiss, J. Rassen, R. Glynn, J. Myers, G. Daniel, J. Singer, D. Solomon et al. Supplementing claims data with outpatient laboratory test results to improve confounding adjustment in effectiveness studies of lipid-lowering treatments. *BMC Medical Research Methodology*, 12:180, 2012.

135. S. Schneeweiss, S. Setoguchi, A. Brookhard, L. Kaci, and P. Wang. Assessing residual confounding of the association between antipsychotic medications and risk of death using survey data. *CNS Drugs*, 23(2):171–180, 2009.

136. A. Serretti and L. Mandelli. Antidepressants and body weight: A comprehensive review and meta-analysis. *The Journal of Clinical Psychiatry*, 71(10):1259–1272, 2010.

137. P. Shafipour, J. Der-Sarkissian, F. Hendee, and K. Coleman. What do I do with my morbidly obese patient? A detailed case study of bariatric surgery in Kaiser Permanente Southern California. *The Permanente Journal*, 13(4):56, 2009.

138. M. Stanfill, M. Williams, S. Fenton, R. Jenders, and W. Hersh. A systematic literature review of automated clinical coding and classification systems. *Journal of the American Medical Informatics Association*, 17(6):646–651, 2010.

139. R. Steinbrook. Health care and the American recovery and reinvestment act. *New England Journal of Medicine*, 360(11):1057–1060, 2009.

140. A. Stunkard, M. Faith, and K. Allison. Depression and obesity. *Biological Psychiatry*, 54(3):330–337, 2003.

141. T. Stürmer, M. Joshi, R. Glynn, J. Avorn, K. Rothman, and S. Schneeweiss. A review of the application of propensity score methods yielded increasing use, advantages in specific settings, but not substantially different estimates compared with conventional multivariable methods. *Journal of Clinical Epidemiology*, 59(5):437–447, 2006.

142. T. Stürmer, S. Schneeweiss, J. Avorn, and R. Glynn. Adjusting effect estimates for unmeasured confounding with validation data using propensity score calibration. *American Journal of Epidemiology*, 162(3):279–289, 2005.

143. T. Stürmer, S. Schneeweiss, K. Rothman, J. Avorn, and R. Glynn. Performance of propensity score calibration? A simulation study. *American Journal of Epidemiology*, 165(10):1110–1118, 2007.

144. Swedish Patient Registry. http://www.socialstyrelsen.se/register/halsodata register/patientregistret/inenglish (accessed December 2, 2013).

145. D. Terris, D. Litaker, and S. Koroukian. Health state information derived from secondary databases is affected by multiple sources of bias. *Journal of Clinical Epidemiology*, 60(7):734–741, 2007.

146. K. Thiru, A. Hassey, and F. Sullivan. Systematic review of scope and quality of electronic patient record data in primary care. *British Medical Journal*, 326(7398):1070, 2003.

147. S. Toh, L. García Rodríguez, and M. Hernán. Confounding adjustment via a semi-automated high-dimensional propensity score algorithm: An application to electronic medical records. *Pharmacoepidemiology and Drug Safety*, 20(8):849–857, 2011.

148. Truven Health Analytics. MarketScan Research. http://marketscan.truven-health.com/? (accessed December 2, 2013).

149. A. Tsiatis. *Semiparametric Theory and Missing Data*. Springer, New York, NY, USA, 2006.

150. US Department of Veteran Affairs. VA Information Resource Center. http://www.virec.research.va.gov/ (accessed December 2, 2013).

151. N. Vogelzangs, S. Kritchevsky, A. Beekman, G. Brenes, A. Newman, S. Satterfield, K. Yaffe, T. Harris, and B. Penninx. Obesity and onset of significant depressive symptoms: Results from a community-based cohort of older men and women. *The Journal of Clinical Psychiatry*, 71(4):391, 2010.

152. C. Wang, G. Parmigiani, and F. Dominici. Bayesian effect estimation accounting for adjustment uncertainty. *Biometrics*, 68(3):661–671, 2012.

153. J. Warren, C. Klabunde, D. Schrag, P. Bach, and G. Riley. Overview of the SEER-medicare data: Content, research applications, and generalizability to the United States elderly population. *Medical Care*, 40(8):IV–3, 2002.

154. M. Weaver and H. Zhou. An estimated likelihood method for continuous outcome regression models with outcome-dependent sampling. *Journal of the American Statistical Association*, 100(470):459–469, 2005.

155. M. Weiner and P. Embi. Toward reuse of clinical data for research and quality improvement: The end of the beginning? *Annals of Internal Medicine*, 151(5):359–360, 2009.

156. N. Weiskopf and C. Weng. Methods and dimensions of electronic health record data quality assessment: Enabling reuse for clinical research. *Journal of the American Medical Informatics Association*, 20(1):144–151, 2013.

157. B. Wells, A. Nowacki, K. Chagin, and M. Kattan. Strategies for handling missing data in electronic health record derived data. *eGEMs*, 1(3):7, 2013.

158. I. White, P. Royston, and A. Wood. Multiple imputation using chained equations: Issues and guidance for practice. *Statistics in Medicine*, 30(4):377–399, 2011.

159. H. Xu and B. Craig. A probit latent class model with general correlation structures for evaluating accuracy of diagnostic tests. *Biometrics*, 65(4):1145–1155, 2009.

160. G. Zhao, E. Ford, C. Li, J. Tsai, S. Dhingra, and L. Balluz. Waist circumference, abdominal obesity, and depression among overweight and obese US adults: National health and nutrition examination survey 2005–2006. *BMC Psychiatry*, 11(1):130, 2011.

161. C. Zigler, K. Watts, R. Yeh, Y. Wang, B. Coull, and F. Dominici. Model feedback in Bayesian propensity score estimation. *Biometrics*, 69(1):263–273, 2013.

15

Evaluating Personalized Treatment Regimes

Eric B. Laber and Min Qian

CONTENTS

ABSTRACT   A treatment regime formalizes personalized treatment selection as a function that maps available patient information to a recommended treatment. Treatment regimes, by recommending if, what, when, and to whom treatment should be applied, have the potential for better patient outcomes as well as lower cost and patient burden. Thus, the goals of treatment regimes are closely aligned with those of comparative effectiveness research. However, many of the practical considerations central to comparative effectiveness research such as clinical impact, cost–benefit analyses, and subgroup identification have received little attention in the treatment regime literature. In this chapter, we review regression-based estimators of optimal treatment regimes. We use this class of estimators to illustrate four key challenges associated with evaluating the clinical and practical benefits of personalized treatment regimes; we offer some preliminary solutions and discuss several pressing open problems.

15.1 Introduction

Personalized medicine takes the perspective that the best possible health care requires that treatment be tailored to individual patient characteristics. This perspective is formalized as a *treatment regime* that is a function that maps up-to-date patient information to a recommended treatment. A treatment regime is said to be optimal if it maximizes the mean outcome if applied to the patients in a population of interest. There has been a recent surge of research on estimating an optimal treatment regime using both randomized and observational studies (Henderson et al., 2010; Orellana et al., 2010; Zhao et al., 2011; Goldberg and Kosorok, 2012; Moodie et al., 2012; Zhao et al., 2012; Zhang et al., 2012a,b; Moodie et al., 2013; Laber et al., 2014b; Kang et al., 2014). However, while many of these estimators have been demonstrated to have strong theoretical properties or good empirical performance in simulated studies, little work has been done on integrating these methods into clinical practice or evaluating their clinical impact. We identify and discuss four current challenges associated with evaluating treatment regimes: (i) evaluating the value added by a personalized treatment regime, say over, a one-size-fits all treatment strategy; (ii) identifying patient subgroups with maximal benefit; (iii) accounting for multivariate outcomes, for example, side effects and efficacy; and (iv) quantifying and communicating uncertainty associated with treatment recommendations. While we discuss some potential solutions to these problems, we believe that these challenges remain open and emphasize the need for more communication between quantitative researchers working in comparative effectiveness research (CER) and personalized medicine. These challenges are not exhaustive and are biased toward our own experiences and preferences.

This chapter is written from the perspective of personalized medicine. However, personalized medicine and CER are connected by the common belief that patients are entitled to the best possible clinical care and the common goal of uncovering the best way to provide care to patients. In personalized medicine, it is believed that, because of high patient heterogeneity, the best care requires tailoring treatment to characteristics of each patient. Thus, personalized medicine utilizes patient heterogeneity to improve the health outcomes of an entire population by identifying if, when, what, and to whom treatment should be applied. In contrast, a common goal of CER is to identify the best single treatment for a large heterogeneous population. Hence, both CER and personalized medicine seek to account for patient heterogeneity. Because CER studies involve a heterogeneous patient population, they may also be amenable to estimation of an optimal personalized treatment regime. The methods presented in this chapter might therefore be integrated into a CER study as a secondary analysis. Heterogeneity of treatment effects is discussed in more detail in Chapter 8.

An outline of the remainder of this chapter is as follows. In Section 15.2, we set up notation and review regression-based estimation of an optimal treatment regime. The following four sections introduce and discuss the challenges listed above. We provide a concluding discussion in the final section.

15.2 Regression-Based Estimators

We assume the available data $\{(\mathbf{X}_i, A_i, Y_i)\}_{i=1}^n$ comprise n independent identically distributed trajectories of the form $(\mathbf{X}, A, Y)$, one for each subject, where $\mathbf{X} \in \mathbb{R}^p$ denotes patient characteristics; $A \in \{-1, 1\}$ denotes binary treatment received; and $Y \in \mathbb{R}$ denotes the outcome of interest, coded so that higher values are better. For simplicity, we assume A is randomly assigned with $P(A = 1) = P(A = -1) = 1/2$. In this context, a treatment regime, say π, maps patient characteristics to a recommended treatment, $\pi : \text{dom}\,\mathbf{X} \mapsto \text{dom}\,A$. Under regime π, a patient presenting with $\mathbf{X} = \mathbf{x}$ is recommended treatment $\pi(\mathbf{x})$. The value of a treatment regime π, denoted $V(\pi)$, is the expected outcome if all subjects in the study population were treated according to π. The optimal treatment regime, say π^{opt}, satisfies $V(\pi^{\text{opt}}) \geq V(\pi)$ for all π. Thus, the perspective taken in the estimation of a personalized treatment regime is that to achieve the best mean performance in a population of interest, one must tailor treatment choice to the individual characteristics of each patient. It can be seen that

$$V(\pi) = \mathbb{E}\left[\mathbb{E}\left\{Y|\mathbf{X}, A = \pi(\mathbf{X})\right\}\right] \leq \mathbb{E}\left[\max_a \mathbb{E}\left\{Y|\mathbf{X}, A = a\right\}\right]. \tag{15.1}$$

Define $Q(\mathbf{x}, a) \triangleq \mathbb{E}(Y|\mathbf{X} = \mathbf{x}, A = a)$. The right-hand side of Equation 15.1 does not depend on π and thus it can be seen that $\pi^{\text{opt}}(\mathbf{x}) = \arg\max_a Q(\mathbf{x}, a)$. Regression-based estimators estimate π^{opt} by first modeling the regression of Y on $\mathbf{X}$ and A to obtain an estimator of $Q(\mathbf{x}, a)$, say $\widehat{Q}_n(\mathbf{x}, a)$, and subsequently the estimator $\widehat{\pi}_n(\mathbf{x}) = \arg\max_a \widehat{Q}_n(\mathbf{x}, a)$. Regression-based estimators are appealing due to their simplicity and familiarity to quantitative researchers. Nevertheless, despite this simple framework and a vast literature on these methods (Qian and Murphy, 2011; Lu et al., 2013), evaluating the clinical impact and benefits of such models is challenging and not well developed. Methods and perspectives from CER may prove useful in addressing some of these challenges.

15.3 Challenge 1: Evaluating the Value Added by a Personalized Treatment Regime

Implementation of a treatment regime may involve substantial logistical cost and patient burden, especially if the characteristics in $\mathbf{x}$ are costly or burdensome to collect (Huang et al., 2014). Thus, a natural question is whether a personalized treatment regime offers a *clinically meaningful* benefit compared with simply recommending the same treatment to all patients. Operationally, the benefit of a personalized treatment in terms of the mean outcome is given by

$$\theta^* = \mathbb{E}\max_a Q(\mathbf{X}, a) - \max_a \mathbb{E}Q(\mathbf{X}, a), \tag{15.2}$$

where $\mathbb{E}\max_a Q(\mathbf{X}, a)$ is $V(\pi^{\mathrm{opt}})$ and $\max_a \mathbb{E}Q(\mathbf{X}, a)$ is the best possible expected outcome achievable by assigning all patients the same treatment. If u denotes a clinically meaningful improvement in the expected outcome, then personalizing treatment might be deemed worthwhile if $\theta^* > u$. One approach to testing $\theta^* > u$ at level $\alpha \in (0, 1)$ is to construct a $(1 - \alpha) \times 100\%$ lower confidence interval of the form $[\widehat{\ell}, \infty)$ for θ^*; if $\widehat{\ell} > u$, then a personalized treatment strategy is deemed worthwhile, otherwise it is not. However, constructing a high-quality confidence interval for θ^* is difficult due to the nonsmooth max-operator appearing in Equation 15.2. For example, one can prove that there is no regular or asymptotically unbiased estimator of θ^* (Hirano and Porter, 2012). We illustrate these issues and discuss potential solutions using a linear working model for $Q(\mathbf{x}, a)$.

We consider a working model of the form $Q(\mathbf{x}, a; \beta) = \mathbf{x}_0^{\mathsf{T}}\beta_0 + a\mathbf{x}_1^{\mathsf{T}}\beta_1$, where $\mathbf{x}_0$ and $\mathbf{x}_1$ are known features constructed from $\mathbf{x}$ and $\beta = (\beta_0^{\mathsf{T}}, \beta_1^{\mathsf{T}})^{\mathsf{T}}$. Let $\mathbb{E}_n$ denote the empirical measure so that $\mathbb{E}_n f(Z) = n^{-1}\sum_{i=1}^n f(Z_i)$. Let $\widehat{\beta}_n = \arg\min_\beta \mathbb{E}_n(Y - Q(\mathbf{X}, A; \beta))^2$ be the ordinary least squares estimator of β. An estimator of θ^* is

$$\widehat{\theta}_n = \mathbb{E}_n \max_a Q(\mathbf{X}, a; \widehat{\beta}_n) - \max_a \mathbb{E}_n Q(\mathbf{X}, a; \widehat{\beta}_n) = \mathbb{E}_n |\mathbf{X}_1^{\mathsf{T}}\widehat{\beta}_{n1}| - |\mathbb{E}_n\mathbf{X}_1^{\mathsf{T}}\widehat{\beta}_{n1}|.$$

$$\tag{15.3}$$

If we assume $Q(\mathbf{x}, a) = Q(\mathbf{x}, a; \beta^*)$ for "true" parameter value β^*, then $\sqrt{n}(\widehat{\theta}_n - \theta^*)$ can be seen to equal $\sqrt{n}(\mathbb{E}_n - \mathbb{E})|\mathbf{X}_1^{\mathsf{T}}\beta_1^*| + \sqrt{n}\mathbb{E}_n(|\mathbf{X}_1^{\mathsf{T}}\widehat{\beta}_{n1}| - |\mathbf{X}_1^{\mathsf{T}}\beta_1^*|) - \sqrt{n}(|\mathbb{E}_n\mathbf{X}_1^{\mathsf{T}}\widehat{\beta}_{n1}| - |\mathbb{E}\mathbf{X}_1^{\mathsf{T}}\beta_1^*|)$. Define $S_1 = (\mathbb{E}\mathbf{X}_1\mathbf{X}_1^{\mathsf{T}})^{-1}$ $A\mathbf{X}_1(Y - \mathbf{X}_0^{\mathsf{T}}\beta_0^* - A\mathbf{X}_1^{\mathsf{T}}\beta_1^*)$, $S_2 = \mathbf{X}_1^{\mathsf{T}}\beta_1^*$, and $S_3 = |\mathbf{X}_1^{\mathsf{T}}\beta_1^*|$. And let $(\mathbb{Z}, \mathbb{W}, \mathbb{U})^{\mathsf{T}} \sim N(0, \Sigma)$, where Σ is the variance–covariance matrix of $(S_1, S_2, S_3)^{\mathsf{T}}$. Then it can be shown (e.g., Laber et al., 2014a) that $\sqrt{n}(\widehat{\theta}_n - \theta^*)$ converges in distribution to

$$\mathbb{U} - |\mathbb{Z}^{\mathsf{T}}\mu_X + \mathbb{W}|1_{\mu_X^{\mathsf{T}}\beta^*=0} - (\mathbb{Z}^{\mathsf{T}}\mu_X + \mathbb{W})[1_{\mu_X^{\mathsf{T}}\beta^*>0} - 1_{\mu_X^{\mathsf{T}}\beta^*>0}]$$

$$+ \mathbb{E}|\mathbf{X}_1^{\mathsf{T}}\mathbb{Z}|1_{\mathbf{X}_1^{\mathsf{T}}\beta_1^*=0} + [\mathbb{E}\mathbf{X}_1^{\mathsf{T}}(1_{\mathbf{X}_1^{\mathsf{T}}\beta_1^*>0} - 1_{\mathbf{X}_1^{\mathsf{T}}\beta_1^*<0})]\mathbb{Z}, \tag{15.4}$$

where μ_X denotes $\mathbb{E}\mathbf{X}_1$ and 1_v denotes the indicator function that evaluates to 1 if v is true and 0 otherwise. The distribution given in Equation 15.4 does not change smoothly with the distribution of $\mathbf{X}_1$ and the true value of β_1^*; thus, in finite samples where neither the distribution of $\mathbf{X}_1$ nor the true value of β_1^* is known, approximating the sampling distribution of $\sqrt{n}(\widehat{\theta}_n - \theta^*)$ is difficult. A consequence is that standard methods for constructing confidence intervals, for example, the bootstrap or Taylor series arguments, are invalid without adjustment (Van Der Vaart, 1991; Dümbgen, 1993; Shao, 1994; Laber and Murphy, 2011; Chakraborty et al., 2013).

A number of methods exist for constructing valid confidence intervals for nonsmooth functionals that could potentially be extended to construct a valid confidence interval for θ^*; we discuss two such methods. The first and potentially the simplest is to use subsampling (Politis et al., 1999). A subsampling confidence interval, say $[\widehat{\ell}^{(b)}, \infty)$, is formed by (i) drawing B samples of size $n_b \ll n$ from the original data set without replacement; (ii) applying Equation 15.3 to each subsampled data set to obtain $\widehat{\theta}_{n_b}^{(1)}, \ldots, \widehat{\theta}_{n_b}^{(B)}$; and (iii) setting $\widehat{\ell}^{(b)}$ to the $(1 - \alpha) \times 100\%$ lower percentile of these values. Subsampling is straightforward to implement for a given subsample size n_b and has been shown to be consistent under very general conditions (Politis and Romano, 1994; Politis et al., 1999); however, n_b is a potentially important tuning parameter. Data-driven methods for choosing n_b can be found in Politis et al. (1999) (see also Bickel and Sakov, 2005; Chakraborty et al., 2013); however, how well these methods apply in this context is currently unknown.

An alternative approach that avoids the use of a tuning parameter is to use a projection interval that treats β_1^* and $\mu_X^\mathsf{T} \beta_1^*$ as nuisance parameters (Berger and Boos, 1994). Define $\theta^*(\beta, \nu) = \mathbb{E} \max_a Q(\mathbf{X}, a; \beta) - |\nu|$ and $\widehat{\theta}_n(\beta, \nu) = \mathbb{E}_n Q(\mathbf{X}, a; \beta) - |\nu|$, then $\theta^* = \theta^*(\beta^*, \mu_X^\mathsf{T} \beta^*)$ and for any fixed $\beta \in \mathbb{R}^p$ $\sqrt{n}(\widehat{\theta}_n(\beta, \nu) - \theta^*(\beta, \nu))$ is asymptotically normal with mean zero and variance $\sigma^2(\beta) = \mathbb{E}(|\mathbf{X}^\mathsf{T} \beta| - \mathbb{E}|\mathbf{X}^\mathsf{T} \beta|)^2$. Define $\widehat{\sigma}^2(\beta) = \mathbb{E}_n(|\mathbf{X}^\mathsf{T} \beta| - \mathbb{E}_n|\mathbf{X}^\mathsf{T} \beta|)^2$ and $\widehat{C}_{1-\alpha}(\beta, \nu) = [\widehat{\theta}_n(\beta, \nu) - z_{1-\alpha} \widehat{\sigma}(\beta)/\sqrt{n}, \infty)$, where $z_{1-\alpha}$ is the $(1 - \alpha)$ percentile of a standard normal distribution. Then, for any $\beta \in \mathbb{R}^p$, $\nu \in \mathbb{R}$, and $\eta \in (0, 1)$, $\widehat{C}_{1-\eta}(\beta, \nu)$ is a valid $(1 - \eta) \times 100\%$ confidence interval for $\theta^*(\beta, \nu)$. In particular, $\widehat{C}_{1-\eta}(\beta^*, \mu_X^\mathsf{T} \beta^*)$ is a valid confidence interval for θ^*. Of course, β^* and $\mu_X^\mathsf{T} \beta^*$ are generally unknown in applications; however, $(\widehat{\beta}_n^\mathsf{T}, \mathbb{E}_n \mathbf{X}^\mathsf{T} \widehat{\beta}_n)^\mathsf{T}$ can be shown to be asymptotically normal using the central limit theorem. Thus, for any $\epsilon \in (0, 1)$, one can construct a $(1 - \epsilon) \times 100\%$ level Wald-type joint confidence interval for $(\beta^{*\mathsf{T}}, \mu_X^\mathsf{T} \beta^*)^\mathsf{T}$, say $\widehat{\Gamma}_{1-\epsilon}$. If $\eta + \epsilon = \alpha$, then the $(1 - \alpha) \times 100\%$ projection confidence interval for θ^* is $\widehat{P}_{1-\alpha} = \bigcup_{\beta, \nu \in \widehat{\Gamma}_{1-\epsilon}} \widehat{C}_{1-\eta}(\beta, \nu)$. Because $P(\theta^* \notin \widehat{P}_{1-\alpha}) \le P((\beta^{*\mathsf{T}}, \mu_X^\mathsf{T} \beta^*)^\mathsf{T} \notin \widehat{\Gamma}_{1-\epsilon}) + P(\theta^* \notin \widehat{C}_{1-\eta}(\beta^*, \mu_X^\mathsf{T} \beta^*)) \le \epsilon + \eta + o_P(1)$, and $\epsilon + \eta = \alpha$, it follows that $\widehat{P}_{1-\alpha}$ is a valid confidence set for θ^*. Recommended practice is to set ϵ to be small relative to η, for example, if $\alpha = 0.05$, then one might choose $\epsilon = 0.001$ and $\eta = 0.049$ (Berger and Boos, 1994). The projection interval can be difficult to implement due to the infinite union over points in $\widehat{\Gamma}_{1-\epsilon}$. A standard approach is to draw a large sample of points from $\widehat{\gamma}_{1-\epsilon}$ and take a finite union over these points. A more sophisticated approach might reformulate the union as a constrained minimization problem that minimizes $\widehat{\theta}_n(\beta, \nu) - z_{1-\eta} \widehat{\sigma}(\beta)/\sqrt{n}$ over $(\beta, \nu) \in \widehat{\Gamma}_{1-\epsilon}$; however, this need not be convex and may require specialized optimization algorithms. Another refinement is to reduce conservatism of the projection interval by making it adaptive using a pretest. Variants of this approach can be found in Robins (2004), Laber et al. (2014a), Laber and Murphy (2011), and Huang et al. (2014), though currently the theory for such adaptive methods is less general, that is, it must be established on a case-by-case basis, and more complicated.

15.4 Challenge 2: Identifying Patient Subgroups with Maximal Benefit

In settings where treatments have substantially different costs, levels of patient burden, or availability, a treatment regime can be used to identify patients that are most likely to benefit from a more costly or intensive treatment. For example, in the treatment of chronic depression, two possible treatments are nefazodone and nefazodone supplemented with cognitive behavioral therapy (CBT). Patients receiving CBT must visit the clinic as often as twice per week, incurring significant additional time and monetary burden compared with nefazodone alone (see Huang and Laber, 2014, for additional examples). For clarity, we assume A is binary and takes values in $\{-1, 1\}$, where -1 corresponds to standard care and 1 corresponds to an alternative treatment that is considered to be more burdensome. Thus, the goal is to identify values of $\mathbf{x}$ for which the expected outcome under treatment 1 is sufficiently larger than the expected outcome under -1 so as to justify the cost of treatment.

Let u denote an improvement that would justify the more costly treatment so that $\pi_u^{\mathrm{opt}}(\mathbf{x}) = \mathrm{sgn}\left(Q(\mathbf{x}, 1) - Q(\mathbf{x}, -1) - u\right)$. We assume that $\mathrm{dom}\,\mathbf{X} = \mathbb{R}^p$. For any estimated treatment regime $\widehat{\pi}_n$, we define the familywise error rate of $\widehat{\pi}_n$ as

$$\mathrm{FWER}(\widehat{\pi}_n) = \sup_{\mathbf{x} \in \mathbb{R}^p\,:\,\pi_u^{\mathrm{opt}}(\mathbf{x}) = -1} P\left(\widehat{\pi}_n(\mathbf{x}) = 1\right),$$

so that $\mathrm{FWER}(\widehat{\pi}_n)$ represents the largest probability of incorrectly assigning a patient to the more burdensome treatment. A conservative approach to subgroup identification is to construct an estimator of π_u^{opt} that (at least asymptotically) satisfies the constraint $\mathrm{FWER}(\widehat{\pi}_n) \leq \alpha$ for some $\alpha \in (0, 1)$. One way to do this is to construct a global $(1 - \alpha) \times 100\%$ lower confidence bound for $Q(\mathbf{x}, 1) - Q(\mathbf{x}, -1)$, say $\widehat{\ell}(\mathbf{x})$, and subsequently

$$\widehat{\pi}_n(\mathbf{x}) = \begin{cases} 1 & \widehat{\ell}(\mathbf{x}) \geq u, \\ -1 & \text{otherwise.} \end{cases}$$

Any $\mathbf{x}$ for which $\pi_u^{\text{opt}}(\mathbf{x}) = -1$ satisfies $Q(\mathbf{x}, 1) - Q(\mathbf{x}, -1) - u < 0$. For such an $\mathbf{x}$,

$$
\begin{aligned}
P(\widehat{\pi}_n(\mathbf{x}) = 1) &= P(\widehat{\ell}(\mathbf{x}) \geq u) \\
&= P\left(\widehat{\ell}(\mathbf{x}) + [Q(\mathbf{x}, 1) - Q(\mathbf{x}, -1) - u] \geq Q(\mathbf{x}, 1) - Q(\mathbf{x}, -1)\right) \\
&\leq P\left(\widehat{\ell}(\mathbf{x}) \geq Q(\mathbf{x}, 1) - Q(\mathbf{x}, -1)\right).
\end{aligned}
$$

Thus,

$$
\begin{aligned}
\text{FWER}(\widehat{\pi}_n) &= \sup_{\mathbf{x} \in \mathbb{R}^p : \pi_u^{\text{opt}}(\mathbf{x}) = -1} P\left(\widehat{\ell}(\mathbf{x}) \geq u\right) \\
&\leq \sup_{\mathbf{x} \in \mathbb{R}^p} P\left(\widehat{\ell}(\mathbf{x}) \geq Q(\mathbf{x}, 1) - Q(\mathbf{x}, -1)\right) \leq \alpha.
\end{aligned}
$$

The policy $\widehat{\pi}_n(\mathbf{x})$ identifies a subgroup of patients that may benefit substantially from a more costly treatment. As the problem of constructing global confidence intervals for regression estimators is well studied (e.g., Sun and Loader, 1994; Faraway and Sun, 1995; Claeskens and Keilegom, 2003), constructing $\widehat{\pi}_n$ should be straightforward in many settings. A drawback of the proposed method is a potential lack of power due to the strict error control imposed by constraining $\text{FWER}(\widehat{\pi}_n)$. An alternative is to control the pointwise error rate $\text{PWER}(\widehat{\pi}_n, \mathbf{x}) = P(\widehat{\pi}_n(\mathbf{x}) = 1)$ for all $\mathbf{x}$ satisfying $\pi_u^{\text{opt}}(\mathbf{x}) = -1$. This can be achieved by replacing $\widehat{\ell}(\mathbf{x})$ with a pointwise confidence band.

We have discussed a crude method for identifying a subgroup with maximal benefit under a costly treatment. However, there are a number of ways in which this result might be refined. First, the global confidence band only needs to hold over the region in $\mathbb{R}^p$ for which $\pi_u^{\text{opt}}(\mathbf{x}) = -1$; thus, one could first construct a conservative estimator of this region and restrict the global confidence band to hold in this region. This approach is similar in spirit to the nuisance-parameter confidence interval approach of Berger and Boos (1994) treating the region $\{\mathbf{x} : \pi_u^{\text{opt}}(\mathbf{x}) = -1\}$ as a nuisance parameter. Another refinement would be to introduce a loss function $\mathcal{L}(\mathbf{x}, a)$ quantifying the loss incurred by assigning treatment a to a patient presenting with $\mathbf{X} = x$. Applying a loss-based framework is complicated by the fact most lost functions of interest would depend on the unobserved optimal decision rule π_u^{opt}. For example, one might consider the loss function $\mathcal{L}(\mathbf{x}, a) = 1_{a \neq \pi_u^{\text{opt}}(\mathbf{x})} \left\{ C_1 1_{\pi_u^{\text{opt}}(\mathbf{x}) = 1} + C_2 1_{\pi_u^{\text{opt}}(\mathbf{x}) = -1} \right\}$, for costs $C_1, C_2 > 0$. A Bayesian approach may be appealing in this framework since the posterior loss of $\mathcal{L}(\mathbf{X}, \pi(\mathbf{X}))$ can be computed and optimized over treatment regimes π.

15.5 Challenge 3: Accounting for Multivariate Outcomes

Data-driven optimal treatment regimes are typically formulated as maximizing $V(\pi)$, the expected value of a single scalar outcome. However, this oversimplifies the goal of clinical decision making, which is often to balance several potentially competing outcomes. The canonical example is the balance of side effects and effectiveness where effective treatments carry the most severe side effect burden, though other considerations like cost, patient preference, patient burden, and so on may also be important. One approach to dealing with multiple outcomes is to form a composite outcome that combines all outcomes into a single scalar summary (e.g., Wang et al., 2012). The appropriateness of this approach depends on the homogeneity of patient preferences across the multiple outcomes. In some contexts, for example, the treatment of severe schizophrenia, patients may have heterogeneous outcome preferences but not be able to effectively communicate these preferences (Laber et al., 2014b); hence, a single composite outcome is not adequate and another strategy must be devised. We describe two approaches to dealing with multiple outcomes that do not require the formation of a single composite outcome or the elicitation of patient preferences.

We will assume the same data-generating structure as used previously except that in this section we will assume that the outcome $\mathbf{Y}$ is multivariate taking values in $\mathbb{R}^q$ and that A takes values in $\{0, 1, \ldots, K\}$ for $K \geq 1$. We assume $\mathbf{Y}_j$ is coded so that higher values are better for each $j = 1, \ldots, q$. Let $\Delta \in \mathbb{R}^q$ denote a vector of clinically meaningful differences so that Δ_j denotes a clinically meaningful difference in the jth component of outcome $\mathbf{Y}$. One approach to dealing with multiple outcomes is to use a set-valued treatment regime $\pi_S : \operatorname{dom} \mathbf{X} \to 2^{\operatorname{dom} A} \setminus \emptyset$, where 2^U denotes the set of all subsets of U, so that a patient presenting with $\mathbf{X} = \mathbf{x}$ is offered treatments $\pi_S(\mathbf{x})$ (Laber et al., 2014b). Furthermore, for each $a \in \pi_S(\mathbf{x})$, the decision maker is given an estimate of $Q(\mathbf{x}, a)$. The motivation for a set-valued treatment regime is to let clinical judgment, patient's individual preference, or other exogenous factors dictate the choice from a set of noninferior treatments.

A natural approach to constructing a set-valued treatment regime is to define a partial ordering on treatments for each $\mathbf{X} = \mathbf{x}$ and let $\pi_S(\mathbf{x})$ be all nondominated (i.e., noninferior) treatments with respect to this ordering. In the context of personalized medicine, the following partial ordering is intuitive: write $a_1 \prec_{\mathbf{x}, Q} a_2$ if $Q_j(\mathbf{x}, a_1) \leq Q_j(\mathbf{x}, a_2) + \Delta_j$ for all j and $Q_k(\mathbf{x}, a_1) < Q_k(\mathbf{x}, a_2)$ for some k. Then, the ideal set-valued treatment regime might be defined as $\pi_S^{\text{Ideal}}(\mathbf{x}) = \{a : \nexists a', \ni a \prec_{\mathbf{x}, Q} a'\}$. An estimator of π_S^{Ideal} can be obtained by using regression to form an estimate of $Q(\mathbf{x}, a)$, say $\widehat{Q}_n(\mathbf{x}, a)$, and then using the approximate partial ordering $\prec_{\mathbf{x}, \widehat{Q}_n}$.

The above formulation of a set-valued treatment regime is appealing due to its conceptual and computational simplicity. However, one (perhaps surprising) drawback of this framework is that the partial ordering $\prec_{\mathbf{x},Q}$ is not transitive. That is, it is possible for $a_1 \prec_{\mathbf{x},Q} a_2$, $a_2 \prec_{\mathbf{x},Q} a_3$, yet it is not true that $a_1 \prec_{\mathbf{x},Q} a_3$. For example, suppose $q = 2$, $\Delta = (0.5, 0.5)$, and that we have three treatments a_1, a_2, a_3. If for $\mathbf{X} = \mathbf{x}$, the Q-functions are $Q(\mathbf{x}, a_1) = (0, 3.7)$, $Q(\mathbf{x}, a_2) = (1, 3.2)$, and $Q(\mathbf{x}, a_3) = (3, 3.1)$, then $a_1 \prec_{\mathbf{x},Q} a_2$, $a_2 \prec_{\mathbf{x},Q} a_3$ yet $a_1 \not\prec_{\mathbf{x},Q} a_3$. Note that due to this lack of transitivity, if the only available treatments were $\{a_1, a_3\}$, then the recommended set would be $\{a_1, a_3\}$, but if one considers a_1, a_2, and a_3, then the recommended treatments are $\{a_3\}$. Thus, *adding* a dominated treatment to the set of possible treatments actually decreased the size of the recommended set! Avoiding this kind of paradoxical behavior requires strengthening the definition of $\prec_{\mathbf{x},Q}$; how to do this in a way that satisfactorily incorporates clinically meaningful differences is, to the best of our knowledge, currently unknown.

Another approach to accommodating multiple outcomes is inverse preference elicitation (Lizotte et al., 2010). The goal of inverse preference elicitation is to communicate to the decision maker the set of all composite outcomes for which each treatment is optimal. Define $\mathcal{S}_q = \left\{ \gamma \in \mathbb{R}^q : \gamma_j \geq 0, j = 1, \ldots, q, \sum_{j=1}^{q} \gamma_j = 1 \right\}$. For illustration, we consider composite outcomes of the form $\gamma^\mathsf{T} \mathbf{Y}$, where $\gamma \in \mathcal{S}_q$. In this case, there is a one-to-one correspondence between elements in $\mathcal{S}_q$ and composite outcomes. Then, for any treatment a and $\mathbf{x}$, define

$$\mathrm{Pref}_Q(a, \mathbf{x}) = \left\{ \gamma \in \mathcal{S}_q : \gamma^\mathsf{T} Q(\mathbf{x}, a) = \max_{a'} \gamma^\mathsf{T} Q(\mathbf{x}, a') \right\}$$

to be the set of composite outcomes for which a is optimal for a patient presenting with $\mathbf{X} = \mathbf{x}$. Given an estimator, say $\widehat{Q}_n(\mathbf{x}, a)$, of $Q(\mathbf{x}, a)$, an estimator of $\mathrm{Pref}_Q(\mathbf{x}, a)$ is given by $\mathrm{Pref}_{\widehat{Q}_n}(\mathbf{x}, a)$. If $\mathrm{Pref}_{\widehat{Q}_n}(\mathbf{x}, a)$ is empty, then we say a is dominated and is not optimal under any composite outcome under consideration; if $\mathrm{Pref}_{\widehat{Q}_n}(\mathbf{x}, a) = \mathcal{S}_q$, then we say a dominates all other treatments; otherwise one can plot $\mathrm{Pref}_{\widehat{Q}_n}(\mathbf{x}, a)$ for each a as a decision aid. Consider an example in which there are $q = 2$ outcomes, say effectiveness (Y_1) and side effect burden (Y_2), and three potential treatments. In this setup, large values of γ_1 (hence small values of $\gamma_2 = 1 - \gamma_1$) correspond to utility functions with large weight on effectiveness whereas small values of γ_1 put a large weight

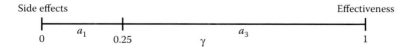

FIGURE 15.1
Schematic for displaying $\mathrm{Pref}_{\widehat{Q}_n}(\mathbf{x}, a)$ for $q = 2$, and three treatments. In this example, we assume the two outcomes are measures of side effect burden and effectiveness, and that $\mathrm{Pref}_{\widehat{Q}_n}(\mathbf{x}, a_1) = [0, 0.25]$, $\mathrm{Pref}_{\widehat{Q}_n}(\mathbf{x}, a_2) = \emptyset$, and $\mathrm{Pref}_{\widehat{Q}_n}(\mathbf{x}, a_3) = [0.25, 1]$.

side effect burden. Figure 15.1 shows a hypothetical display of $\text{Pref}_Q(\mathbf{x}, a)$; in this example, it can be seen that treatment a_2 is dominated; treatment a_1 is consistent with utilities strongly weighting side effects; and treatment a_3 is consistent for all other utilities. In the case of $q = 3$, one can plot $\text{Pref}_{\widehat{Q}_n}(\mathbf{x}, a)$ across values of a as regions inside of a triangle. For example, suppose we are considering three potential medications for the treatment of schizophrenia and that we are interested in two side effect measures, say weight gain (BMI), and lethargy, and a symptom severity measure, say on the positive and negative syndrome scale (PANSS). The left-hand side of Figure 15.2 shows a display of $\text{Pref}_{\widehat{Q}_n}(\mathbf{x}, a)$ when $\widehat{Q}_n(\mathbf{x}, a_1) = (0, 0, 5)$, $\widehat{Q}_n(\mathbf{x}, a_2) = (1, 2, 3)$, and $\widehat{Q}_n(\mathbf{x}, a_3) = (2, 0, 1)$. The figure shows that a_1 consistent with utilities putting large weight on PANSS; a_2 is consistent with utilities emphasizing side effects; and a_3 is consistent only with utilities putting almost all weight on BMI. This plot is created by mapping the three-dimensional probability simplex $\mathcal{S}_3$ onto an equilateral triangle in $\mathbb{R}^2$ with vertices at v_1, v_2, and v_3 via the mapping $\gamma \mapsto \sum_{j=1}^{3} \gamma_j v_j$; the right-hand side of Figure 15.2 shows this triangle. Thus, there is a one-to-one correspondence between points in $\mathcal{S}_3$ and points in the triangle formed by v_1, v_2, and v_3 with the vertex v_j corresponding to utility that places weight solely on the jth outcome. For each point in the triangle, we compute the corresponding utility vector γ and label that point with $\arg\max_a \gamma^{\mathsf{T}} \widehat{Q}_n(\mathbf{x}, a)$.

It is not clear how to extend the above displays to account for $q > 3$, nor is it clear that the above displays are the best possible for $q \leq 3$. Furthermore, the above displays do not convey any of the uncertainty in $\widehat{Q}_n$. Tools to effectively communicate trade-offs among multiple outcomes across potential treatments for each set of patient characteristics are an important tool for closing the gap between statistical methodology for personalized medicine and clinical decision making.

15.6 Challenge 4: Quantifying and Communicating Uncertainty Associated with Treatment Recommendations

A data-driven treatment recommendation $\widehat{\pi}_n(\mathbf{x})$ is a point estimate of $\pi^{\text{opt}}(\mathbf{x})$ and thus fails to communicate two important sources of variation: (E1) variation of $\widehat{\pi}_n(\mathbf{x})$ about $\pi^{\text{opt}}(\mathbf{x})$, and (E2) variation of Y about $Q(\mathbf{x}, a)$ under treatment assignment a. For simplicity, we are assuming that $\widehat{Q}_n(\mathbf{x}, a)$ is a consistent estimator of $Q(\mathbf{x}, a)$ so that there is no approximation error. Quantifying and communicating these two types of uncertainty can serve different purposes. For example, (E1) is useful for clinical or intervention scientists, as well as policy makers to understand the strength of evidence associated with

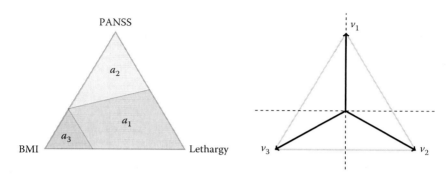

FIGURE 15.2

Left: Plot of $\text{Pref}_{\widehat{Q}_n}(\mathbf{x}, a)$ across values of a for a hypothetical subject with $\widehat{Q}_n(\mathbf{x}, a_1) = (0, 0, 5)$, $\widehat{Q}_n(\mathbf{x}, a_2) = (1, 2, 3)$, and $\widehat{Q}_n(\mathbf{x}, a_3) = (2, 0, 1)$. Right: Vectors forming an equilateral triangle. These vectors are used to map the three-dimensional probability simplex into the triangle via the map $\gamma \mapsto \sum_{j=1}^{3} \gamma_j \nu_j$.

the recommendation $\widehat{\pi}_n(\mathbf{x})$, whereas (E2) is useful for communicating to a patient presenting with $\mathbf{X} = \mathbf{x}$ a plausible range of outcomes they may experience under each treatment recommendation (including $\widehat{\pi}_n(\mathbf{x})$). We present two simple approaches to communicating (E1) and (E2). We regard $\mathbf{X} = \mathbf{x}$ as fixed throughout.

One approach to quantifying (E1) is to construct a confidence interval for $\pi^{\text{opt}}(\mathbf{x})$. As $\widehat{\pi}_n(\mathbf{x}) = \arg\max_a \widehat{Q}_n(\mathbf{x}, a)$ is not a smooth function of the data, it is difficult to directly approximate the sampling distribution of $\widehat{\pi}_n(\mathbf{x})$ (Van Der Vaart, 1991; Laber and Murphy, 2011; Hirano and Porter, 2012). An alternative is to first construct a $(1 - \alpha) \times 100\%$ joint confidence region for the differences $\{Q(\mathbf{x}, a) - Q(\mathbf{x}, a_0) : a \neq a_0\}$ for some baseline treatment a_0, say $\mathcal{C}_{n,1-\alpha}$, and then use a projection confidence interval for $\pi^{\text{opt}}(\mathbf{x})$. Assume the treatments available for a patient presenting with $\mathbf{X} = \mathbf{x}$ are coded to take values in $\{0, 1, \dots, K\}$ with a_0 coded as 0. Define $q_j = Q(\mathbf{x}, j) - Q(\mathbf{x}, 0)$, and write $q = (q_0, q_1, \dots q_K)^{\mathsf{T}}$. Then, $\pi^{\text{opt}}(\mathbf{x}) = \arg\max_j q_j$, and $\bigcup_{r \in \mathcal{C}_{n,1-\alpha}} \arg\max_j r_j$ is a $(1 - \alpha) \times 100\%$ confidence interval for $\pi^{\text{opt}}(\mathbf{x})$ as

$$P\left(\pi^{\text{opt}}(\mathbf{x}) \in \bigcup_{r \in \mathcal{C}_{n,1-\alpha}} \arg\max_j r_j\right) \geq P\left(q \in \mathcal{C}_{n,1-\alpha}\right) \geq 1 - \alpha.$$

Because q is a difference of conditional means, it is a smooth functional of the underlying generative distribution and therefore standard methods can be applied to construct $\mathcal{C}_{n,1-\alpha}$. For example, suppose $Q(\mathbf{x}, a) = \mathbf{x}_0^{\mathsf{T}} \beta_0 + \sum_{j=1}^{K} 1_{a=j} \mathbf{x}_1^{\mathsf{T}} \beta_j$ so that $q = (\mathbf{x}^{\mathsf{T}} \beta_1, \dots, \mathbf{x}^{\mathsf{T}} \beta_K)^{\mathsf{T}}$. Define $\widehat{q}_n =$

$(\mathbf{x}^\mathsf{T}\widehat{\beta}_{n1}, \ldots, \mathbf{x}^\mathsf{T}\widehat{\beta}_{nk})^\mathsf{T}$ where the estimated coefficients are obtained using ordinary least squares. Then, $\sqrt{n}(\widehat{q}_n - q)$ is asymptotically normal and standard methods can be used to construct $\mathcal{C}_{n,1-\alpha}$.

The confidence interval for $\pi^{\mathrm{opt}}(\mathbf{x})$ can be viewed as another type of set-valued dynamic treatment regime. A decision maker can select from among the confidence interval using things like patient individual preference, cost, availability, and clinical judgment as "tie breakers." However, to help the patient understand how the treatments differ, one must address (E2).

One way to do this is to construct prediction intervals for Y for a patient presenting with $\mathbf{X} = \mathbf{x}$ and assigned treatment a across all values of a. The construction of pointwise prediction intervals for regression problems is well studied, so we do not discuss specifics here (e.g., Ruppert et al., 2003; Shafer and Vovk, 2008; Seber and Lee, 2012). The left-hand side of Figure 15.3 shows a simple display of prediction intervals across three treatments. In this hypothetical example, treatment a_3 yields the highest mean outcome but the prediction interval is twice as wide under a_3 as it is under a_1. In this case, a decision maker may choose treatment a_1 over a_3 due to the reduced uncertainty. Displaying prediction intervals can also help to set up realistic expectations for the patient receiving treatment.

Prediction regions can be used to convey information in settings with more than one outcome. The right-hand side of Figure 15.3 shows joint prediction regions for a hypothetical example with two outcomes Y_1 and Y_2 and two treatments a_1 and a_2. From this figure, it can be seen that Y_1 is higher on average and the prediction interval is slightly less variable under a_2 than under a_1. On the other hand, Y_2 is higher on average and the prediction interval is significantly wider under a_1 than under a_2.

We have presented simple displays that might be used to convey uncertainty to decision and policy makers in the context of personalized medicine.

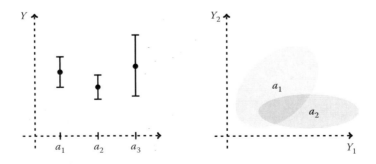

FIGURE 15.3
Left: Prediction intervals for Y given a patient presents with $\mathbf{X} = \mathbf{x}$ and is treated with a_1, a_2, or a_3. Right: Prediction in the $\mathbf{Y} = (Y_1, Y_2)$ plane for a patient presenting with $\mathbf{X} = \mathbf{x}$ and treated according to a_1 or a_2.

We believe that decision aids, such as visual displays, are essential for integrating data-driven treatment regimes into clinical decision making. This seems especially important as statistical methods for estimating treatment regimes grow more complex (Zhao et al., 2011, 2012; Zhang et al., 2012a,b).

15.7 Discussion

Comparative effective research and personalized medicine are closely linked by the common goal of providing patients with the best possible health care. We identified four challenges associated with estimating and evaluating personalized treatment regimes that are particularly relevant for informing clinical and policy decisions. A common theme in these challenges is the communication of statistical evidence and uncertainty. While we discussed first-pass solutions to some of these questions raised, we believe that all of these questions are currently open and best addressed by an interdisciplinary research team, including clinicians, statisticians, policy makers, and other stakeholders.

We focused on regression-based estimators for illustration. There is an emerging interest in policy search or classification-based estimators (Orellana et al., 2010; Zhao et al., 2012; Zhang et al., 2012a,b). These estimators do not rely on high-quality outcome models and are thereby potentially more robust than regression-based estimators. However, the lack of an outcome model can complicate prediction of patient outcomes and the formation of valid confidence intervals. Thus, classification-based methods may introduce additional methodological obstacles to those presented here and may be more difficult to communicate to patients and decision makers than regression-based estimators. Nevertheless, we believe that the challenges presented here must be addressed regardless of the estimation method.

References

Berger, R. L. and Boos, D. D. P values maximized over a confidence set for the nuisance parameter. *Journal of the American Statistical Association*, 89(427): 1012–1016, 1994.

Bickel, P. J. and Sakov, A. On the choice of m in the m out of n bootstrap and its application to confidence bounds for extreme percentiles. *Statistica Sinica*, 18:967–985, 2008.

Chakraborty, B., Laber, E. B., and Zhao, Y. Inference for optimal dynamic treatment regimes using an adaptive m-out-of-n bootstrap scheme. *Biometrics*, 69(3):714–723, 2013.

Claeskens, G. and Keilegom, I. v. Bootstrap confidence bands for regression curves and their derivatives. *The Annals of Statistics*, 31(6):1852–1884, 2003.

Dümbgen, L. On nondifferentiable functions and the bootstrap. *Probability Theory and Related Fields*, 95(1):125–140, 1993.

Faraway, J. J. and Sun, J. Simultaneous confidence bands for linear regression with heteroscedastic errors. *Journal of the American Statistical Association*, 90(431):1094–1098, 1995.

Goldberg, Y. and Kosorok, M. R. Q-learning with censored data. *Annals of Statistics*, 40(1):529, 2012.

Henderson, R., Ansell, P., and Alshibani, D. Regret-regression for optimal dynamic treatment regimes. *Biometrics*, 66(4):1192–1201, 2010.

Hirano, K. and Porter, J. R. Impossibility results for nondifferentiable functionals. *Econometrica*, 80(4):1769–1790, 2012.

Huang, Y. and Laber, E. Personalized evaluation of biomarker value: A cost-benefit perspective. *Statistics in Biosciences*, 8:43–65, 2016.

Huang, Y., Laber, E., and Janes, H. Characterizing expected benefits of biomarkers. *Biostatistics*, 2014, doi: 10.1093/biostatistics/kxu039.

Kang, C., Janes, H., and Huang, Y. Combining biomarkers to optimize patient treatment recommendations. *Biometrics*, 70(3):695–707, 2014.

Laber, E.B., Lizotte, D.J., Qian, M., Pelham, W.E., and Murphy, S.A. Dynamic treatment regimes: Technical challenges and applications. *Electronic Journal of Statistics*, 8(1):1225–1272, 2014a.

Laber, E. B., Lizotte, D. J., and Ferguson, B., Set-valued dynamic treatment regimes for competing outcomes. *Biometrics*, 70(1), 53–61, 2014b.

Laber, E. B. and Murphy, S. A. Adaptive confidence intervals for the test error in classification. *Journal of the American Statistical Association*, 106(495):904–913, 2011.

Lizotte, D. J., Bowling, M. H., and Murphy, S. A. Efficient reinforcement learning with multiple reward functions for randomized controlled trial analysis. In *Proceedings of the 27th International Conference on Machine Learning (ICML-10)*, Haifa, 695–702, 2010.

Lu, W., Zhang, H. H., and Zeng, D. Variable selection for optimal treatment decision. *Statistical Methods in Medical Research*, 22:493–504, 2013.

Moodie, E. E., Chakraborty, B., and Kramer, M. S. Q-learning for estimating optimal dynamic treatment rules from observational data, *Canadian Journal of Statistics*, 40(4):629–645, 2012.

Moodie, E. E., Dean, N., and Sun, Y. R. Q-learning: Flexible learning about useful utilities. *Statistics in Biosciences*, 6(2):1–21, 2013.

Orellana, L., Rotnitzky, A., and Robins, J. M. Dynamic regime marginal structural mean models for estimation of optimal dynamic treatment regimes, part I: main content. *The International Journal of Biostatistics*, 6(2):1–49, 2010.

Politis, D., Romano, J., and Wolf, M. Subsampling. Springer, New York, 1999.

Politis, D. N. and Romano, J. P. Large sample confidence regions based on subsamples under minimal assumptions. *The Annals of Statistics*, 22(4):2031–2050, 1994.

Qian, M. and Murphy, S. A. Performance guarantees for individualized treatment rules. *Annals of Statistics*, 39(2):1180, 2011.

Robins, J. M. Optimal structural nested models for optimal sequential decisions. In *Proceedings of the Second Seattle Symposium in Biostatistics*, 189–326, Springer, New York, 2004.

Ruppert, D., Wand, M. P., and Carroll, R. J. *Semiparametric Regression*, volume 12, Cambridge University Press, New York, 2003.

Seber, G. A. and Lee, A. J. *Linear Regression Analysis*, volume 936, John Wiley & Sons, Hoboken, 2012.

Shafer, G. and Vovk, V. A tutorial on conformal prediction. *The Journal of Machine Learning Research*, 9:371–421, 2008.

Shao, J. Bootstrap sample size in nonregular cases. *Proceedings of the American Mathematical Society*, 122(4):1251–1262, 1994.

Sun, J. and Loader, C. R. Simultaneous confidence bands for linear regression and smoothing. *The Annals of Statistics*, 22(3):1328–1345, 1994.

Van Der Vaart, A. On differentiable functionals. *The Annals of Statistics*, 19(1):178–204, 1991.

Wang, L., Rotnitzky, A., Lin, X., Millikan, R. E., and Thall, P. F. Evaluation of viable dynamic treatment regimes in a sequentially randomized trial of advanced prostate cancer. *Journal of the American Statistical Association*, 107(498):493–508, 2012.

Zhang, B., Tsiatis, A. A., Davidian, M., Zhang, M., and Laber, E. Estimating optimal treatment regimes from a classification perspective. *Stat*, 1(1):103–114, 2012a.

Zhang, B., Tsiatis, A. A., Laber, E. B., and Davidian, M. A robust method for estimating optimal treatment regimes. *Biometrics*, 68(4):1010–1018, 2012b.

Zhao, Y., Zeng, D., Rush, A. J., and Kosorok, M. R. Estimating individualized treatment rules using outcome weighted learning. *Journal of the American Statistical Association*, 107(499):1106–1118, 2012.

Zhao, Y., Zeng, D., Socinski, M. A., and Kosorok, M. R. Reinforcement learning strategies for clinical trials in nonsmall cell lung cancer. *Biometrics*, 67(4):1422–1433, 2011.

16

Early Detection of Diseases

Sandra Lee and Marvin Zelen

CONTENTS

ABSTRACT In this chapter, we present an overview of comparative effectiveness research in the area of early detection of diseases. The screening of asymptomatic individuals for chronic disease is a public health initiative that is rapidly growing. This is especially true in cancer where there are expanding early detection programs in breast, cervical, colorectal, lung, prostate and stomach cancers. The basic idea motivating the screening of asymptomatic populations is that diagnosing the disease early before it becomes symptomatic may result in better prognosis. Mathematical and simulation models are available to evaluate early detection programs. Model-based comparative effectiveness research provides insights into expected outcomes, positive and negative, from early detection programs. An exemplar mathematical model was introduced and an outcome-generating process was described.

Examples of comparative effectiveness research conducted by the Cancer Intervention and Surveillance Modeling Network (CISNET) working groups are presented.

16.1 Introduction

Comparative effectiveness research (CER) is the field of research designed to compare the effectiveness of two or more approaches to health care evaluating their benefits and harms. In 2009, the Institution of Medicine defined CER as the generation and synthesis of evidence that compares benefits and harms of alternative methods to prevent, diagnose, and monitor a clinical condition or to improve the delivery of care. The purpose of CER is to assist consumers, clinicians, purchasers, and policy makers to make informed decisions that will improve health care at both the individual and population levels.

Before this national initiative on CER was formally introduced, model-based research in comparing the benefits and harms of screening strategies targeted at the early detection of chronic diseases had been actively pursued. The mathematical models that describe the disease progression and early detection process can be used to characterize early detection programs. Chapter 9 discusses the hierarchy of evidence in the context of CER in general. Many investigators may believe that a randomized early detection trial is the "gold standard" for generating scientific evidence of the advantage of an intervention on a patient population. However, as also noted in Chapter 17, it is difficult to conduct such randomized screening trials and often is not feasible. Similar issues are discussed in the context of treatment studies in Chapter 3 and in the context of mathematical modeling in Chapter 13. Conducting CER in the early detection of disease using models allows a comparison of two or more screening strategies and could provide guidance on selecting the most effective screening program from individual or population perspectives.

In this chapter, we introduce CER in the early detection of diseases, especially in cancer. The chapter is organized as follows. Section 16.1.1 provides the rationale for the early detection of diseases and potential implications in public health. Section 16.1.2 describes randomized screening trials and practical issues in conducting these trials. Section 16.1.3 introduces a concept of using mathematical models in CER of the early detection of diseases. Section 16.2 provides an overview of mathematical models for the early detection of diseases: Section 16.2.1 introduces mathematical models in the early detection of diseases, Section 16.2.2 uses an exemplar model to describe the model elements and mortality modeling process; Section 16.2.3 describes an event of overdiagnosis and its definition. Section 16.3 provides various examples of CER in the early detection of cancer from the Cancer Intervention and Surveillance Modeling Network (CISNET) Working Groups. The CISNET has been conducting the model-based CER of cancer control interventions since 2000 and made significant contributions in addressing important public health questions. Section 16.4 concludes the chapter with general remarks.

16.1.1 Background: Early Detection of Diseases

During the last several decades, there has been a growth in programs aimed at diagnosing chronic diseases before they appear as clinical disease. This is especially true in cancer where there are expanding early detection programs in breast, cervical, ovarian, colorectal, lung, prostate, and stomach cancers. Individuals are also being screened for HIV-related diseases as AIDS has many of the manifestations of a chronic disease. The Center for Disease Control (CDC) in the United States has recommended that HIV testing should be a routine part of medical care for people in the 13–64 year age group (CDC 2006). Other examples include hypertension, coronary artery disease, and osteoporosis.

A screening program for a particular chronic disease usually consists of administering a special screening test to a population of individuals who have no symptoms of the disease. The rationale is that if the disease is diagnosed earlier, compared to usual care, then the benefit from therapy may be enhanced. This can potentially lead to a higher cure rate or reduce mortality. In order to consider an effective early detection program, it is essential to have a highly sensitive and specific screening test and beneficial therapy, which can be applied at an earlier stage.

16.1.2 Randomized Screening Trials for Early Detection of Diseases

Randomized clinical trials form part of the foundation of the practice of modern "evidence-based" medicine. They often serve as the main means of synthesizing scientific evidence of the benefit for a new intervention. In this section, we present the difficulty of conducting a randomized early detection trial to evaluate effective screening interventions.

In an early detection trial, one can only evaluate the potential benefit from individuals who will eventually be diagnosed with a disease. As a result, many more individuals must be entered on early detection trials as the incidence of many chronic diseases is relatively low. This can be contrasted to a therapeutic trial where all individuals provide evidence for treatment comparisons. For example, the incidence of female breast cancer is approximately 100–400 per 100,000 women per year depending on age. Consequently, most of the individuals on early detection trials do not ever get the disease and do not contribute information on the benefit of early detection.

Mortality benefit is often the primary end point in the early detection trial and this requires that the individuals enrolled in an early detection trial be followed for many years in order to monitor their outcomes. During this time, there are many opportunities for individuals to violate the rules of the study. For example, some individuals in the control group may receive early detection tests as part of their usual medical care. Others in the early detection group may not cooperate if it is necessary to have periodic exams over a period of time; that is, they will not show up for scheduled exams. The longer the follow-up period, the more opportunities for noncompliance with the clinical trial. An example of noncompliance occurs in prostate cancer screening trials, based on a biomarker, prostate-specific antigen (PSA). Individuals assigned to a control group may have a routine digital rectal exam as part of an annual physical or even have a PSA measurement when a blood sample is routinely drawn. Hence, it is possible for prostate cancer diagnoses to be made for men in the control group, who have no signs/symptoms of prostate cancer. These noncompliance incidents will dilute the scientific comparisons of benefit. If the average compliance is 80%, the efficiency of the trial is 64%. This means that if one has 100 individuals in a trial and the average compliance is 80%, it is equivalent to having 64 individuals in the trial having 100% compliance (cf. Lachin and Foulkes 1986).

Another issue that serves to dilute the outcomes of early detection trials arises when the individuals in a trial are relatively old and possibly may die of other causes. The most notable of these is prostate cancer, which has the bulk of the incidence with older men. A man may be diagnosed early by an early detection exam, but may die of other causes (e.g., cardiovascular disease) before the disease would ever present with clinical symptoms. Consequently, we do not know if there is overdiagnosis or that the earlier diagnosis of the specific chronic disease would have resulted in a cure or longer survival as the natural history of the disease has been interrupted by a death due to other causes.

Lastly, there are ethical considerations. For example, there had been nine randomized screening trials to evaluate the benefit of mammography in the past (cf. Shapiro et al. 1982, 1988; Tabar et al. 1985; Frisell et al. 1986; Andersson et al. 1988; Roberts et al. 1990; Miller et al. 1992a,b; Tabar et al. 1992; Bjurstam et al. 1997; Moss et al. 2006). These early trials have led to the belief that earlier diagnosis by mammography is associated with lower mortality, but debates over the benefits and harms of mammography continue. It would not be feasible to initiate a new trial as very few women are likely to give their consent to enter such a trial. Even if some of the ethical concerns and recruitment can be solved, the trials would require a relatively long time to reach fruition due to the principal end point being mortality. During this period, the technology for the early detection of disease may advance, making the old early detection tests outmoded.

In general, conducting randomized early detection trials is challenging (Hu and Zelen 1997, 2002, 2004). It requires a larger number of trial participants and longer follow-up time, thus a larger budget. These execution aspects of early detection trials make it more difficult to assess the benefits of early detection by conducting randomized trials.

16.1.3 Role of Mathematical Models

A successful intervention in early detection is likely to be adopted to a public health program. There are a number of key factors to consider in planning a public health program for the early detection of diseases. For example, issues such as (i) target population for screening, (ii) initial age to begin screening, (iii) intervals between consecutive exams if there will be more than one exam, and (iv) total number of exams to be administered need to be taken into considerations. For the reasons stated in Section 16.1.2, it is not feasible to evaluate these issues (such as annual vs. biennial mammography, starting at age 45 vs. 50, stop screening at age 74 vs. no upper age limit, etc.) by conducting screening trials. There are too many combinations of issues and it is not simply realistic to evaluate them all by conducting screening trials. One reasonable approach is to develop mathematical models that describe the early detection of the disease process and evaluate the benefits and harms of various early detection scenarios using the models. Mathematical models may play a significant role in this setting. Henceforth, we will focus on CER in the early detection of cancer based on the mathematical models.

16.2 Model-Based Approaches in Comparative Effectiveness Research

16.2.1 Models for Early Detection of Diseases

Many models have been developed to evaluate the early detection process. One general model describing the early disease process, which is in wide use, is that put forth by Zelen and Feinleib (1969). Other models include the work by Albert et al. (1978), Baker and Chu (1990), Chen et al. (1996, 1997), Day and Walter (1984), Duffy et al. (1995), Dubin (1981), Eddy (1980, 1983), Eddy and Shwartz (1982), Kirch and Klein (1974), Lee and Zelen (1998, 2008), Lincoln and Weiss (1964), Parmigiani (1993, 1997), Prorok (1976a,b), Shwartz (1978), Shwartz and Plough (1984), and Zelen (1993). These models are purely analytical. Some analytical models have simulation components. Such simulation models include the work developed by Knox (1973), Habbema et al. (1985), Berry et al. (2006), Fryback et al. (2006), Hanin et al. (2006), Mandelblatt et al. (2006), and Prevritis et al. (2006).

The basic goal of using models is to make predictions on how outcomes change with changing inputs. This feature enables generating outcomes under various screening scenarios. The input information may be (i) different populations characterized by age, (ii) different exam schedules, (iii) screen tool parameters such as sensitivity and specificity of the screening test, (iv) disease stage, (v) disease sojourn time in various disease stages, and (vi) efficacy of treatment. There are two classes of outcomes generated by models. The first class of outcomes captures the benefits of early detection. The mortality, mortality reduction attributed to the screening process, deaths averted, and years of life saved are the common measures of the benefit. The other class of outcomes captures the harms of early detection. The commonly used items in this category include false-positive findings and overdiagnosis. Overdiagnosis of disease may occur when a screening examination detects a disease early (relative to usual care) in the preclinical state, but the disease would have never exhibited clinical symptoms in a person's remaining lifetime. Thus, finding these cases early through screening does not yield any benefit, but could be potentially harmful since these cases could be overtreated.

All models have assumptions and require input parameters. The chapter on mathematical modeling (Chapter 13) provides a general discussion of these challenges. In the context of screening, input parameters such as the sensitivity, specificity, disease sojourn time, and the distribution of disease stages by the mode of detection (screen-detected, clinically detected, diagnosed between two screening examinations, etc.) are essential in mathematical models. Such model parameters need to be estimated from real data sources. This aspect of estimating the model parameters accurately could be challenging as the real data sources are limited. In general, the National Cancer Institute-sponsored registry studies, such as Breast Cancer Surveillance Consortium (BCSC, http://breastscreening.cancer.gov) and Population-based Research Optimizing Screening through Personalized Regimens (PROSPR, http://appliedresearch.cancer.gov/prospr) are valuable data sources. Surveillance, Epidemiology and End Results (SEER, http://seer.cancer.gov) is another great source for cancer statistics in the U.S. population. Data from randomized screening trials or registration studies are also used.

16.2.2 Exemplar Model

In this section, we describe a mathematical model developed by Lee and Zelen as an example. The model assumptions, model component, and the process of generating mortality outcome are illustrated. The Lee–Zelen model (Lee and Zelen 1998, 2006, 2008) is a stochastic model that depicts the early detection process of screening. The model has been developed for screening of chronic diseases. It has mainly been applied to the early detection of breast cancer (Berry et al. 2005; Lee and Zelen 2006; Mandelblatt et al. 2009; van Ravensteyn et al. 2012; Stout et al. 2014), but is a general model that can be applied to other disease sites as long as the model assumptions are satisfied.

16.2.2.1 Overview of Model: Natural History of Disease

One approach of developing mathematical models for the early detection of disease is using the natural history of disease. The natural history of disease model assumes that there are several health states. The health states are designated by S_0, S_p, S_c, and S_d. S_0 refers to an individual being disease free or if he/she has the disease, there are no signs/symptoms and the disease cannot be diagnosed by any known test; S_p (preclinical state) refers to an individual having disease, but there are no symptoms; however, the disease may be diagnosed by screening tests; S_c (clinical state) refers to the disease having clinical signs/symptoms leading to diagnosis by usual medical care; S_d (disease-specific death state). The aim of an early detection program is to diagnose disease while it is in the preclinical state (S_p).

There are several disease natural histories that can be described by these four states. A progressive disease is characterized by an individual moving from S_0 to S_p to S_c as time progresses and some will continue to S_d and eventually die of the disease. This model is assumed to characterize breast cancer. A modification of the progressive disease model is that not all individuals progress to clinical disease, but stay in S_0 indefinitely. This model may describe prostate cancer and allows for overdiagnosis, that is, it is not known if a person diagnosed in S_p would eventually enter eS_c. Another natural history model may permit a transition from S_p to S_0 reflecting the possibility that host defensive mechanisms may result in a cure. This natural history is designated as a nonprogressive disease natural history.

Whatever natural history model is adopted, it must allow for the length-biased sampling, transition probabilities of entering the preclinical and clinical states, sojourn time in the preclinical state, exam sensitivity, the role of treatment in extending survival, and how prognosis depends on the disease stage at the time of diagnosis. Furthermore, all of these features may be age and stage related. Available data may be used to estimate these aspects of the model and provide for inputs to the model.

16.2.2.2 Mortality Modeling with No Screening

The major components of the model to estimate mortality are as follows. First assume there is no screening and the output is generated for a specific birth cohort or multiple birth cohorts. Define (i) v = year of birth cohort; (ii) τ = age at disease incidence; (iii) T = age at death; (iv) $S_v(t)$ = probability distribution of normal population surviving up to age t; (v) $I_v(\tau)$ = age-specific disease incidence; and (vi) $g(t|\tau)$ = probability density function (pdf) of disease-specific survival for subject incident at age τ. The probability density function (pdf) $g(t|\tau)$ is a mixture of distributions weighted by the probability of being diagnosed in a particular stage. Specifically, $g(t|\tau) = \sum_{i=1}^{k} \theta_i g_i(t|\tau)$, where θ_i is the probability of being diagnosed in stage i ($i = 1, 2, \ldots, k$) and $g_i(t|\tau)$ is the survival distribution pdf for stage i for a subject incident at age τ.

Note that "stage" can be represented by any set of prognostic factors, such as SEER historic stage, AJCC (American Joint Committee on Cancer) stage, categorized values of tumor thickness or size, etc. Define the probability of disease-specific death at age T for birth cohort v as

$$\mathbf{d_v(T)} = \int\limits_{T}^{T+1} \left\{ \int\limits_{0}^{y} S_v(\tau) I_v(\tau) g(y - \tau | \tau) d\tau \right\} dy. \tag{16.1}$$

The sequence of events in the inner integral is (i) normal population surviving to age τ, (ii) conditional on being alive at age τ, to become incident with disease in the age interval $(\tau, \tau + d\tau)$, and (iii) dying in the interval $(y - \tau, y - \tau + dy)$. The outer integral restricts the survival function $g(y)$ to the age interval $(T, T + 1)$.

16.2.2.3 Mortality Modeling with Screening

Subjects undergoing screening require a more complex model, distinguishing between cases diagnosed at a screening examination (screen-detected cases) and those diagnosed at other than a screening exam (interval cases).

Figure 16.1 displays the process of case finding with screening. Suppose a subject from cohort year v follows n screening exams at ages $t_0 < t_2 < \cdots < t_{n-1}$. Let t be the age of detection. Interval cases get diagnosed in between exams (t_i, t_{i+1}) for $i = 0, \ldots, n - 2$ or after the last exam at t_{n-1}. The probability of disease-specific death at age T for birth cohort v who has a screening history H (i.e., exams at $t_0, t_1, \ldots, t_{n-1}$) has a more complicated expression

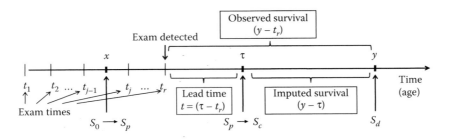

FIGURE 16.1
Early detection of the disease process. This figure describes the dynamics of case finding in early detection programs. The lead time is denoted by $t = (\tau - t_r)$, where τ is not observed among screen-detected cases. It is important to adjust for the lead time when the mortality benefit from screening program is assessed. Health states are defined as S_0 (disease-free state), S_p (preclinical state, early stage of disease with no symptoms), S_c (clinical state with symptomatic disease), and S_d (death due to disease).

that can be written as

$$d_v(T|H) = \int\limits_{T}^{T+1} \left\{ \int\limits_{0}^{y} D_v(t|H) + I_v(t|H)dt \right\} dy, \qquad (16.2)$$

where $D_v(t|H)$ is the probability of disease-specific death for screen-detected cases with a screening history H and $I_v(t|H)$ is the probability of disease-specific death for interval cases with a screening history of H. These probabilities are a function of many parameters involved in the case finding process and have complicated expressions (cf. Lee and Zelen 2006, 2008). They include transition probabilities from S_0 to S_p, sojourn time distribution in S_p, and the sensitivity of the screening test. Since $I_v(\tau)$ in Equation 16.1 is not observed in the screen-detected or interval-detected cases, this has to be estimated by a function of $w(x)q(t - x)$, where x is the time entering S_p and $w(x)dx$ denotes the transition probability $(S_0 \rightarrow S_p)$ in the age interval $(x, x + dx)$, and $q(t)$ is the pdf of the sojourn time distribution in S_p.

The stage shift for screen-detected cases is represented by the new values of θ_i^* and better prognostic stages are expected for screen-detected cases. Note that the lead time $(\tau - t)$, which is defined to be the difference between the age transitioning into the clinical state and the age of earlier diagnosis, is a random variable, which is not observed. For screen-detected cases, the lead time is adjusted by using the imputed survival $(y - \tau)$ as shown in Figure 16.1 when computing the mortality for screen-detected cases. The proportional mortality reduction (MR%) from screening (compared to no screening) for a specified age interval (AI) then can be estimated using the Equations 16.1 and 16.2, that is,

$$\text{MR\%} = \frac{\sum_{T=AI}\{d_v(T)S_v^*(T) - d_v(T|H)S_v^{**}(T)\}}{\sum_{T=AI} d_v(T)S_v^*(T)} \times 100, \qquad (16.3)$$

where $S_v^*(T)$ is the probability of being free of breast cancer and surviving up to age T without screening and $S_v^{**}(T)$ with screening. Note that AI can be any age intervals, such as [40, 74] or entire lifetime [0, 100]. MR% enables us to quantify the benefits associated with a screening strategy and compare various screening strategies.

16.2.3 Overdiagnosis

Overdiagnosis of disease may occur when a screening examination detects a disease early (relative to usual care) in the preclinical state, but the disease would have never exhibited clinical symptoms in a person's remaining lifetime. Figure 16.2 depicts an event of overdiagnosis. Davidov and Zelen (2004) have formulated this problem and have made calculations for prostate cancer. In most diseases with a progressive nature, the event of overdiagnosis can

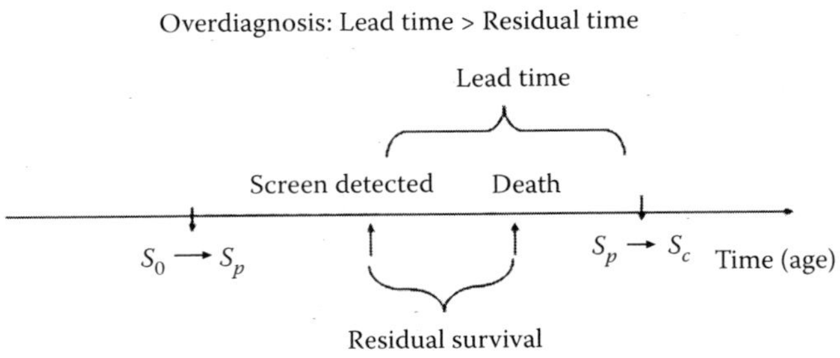

Overdiagnosis: Lead time > Residual time

FIGURE 16.2
Overdiagnosis. Overdiagnosis refers to the situation that the lead time generated by an early detection of disease is being longer than the remaining lifetime (i.e., residual survival time). This implies that one would not have diagnosed with disease under usual care in one's lifetime. Health states are defined as S_0 (disease-free state), S_p (preclinical state, early stage of disease with no symptoms), and S_c (clinical state with symptomatic disease).

be defined as the lead time being greater than a person's remaining lifetime, given the age of early diagnosis. Overdiagnosis is an important parameter as it measures potential harms of early detection programs. However, it is not straightforward to quantify overdiagnosis as the lead time is not directly observable. Many authors have derived the theoretical lead time distribution and their derivations can be adopted to quantify overdiagnosis (cf. Prorok 1982; Kafadar and Prorok 2003; Wu et al. 2007).

16.3 Examples of CER in Early Detection of Cancer

The CISNET was founded in 2000 by the National Institute of Health/ National Cancer Institute (cf. http://cisnet.cancer.gov). The main purpose was to improve our understanding of the impact of cancer control interventions on population trends in cancer incidence and mortality using modeling. There are a number of independent models to conduct CER of the cancer control interventions in the area of breast, colon, prostate, lung, and esophagus cancers. The work conducted by the CISNET constitutes great examples of model-based CER in the early detection of cancer. One noteworthy accomplishment of the CISNET was providing the model-generated outcome of various screening strategies to the U.S. Preventive Services Task Force. The U.S. Preventive Services Task Force is a panel of experts in prevention and evidence-based medicine. They make recommendations about the clinical preventive services including screening. The model-based data from the CISNET was utilized in evaluating the benefits and harms of screening strategies by the U.S. Preventive Services Task Force. This section summarizes various modeling works of CER in the early detection of cancer by the CISNET.

16.3.1 CER in Mammography Screening

Although the benefits of mammography screening are well established through the randomized screening trials, at least for women 50–65 years of age, there are many controversial topics that are being debated continuously. The most common topics of debate are how to choose an efficient screening program balancing the benefits and harms, whether to screen women under age 50 years or not and the degree of overdiagnosis from mammography screening. CER of mammography screening generates potential outcomes (including mortality reduction, overdiagnosis) under various screening scenarios. This allows a comparison of different screening scenarios with respect to the benefits and harms.

The CISNET Breast Working Group consists of multiple independent modeling groups—each with a unique model for breast cancer progression and early detection process. Model description details are provided on the CIS-NET website and in the JNCI Monographs, the impact of mammography and adjuvant therapy on U.S. breast cancer mortality (1975–2000): collective results from the CISNET (JNCI Monographs 2006).

One fundamental issue evaluated by the CISNET Breast Working Group was assessing the relative and absolute contributions of screening mammography and adjuvant treatment to the reduction in breast cancer mortality in the United States from 1975 to 2000 (Berry et al. 2005). The breast cancer mortality rate for women 30–79 years of age in 1997 was 48.3 per 100,000. This rate remained unchanged until 1990 and then started to decrease over time. By 2000, the breast cancer mortality rate was 38.0 per 100,000 (24% decrease from 1990). Mammography and adjuvant treatments became available in the United States since 1980. This led to a question of the relative and absolute contributions of screening mammography versus adjuvant treatment. Common input sources were prepared for the models, including the mammography and adjuvant treatment dissemination in the United States (Cronin et al. 2006; Mariotto et al. 2006; JNCI Monographs 2006) and each model projected the mortality reduction explained by screening mammography versus adjuvant treatment.

The results from the modeling groups led to a conclusion that both screening mammography and treatment played a role in reducing the death from breast cancer in the United States. The relative contribution from screening varied from 28% to 65%, with a median of 46%. The rest was attributed to the adjuvant treatment. This was a huge undertaking from a perspective of preparing common input data (JNCI Monographs 2006) and addressing a complex public health question through the collaborative modeling approach from seven modeling groups.

Another notable contribution from the modeling effort was collaborations with organizations involved in making public health recommendations about the screening policies. The CISNET Breast Working Group evaluated the effect of mammography screening under different screening schedules and quantified the potential benefits and harms of mammography (Mandelblatt et al. 2009). Using a contemporary population cohort, 20 different screening strategies with varying initiation and stopping ages and two different screening intervals (annual vs. biennial) were evaluated and compared. For each screening scenario, number of mammograms conducted, reduction of breast cancer mortality or life-years gained (vs. no screening), false-positive mammograms, unnecessary biopsies, and overdiagnosis from screening were estimated. Screening programs with starting ages of 40, 45, 50, 55, 60 and stopping ages of 69, 74, 79, 84 were considered. Each screening scenario consisted of different combinations of starting and stopping mammography ages and screening interval.

Efficiency frontier plots, which evaluate the mortality reduction as a function of total mammograms conducted in 1,000 women under different screening scenarios and allow a ranking of the efficiency of the screening strategies, were generated. Six CISNET models produced consistent rankings of screening strategies. Biennial screening was efficient in maintaining 81% of the benefit from annual screening (model results varied from 67% to 99%) with almost half the number of false-positive results. Biennial screening program screening of women 50–69 years achieved a median of 16.5% breast cancer mortality reduction (range 15%–23%) compared to no screening. There was a small gain by starting screening at 40 versus 50, with an additional mortality reduction of 3% (range 1%–6%). Biennial screening after age 69 resulted in additional mortality reduction, but overdiagnosis was substantially increased at older ages. These modeling results were independently reviewed by the U.S. Preventive Services Task Force in updating their screening mammography guidelines (U.S. Preventive Services Task Force 2009).

The last example of the modeling work is addressing mammography screening in women in their forties. Women in their forties have the smallest benefit from screening, yet have the largest degree of harms. For example, to save one life, 1,900 women in their forties need to be screened over 10 years in comparison to 1,300 women in their fifties (Nelson et al. 2009). False-positive rates are higher in women in their forties. Following the U.S. Preventive Services Task Force recommendation in 2009 (biennial screening for 50–74 years of age), one consideration for women in their forties is only to screen if they are at a higher risk of developing breast cancer. This rationale led to the work in tipping the balance of benefits and harms to favor screening mammography starting at age 40 years (van Ravensteyn et al. 2012). Four of the CISNET breast modeling groups jointly worked on this problem. The main goal was to determine the threshold relative risk at which the harm–benefit ratio of screening women in 40–49 years of age is equivalent to the harm–benefit ratio of screening women in 50–74 years of age. The harm–benefit ratio was defined as the ratio of false-positive findings/life-years gained and false-positive rates/deaths averted. The comparator group of 50–74 biennial screening was chosen as this was the U.S. Preventive Services Task Force recommendation (2009) for average-risk U.S. women. The modeling result suggested that if women in their forties have a twofold increased risk, then it is expected their harm–benefit ratio from biennial mammography screening is the same as women following biennial mammography screening during 50–74 years of age. This implies that if women in their forties desire to have a balanced screening program and expect to have the same harm–benefit ratio as women in their fifties, they could start screening in their forties only if they are at least twice as likely to develop breast cancer.

16.3.2 CER in Early Detection of Other Cancer

The CISNET has other disease sites including colorectal, esophagus, lung, and prostate cancers. The highlights of their CER are summarized in this section.

The CISNET Colon Working Group has three independent modeling groups where models incorporate the adenoma–carcinoma sequence and potential multiplicity of polyps. They have been focusing on investigating the potential benefits and costs of different screening modalities and regimens of screening. The impact of risk factor modification and treatment advances on population incidence and mortality trend is another area of research. The CISNET Colon Working Group has collaborated with the U.S. Preventive Services Task Force to evaluate test strategies for colorectal cancer screening (Zauber et al. 2008). The main goal was to assess life-years gained and colonoscopy requirements for colorectal cancer screening strategies and identify a set of recommendable screening strategies. Both colonoscopy and noncolonoscopy tests (fecal occult blood tests [FOBT], flexible sigmoidoscopy) were considered with various starting and stopping ages and screening intervals. The modeling results support colorectal cancer screening with colonoscopy every 10 years plus annual screening with a sensitive FOBT or flexible sigmoidoscopy every 5 years plus a midinterval sensitive FOBT from age 50 to 75 years.

The CISNET Lung Working Group consists of five independent modeling groups. The main interests of the CISNET Lung Working Group include tobacco control policies, screening, and genetic susceptibility. Recently, they evaluated the tobacco control and reduction in smoking-related premature deaths in the United States between 1964 and 2012 (Holford et al. 2014). January 2014 was the 50th anniversary of the first surgeon general's report on smoking and health. The models evaluated the reduction in smoking-related mortality associated with implementation of tobacco control since 1964. Their work indicates that tobacco control is estimated to be associated with avoidance of 8 million premature deaths and extended life span of 19–20 years. This marks an important public health achievement, but tobacco control effort must continue.

Another important contribution of this group is their collaboration with the U.S. Preventive Services Task Force on optimum screening policy for lung cancer. The National Lung Screening Trial (NLST) demonstrated that three annual computed tomography (CT) screening examinations reduced lung cancer mortality by 20% relative to three annual chest radiography screening examination in current and former smokers (Aberle et al. 2011). However, this study did not directly evaluate the effects of additional rounds of screening, long-term benefits and harms, or multiple alternative screening policies with different screening intervals. These questions were addressed by CER. The modeling work concluded that annual CT screening for lung cancer has a favorable benefit–harm ratio for individuals from 55 to 80 years of age with 30 or more pack-years' exposure of smoking.

The CISNET Prostate Working Group has three independent modeling teams. The group has been focusing on evaluating the natural history of prostate cancer and its potential implications for the efficacy of the PSA screening test, screening policy, overdiagnosis, novel prostate cancer biomarkers, patterns and outcomes of prostate cancer care, and health disparities in prostate screening and treatment. The survival benefit from PSA screening for prostate cancer has been controversial. Two ongoing studies of PSA screening, the European Randomized Study of Screening for Prostate Cancer (ERSPC), and the U.S.-based Prostate, Lung, Colorectal, and Ovarian (PLCO) cancer screening trial reported conflicting conclusions. ERSPC (Schroder et al. 2009) reported a mortality rate ratio of 0.80 after a median of 9-year follow-up, whereas PLCO (Andriole et al. 2012) reported the corresponding ratios of 1.15 after 10 year and 1.09 after 13-year follow-ups. These conflicting results have been evaluated by the CISNET Prostate Working Group. By conducting modeling work, the Prostate Working Group identified that contamination in the PLCO control group substantially limited the PLCO to identify a clinically significant screening benefit (Gulati et al. 2012).

Another important area of debate in prostate cancer screening is overdiagnosis. That is, screening finding cases that would have never been diagnosed in the remaining lifetimes of the patients. In 2011, the U.S. Preventive Services Task Force recommendation highlights the potential harms associated with PSA screening. The main harms under discussion included potential overdiagnosis and treatment of overdiagnosed cancers. The CISNET Prostate Working Group conducted a modeling work to evaluate the level of overdiagnosis from PSA screening based on age, Gleason score, and PSA at diagnosis. They concluded that the level of overdiagnosis varies widely (2.9%–88%) depending on age, Gleason score, and PSA at diagnosis (Gulati et al. 2014).

16.4 General Remarks

Although proponents of evidence-based modern medicine may insist on randomized screening trials to demonstrate the benefit of early detection, such trials are very costly and are fraught with many issues that tend to dilute the outcomes. Furthermore, many trials may not be feasible due to ethical concerns. Early detection trials are much more difficult to plan, carry out, and analyze than therapeutic trials. Furthermore, even if there is general scientific agreement on benefit, transferring the benefit to a larger population through a public health program may be very costly and require decisions on eligible individuals and exam schedules. Empirical data may not be available to decide on "optimal schedules."

There are thousands of therapeutic trials being carried out today, but only a handful of early detection clinical trials in existence. What can be done? Model-based CER of screening strategies provides an attractive solution. Models can be built based on existing data and further utilized to answer many questions that cannot be obtained from any real screening studies. Modeling approaches taken in CER of early detection strategies, however, face challenges. Models should be built so that they reflect the disease progression, early detection process, and benefits and harms associated with early detection accurately. It is important to validate model assumptions and model results against the real data. For example, Lee and Zelen (2003) used their model to project the results published from the breast cancer screening trials and validated their model assumptions. Another challenging aspect of using models is the limitation of available data to estimate model parameters accurately. The model input parameters themselves are often estimates with their uncertainties. These uncertainties are reflected in the model outputs (such as mortality, overdiagnosis, false positivity). Consequently, the model predictions have to be judged on the limitation of the inputs and how the outputs would change with modifications of the inputs.

Despite the challenges, model-based CER of the early detection of cancer has been useful in evaluating the benefits and harms of various screening programs and made significant contributions in addressing important public health questions.

References

Aberle DR et al. National Lung Screening Trial Research Team. Reduced lung-cancer mortality with low-dose computed tomographic screening. *N Engl J Med* 2011;365(5):395–409.

Albert A, Gertman PM, Lois T, Liu S. Screening for the early detection of cancer II. The impact of screening in the natural history of the disease. *Math Biosci* 1978;40:61–109.

Andersson I et al. Mammographic screening and mortality from breast cancer: The Malmo, mammographic screening trial. *BMJ* 1988;30:943–8.

Andriole GL et al. Prostate cancer screening in the randomized prostate, lung, colorectal, and ovarian cancer screening trial: Mortality results after 13 years of follow-up. *J Natl Cancer Inst* 2012;104:1–8.

Baker SG, Chu KC. Evaluating screening for the early detection and treatment of cancer without using a randomized control group. *J Am Stat Assoc* 1990;85:321–27.

Berry DA, Cronin KA, Plevritis SK, Fryback DG, Clarke L, Zelen M, Mandelblatt JS, Yakovlev AY, Habbema DF, Feuer EJ (CISNET Collaborators: Gelman R; Lee SJ). Effect of screening and adjuvant therapy on mortality from breast cancer. *N Engl J Med* 2005;353:1784–92.

Berry DA, Inoue L, Shen Y, Venier J, Cohen D, Bondy M, Theriault R, Munsell MF. Modeling the impact of treatment and screening on U.S. breast cancer mortality: Bayesian approach. *J Natl Cancer Inst Monogr* 2006;(36):30–6.

Bjurstam N et al. The Gothenburg breast screening trial: First results on mortality, incidence, and mode of detection for women ages 39–49 years at randomization. *Cancer* 1997;80:2091–9.

CDC. Revised Recommendations for HIV Testing of Adults, Adolescents and Pregnant Women in Health Care, MMWR 2006, 55, RR14; 1–17.

Chen HH, Duffy DW, Tabar L. A Markov chain method to estimate the tumor progression rate from preclinical to clinical phase, sensitivity and positive predictive value for mammography in breast cancer screening. *Statistician* 1996;45:307–17.

Chen HH, Duffy DW, Tabar L, Day NE. Markov chain models for progression of breast cancer—Part I: Tumor attributes and the preclinical screen-detectable phase. *J Epidemiol Biostat* 1997;2:(1):9–23.

Cronin KA, Mariotto AB, Clarke LD, Feuer EJ. Additional common inputs for analyzing impact of adjuvant therapy and mammography on U.S. mortality. *J Natl Cancer Inst Monogr* 2006;(36):26–9.

Davidov O, Zelen M. Overdiagnosis in early detection programs. *Biostatistics* 2004; 5:603–13.

Day NE, Walter SD. Simplified models of screening of chronic disease: Estimation procedures from mass screening programs. *Biometrics* 1984;40:1–13.

Duffy SW, Chen HH, Tabar L, Day NE. Estimation of mean sojourn time in breast cancer screening using a Markov chain model of both entry to and exit from the preclinical detectable phase. *Stat Med* 1995;14:1531–43.

Dubin N. Predicting the benefit of screening for disease. *J Appl Probab* 1981;18:348–60.

Eddy DM. *Screening for Cancer: Theory, Analysis and Design*. 1980. Englewood Cliffs, NJ: Prentice-Hall.

Eddy DM. A mathematical model for timing repeated medical tests. *Med Decis Making* 1983;3:34–62.

Eddy DM, Shwartz M. Mathematical models in screening. In: Schottenfeld D, Fraumeni J eds. *Cancer Epidemiology and Prevention*. 1982. Philadelphia: W.B. Saunders, 1075–90.

Frisell J et al. Randomized mammographic screening for breast cancer in Stockholm. *Breast Cancer Res Treat* 1986;8:45–54.

Fryback DG, Stout NK, Rosenberg MA, Trentham-Dietz A, Kuruchittham V, Remington PL. The Wisconsin breast cancer epidemiology simulation model. *J Natl Cancer Inst Monogr* 2006;(36):37–47.

Gulati R, Inoue LY, Gore JL, Katcher J, Etzioni R. Individualized estimates of overdiagnosis in screen-detected prostate cancer. Individualized estimates of overdiagnosis in screen-detected prostate cancer. *J Natl Cancer Inst* 2014;106(2):1–5.

Gulati R, Tsodikov A, Wever EM, Mariotto AB, Heijnsdijk EA, Katcher J, de Koning HJ, Etzioni R. The impact of PLCO control arm contamination on perceived PSA screening efficacy. *Cancer Causes Control* 2012;23(6): 827–35.

Habbema JDF, Van Oortmarssen GJ, Lubbe JTN, van derMass PJ. The MISCAN simulation program for the evaluation of screening for disease. *Comput Programs Biomed* 1985;20:79–83.

Hanin LG, Miller A, Zorin V, Yakovlev Y. The University of Rochester model of breast cancer detection and survival. *J Natl Cancer Inst Monogr* 2006;(36):66–78.

Holford TR, Meza R, Warner KE, Meernik C, Jeon, J, Moolgavkar SH, Levy DT. *JAMA* 2014;311(2):164–71.

Hu P, Zelen M. Planning clinical trials to evaluate early detection programs. *Biometrika* 1997;84(4):817–29.

Hu P, Zelen M. Experimental design issues for the early detection of disease: Novel designs. *Biostatistics* 2002;3(3):299–313.

Hu P, Zelen M. Planning of randomized dearly detection trials. *Stat Methods Med Res* 2004;13(6):491–506.

Kafadar K, Prorok PC. Alternative definitions of comparable case groups and estimates of lead time and benefit time in randomized cancer screening trials. *Stat Med* 2003;22:83–111.

Kirch RLA, Klein M. Examination schedules for breast cancer. *Cancer* 1974;33;1444–50.

Knox EG. A simulation system for screening procedures. In: McLachlan G ed. *The Future and Present Indicatives, Problems and Progress in Medical Care, Ninth Series*, Nuffield Provincial Hospitals Trust. 1973. London: Oxford University Press, 17–55.

Lachin JM, Foulkes MA. Evaluation of sample size and power for analyses of survival with allowance for nonuniform patient entry, losses to follow-up, noncompliance, and stratification. *Biometrics* 1986;42(3):507–19.

Lee SJ, Zelen M. Scheduling periodic examinations for the early detection of disease: Applications to breast cancer. *J Am Stat Assoc* 1998;93:1271–81.

Lee SJ, Zelen M. Modeling the early detection of breast cancer. *Ann Oncol* 2003;14:1199–202.

Lee SJ, Zelen M. A stochastic model for predicting the mortality of breast cancer. *J Natl Cancer Inst Monogr* 2006;(36):79–85.

Lee SJ, Zelen M. Mortality modeling of early detection program. *Biometrics* 2008;64(2):386–95.

Lincoln TL, Weiss GH. A statistical evaluation of recurrent medical examinations. *Oper Res* 1964;12:187–205.

Mandelblatt JS et al. Effects of mammography screening under different screening schedules: Model estimates of potential benefits and harms. *Ann Intern Med* 2009;151(10):738–48.

Mandelblatt JS, Schechter CB, Lawrence W, Yi B, Cullen J. The SPECTRUM population model of the impact of screening and treatment on U.S. breast cancer trends from 1975 to 2000: Principles and practice of the model methods. *J Natl Cancer Inst Monogr* 2006;(36):47–55.

Mariotto AB, Feuer EJ, Harlan LC, Abrams J. Dissemination of adjuvant multiagent chemotherapy and tamoxifen for breast cancer in the United States using estrogen receptor information: 1975–1999. *J Natl Cancer Inst Monogr* 2006;(36):7–15.

Miller AB, Baines CJ, To T, Wall C. Canadian National Breast Screening Study: 1. Breast cancer detection and death rates among women aged 40–49 years. *Can Med Assoc J* 1992a;147(10):1459–76.

Miller AB, Baines CJ, To T, Wall C. Canadian National Breast Screening Study: 2. Breast cancer detection and death rates among women aged 50–59 years. *Can Med Assoc J* 1992b;147(10):1477–88.

Moss SM, Cuckle H, Johns L, Waller M, Bobrow L and Trial Management Group. Effects of mammographic screening from age 40 years on breast cancer mortality at 10 years follow-up: A randomized controlled trial. *Lancet* 2006;368:2053–60.

Nelson HD, Tyne K, Naik A, Bougatsos C, Chan BK, Humphrey L. Screening for breast cancer: An update for the U.S. Preventive Services Task Force. *Ann Intern Med* 2009;151(10):727–37.

Parmigiani G. On optimal screening ages. *J Am Stat Assoc* 1993;88:622–8.

Parmigiani G. Timing medical examinations via intensity functions. *Biometrika* 1997;84:803–16.

Prevritis SK, Sigal M, Salzman P, Rosenberg J, Glynn P. A stochastic simulation model of U.S. breast cancer mortality trends from 1975 to 2000. *J Natl Cancer Inst Monogr* 2006;(36):86–95.

Prorok PC. The theory of periodic screening I. Lead time and proportion detected. *Adv Appl Probab* 1976a;8:127–43.

Prorok PC. The theory of periodic screening II. Doubly bounded recurrence times and mean lead time and detection probability estimation. *Adv Appl Probab* 1976b;8:460–76.

Prorok PC. Bounded recurrence times and lead time in the design of a repetitive screening program. *J Appl Probab* 1982;19:83–111.

Roberts MM et al. Edinburgh trial of screening for breast cancer: Mortality at seven years. *Lancet* 1990;335:241–6.

Schroder FH et al. Screening and prostate-cancer mortality in a randomized European study. *N Engl J Med* 2009;360(13):1320–8.

Shwartz M. An analysis of the benefits of serial screening for breast cancer based upon a mathematical model of the disease. *Cancer* 1978;41:1550–64.

Shwartz M, Plough AL. Models in planning cancer programs. In Cornell RG ed. *Statistical Methods for Cancer Studies*. 1984. New York: Marcel Dekker, pp. 329–416.

Shapiro S et al. *Periodic Screening for Breast Cancer: The Health Insurance Plan Project and Its Sequelae, 1963–1986*. 1988. Baltimore, MD: The Johns Hopkins University Press.

Shapiro S, Venet W, Strax PH, Venet L, Rosener R. Ten to fourteen year effect of screening on breast cancer mortality. *J Natl Cancer Inst* 1982;69:349–55.

Stout NK et al. Benefits, harms, and costs for breast cancer screening after U.S. implementation of digital mammography. *J Natl Cancer Inst* 2014 May 28;106(6). Doi:10.1093/jnci/dju092.

Tabar L et al. Reduction in mortality from breast cancer after mass screening with mammography. *Lancet* 1985;1:829–32.

Tabar L et al. Update of the Swedish two-county program of mammographic screening for breast cancer. *Radiol Clin North Am* 1992;30:187–210.

U.S. Preventive Services Task Force. Screening for breast cancer: U.S. Preventive Services Task Force recommendation statement. *Ann Intern Med* 2009;151(10):716–26.

van Ravensteyn NT et al. Tipping the balance of benefits and harms to favor screening mammography starting at age 40 years: A comparative modeling study of risk. *Ann Intern Med* 2012;156(9):609–17.

Wu D, Rosner GL, Broemeling L. Bayesian inference for the lead time in periodic cancer screening. *Biometrics* 2007;63:873–80.

Zauber AG, Lansdorp-Vogelaar I, Knudsen AB, Wilschut J, van Ballegooijen M, Kuntz KM. Evaluating test strategies for colorectal cancer screening: A decision analysis for the U.S. Preventive Services Task Force. *Ann Intern Med* 2008;149(9):659–69.

Zelen M. Optimal scheduling of examinations for the early detection of disease. *Biometrika* 1993;80:279–93.

Zelen M, Feinleib M. On the theory of screening for chronic diseases. *Biometrika* 1969;56:601–14.

17

Evaluating Tests for Diagnosis and Prediction

Constantine Gatsonis

CONTENTS

ABSTRACT   The evaluation of a diagnostic test addresses three major questions: (a) how accurate is the test in diagnosis and/or prediction?; (b) what is the effect of the test on subsequent healthcare decisions and choices?; and (c) what is the effect of the test on patient outcomes? Among these three questions, the assessment of accuracy has received the most extensive attention in the literature. However, comparative effectiveness research calls for the comparison of the impact of different diagnostic tests on subsequent care and patient outcomes. This is a challenging task because the main function of tests is to provide information, which is subsequently incorporated into further diagnostic and therapeutic decision making. Thus, the impact of tests on patient outcomes is mediated by the intervening decisions about medical care. In this chapter, we discuss the methodologic challenges in the evaluation of the downstream consequences of tests, emphasizing the potential role of studies with observational data and simulation modeling.

17.1 Introduction: Diagnosis versus Therapy

The effectiveness of test modalities for diagnosis and prediction is a broadly shared concern in health care, at a time when the utilization of tests is growing and their role is becoming even more central than before with the advent of precision medicine. The discussion and surrounding controversies have gone on for decades (Fryback and Thornbury 1991; Gatsonis 2000). In recent years, the discussion has addressed the potential overutilization of tests (Hendee et al. 2010), the need to assess and quantify the value of tests to patients (Carlos et al. 2012; Shyu et al. 2014; Durand et al. 2015), the need for comparative effectiveness research (CER) of diagnostic tests (Gatsonis 2010; Gazelle et al. 2011), and the emerging reduction in the use of some of the more expensive tests (Sharpe et al. 2013). A recent effort by the Centers for Medicare and Medicaid Services to reign in on spending for diagnostic laboratory tests has created a wave of reaction and calls for CMS to cover new tests, while possibly requiring the collection of data on their use through national registries (CMS 2015, Cancer Letter Oct 2, 2015; Goozner 2015).

The particularity of the role of tests for diagnosis and prediction in health care leads to a cascade of questions that need to be answered in order to understand the impact of tests:

a. How accurate is a test in its diagnostic or predictive task?

b. Does the information obtained from a test influence subsequent diagnostic workups and therapeutic interventions?

c. Can the use of a test be linked to patient-level outcomes, such as those assessed in studies of therapy?

These questions can be asked about individual tests and, more importantly for CER, about alternative tests that can be used in a specific context. Although much of diagnostic test evaluation has been concerned with diagnostic or predictive accuracy, it is fair to say that the main interest in CER is on the impact of tests on subsequent care and patient outcomes. Thus, this chapter will mainly be concerned about methods for addressing comparative questions in these two areas.

The CER paradigm has been largely developed on the basis of experience from the assessment of therapeutic interventions. This can be seen in the material of Chapters 1 through 15 of this book. However, tests have a different role in medical care, especially in their relation to patient outcomes. The primary role of tests is to provide *information* for use in deciding subsequent care (Figure 17.1). However, the precise way to use this information is often not specified.

When examining the impact of tests on outcomes, it is important to note that the short- and long-term effects of tests materialize in the context

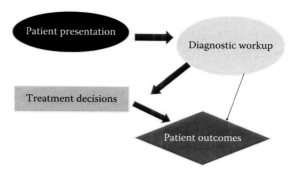

FIGURE 17.1
The role of testing in the process of health care.

of the available healthcare options, such as further tests and therapeutic interventions. Fundamentally then, it is not possible to define and measure test effects outside the particular healthcare context in which the test will be used. For example, the utility of the information of a test that has perfect accuracy in diagnosing a particular kind of cancer may be nil in the absence of any effective therapy for this cancer. The information from the same testing modality may have considerably more utility in a different cancer setting for which effective therapy options are available.

Situations in which diagnosis is ahead of therapy present a difficult challenge for the evaluation of tests. Current examples include imaging tests for diagnosing breast ductal carcinoma *in situ* and imaging tests for detecting amyloid plaques in the brain of individuals with cognitive decline. The presence of such plaques is a strong predictor of the eventual onset of Alzheimer's dementia, a disease for which therapies are not currently available.

In this chapter, we survey and comment on methodologic approaches to CER for diagnosis and prediction. The list includes several of the options discussed in other chapters of this book, notably randomized studies, registries, and observational studies using large administrative databases such as electronic health records (EHRs), Medicare claims data, and health insurance claims. We also comment briefly on the potential for modeling to span the gap between diagnosis and patient-level outcomes.

17.2 Randomized Studies of Tests

Randomized trials to evaluate tests in terms of their impact on subsequent care and outcomes are few in comparison to similar trials of therapy interventions (Bossuyt et al. 2000; Ferrante di Ruffano et al. 2012). Insofar as they exist, randomized test comparisons have been done more frequently to evaluate tests in screening and early detection (NLST 2011a,b; Gohagan et al. 2015) but less so in other contexts, such as diagnosis, staging, and guiding therapy (Jarvik et al. 2003; Turnbull et al. 2010; Douglas et al. 2015; Stillman et al., 2016). Chapter 16 provides a detailed discussion of design considerations for screening trials.

17.2.1 A Heuristic for the Simple Randomized Design

We begin this section with a heuristic analysis of a simplified but often relevant randomized design used to compare two tests. In this design, alternative tests A and B for a particular condition are compared in terms of the outcomes of individuals in a cohort of interest (Figure 17.2). The test results are binary ("positive"/"negative") and the choice of subsequent care involves two alternative approaches ("Tx1" and "Tx2"). A positive test result would imply a recommendation for Tx1 while a negative test result would imply a recommendation for Tx2.

The setting of this design is applicable to many comparisons of tests in the diagnostic or the screening context. To fix ideas, the National Lung Screening Trial, a comparative study of 53,546 participants randomized to low-dose computed tomography (CT) or x-ray screening for lung cancer, can be cast in this framework (NLST 2011a,b). In particular, test A would be the performance of three annual screens with low-dose CT; test B would be the performance of three annual screens with x-ray; Tx1 would be the diagnostic workup following a positive screening result together with subsequent therapeutic interventions as needed; and Tx2 would be no further intervention. The outcome in both arms would be lung cancer-specific mortality.

For purposes of this heuristic argument, assume for simplicity that the outcome at the patient level is binary ("success"/"failure"). Under these

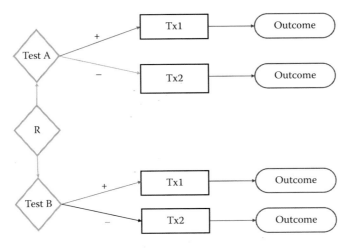

FIGURE 17.2
Simple randomized design for comparing two tests.

assumptions, the difference in success rates between the two arms is the following function of the sensitivity and specificity of the two tests and the success rates of subsequent care:

$$D = r^A - r^B = (r_{21} - r_{11}) \times p \times (Se_B - Se_A)$$
$$+ (r_{22} - r_{12}) \times (1 - p) \times (Sp_A - Sp_B) \qquad (17.1)$$

In the above notation, p denotes the prevalence of the condition, and r_{ij} the success rate when disease status is j ($1 = $ positive, $2 = $ negative) and the healthcare intervention is Tx_i.

Assume further that the two tests have the same specificity but different sensitivities. It can then be seen from Equation 17.1 that the difference in success rates between the two arms depends on the difference in the effectiveness of the Tx1 and Tx2 when applied to appropriate individuals, the prevalence of the condition, and the difference in the sensitivity of the two tests. In particular, the difference in success rates between the arms is only a fraction of the success rates between Tx1 and Tx2. This fraction can be very small when the prevalence of the condition is small and/or when the sensitivities of the two tests are similar. For example, when the prevalence of the condition is 10% and the difference in sensitivities is also 10%, the difference in success rates between the two arms of the randomized design is 1% of the difference between the success rates of Tx1 and Tx2. In such a setting, the sample size for a study comparing test A to test B would be considerably larger than the corresponding sample size for comparing Tx1 to Tx2.

The heuristic analysis of the simple randomized design points to an important concern about sample size considerations in randomized trials of tests. With the exception of the large screening trials, many randomized comparisons of tests may be criticized for assuming unrealistically large effect sizes and thus setting too low sample size requirements. A careful modeling analysis of the testing and outcomes cascade would be an effective way to prevent the ultimate conduct of underpowered randomized test comparisons.

17.2.2 Other Designs

Alternatives to the potentially inefficient simple randomized design have been discussed in the literature (Bossuyt et al. 2000; de Graaff et al. 2004; Lu and Gatsonis 2012). In particular, Lu and Gatsonis (2012) discuss properties of the "discordant pairs design" in which both tests are performed on all individuals in the study, but only cases in which the two tests disagree are randomized. Such a design can be considerably more efficient but has not yet been used extensively in practice. A recent example of its use is the *MINDACT* study comparing clinical to genomic risk assessment as a guide for the selection of breast cancer patients for adjuvant chemotherapy (Bogaerts et al. 2006; Rutgers et al. 2011).

17.2.3 Randomization of Tests or Strategies?

An important tenet of CER studies of tests is to assess the impact of the use of alternative tests in conditions that reflect medical practice in the field. A key choice to be made in the design of such studies relates to the linkage of test results to downstream decision making about the care of the individual. In situations when strong clinical practice guidelines have been developed and are generally accepted, the design may require that test results lead to specific decisions according to the guidelines. When guidelines are not available or not broadly used, the protocol of the trial may offer only broad guidance on how test results should be used and not require specific actions to be taken. The first scenario leads to studies in which tests are very closely linked to downstream actions while the second leads to studies in which such close linkage does not exist. The first scenario would ordinarily be expected to lead to more efficient study designs than the second.

Another setting that leads to close linkage of tests and downstream actions is when tests are embedded in alternative healthcare *strategies* that need to be compared. These strategies involve diagnostic and therapeutic interventions and may include alternative guidelines. The care of patients with stable angina provides a good illustration of this situation. In this setting, two alternative strategies of care are available. The first strategy begins with the use of anatomic imaging (CT angiography) followed by angiography if the percent of stenosis is high or optimal medical care (OMT) if the percent of stenosis is low. The alternative strategy begins with functional imaging (SPECT) and proceeds to angiography or follow-up according to SPECT findings. The results of angiography may be used to recommend OMT for a patient. Randomization to one of these two strategies was performed by the RESCUE trial, which had a projected sample size of 4,300 participants (Stillman et al. 2016). An alternative approach was taken in the PROMISE trial, in which 10,003 patients were randomized to anatomic (CTA) versus functional testing (e.g., SPECT) but subsequent decision making was not precisely specified without specified follow-up (Douglas et al. 2015).

From a design standpoint, the choice of randomization to "test only" or to test as part of a strategy presents a trade-off between generalizability and efficiency. The "test only" design controls for fewer confounders and hence can lead to larger sample sizes. However, it can be argued that it can also lead to a more "pragmatic" trial and hence provide more generalizable conclusions. The "test as part of a strategy" design would be expected to be more efficient. However, the results of such a study would apply only to the comparison of the specific strategies. In practice, the choice of the design would be primarily guided by the clinical or health care policy question that needs to be addressed. Naturally, it is essential that both types of designs should be powered appropriately.

17.3 Beyond Randomized Trials

Randomized comparisons of tests or strategies are generally challenging to organize and implement and often require significant resources and time. As noted earlier, these challenges have resulted in far fewer published randomized trials of diagnostic tests compared to trials of therapeutic interventions. Alternative approaches include several types of observational studies, notably prospective registry studies, as well as studies using administrative databases such as EHRs, Medicare claims data, and health insurance claims data. They also include modeling and simulation studies.

17.3.1 Large Databases

A growing number of studies of diagnostic tests in recent years utilize information from large administrative databases. The general approach is to construct a cohort of clinical interest, with longitudinal records including test and outcome information, and to utilize methods for observational data to make comparisons of interest. Methods for causal inference discussed in this book are applicable in these studies.

In a recent example of such a study, Shreibati et al. (2014) used propensity score matching with Medicare claims data from a 20% sample of beneficiaries to compare healthcare utilization and outcomes in patients who received coronary artery calcium testing or high-sensitivity c-reactive protein testing. They selected a cohort of beneficiaries who had undergone such testing but did not have cardiovascular disease claims in the previous 6 months. In another example, Foy et al. (2015) used Marketscan records from over 420,000 patients who arrived at an ER with chest pain to compare diagnostic testing strategies. They classified the patients into five testing strategies and used regression analysis to compare subsequent medical outcomes and resource utilization across the five groups.

Although EHR and claims databases offer major opportunities for CER of diagnostic tests, they also present significant challenges to the analyst. In addition to the general problems with secondary databases, as discussed for example in Chapter 14 for EHRs, secondary databases can be deficient in the availability of important information for the evaluation of diagnostic tests. In particular, deficiencies have been reported in the availability of information about the context in which a test was performed (indication, patient filtering, and previous tests), the clinical characteristics of the patients (especially in claims databases), the results of the test, and the role of the test in subsequent diagnostic and therapeutic decisions. These challenges are compounded by "defensive medicine" practices, which can result in a preponderance of unnecessary testing, and by "creative" coding practices of healthcare providers.

In some settings, suitable proxy information has been defined that can be used in subsequent studies. For example, algorithms for identifying screening mammograms and evaluating cancer detection rates using CMS claims data have been developed (Hubbard et al. 2015; Fenton et al. 2016). However, a lot of work remains to be done to develop similar methods for other diagnostic tests. Progress in this effort will depend on the speed with which EHR and large administrative databases can evolve to incorporate critically needed data elements.

17.3.2 Prospective Registries

The development of prospective registries is a particularly attractive approach for the evaluation of the impact of diagnostic tests in the field. Indeed, the use of registries in this area of CER is becoming widespread, especially in the evaluations of modalities for screening and early detection. For example, the recent CMS call for Coverage with Evidence studies of CT screening for lung cancer has given rise to registries collecting data on individuals undergoing such screening across the country (CMS 2016, Lung cancer registries). As another example, a long-standing registry in the area of breast cancer was organized by the Breast Cancer Screening Consortium and led to a wealth of information about the accuracy and outcomes of mammography screening (BCSC website, Ballard-Barbash et al. 1997).

Registries by necessity collect narrowly defined information on their participants and do not generally contain the level of clinical detail that exists in EHRs. In addition, registries do not achieve the broad population coverage that can be achieved by claims databases. However, registries can serve as the core of an ecosystem of studies that link information on registry participants that exists in other sources (such as insurance claims, EHR, and other registries).

Here, we discuss two recent examples of prospective registry-based studies that address questions outside cancer screening. The first is the National Oncologic PET Registry (NOPR), which was used to study the impact of positron emission tomography (PET) for cancer patients. The second is the IDEAS study, which includes a prospective registry of Medicare beneficiaries with mild cognitive decline who undergo brain amyloid plaque scanning with PET.

17.3.3 National Oncology PET Registry: A Study of the Effectiveness of PET for Cancer Patients

The NOPR was a public–private collaboration organized to assess the effect of PET on referring physicians' plans of intended cancer patient management (NOPR web site, Hillner et al. 2007). The impetus was a Coverage with Evidence Decision (CED) by CMS, which called for evidence on the impact of PET on the care of patients across a wide spectrum of cancer indications for

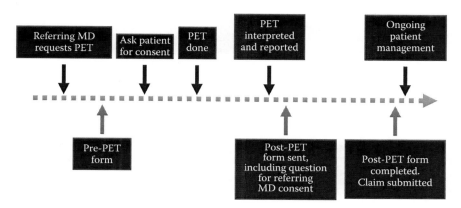

FIGURE 17.3
NOPR workflow.

PET, not covered by the Medicare program at the launch of the registry. The goal of NOPR was to assess the impact of PET by cancer type, indication (diagnosis, staging, restaging, and recurrence), patient performance status, physician's role in management, and type of particular PET scan. A large number of patients (in excess of 200,000) were accrued to the NOPR within a 3-year period, providing national coverage, as needed for a CED study.

The primary assessment of PET impact in NOPR was made by determining whether the information from the PET scan led to a change in management plans for the patient. To make this assessment, the registry collected information on patient management plans before and after the PET scan. The workflow in NOPR is summarized in Figure 17.3. Ultimately the registry data showed that the PET scan was followed by a change in intended management for 36.5% of registry participants, across all indications (Hillner et al. 2008). Several publications from the study report on particular aspects such as the impact on patient management by cancer type, and the impact on monitoring treatment decisions (Hillner et al. 2008, 2009).

As noted above, information from registries can be linked to information from other sources to study aspects of care and outcome that are not covered in the narrow focus of the registry. In the case of NOPR, data on registry participants who were Medicare beneficiaries were linked with CMS claims information on these participants. This linkage made it possible to address a key question about NOPR, namely whether the change in intended care assessed by the registry actually agreed with patient management as determined by CMS claims data. The results of this comparison showed moderate concordance between intended and actual treatment (Hillner et al. 2013). Interestingly, the NOPR results are generally in agreement with those from prospective clinical studies of the impact of PET conducted in Australia (Scott et al. 2008; Fulham et al. 2009).

The potential strengths of NOPR and other similar, pragmatic, prospective registries are important. Such registries can provide extensive, timely, "real world" data that are very difficult and expensive to collect in clinical trials. It is relatively easy to organize and control the collection of registry data prospectively. It is also possible to link registry data to data from other information sources and expand the scope of the study that can be done by the registry alone.

The potential weaknesses are many and flow mainly from the narrow range of information that can be efficiently collected and the corresponding narrow focus of the questions that can be addressed in a pragmatic registry. In particular, (a) NOPR evidence documents change in *intended* patient management but not *actual* management; (b) there was no assessment of whether intended management changes were actually appropriate; (c) there was no information on whether the use of PET improved long-term outcomes for cancer patients; (d) the registry was useful in assessing the impact of a particular test but could not address the broader question of how PET should be used in the *flow* of cancer patient care; and (e) the NOPR registry did not include a control arm in which cancer patients did not undergo PET testing. These weaknesses stemming from the particular approach in the NOPR registry should be added to the broader concerns about the potential for selection and bias in data obtained from these observational registries.

17.3.4 Adding a Control Arm to a Registry Study: The IDEAS Study

The IDEAS study is a recently launched effort to assess aspects of the effectiveness of amyloid plaque PET imaging in patients with mild cognitive impairment who are at risk of developing Alzheimer's disease (AD). As in the case of NOPR, the impetus for the study was a CED announcement from CMS. The protocol and other details of the study are available from its website (IDEAS website).

As noted earlier in this chapter, a positive amyloid PET test result is strongly predictive of the eventual onset of AD. However, approved therapies for AD are not currently available. There are few established guidelines on how to use the amyloid test results and the onset of AD may take a considerable period of time after the amyloid scan. This is a classic situation in medicine where diagnosis is ahead of therapy and where CER studies of diagnosis are particularly challenging.

Although the evaluation of the impact and effectiveness of amyloid PET is difficult, there is still potentially significant value in the information from an amyloid plaque test. On the one hand, the test result may be used to exclude other types of cognitive disease and thus help avoid unnecessary medications. On the other, the test result may help the clinician formulate appropriate patient-counseling strategies that could ameliorate the effects of the eventual onset of AD. Thus, the IDEAS study chose to evaluate two separate endpoints, (a) the impact of the test on the planned care of patients and

(b) the impact of the test on downstream healthcare utilization as assessed by Emergency Department visits and hospitalizations in the period following the test. The current design calls for 18,500 participants to be enrolled in the registry arm of the IDEAS study.

The assessment of the first endpoint is being done via a prospective registry of patients who fulfill appropriate use criteria for amyloid plaque scanning (Johnson et al. 2013). As in NOPR, this is a pre- to post-test comparison of patient management plans reported by the treating physicians. Importantly, the registry is already linked to CMS claims data, and such data will be used to ascertain what the actual care and the course of the disease will be on the registry participants.

The assessment of the second endpoint requires a control group of patients who do not undergo amyloid plaque testing. The IDEAS study plan is to develop such a control group by matching registry patients to control patients selected on the basis of their longitudinal profile as constructed from CMS records. An elaborate matching algorithm has been developed requiring access to 100% Medicare claims data as nearly concurrent as possible to the timeframe of the registry. Propensity scores and other methodology described in Chapters 1–4 will be used in the comparative analysis of the registry to the control arm.

17.3.5 The Role of Modeling

Decision modeling and simulation analysis, notably microsimulation, have significant promise as CER methodologies for both therapy and diagnosis. Chapter 14 provides a detailed account and examples. In the context of diagnosis and prediction, modeling is used to link test and outcome by making use of available information in a systematic and transparent way.

To build the bridge from tests to outcomes, modeling utilizes and integrates information from empirical studies on test accuracy, course of the disease, effectiveness of therapeutic interventions, utilities, and costs. A major capability of modeling is that, in contrast to prospective trials that are bound to the narrow confines of the design of the protocol, modeling analysis can assess a range of scenarios, with different assumptions about each of the particular components of the model. Thus, modeling can be a realistic approach to develop information for clinical and health policy questions about the use of tests.

A recent example of a major modeling initiative in cancer screening is the Cancer Intervention and Surveillance Modeling Network (CISNET), organized by National Cancer Institute (NCI) (CISNET web site, CISNET 2012). CISNET collaborators developed and compared models for assessing the impact of several cancers, including breast, lung, and colorectal cancer (CISNET Breast Cancer Collaborators 2006; Habbema et al. 2006; Zauber et al. 2008). Full-scale modeling analyses of the impact of tests in other healthcare contexts such as diagnosis, staging, and prediction have been less common.

17.4 Discussion

This chapter's survey of potential options for CER studies of tests for diagnosis and prediction, on the one hand, identified significant methodologic and pragmatic challenges in this area and, on the other, highlighted several potential approaches that hold promise to provide useful information. Importantly, the survey also highlighted the need for methodological flexibility that would allow the effective use of analytic tools and databases.

Randomized studies are feasible in this space but it is not difficult to argue on pragmatic grounds that such studies will continue to be far less prevalent than randomized studies in CER of therapeutic interventions. Large secondary databases hold great promise but, currently, they may lack key portions of the specific information needs for studies of diagnosis. The use of prospective registries has significant merit in this area of CER, especially when registry information can be combined with other sources.

The ability to conduct empirical studies of diagnostic tests will undoubtedly be enhanced in the environment of the emerging organizational structures in health care. The growth of integrated healthcare systems and Accountable Care Organizations, on the one hand, makes it easier to collect and integrate data collection systems and processes that cover the continuum of care and, on the other, aligns diverse interests and incentives for supporting CER studies.

Finally, the evaluation of the impact and effectiveness of modalities for diagnosis and prediction is particularly suitable for modeling analyses, as has been demonstrated in the screening context. The role of modeling in the effort to link diagnosis and prediction to outcomes can only grow.

References

Ballard-Barbash R, Taplin SH, Yankaskas BC et al. 1997. Breast Cancer Surveillance Consortium: A national mammography screening and outcomes database. *AJR American Journal of Roentgenology*, 169(4):1001–8.

BCSC website: http://breastscreening.cancer.gov/ (Last accessed, Aug 8 2016).

Bogaerts J, Cardoso F, Buyse M et al. 2006. TRANSBIG Consortium. Gene signature evaluation as a prognostic tool: Challenges in the design of the MINDACT trial. *National Clinical Practice Oncology*, 3:540–51.

Bossuyt P, Lijmer J, Mol B. 2000. Randomised comparison of medical tests: Sometimes invalid, not always efficient. *Lancet*, 356:1844–7.

Carlos RC, Buist DS, Wernli KJ, Swan JS. 2012. Patient-centered outcomes in imaging: Quantifying value. *Journal of the American College of Radiology*, 9(10):725–8.

CISNET. 2012. The impact of the reduction in tobacco smoking on U.S. lung cancer mortality (1975–2000): Collective results from the Cancer Intervention and

Surveillance Modeling Network (CISNET). *Risk Analysis,* Special Issue, Vol 32, Suppl 1.

CISNET Breast Cancer Collaborators. 2006. The impact of mammography and adjuvant therapy on U.S. breast cancer mortality (1975–2000): Collective results from the Cancer Intervention and Surveillance Modeling Network. *Journal of the National Cancer Institute Monographs,* 36:1–126.

CISNET. web page: http://cisnet.cancer.gov/ (Last accessed August 8 2016).

CMS. 2015. Medicare Clinical Diagnostic Laboratory Tests Payment System Proposed Rule: https://www.cms.gov/Newsroom/MediaReleaseDatabase/Factsheets/2015-Fact-sheets-items/2015-09-25-2.html (Last accessed Aug 8 2016).

CMS. 2016. Lung cancer registries: https://www.cms.gov/Medicare/Medicare-General-Information/MedicareApprovedFacilitie/Lung-Cancer-Screening-Registries.html (Last accessed Aug 8 2016).

de Graaff JC, Ubbink DT, Tijssen JGP, Legemate DA. 2004. The diagnostic randomised clinical trial is the best solution for management issues in critical limb ischemia. *Journal of Clinical Epidemiology,* 57:1111–8.

Douglas PS, Hoffmann U, Patel MR et al. 2015. Outcomes of anatomical versus functional testing for coronary artery disease. *New England Journal of Medicine,* 372:1291–300.

Durand DJ, Narayan AK, Rybicki FJ, Burleson J, Nagy P, McGinty G, Duszak R Jr. 2015. The health care value transparency movement and its implications for radiology. *Journal of the American College of Radiology,* 12:51–8.

Fenton JJ, Onega T, Zhu W, Balch S, Smith-Bindman R, Henderson L, Sprague BL, Kerlikowske K, Hubbard RA. 2016. Validation of a Medicare claims-based algorithm for identifying breast cancers detected at screening mammography. *Medicine Care,* 54(3):e15–22.

Ferrante di Ruffano L, Davenport C, Eisinga A, Hyde C, Deeks JJ. 2012. A capture–recapture analysis demonstrated that randomized controlled trials evaluating the impact of diagnostic tests on patient outcomes are rare. *Journal of Clinical Epidemiology,* 65:282–7.

Foy AJ, Liu G, Davidson WR Jr, Sciamanna C, Leslie DL. 2015. Comparative effectiveness of diagnostic testing strategies in emergency department patients with chest pain: An analysis of downstream testing, interventions, and outcomes. *JAMA Internal Medicine,* 175(3):428–36. doi:10.1001/jamainternmed.2014.7657.

Fryback DG, Thornbury JR. 1991. Efficacy of diagnostic imaging. *Medical Decision Making,* 11:88–94.

Fulham MJ, Carter J, Baldey A et al. 2009. The impact of PET–CT in suspected recurrent ovarian cancer: A prospective multi-centre study as part of the Australian PET Data Collection Project. *Gynecologic Oncology,* 112:462–8.

Gatsonis C. 2010. The promise and realities of CER. *Statistics in Medicine,* 29(19):1977–81.

Gatsonis CA. 2000. Design of evaluations of imaging technologies: Development of a paradigm. *Academic Radiology,* 7:681–3.

Gazelle GS, Kessler L, Lee DW, McGinn T, Menzin J, Neumann PJ, van Amerongen D, White LA. 2011. Working Group on Comparative Effectiveness Research for Imaging. A framework for assessing the value of diagnostic imaging in the era of comparative effectiveness research. *Radiology,* 261(3):692–8.

Gohagan JK, Prorok PC, Greenwald P, Kramer BS. 2015. The PLCO cancer screening trial: Background, goals, organization, operations, results. *Review of Recent Clinical Trials*, 10(3):173–80.

Goozner, Mel CMS's PET peeve. Editorial. Modern Healthcare Sept 15, 2016.

Habbema JD, Schechter CB, Cronin KA, Clarke LD, Feuer EJ. 2006. Modeling cancer natural history, epidemiology, and control: Reflections on the CISNET breast group experience. *Journal of the National Cancer Institute Monographs*, (36):122–6. DOI: 10.1093/jncimonographs/lgj017.

Hendee WR1, Becker GJ, Borgstede JP, Bosma J, Casarella WJ, Erickson BA, Maynard CD, Thrall JH, Wallner PE. 2010. Addressing overutilization in medical imaging. *Radiology*, 257:240–5. PMID 20736333.

Hillner B, Siegel B, Liu D et al. 2008. Impact of positron emission tomography/computed tomography and positron emission tomography (PET) alone on expected management of patients with cancer: Initial results from the National Oncologic PET Registry. *Journal of Clinical Oncology*, 26:2155–61.

Hillner BE, Siegel BA, Shields AF, Liu D, Gareen IF, Hanna L, Stine SH, Coleman RE. 2009. The impact of positron emission tomography (PET) on expected management during cancer treatment: Findings of the National Oncologic PET Registry. *Cancer*, 115(2):410–8.

Hillner BE, Tosteson TD, Tosteson AN, Wang Q, Song Y, Onega T, Hanna LG, Siegel BA. 2013. Intended versus inferred management after PET for cancer restaging: Analysis of Medicare claims linked to a coverage with evidence development registry. *Medical Care*, 51:361–7.

Hillner BE, Liu D, Coleman RE, Shields AF, Gareen IF, Hanna L, Stine SH, Siegel BA. 2007. The National Oncologic PET Registry (NOPR): Design and analysis plan. *Journal of Nuclear Medicine*, 48(11):1901–8.

Hubbard RA, Benjamin-Johnson R, Onega T, Smith-Bindman R, Zhu W, Fenton JJ. 2015. Classification accuracy of claims-based methods for identifying providers failing to meet performance targets. *Statistics in Medicine*, 34(1):93–105.

IDEAS Study Clinical Trials listing: https://clinicaltrials.gov/ct2/show/NCT 02420756?term=IDEAS&rank=1

IDEAS Study website: http://www.ideas-study.org/ (Last accessed Aug 8 2016).

Jarvik JG, Hollingworth W, Martin B et al. 2003. Rapid magnetic resonance imaging vs radiographs for patients with low back pain: A randomized controlled trial. *Journal of American Medical Association*, 289(21):2810–8.

Johnson KA, Minoshima S, Bohnen NI et al. 2013. Alzheimer's Association; Society of Nuclear Medicine and Molecular Imaging; Amyloid Imaging Taskforce. Appropriate use criteria for amyloid PET: A report of the Amyloid Imaging Task Force, the Society of Nuclear Medicine and Molecular Imaging, and the Alzheimer's Association. *Alzheimer's and Dementia*, 9(1):e-1–16.

Lu B, Gatsonis C. 2012. Efficiency of study designs in diagnostic randomized clinical trials. *Statistics Medicine*, 32(9):1451–66.

NLST. 2011a. The National Lung Screening Trial Research Team. The National Lung Screening Trial: Overview and study design. *Radiology*, 258:243–53.

NLST. 2011b. National Lung Screening Trial Research Team. In: Aberle DR, Adams AM, Berg CD, Black WC, Clapp JD, Fagerstrom RM, Gareen IF, Gatsonis C, Marcus PM, Sicks JD. Reduced lung-cancer mortality with low-dose computed tomographic screening. *New England Journal of Medicine*, 365(5):395–409.

NOPR website: https://www.cancerpetregistry.org/ (Last accessed, Aug 8 2016).

RESCUE trial http://www.acrin.org/PROTOCOLSUMMARYTABLE/ACRIN4701 RESCUE/tabid/747/Default.aspx (Last accessed Aug 8 2016).

Rutgers E, Piccart-Gebhart MJ, Bogaerts J et al. 2011. The EORTC 10041/BIG 03-04 MINDACT trial is feasible: Results of the pilot phase. *European Journal of Cancer*, 47:2742–9.

Scott AM, Gunawardana DH, Kelley B et al. 2008. PET changes management and improves prognostic stratification in patients with recurrent colorectal cancer: Results of a multicenter prospective study. *Journal of Nuclear Medicine*, 49:1451–7.

Sharpe RE Jr, Levin DC, Parker L, Rao VM. 2013. The recent reversal of the growth trend in MRI: A harbinger of the future? *Journal of the American College of Radiology*, 10:770–3.

Shreibati JB1, Baker LC2, McConnell MV2, Hlatky MA. 2014. Outcomes after coronary artery calcium and other cardiovascular biomarker testing among asymptomatic Medicare beneficiaries. *Circulation, Cardiovascular Imaging*, 7(4):655–62. doi:10.1161/CIRCIMAGING.113.001869.

Shyu Y-L, Burleson J, Tallant C, Seidenwurm D, Rybicki FJ. 2014. Performance measures in radiology. *Journal of the American College of Radiology*, 11:456–63.

Stillman AE, Gatsonis C, Lima JA et al. 2016. Rationale and design of the randomized evaluation of patients with stable angina comparing utilization of noninvasive examinations (RESCUE) trial. *American Heart Journal*, 179:19–28.

Turnbull L, Brown S, Harvey I, Olivier C, Drew P, Napp V, Hanby A, Brown J. 2010. Comparative effectiveness of MRI in breast cancer (COMICE) trial: A randomised controlled trial. *Lancet*, 375:563–71.

Zauber A, Lansdorp-Vogelaar I, Knudsen A, Wilschut J, van Ballegooijen M, Kuntz K. 2008. Evaluating test strategies for colorectal cancer screening: A decision analysis for the U.S. Preventive Services Task Force. *Annals of Internal Medicine*, 149:659–69.

Index